T0320577

Clinical Handbook for the Management of Mood Disorders

Clinical Handbook for the Management of Mood Disorders

Edited by

J. John Mann
New York State Psychiatric Institute,
and College of Physicians and Surgeons of Columbia University,
New York, New York, USA

Patrick J. McGrath
New York State Psychiatric Research Institute,
and College of Physicians and Surgeons of Columbia University,
New York, New York, USA

Steven P. Roose
New York State Psychiatric Institute,
and College of Physicians and Surgeons of Columbia University,
New York, New York, USA

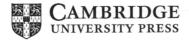
CAMBRIDGE
UNIVERSITY PRESS

CAMBRIDGE
UNIVERSITY PRESS

University Printing House, Cambridge CB2 8BS, United Kingdom

One Liberty Plaza, 20th Floor, New York, NY 10006, USA

477 Williamstown Road, Port Melbourne, VIC 3207, Australia

314-321, 3rd Floor, Plot 3, Splendor Forum, Jasola District Centre, New Delhi - 110025, India

103 Penang Road, #05-06/07, Visioncrest Commercial, Singapore 238467

Cambridge University Press is part of the University of Cambridge.

It furthers the University's mission by disseminating knowledge in the pursuit of education, learning and research at the highest international levels of excellence.

www.cambridge.org
Information on this title: www.cambridge.org/9781107024632

First published 2013

A catalogue record for this publication is available from the British Library

Library of Congress Cataloging in Publication data
Clinical handbook for the management of mood disorders /
[edited by] J. John Mann, Steven P. Roose, Patrick J. McGrath.
  p. ; cm.
Includes bibliographical references and index.
ISBN 978-1-107-02463-2 (hardback)
I. Mann, J. John (Joseph John)   II. Roose, Steven P., 1948–
III. McGrath, Patrick J.
[DNLM: 1. Mood Disorders – therapy.   2. Behavior Therapy –
methods. WM171]
616.85′27 – dc23   2013001655

ISBN 978-1-107-02463-2 Hardback

Contents

v

Contributors

Jimmy N. Avari, MD
Instructor in Psychiatry, Weill Cornell Medical College, and Assistant Attending Psychiatrist, New York Presbyterian Hospital, New York, NY, USA

Joshua Berman, MD
Assistant Professor of Clinical Psychiatry, Columbia University, New York State Psychiatric Institute, New York, NY, USA

David A. Brent, MD
Professor, University of Pittsburgh School of Medicine, Pittsburgh, PA, USA

Benjamin D. Brody, MD
Attending Psychiatrist at New York Presbyterian Hospital and Instructor in Psychiatry at Weill Cornell Medical College, New York, NY, USA

Carolyn Broudy, MD
Practicing Psychiatrist, Northampton, MA, USA

Gerard E. Bruder, PhD
Professor of Clinical Psychology (in Psychiatry) Columbia University, New York State Psychiatric Institute, New York, NY, USA

Deborah L. Cabaniss, MD
Clinical Professor of Psychiatry, Director of Psychotherapy Training, Department of Psychiatry, Columbia University, New York, NY, USA

Megan S. Chesin, MA
Columbia University, New York State Psychiatric Institute, New York, NY, USA

Melissa P. DelBello, MD, MS
Professor of Psychiatry and Pediatrics, Vice Chair of Clinical Research, Co-Director, Division of Bipolar Disorders Research, Department of Psychiatry and

Behavioral Neuroscience, University of Cincinnati College of Medicine, Cincinnati, OH, USA

Davangere P. Devanand, MD
Professor of Clinical Psychiatry and Neurology and Director, Division of Geriatric Psychiatry, Columbia University, New York State Psychiatric Institute, New York, NY, USA

Jordan W. Eipper, BA
MD Candidate, 2016 Suny Downstate College of Medicine, Brodelyn, NY, USA

Jean Endicott, PhD
Professor of Clinical Psychology (in Psychiatry), Director, Research Assessment and Training, Columbia University, New York State Psychiatric Institute, New York, NY, USA

Eric A. Fertuck, PhD
Assistant Professor of Clinical Psychology (in Psychiatry), Columbia University, New York State Psychiatric Institute, New York, NY, USA

Michael B. First, MD
Professor of Clinical Psychiatry, Columbia University, New York State Psychiatric Institute, New York, NY, USA

Benicio N. Frey, MD, PhD
Assistant Professor, Psychiatry and Behavioural Neurosciences, McMaster University, Hamilton, ON, Canada

Emily Gastelum, MD
Fellow, Psychosomatic Medicine, Department of Psychiatry, Columbia University, New York, NY, USA

Lucas Giner
Assistant Professor, University of Seville, Seville, Spain

Barbara L. Gracious, MD

Jeffrey Research Fellow, Center for Innovations in Pediatric Practice, The Research Institute, Nationwide Children's Hospital and Associate Professor of Psychiatry, The Ohio State University, Columbus, OH, USA

David J. Hellerstein, MD

Professor of Clinical Psychiatry, Columbia University, New York State Psychiatric Institute, New York, NY, USA

Aerin M. Hyun, MD, PhD

Psychiatry Resident, Columbia University, New York State Psychiatric Institute, New York, NY, USA

David A. Kahn, MD

Professor of Clinical Psychiatry, Presbyterian Hospital, Ph-Psych Serve, New York, NY, USA

Jürgen Kayser, PhD

Associate Professor of Clinical Neuroscience (in Psychiatry) Columbia University, New York State Psychiatric Institute, New York, NY, USA

S. Aiden Kelly, BA

Columbia University, New York State Psychiatric Institute, New York, NY, USA

James H. Kocsis, MD

Professor of Psychiatry, Weill Cornell Medical College and Attending Psychiatrist, New York Presbyterian Hospital, New York, NY, USA

Robert A. Kowatch, MD, PhD

Professor of Psychiatry, Ohio State Medical Center, Nationwide Children's Hospital, Columbus, OH, USA

Gonzalo Laje

Assistant Clinical Professor of Psychiatry and Behavioral Sciences, George Washington University, Washington DC, USA

Martin J. Lan, MD, PhD

Research Fellow in Affective Disorders, Molecular Imaging and Neuropathology Divison, Department of Psychiatry, Colombia University, NY, USA

Kyle A. B. Lapidus, MD, PhD

Associate in Psychiatry, Mount Sinai School of Medicine, New York, NY, USA

Frances R. Levin, MD

Kennedy-Leavy Professor of Clinical Psychiatry, Columbia University, New York State Psychiatric Institute, New York, NY, USA

Sarah H. Lisanby, MD

Lawrance C. Katz Professor and Chair, Department of Psychiatry and Behavioral Sciences, and Director, Brain Stimulation and Neurophysiology Divison, Duke University School of Medicine, Durham, NC, USA

J. John Mann, MD

Paul Janssen Professor of Translational Neuroscience and Director, Molecular Imaging and Neuropathology, Columbia University, New York State Psychiatric Institute, New York, NY, USA

Sanjay J. Mathew, MD

Brown Foundation Chair of Psychopharmacology of Mood Disorders and Associate Professor, Meuninger Department of Psychiatry and Behavioral Sciences, Baylor College of Medicine, Houston, TX, USA

Patrick J. McGrath, MD

Professor of Clinical Psychiatry, Columbia University, New York State Psychiatric Institute, New York, NY, USA

Francis J. McMahon, MD

Chief of Genetic Basis of Mood and Anxiety Disorders, National Institute of Mental Health, Bethesda, MD, USA

Barnett S. Meyers, MD

Professor of Psychiatry – Clinical Epidemiology, Weill Cornell Medical College and Attending Psychiatrist, New York Presbyterian Hospital, New York, NY, USA

Luciano Minuzzi, MD, PhD

Clinical Fellow, Psychiatry and Behavioural Neurosciences, McMaster University, Hamilton, ON, Canada

Diana E. Moga, MD

Psychiatrist, New York Presbyterian Hospital, New York, NY, USA

Philip R. Muskin, MD
Professor of Clinical Psychiatry, Columbia University, New York State Psychiatric Institute, New York, NY, USA

Edward V. Nunes Jr, MD
Professor of Clinical Psychiatry, Columbia University, New York State Psychiatric Institute, New York, NY, USA

Maria A. Oquendo, MD
Professor of Clinical Psychiatry and Vice Chair of Education, Director of Residency Training, Columbia University, New York State Psychiatric Institute, New York, NY, USA

Ramin V. Parsey, MD, PhD
Clinical Professor of Psychiatry, Columbia University, New York State Psychiatric Institute, New York, NY, USA

Joan Prudic, MD
Clinical Professor of Psychiatry, Columbia University, New York State Psychiatric Institute, New York, NY, USA

Annie E. Rabinovitch, MA
Teachers College, Columbia University, New York, NY, USA

Drew Ramsey, MD
Assistant Clinical Professor of Psychiatry, Columbia University, New York, NY, USA

Steven P. Roose, MD
Professor of Clinical Psychiatry, Columbia University, New York State Psychiatric Institute, New York, NY, USA

Moacyr A. Rosa, PhD
Afíliate Professor, Institute for Advanced Research in Neurostimulation, São Paulo, Brazil

Bret R. Rutherford, MD
Assistant Professor of Clinical Psychiatry, Columbia University, New York State Psychiatric Institute, New York, NY, USA

Roberto Sassi, MD, PhD
Assistant Professor, Psychiatry and Behavioural Neurosciences, McMaster University, Hamilton, ON, Canada

Peter A. Shapiro, MD
Professor of Clinical Psychiatry, Columbia University, New York State Psychiatric Institute, New York, NY, USA

Margaret G. Spinelli, MD
Associate Professor of Clinical Psychiatry, Columbia University, New York State Psychiatric Institute, New York, NY, USA

Barbara H. Stanley, PhD
Lecturer in Psychiatry, Columbia University, New York State Psychiatric Institute, New York, NY, USA

Meir Steiner, MD, PhD, FRCPC
Professor Emeritus, Departments of Psychiatry and Behavioural Neurosciences and Obstetrics and Gynecology, McMaster University, Hamilton, ON and Professor, Department of Psychiatry and Institute of Medical Sciences, University of Toronto, Toronto, ON, Canada

Jonathan W. Stewart, MD
Professor of Clinical Psychiatry, Columbia University, New York State Psychiatric Institute, New York, NY, USA

M. Elizabeth Sublette, MD, PhD
Assistant Professor of Clinical Psychiatry, Columbia University, New York State Psychiatric Institute, New York, NY, USA

Craig E. Tenke, PhD
Research Scientist, Columbia University, New York State Psychiatric Institute, New York, NY, USA

Jiuan Su Terman, PhD
Research Psychologist, Department of Psychiatry, Columbia University, New York, NY, USA

Michael Terman, PhD
Professor of Clinical Psychology in Psychiatry, Columbia University, New York State Psychiatric Institute, New York, NY, USA

Michael E. Thase, MD
Professor of Psychiatry, Philadelphia VA Medical Center, Department of Psychiatry, Mood and Anxiety Disorders Treatment and Research Program, Philadelphia, PA, USA

Helen Verdeli, PhD

Assistant Professor of Clinical Psychology, Teachers College, Columbia University, New York, NY, USA

Myrna M. Weissman, PhD

Professor of Psychology / Epidemiology (in Psychiatry), Columbia University, New York State Psychiatric Institute, New York, NY, USA

Models of depression

Steven P. Roose, Patrick J. McGrath, and J. John Mann

Explanatory models of depression are constructed to serve multiple purposes including: (1) helping clinicians organize a body of knowledge to help in patient evaluation and treatment planning, (2) guiding research, and (3) informing about treatment outcome. Models are judged based on various types of validity, including predictive validity regarding prognosis and treatment outcome. Models exist at different levels, from more broad models that apply to all depressed patients, e.g., the gene–environment interaction, to the more specific that explain a particular dimension of the illness, e.g., the association between depression and ischemic heart disease. A model does not have to be comprehensive to be useful; a model may be constructed to understand treatment response or course of illness and have little if any explanatory value with respect to gender difference in rates of illness. A problem for all models of depression is the heterogeneity of the clinical picture of depression, raising the question as to what "depression" or subtype does the model apply? Patients who meet criteria for major depressive disorder (MDD) comprise a heterogeneous group that may share some phenomenology, but probably have disparate illnesses with multiple pathophysiologies. Indeed, biological abnormalities that have been shown to be associated with depression are present in only a moderate proportion of cases, indicating biologic heterogeneity. A model that is relevant for early-onset chronic depression may not be useful when applied to melancholia or "vascular depression." In this chapter we will discuss models of unipolar mood disorder that incorporate both current neuroscience and clinical research. It is hoped that these models will help the clinician both conceptualize the illness of a particular patient and formulate an effective individualized treatment plan.

There has been a long search for the gene or genes that carry the risk of depressive illness and though the research results have, to date, fallen short of this goal, they still have been illuminating and serve as a cornerstone for understanding the genesis of depression. Data come from adoption, twin, family, and population studies. In a meta-analysis of genetic studies of unipolar depression, Sullivan *et al.* (2000) estimated that 37% of the illness is accounted for by genetic factors and other compelling data suggest that the genetic contribution to bipolar disorder is greater than that for unipolar depression. Twin studies consistently report greater concordance rate for monozygotic vs. dizygotic twins, but even in the studies reporting the highest rates of concordance for bipolar disorder in monozygotic twins, they never report 100% concordance (Kendler *et al.* 1993), indicating that epigenetic modification, environment, or a gene interaction with environment must play a significant role in both unipolar and bipolar disorders.

Although genes are an important cause of major depression and bipolar disorder, we have not confirmed the identity of the responsible genes. For example, does genetic vulnerability produce a heightened sense of fear and anxiety so that life is experienced as a series of "stresses," i.e., events, including interpersonal failures and rejections, are experienced as overwhelming and as such ultimately lead to depressive illness? Depression could also result from early environmental deprivation or abusive experiences that produce epigenetic changes and recalibrate stress response systems to be hyper-reactive to stress in adult life. Perhaps the most compelling model is one in which genes and childhood adverse environmental conditions produce a gene–environment interaction that results in a diathesis for a mood disorder.

Clinical Handbook for the Management of Mood Disorders, ed. J. John Mann, Patrick J. McGrath, and Steven P. Roose.
Published by Cambridge University Press. © Cambridge University Press 2013.

There are considerable animal data to support variants of this model. During a critical period in early life, the experience of significant environmental stress, and in early life this primarily means some form of maternal deprivation, induces changes in brain structure that result in a demonstrable heightened reactivity to adverse conditions and specific patterns of behavior throughout adulthood (Hofer, 2003). There are genetic strains of mice that have the vulnerability to anxiety behaviors that are more intensely expressed in adverse environmental conditions. These consequences are reversed in adult mice by the administration of antidepressant medications, most specifically SSRIs (McEwen, 2003).

A major stress response system is the hypothalamic pituitary adrenal (HPA) axis. It is well documented that many patients with severe depression, in particular patients with melancholia or delusional depression, have marked dysfunction in the HPA axis, including loss of normal circadian rhythm of cortisol excretion and high cortisol levels (Nemeroff et al. 2002). Furthermore, genes and childhood adverse life events recalibrate such stress response systems in the brain and their components outside the brain. Maternal deprivation in lab animals is a model of early childhood stress and results in hypersensitivity in stress response systems that can persist into adulthood (Gutman and Nemeroff, 2002).

Cross-sectional studies in depressed patients reporting childhood physical or sexual abuse suggest such hyperactive stress responses may also be found in depressed patients (Heim et al. 2000, 2001). Severe MDD is associated with higher basal cortisol secretion and higher peak levels, as well as dexamethasone resistance, indicating failure of feedback inhibition at both the higher stimulated cortisol levels and the lower resting cortisol levels. Interestingly, post-traumatic stress disorder (PTSD) is associated with lower basal cortisol and increased glucocorticoid receptor (GCR) expression, indicating that the response to stress can be different in different disorders. In rodent models stress and glucocorticoids reduce neurogenesis and this can be reversed by antidepressant medication administration. Persistently elevated cortisol levels in rodents lead to hippocampal atrophy and both of these phenotypes are seen in moderate to severe depressions in humans. Therefore enhanced cortisol release in MDD may explain smaller hippocampal volume, which in turn has been reported to be proportional to duration of untreated depression lifetime, and progresses with lack of remission of depression (Sheline et al. 1999).

Another line of support for this model comes from the studies of humans that appear to demonstrate a gene–environment interaction that results in depression. The best-known example is the report that children exposed to childhood adversity who also carry the lower expressing gene variants of the promoter or regulatory region of the serotonin transporter gene (the target of SSRIs) have an elevated risk of major depression when exposed to stress in their midtwenties (Caspi et al. 2003). Although the finding by Caspi has been both replicated and challenged, it is a compelling illustration of a gene–environment interaction.

The same variant of the serotonin transporter gene favors hyper-responsiveness of the amygdala when matching fearful or angry faces on functional magnetic resonance imaging. A hyperactive amygdala is also reported in PET studies of major depression and this over activity may facilitate encoding of painful memories contributing to stress sensitivity in adulthood and greater likelihood of depression when stressed (Hariri et al. 2005). The amygdala is the site where memories and associated affects are encoded. In nonhuman primates lower expressing serotonin transporter gene variants are associated with reduction of serotonin function in response to maternal deprivation, an effect that persists into adulthood and may explain part of the biologic impact of childhood adversity in the genetically susceptible individuals who are more prone to depression in adulthood (Bennett et al. 2002). Patients with MDD, who report childhood adversity, also have lower serotonin transporter binding on PET scanning, and this may be a biological endophenotype associated with a vulnerability to stress-induced MDD.

The fundamental concept of the gene–environment interaction model is that whether a result of genes or early environmental trauma, or both, early life stress results in functional and structural changes in the brain that confer a life-long hyperactive stress response mediated by the HPA axis. Direct genetic effects or purely environmental effects may result in depressions. For example, genes are associated with internalizing disorders or excessive sensitivity to the environment, and the experience of life events as more stressful, reinforcing a negative life experience whose final result is helplessness and despair, i.e., depression. Though much attention has been given to the enduring impact of early stressful experiences, there are animal models and human stories in which conditions of repeated and unpredictable frustrations result in a state of "learned helplessness," a state that is characterized by behaviors that are associated with depression (Maier, 1984). This represents a model in which depression can result from external or interpersonal experiences in a person who does or does not have a genetic vulnerability to a mood disorder.

Another model of depression focuses on brain structure and neural circuits and asks the question, where in the brain does depression occur? Imaging studies of the depressed brain at baseline (MRI and PET studies), in response to stimuli (fMRI studies), and after treatment (PET and fMRI) have found alterations in structure and/or activity in a number of brain regions in major depression. Mayberg and others have found that MDD is characterized by increased brain activity in many ventral brain structures, including limbic structures, and hypoactivity in dorsal and lateral prefrontal cortex (Mayberg et al. 1999). Recovery from an episode of major depression is associated with reversal of much of this picture with changes in brain activity in the direction of that found in healthy volunteers. The disordered neurocircuitry of major depression more specifically includes hypoactivity in the ventral, medial, and dorsolateral prefrontal cortex, the anterior insula, the ventral striatum, the posterior cingulate gyrus, and hippocampus, and hyperactivity in the anterior cingulate cortex (ACC), medial thalamus, amygdala, and brainstem (Milak et al. 2005). These brain areas regulate emotional, cognitive, autonomic, sleep, and stress response behaviors, which are all impaired in MDD. Perhaps most intriguing is that a recent study found that children at risk for MDD by virtue of both parents having the illness had characteristic changes in brain structure, specificially cortical thinning (Peterson et al. 2009). Most recently deep brain stimulation treatments of patients with treatment-resistant MDD have focused interest on Brodmann area 25. The stimulation of this area by implanted electrodes can have a very swift and remarkable antidepressant effect (Mayberg et al. 2005).

Of course locating the areas in the brain that have altered activity in a patient with MDD still leaves unanswered the question of what is dysfunctional in these regions with respect to neurotransmitters, signal transduction, and circuitry. Perhaps the first compelling model of depression was the chatecholamine hyothesis (later extended to the biogenic amine hypothesis) that was formulated based on a limited understanding of the effects of antidepressant medications available in the 1960s (Schildkraut, 1965). This model postulates that depression is caused by a functional decrease in norepinephrine and/or serotonin activity in critical areas of the brain. This decrease may result from a deficiency in the amount of neurotansmitter available, abnormalities in metabolism and/or inadequete receptor response due to fewer receptors or lower receptor sensitivity. The longevity and popularity of this model may be due in large part because it offered an explanation of how antideprenant medications work, that is, TCAs and SSRIs block the reuptake of neurotransmitter from the synaptic cleft and MAOIs block the breakdown of monoamines and both thereby increase activation of postsynaptic receptors. There is a significant body of data that monoamine alterations characterize some depressions and that drugs raising monoamines are therapeutic, whereas depletion of monoamines reverses antidepressant effects, thus supporting the hypothesis. However, the biogenic amine hypothesis as originally stated posits that only two neurotransmitters are involved in MDD, norepinephrine and serotonin, and ignores dopamine, GABA, glutamate, neuropepetides, hormones, etc., and though blockade of neurotransmitter reuptake is an effect of some antidepressant medications, it is only one of several potential antidepressant mechanisms of action. This model also illustrates a potential negative consequence of a model if it is treated as "fact" rather than a useful paradigm. The development of new pharmacological treatments has probably been delayed because this model dictated looking for compounds that block the reuptake of serotonin or norepinephrine (Berton and Nestler, 2006). New antidepressants, such as ketamine, most likely act on other neurotransmitter systems and/or work through novel pathways to achieve antidepressant effects, raising questions about extrapolating from the presumed mechanism of action of a treatment to the pathogenesis of mood disorders. Nonetheless, regardless of how limited or inaccurate, the biogenic monoamine model of depression and the related view of antidepressant action continues to be a useful organizing and testable model that has been the stimulus for much valuable research.

Antidepressants are not the only treatments linked to a model of depression. Effective psychotherapies, whether CBT, IPT, or DBT, all offer a model of depression based on dysfunctional cognitions, relationships or self-identity as outlined in Chapters 19, 20, and 21 respectively. Results of neuroimaging studies of depressed patients done pre- and post-treatment have led to a model that proposes that psychotherapy treatments for depression work "from top (cortex) down (amagdyla, hippocampus, and other structures) and medications the opposite" (Martin *et al.* 2001, Goldapple *et al.* 2004). Pre- and post-studies of different types of treatment, e.g., medication, psychotherapy, ECT, can provide persuasive data to support models of depressive illness when they can identify changes that only occur in responders, thereby deconstructing a general effect of treatment from the antidepressant mechanism of action. A caveat is that given the presumed heterogeneity in etiology among a group of patients, all of whom meet criteria for MDD, there may be an effect of medication that occurs in all patients, but only has an anitdepressant effect in a sub-group.

Another example of model building is the attempt to understand the relationship between depression and vascular disease. A replicated finding from multiple longitudinal studies is that depression early in life is a risk factor for development of coronary heart disease, the rate of depression in patients following myocardial infarction (MI) is approximately 20%, and an additional 20–25% have significant depressive symptoms (Roose and Krishnan, 2004).

One model has focused on the role of insulin resistance as an important mechanism to explain depression as a risk factor for vascular disease (Musselman *et al.* 2003). The hypercortisolemia associated with depression can induce hyperglycemia and insulin resistance. Furthermore, increased plasma cortisol, as well as other hormone abnormalities associated with depression, specifically decreases secretion of growth hormone and sex steroids, and can lead to increased visceral fat that subsequently contributes to insulin resistance. Once established, insulin resistance promotes hypertension through multiple mechanisms including: (1) increased renal tubular reabsorption of sodium, (2) increased sympathetic activity, and (3) proliferation of vascular smooth muscle. Independent of its stimulation of insulin resistance, visceral fat further promotes vascular damage by activating hepatic secretion of tumor necrosis factor that ultimately leads to an inflammatory process now recognized as a critical component in the pathogenesis of atherosclerosis (Troxler *et al.* 1977, Gold *et al.* 1999). Thus, the physiology of depression, specifically increased cortisol leading to insulin resistance, contributes to vascular damage, which in turn explains why patients with depression are at increased risk for myocardial infarction and stroke.

Although it has long been assumed that the depression follows the cardiac event as reflected in the phrase, "post-MI depression," Glassman *et al.* reported that in 50% of patients the depressive episode preceded the MI (Glassman *et al.* 2000). The physiology of depression may significantly contribute to the development of an ischemic event. Patients with depression have hyperactive platelets. When injury to blood vessel endothelium occurs, such as in patients with atherosclerosis, both platelets and circulating leukocytes attach to exposed sub-endothelial layers. This begins a cascade of events that includes conversion of platelet membrane GPIIB/IIIa complexes into receptors for fibrinogen and release from storage granules of chemotactic factors such as platelet factor 4, beta-thyroglobulin, and serotonin that stimulate other platelets and thereby induce the process of platelet aggregation. Mechanical obstruction secondary to platelet aggregation can play a central role in the development of acute ischemia in patients with atherosclerosis resulting in either MI or stroke. Thus depression can induce platelet activity that in turn contributes to an ischemic event. This sequence is a building block of a model of the relationship between depression and vascular disease in which the stress associated with an MI can lead to depression and equally depression can lead to an MI.

There is also a model of the relationship between late-life depression and cerebrovascular disease that hypothesizes that sub-clinical vascular disease is critical in the genesis of depression in late life (Krishnan *et al.* 2004). The vascular depression hypothesis (see Chapter 9) is that depression can occur as a consequence of structural damage in cortico-striatal circuits due to cerebral ischemia. Structural damage creates a vulnerability to depression and this vulnerability is further influenced by psychosocial risk factors, including negative life events and lack of social support.

Ideally models of mood disorders should have explanatory power, be able to be tested and disproven, help identify potential new treatment targets, and have predictive value for treatment response and prognosis. Perhaps most important, models should advance research and clinical care without inhibiting innovative thinking to better understand disease pathophysiology, help develop treatments and prevention strategies, and stimulate the formulation of new models.

References

Bennett A.J., Lesch K.P., Heils A., *et al.* (2002). Early experience and serotonin transporter gene variation interact to influence primate CNS function. *Molecular Psychiatry*, 7(1), 118–122.

Berton, O. and Nestler, E.J. (2006). New approaches to antidepressant drug discovery: Beyond monoamines. *Nature Reviews Neuroscience*, 7, 137–151.

Caspi, A., Sugden, K., Moffitt, T.E., *et al.* (2003). Influence of stress on depression: Moderation by a polymorphism in the 5-HTT gene. *Science*, 301, 386–389.

Glassman, A.H., O'Connor, C.M., Califf, R.M., *et al.* (2000). Sertraline treatment of major depression in patients with acute MI or unstable angina. *Journal of the American Medical Association*, 288(6), 701–709.

Gold, P.W. and Chrousos, G.P. (1999) The endocrinology of melancholic and atypical depression: Relation to neurocircuitry and somatic consequences. *Proceedings of the Association of American Physicians*, 111(1), 22–34.

Goldapple, K., Segal, Z., Garson, C., *et al.* (2004). Modification of cortical-limbic pathways in major depression. *Archives of General Psychiatry*, 61, 34–41.

Gutman, D. and Nemeroff, C.B. (2002). Neurobiology of early life stress: Rodent studies. *Seminars in Clinical Neuropsychiatry*, 7, 89–95.

Hariri, A.R., Drabant, E.M., Munoz, K.E., *et al.* (2005). A susceptibility gene for affective disorders and the response of the human amygdala. *Archives of General Psychiatry*, 62, 146–152.

Heim, C., Newport, D.J., Bonsall, R., Miller, A.H., and Nemeroff, C.B. (2001). Altered pituitary-adrenal responses to provocative challenge tests in adult survivors of childhood abuse. *American Journal of Psychiatry*, 158, 575–581.

Heim, C., Newport, D.J., Heit, S., *et al.* (2000). Pituitary-adrenal and autonomic responses to stress in women after sexual and physical abuse in childhood. *Journal of the American Medical Association*, 284, 592–597.

Hofer, M.A. (2003). Studies on how early maternal separation produces behavioral change in young rats. *Psychosomatic Medicine*, 37(3), 245–264.

Kendler, K.S., Pedersen, N., Johnson, L., *et al.* (1993). A pilot Swedish twin study of affective illness, including hospital- and population-ascertained subsamples. *Archives of General Psychiatry*, 50(9), 699–706.

Krishnan, K.R., Taylor, W.D., McQuoid, D.R., *et al.* (2004). Clinical characteristics of magnetic resonance imaging-defined subcortical ischemic depression. *Biological Psychiatry*, 55, 390–397.

Maier, S.F. (1984). Learned helplessness and animal models of depression. *Progress in Neuro-Psychopharmacology and Biological Psychiatry*, 8(3), 435–446.

Martin, S.D., Martin, E., Rai, S.S., Richardson, M.A., and Royall, R. (2001). Brain blood flow changes in depressed patients treated with interpersonal psychotherapy or venlafaxine hydrochloride. *Archives of General Psychiatry*, 58, 641–648.

Mayberg, H.S., Liotti, M., Brannan, S.K., *et al.* (1999). Reciprocal limbic-cortical function and negative mood: Converging PET findings in depression and normal sadness. *American Journal of Psychiatry*, 156, 675–682.

Mayberg, H.S., Lozano, A.M., Voon, V., *et al.* (2005). Deep brain stimulation for treatment-resistant depression. *Neuron*, 45, 651–660.

McEwen, B.S. (2003). Stress and neuroendocrine function: individual differences and mechanisms leading to disease. In Wolkowitz, O.M. and Rothschild, A.J., eds., *Psychoneuroendocrinology: The Scientific Basis of Clinical Practice*. Washington, DC: American Psychiatric Publishing, 513–546.

Milak, M.S., Parsey, R.V., Keilp, J., *et al.* (2005). Neuroanatomic correlates of psychopathologic components of major depressive disorder. *Archives of General Psychiatry*, 62, 397–408.

Musselman, D.L., Betan, E., Larsen, H., and Phillips, L.S. (2003). The relationship of depression to diabetes – Type 1 and Type 2: Epidemiology, biology, and treatment. *Biological Psychiatry*, 54, 317–329.

Nemeroff, C.B., Widerlov, E., Bissette, G., *et al.* (2002). Elevated concentration of CSF corticotropin-releasing factor-like immunoreactivity in depressed patients. *Science*, 226, 1342–1344.

Peterson, B.S., Warner, V., Bansal, R., *et al.* (2009). Cortical thinning in persons at increased familial risk for major depression. *Proceedings of the National Academy of Sciences USA*, 106(15), 6273–6278.

Roose, S.P. and Krishnan, R. (2004). Depression comorbid with other illness. In Charney D.S. and Nestler, E.J., eds., *Neurobiology of Mental Illness Second Edition*. New York: Oxford University Press.

Schildkraut, J.J. (1965). The catecholamine hypothesis of affective disorders: A review of supporting evidence. *Journal of Neuropsychiatry and Clinical Neurosciences*, 7, 524–533.

Sheline, Y.I., Sanghavi, M., Mintun, M.A., and Gado, M.H. (1999). Depression duration but not age predicts hippocampal volume loss in medically healthy women with recurrent major depression. *Journal of Neuroscience*, 19, 5034–5043.

Sullivan, P.F., Neale, M.C., and Kendler, K.S. (2000). Genetic epidemiology of major depression: Review and meta-analysis. *American Journal of Psychiatry*, 157(10), 1552–1562.

Troxler, R.G., Sprague, E.A., Albanese, R.A., Fuchs, R., Thompson, A.J. (1977) Association of elevated plasma cortisol and early atherosclerosis demonstrated by coronary angiography. *Atherosclerosis*, 26, 151–162.

Chapter

2

The diagnosis of mood disorders

Michael B. First and Jean Endicott

Introduction

The diagnosis of mood disorders, like the diagnosis of every other type of mental disorder, is based on a determination of whether a patient's presenting and lifetime symptomatology conforms to the standardized definitions of the various mood disorders included in one of the field's descriptive psychiatric nomenclatures: either the *Diagnostic and Statistical Manual of Mental Disorders – Fourth Edition – Text Revision* (DSM-IV-TR) (American Psychiatric Association, 2000) or the *International Classification of Diseases, Tenth Edition* (ICD-10) (World Health Organization, 1992). Clinicians working in the United States invariably rely on the DSM-IV-TR definitions, whereas clinicians working in most parts of the rest of the world use the definitions contacted in the ICD-10 (Reed *et al.* 2011). Researchers, regardless of where they are working, generally use the DSM-IV-TR definitions. Mood disorders in both of these systems are defined in terms of "syndromes," i.e., clusters of symptoms that co-occur. An overarching presumption has been that symptom co-occurrence within a syndrome reflects a common underlying pathophysiological process (or processes) that, with sufficient research efforts, can be elucidated and that will eventually form the basis for a more "objective" method for diagnosing mood disorders. Unfortunately, despite great efforts over the past 30 years and despite several initially promising candidates, such as the dexamethasone suppression test (The APA Task Force on Laboratory Tests in Psychiatry, 1987), not a single biomarker has been found that is useful in making a mood disorder diagnosis. Thus, for now and the foreseeable future, the diagnosis of mood disorders will continue to rely on a careful clinical assessment of the patient's signs, symptoms, and past history.

Basis for the organization of mood disorders in DSM

Unlike most other disorders which are defined in terms of self-contained criteria sets in DSM-IV-TR, the diagnostic criteria for mood disorders include separate uncoded criteria sets for mood episodes (i.e., major depressive episode, hypomanic episode, manic episode, and mixed episode) and coded criteria sets for mood disorders (i.e., major depressive disorder, dysthymic disorder, bipolar I disorder, bipolar II disorder, cyclothymic disorder, substance-induced mood disorder, and mood disorder due to a general medical condition), which for the most part are expressed in terms of the mood episode criteria sets. Moreover, the adoption of a "lumping" rather than "splitting" strategy for the mood disorders (a strategy which is being continued in DSM-5) involves the extensive use of specifiers in order to define sub-groups of patients with mood disorders that might share a common treatment response pattern (e.g., seasonal pattern to indicate efficacy of light therapy) or possibly common pathophysiology (e.g., melancholic features).

Episodes vs. disorders

Historically, mood disorders occur in episodes of mood disturbance that are punctuated by periods of relatively symptom-free intervals of high functioning. Largely based on common treatment response patterns and family history, mood disorders have been divided into those that are characterized exclusively by episodes of depressed mood (so-called "unipolar depression") and those characterized by episodes of both depressed mood and mania ("bipolar depression"). Given the episodic nature of mood disorders, the basic "building blocks" of the mood disorders are

Clinical Handbook for the Management of Mood Disorders, ed. J. John Mann, Patrick J. McGrath, and Steven P. Roose.
Published by Cambridge University Press. © Cambridge University Press 2013.

mood episodes, as these embody the syndromal nature of these disorders. Accordingly, the major organizational division in the Mood Disorders chapter in DSM-IV is between Mood Episodes, which come first, followed by Mood Disorders. Reflecting its position as one of the most common psychiatric presentations seen by mental health professionals, the criteria for major depressive episode come first, followed by the criteria for manic episode, mixed episode, and hypomanic episode. The definitions of mood episodes are then followed by the definitions of the mood disorders, with depressive disorders coming first (again reflecting their relative commonality), followed by the criteria sets for bipolar disorders, substance-induced mood disorder and mood disorder due to a general medical condition. Since the mood episodes cannot be diagnosed on their own as free-standing diagnostic entities, there are no diagnostic codes associated with them.

Extensive use of specifiers for diagnostic homogeneity

There are two basic classificatory strategies that apply when deciding on the organization of diagnostic entities "lumping" and "splitting." A "lumping" strategy prefers relatively fewer diagnostic entities that are defined relatively broadly and heterogeneously, with the assumption that differences among cases are not as important as their commonalities in terms of understanding their etiology or selecting treatment. In contrast, a "splitting" strategy favors many more narrowly defined entities, with the assumption that the differences between cases are more important than their similarities in terms of defining etiologically and therapeutically homogeneous entities.

The adoption of a lumping strategy for mood disorders, particularly for classifying depressive disorders, reflects the perspective of depression as a unitary construct that represents a final common pathway derived from a variety of etiological and pathophysiological sources (Akiskal and McKinney, 1975), which "accounts for the shared clinical features seen in the heterogeneous groups of depressive disorders" (p. 300). Thus, starting with the first set of diagnostic criteria proposed for research (Feighner *et al.* 1972), continuing with the DSM-III (American Psychiatric Association, 1980), and subsequent DSM revisions, all episodes of clinical depression are defined using the same set of descriptive criteria, even

those occurring in the context of bipolar disorder as opposed to major depressive disorder, despite evidence of heterogeneity in terms of pathophysiological mechanisms and treatment response.

As noted in the introduction to the DSM, its "highest priority has been to provide a helpful guide to clinical practice" (American Psychiatric Association, 2000, p. xxiii). One of the most important aspects of clinical utility is facilitating treatment selection. If it were the case that simply meeting the diagnostic criteria for a disorder like depression or bipolar disorder would be sufficient to determine the optimal treatment, then having a single unitary diagnosis of major depression or bipolar disorder would suffice. However, the long-recognized inconsistent response to various treatment options suggests the value of identifying sub-groups of cases that are more likely to respond to a specific treatment based on severity, phenomenological course, and other factors. DSM-IV thus encourages the use of multiple specifiers to describe the various aspects of the patient's mood disorder presentation in order to help with treatment selection. Fifteen different specifiers are provided in DSM-IV, more than for any other section of the DSM, with several additional specifiers (e.g., with mixed features, with anxious distress level of concern for suicide planned for DSM-5. While this approach has the advantage of providing clinicians with maximum flexibility in terms of allowing them to optionally specify the various important clinical features of the mood presentation, it has the disadvantage that, with the exception of severity, psychosis, and episode type, these specifiers cannot be reflected in the diagnostic coding system so that there is no way this information can be captured in most data systems.

Definitions of mood episodes in DSM-IV
Major depressive episode

A diagnosis of a major depressive episode (MDE) is made by recognizing the characteristic syndrome of symptoms that cluster together during the same period of time. There are two orthogonal dimensions to the major depressive syndrome: the number of characteristic symptoms and the duration/persistence of these symptoms. Nine symptom criteria are included in the syndrome, some of which are compound in the sense that they include several different possible symptoms, only one of which is required for that criterion to be met: (1) depressed mood, (2) diminished interest or pleasure in all or almost all activities, (3) significant increase in appetite or increase in weight or significant decrease in appetite or weight, (4) insomnia or hypersomnia, (5) psychomotor agitation or psychomotor retardation, (6) fatigue or low energy, (7) feelings of worthlessness or excessive or inappropriate guilt, (8) diminished ability to think or indecisiveness, and (9) recurrent thoughts of death, suicidal ideation, or a suicide attempt. DSM-IV sets a diagnostic threshold of at least five out of these nine criteria, which must co-occur during the same period of time. Moreover, DSM-IV elevates two of these symptoms, depressed mood and diminished interest or pleasure to a position of special importance in the diagnosis of a depressive episode; one of these two must be part of the syndrome. This reflects the conventional wisdom that depressed mood should be a required element of a depressive episode. However, given that some individuals with depression (around 20%) do not report feeling sad, depressed, or tearful during an episode, a "depressive-equivalent," i.e., diminished interest in activities, is offered as an alternative. For the temporal dimension, 2 weeks has been chosen as the minimum duration for the symptoms in order to be considered an episode of clinical depression. Moreover, the symptoms have to be present nearly every day during this minimum 2-week period.

The individual symptom criteria in DSM-IV have purposely been worded in such a way as to emphasize the severity of each item. For example, the diminished interest or pleasure in criterion (2) must be "marked," weight loss or gain in criterion (3) must be "significant," psychomotor agitation or retardation in criterion (5) must be sufficiently severe to be noticeable to others, and the feelings about oneself in criterion (7) have to rise to the level of worthlessness. A common error in the diagnosis of a major depressive episode is to stretch the diagnostic threshold so that it includes milder cases than intended by the diagnostic criteria; this has potential clinical implications, given the evidence that somatic treatments tend to be effective in more severe cases.

It should be noted that the threshold of five symptoms and the duration requirement of 2 weeks were not based on empirical evidence of any kind of discontinuity of zone or rarity (Kendell, 1989) that demarcates cases with four or fewer symptoms vs. five or more symptoms, or episodes of less than 2 weeks duration vs. episodes of more than 2 weeks duration. These

thresholds were based on expert consensus that these thresholds defined a level of severity and persistence that would be reasonable to consider "disordered." However, many cases with three or four symptoms may be as ill as cases with five or more symptoms. Further complicating matters, doing a straight symptom count to define disorder as the DSM calls for ignores the reality that different symptoms may have inherently different severities or have differential impact on the need for treatment. For example, a case with only three symptoms but each one at a severe level (e.g., severe suicidal ideation, depressed mood, and inability to sleep) may be more severe than another case with five symptoms, but each of lesser severity. However, despite the potential negative impact of fixed thresholds on validity, their use has been shown to improve diagnostic reliability, especially in research settings. Clinicians using the DSM thresholds should exercise clinical judgment in their application and should view the duration and severity thresholds more as rules of thumb rather than as strict cutoffs to be applied rigidly. As noted in the introductory sections of the DSM-IV-TR, "the specific diagnostic criteria included in DSM-IV are meant to serve as guidelines to be informed by clinical judgment and are not meant to be used in a cookbook fashion. For example, the exercise of clinical judgment may justify giving a certain diagnosis to an individual even though the clinical presentation falls just short of meeting the full criteria for the diagnosis as long as the symptoms that are present are persistent and severe" (p. xxxii).

In addition to the syndromal requirements, the DSM-IV-TR definition has additional requirements to help differentiate between normal sadness and clinical depression. The first requirement is that the cluster of symptoms "cause clinically significant distress or impairment in social, occupational, or other important areas of functioning" (p. 356). Given that many of the symptoms that comprise a major depressive episode (e.g., insomnia, depressed mood, difficulty concentrating) can occur in individuals experiencing normal sadness, this "clinical significance criterion" has been added to the criteria set for a major depressive episode (as well as over 70% of the other disorders in DSM-IV) to help communicate to the clinician that the symptoms should be sufficiently severe so as to have a significant negative impact on the person's life. The other criterion that is intended to avoid inappropriately diagnosing normal individuals as suffering from clinical depression is known as the "bereavement exclusion," which has been a part of the definition since DSM-III. It has long been recognized that individuals experiencing a normal grief reaction may experience many of the nine symptoms included in the definition of a major depressive episode (Clayton *et al.* 1971). In order to prevent normally grieving individuals who happen to have enough major-depressive-like symptoms to meet criteria for an MDE from being diagnosed as clinically depressed, the clinician is instructed *not* to give the diagnosis of MDE to such individuals unless there is evidence that the pattern or duration of the depressive symptoms is no longer consistent with a normal grief reaction, i.e., if the episode persists for longer than two months or certain uncharacteristic features such as morbid preoccupation with worthlessness, psychosis, suicidal ideation, psychomotor retardation, or marked functional impairment are present. This "exception" to the bereavement exclusion is important because for susceptible individuals, the loss of a loved one can trigger the development of a bona fide depressive episode needing psychiatric management.

One of the more controversial changes for DSM-5 is the elimination of the bereavement exclusion so that all cases that meet the syndromal requirement for a major depressive episode be given the diagnosis regardless of the context. This change was put forth on two grounds. First of all, several studies (Wakefield *et al.* 2007, Kendler *et al.* 2008) have suggested that episodes meeting syndromal criteria for a major depressive episode following loss of the loved one are no different than episodes following other severe losses such as divorce or job termination. Secondly, the validity of the bereavement exclusion has been challenged based on review articles which contend that bereavement-related depression is no different than other types of depression (Zisook *et al.* 2007, Lamb *et al.* 2010). Wakefield and First (2012), however, challenged the validity of these review articles, noting that the studies cited in the review article do not actually support the lack of validity of the bereavement exclusion and that two reanalyses of large epidemiological studies (Mojtabai, 2011, Wakefield and Schmitz, 2012) actually support its validity.

Two additional requirements are included in the definition to help differentiate a major depressive episode from other DSM-IV conditions also characterized by clinically significant depressed mood. First of all, following a system-wide DSM convention requiring that psychiatric symptoms that are due to a neurological or systemic general medical condition or that are due to the direct effects of a substance on the central nervous system be given a different diagnosis, the definition of an MDE has a criterion which excludes these etiologies ("the symptoms are not due to the direct physiological effects of a substance (e.g., a drug of abuse, a medication) or a general medical condition (e.g., hypothyroidism)"). In such situations the diagnosis would be a substance-induced mood disorder or a mood disorder due to a general medical condition. Finally, the definition also requires that the "criteria not be met for a mixed episode," which is a type of manic episode in which the criteria are simultaneously met for a manic and major depressive episode at the same time (see Mixed episode below). This is needed to prevent the clinician from mistakenly making the diagnosis of a major depressive episode without considering whether the criteria are also simultaneously met for a manic episode, thus justifying a diagnosis of mixed episode.

Manic episode/hypomanic episode

The hallmark of manic and hypomanic episodes is a discrete period of abnormally elevated, euphoric, expansive, or irritable mood that persists for at least a week in the case of mania or at least 4 days in the case of hypomania. Accompanying the elevated or irritable mood are a set of symptoms including inflated self-esteem or grandiosity, decreased need for sleep (for example, sleeping less than 3 hours yet still feeling rested), pressured speech, flight of ideas, distractibility to external stimuli, increase in social/sexual or occupational/academic activities or psychomotor agitation, and excessive involvement in pleasurable activities that have a high potential for painful consequences that the person ignores (e.g., making foolish business investments, going on unrestrained buying sprees). Unusual for DSM-IV, two different symptom thresholds are offered, depending on whether the mania is characterized by euphoric mood, in which case at least three symptoms must co-occur, or whether there is only irritable mood in which case a minimum of four symptoms are needed for the diagnosis. This requirement for an additional symptom was put into place to help differentiate irritable forms of mania from the irritability that often accompanies a depressive episode. In particular, while it is conceivable that an individual in a depressive episode might experience distractibility, psychomotor agitation, and the subjective experience of racing thoughts (negative brooding thoughts in particular), thus meeting three of the criteria for mania or hypomania, it is unlikely that any of the remaining four symptoms would be present in a bona fide non-mixed major depressive episode (i.e., inflated self-esteem, decreased need for sleep, pressured speech, and excessive involvement in pleasurable activities).

While both mania and hypomania are phenomenologically similar in that they occur as discrete episodes characterized by the same collection of symptoms, they differ primarily in terms of severity. In order for the symptoms to be considered evidence of a manic episode, they must be sufficiently severe so as to cause marked impairment in occupational functioning (e.g., leading to being fired from work) or in usual social activities or relationships with others (e.g., result in termination of friendships or breakup of a relationship), or to necessitate hospitalization in order to prevent self-harm or violence to others, or include psychotic features such as grandiose delusions and hallucinations. Episodes that are not severe enough to cause marked impairment, but that are still pronounced enough to be observable by others are considered to be hypomanic episodes. Given their lack of impairment, hypomanic episodes on their own are not evidence of the presence of a mental disorder in DSM-IV; they are only of psychopathological significance insofar that they occur along with depressive episodes, in which case their presence would justify a diagnosis of bipolar II disorder rather than major depressive disorder.

As with the criteria set for a major depressive episode, an individual would not be diagnosed with a manic or hypomanic episode if the manic/hypomanic symptoms are due to the direct physiological efforts of a substance or a general medical condition. One exception is with manic or hypomanic symptoms that occur in the context of treatment with an antidepressant or other somatic treatment for depression. Although in DSM-IV such episodes were considered to be examples of a substance-induced mood disorder and would not count as manic or hypomanic episodes for the purposes of determining whether the diagnosis is bipolar vs. major depressive disorder, starting with DSM-5 manic- or hypomanic-like episodes that are triggered by antidepressant treatment and that persist after the treatment is stopped are considered to be true manic or hypomanic episodes, justifying a diagnosis of bipolar disorder in such individuals.

Mixed episode

This third variety of mood episode is characterized by the simultaneous presence of symptoms characteristic of a manic and major depressive episode, occurring every day for at least a 1-week period. The major depressive and manic symptoms can be intermixed, or else the person may instead experience rapidly alternating mood states, such as depression giving way to irritability, and then euphoria. Functionally, DSM-IV considers a mixed episode to be a variety of manic episode, in that, like a manic episode, the presence of a mixed episode is sufficient to make a diagnosis of bipolar I disorder. DSM-5 is replacing the concept of a mixed episode by including a "mixed features" specifier that can apply to either a manic episode or a depressive episode in cases in which there are co-occurring features characteristic of the episode of the opposite polarity. In the case of a manic episode, the mixed features specifier would apply if during the manic episode, three or more depressive symptoms were present every day, and in the case of a major depressive episode, the specifier would apply if during the major depressive episode, at least three manic symptoms were present nearly every day. One potential problem with using the mixed features specifier for a major depressive episode occurring in the context of a diagnosis of major depressive disorder is that the co-occurring manic symptoms may more reasonably suggest that the individual is in the bipolar spectrum (Sato *et al.* 2003), but DSM-5 will continue to consider such individuals as having unipolar depression.

Definitions of mood disorders in DSM-IV

Mood disorders in DSM-IV are sub-divided into two sections: depressive disorders and bipolar disorders, based on differences in management, pathophysiology, and genetics.

Major depressive disorder

Major depressive disorder is characterized by one or more major depressive episodes. Required elements of the diagnostic coding include indicating whether there has been only a single episode of depression or whether there have been multiple episodes, in which case the major depressive disorder is considered to be recurrent. Because the severity of depression can wax and wane over time, it is sometimes not so straightforward to determine whether a person has had an extended single episode with periods of mild improvement or whether periods of worsening mood separated by periods of relative improvement count as separate episodes.

Moreover, the severity of the current episode is also part of the diagnostic coding. If the patient is currently in the midst of a full depressive episode, the clinician is asked to indicate the current severity, ranging from mild (for episodes in which five or six of the nine items are present and for which the symptoms result in only minor impairment in social or occupational functioning), moderate (for episodes in which the symptoms or functional impairment is in between mild and severe), severe without psychotic features (for episodes with seven or more items and for which the symptoms markedly interfere with social or occupational functioning), and severe with psychotic features (for episodes in which there are delusions or hallucinations). If the patient with major depressive disorder is not currently in the midst of a full depressive episode, the clinician should indicate whether the disorder is in partial or full remission. The disorder is considered to be in full remission if the patient has been free of any significant mood symptoms for at least the past 2 months. The disorder is in partial remission if either the person has recently been without significant symptoms, but for less than 2 months, or there are some symptoms of major depression that persist, but not enough to meet the diagnostic threshold of five symptoms.

The inclusion of recurrence and severity in the diagnostic coding structure reflects the particular clinical importance of these factors. The determination of whether there has been more than one episode is relevant to decisions regarding the need for ongoing maintenance treatment. In general, the risk of having a future episode is related to the number of past episodes. According to the DSM-IV, although individuals with a single episode have a 60% chance of developing a second episode, those with two episodes have a 70% chance of a third and those with three episodes have a 90% chance of developing a fourth. The severity/psychosis/remission coding is also important with regard to management. Whereas individuals with mild or moderate depression will generally do well with either psychotherapy or somatic treatment, individuals with severe depression usually need somatic treatment. Those with psychotic features invariably need antipsychotic medication or electroconvulsive therapy to treat the psychosis.

Dysthymic disorder (called persistent depressive disorder in DSM-5)

Dysthymic disorder is characterized by a chronic persistent period of depressed mood that remains below the symptom severity threshold of a major depressive episode. The chronic and persistent depressed mood is operationalized in the DSM-IV as having depressed mood, more days than not, for at least 2 years. While some gaps in the chronic depression may still be consistent with the diagnosis, none of those symptom-free periods can have lasted for as long as 2 months. Both major depressive disorder and dysthymic disorder can be diagnosed co-morbidly (also known as "double depression") for situations in which major depressive episodes are superimposed on a mild chronic depression.

Bipolar I disorder

Bipolar I disorder is typically characterized by manic or mixed episodes, plus major depressive episodes. Definitionally, however, bipolar I disorder is diagnosed after only one manic or mixed episode. Because the type of the current episode is so relevant for current management decisions, in order to select the right ICD-9-CM diagnostic code, the clinician needs to indicate the type of the current episode, or, if the patient is no longer currently in a full episode (i.e., the disturbance is in partial or full remission), the type of the most recent episode. As with major depressive disorder, the fifth digit in the diagnostic code is used to indicate the severity of the current mood episode (i.e., mild, moderate, severe without psychotic features, severe with psychotic features) or else to indicate that the bipolar I disorder is currently in partial or full remission. Major depressive episodes occurring in the context of bipolar I disorder phenomenologically look the same as those that occur in the context of major depressive disorder; accordingly, the definitions of mild, moderate, and severe are the same as for major depressive episodes occurring in major depressive disorder. Definitions for the severity specifiers for a manic and mixed episode differ from those of a major depressive episode. A manic episode is considered to be mild if only minimum symptom criteria are met (i.e., three to four symptoms), moderate if there is an extreme increase in activity or impairment in judgment, severe without psychotic features if almost continual supervision is required to prevent harm to self or others, and severe with psychotic features if delusions or hallucinations are present during the episode. As might be expected, the severity specifiers of a mixed episode are a hybrid of those for a major depressive and manic episode. A mixed episode is considered to be mild if no more than minimum symptom criteria are met for both a manic and major depressive episode, moderate if symptoms or functional impairment are between mild and severe, severe with psychotic features if almost continual supervision is required to prevent harm to self or others, and severe with psychotic features if delusions or hallucinations are present.

Bipolar II disorder

Bipolar II disorder is a variant of bipolar disorder in which the patient has had one or more hypomanic episodes and one or more major depressive episodes, but has never had any full-blown manic or mixed episodes. As with bipolar I disorder, it is recommended for the clinician to indicate whether the current or most recent episode is a hypomanic or major depressive episode; unlike bipolar I disorder, this specification is not reflected in the diagnostic coding, so it is likely rarely used by clinicians, especially since the vast majority of patients with bipolar II disorder will be seen clinically when they are suffering from a major depressive episode.

Cyclothymic disorder

Analogous to the relationship between dysthymic disorder and major depressive disorder, cyclothymic disorder is a chronic mild version of bipolar I disorder, with numerous periods of hypomania and mild depression that do not meet criteria for a full-blown manic or major depressive episode. Almost like dysthymic disorder, manic and major depressive episodes may be superimposed on the persistent cyclothymic pattern, justifying a co-morbid diagnosis of bipolar I disorder (in the case of manic episodes) or bipolar II disorder (in the case of superimposed major depressive, but no superimposed manic episodes).

Bipolar disorder not otherwise specified

Epidemiological data suggests that manic-like episodes of briefer duration and fewer symptoms may be common (Angst *et al.* 2011). Patients with recurrent briefer episodes would be classified under the bipolar NOS category so long as these episodes cause a significant degree of distress or impairment.

Substance-induced mood disorders

Mood symptoms that are due to the direct physiological effects of a substance on the central nervous system are diagnosed as a substance-induced mood disorder. It is important to understand that co-morbid substance use and mood symptomatology do not necessarily indicate the presence of a substance-induced mood disorder. In such situations, three explanatory diagnostic scenarios are possible and must be considered. First, the mood symptoms could be primary and result in substance abuse (e.g., as a form of self-medication). In such cases, the diagnosis would be the primary mood disorder plus a co-morbid diagnosis of a substance-use disorder. Second, the mood symptoms could be a direct consequence of the substance use, i.e., were it not for the substance use, the patient would not be suffering from the mood symptoms. In such cases, the diagnosis is substance-induced mood disorder. In the third scenario, the patient could have a primary mood disorder (e.g., depression), which predisposes the patient to abuse a substance, which then produces a different type of mood symptom through the substance's action on the central nervous system (e.g., manic symptoms). In such cases, both the primary mood disorder and substance-induced mood disorder would be diagnosed. Determining the causal relationship between the mood symptoms and the substance use usually depends on the temporal relationship between the two: if the person only experienced the mood symptoms in the context of substance use, then it is a substance-induced mood disorder. If the mood symptoms are present either prior to substance use or persist long after the person is abstinent, then the diagnosis is a primary mood disorder. It should be noted that in actual practice settings, it is often impossible to ascertain the temporal relationship between the mood symptoms and substance use (see Chapter 17 by Nunes and Levin for a more extensive discussion of this issue).

Mood disorder due to a general medical condition

Mood symptoms can also arise as a direct result of a neurological condition involving the CNS (e.g., brain

Table 2.1 Specifiers (excluding severity/psychosis/remission) that apply to current mood episode or disorder

Specifier	Definition	Applicable to:	Potential Clinical Utility
Chronic	Criteria have been made continuously for 2 years	Major depressive episodes	Likely more difficult to treat
With catatonic features	Clinical picture dominated by motor abnormalities such as motoric immobility, excessive motor activity, negativism, peculiar movements, echolalia, or echopraxia	Manic episodes, mixed episodes, or major depressive episodes	Treatment implications (ECT, benzodiazipines)
With melancholic features	Ahhedona or lack of mood reactivity accompanied by other symptoms such as distinct quality of mood, mood worse in AM, early morning awakening, marked psychomotor agitation or retardation, significant anorexia or weight loss, excessive guilt	Major depressive episodes	Indicates need for somatic treatment as opposed to psychotherapy alone
With atypical features	Mood reactivity accompanied by other symptoms such as increased appetite or weight gain, hypersomnia, leaden paralysis, interpersonal rejection sensitivity	Major depressive episodes, dysthymic disorder	Indicates lack of responsiveness to tricyclic antidepressants, responsiveness to MAO inhibitors
Post-partum onset	Onset within 4 weeks post-partum	Manic episodes, mixed episodes, or major depressive episodes	Current management (supervision for infant care) and future prognosis

tumor, stroke, Parkinson's disease) or due to the systemic effects of a general medical condition on the central nervous system (e.g., hypothyroidism). In such cases, a diagnosis of mood disorder due to a general medical condition is made. A presentation in which mood symptoms develop as a psychological reaction to some aspect of a medical condition (e.g., depressive reaction to the physical disability resulting from a stroke) is not diagnosed as a mood disorder due to a general medical condition, but instead as a primary mood disorder (if the full syndromal criteria are met) or an adjustment disorder.

Mood specifiers

As noted in the beginning of this chapter, specific information about the mood disorder that is treatment-relevant can be indicated using one or more of the many available specifiers. Specifiers can be applied either to the current mood episode (for example, "with melancholic features" to indicate the characteristic symptom pattern of melancholia), or to the overall longitudinal pattern of the episodes (for example, "with rapid cycling" for bipolar disorder to indicate the presence of four or more mood episodes in the past 12 months). Table 2.1 indicates those specifiers (excluding the severity/psychosis/remission specifiers already discussed) that apply to the current mood episode and summarizes their definitions,

indicates those types of episodes to which the specifier applies, and then notes its potential clinical utility in the management of the disorder. Table 2.2 indicates those specifiers that apply to the longitudinal course of the disorders, summarizes their definitions, indicating the disorders to which the specifier might apply, and notes its potential clinical utility as well.

Assessment procedures used as aids in making diagnoses and evaluating levels of severity

Clinicians are usually (if not always) pressed for time when they evaluate patients diagnostically or monitor their clinical status. Fortunately, there are a number of procedures that can help in obtaining the needed clinical information in an efficient manner. Detailed descriptions of the assessment procedures noted below are available elsewhere (Rush *et al.* 2008).

Diagnostic aids

A good diagnostic evaluation requires clinicians to establish the symptoms experienced by the patient currently and in the past, and also to be attentive to differential diagnostic issues and identification of possible clinically relevant co-morbid conditions. Two types of diagnostic assessment procedures are available, clinical interview guides and self-report questionnaires.

Table 2.2 Specifiers that apply to longitudinal course of mood disorders

Specifier	Definition	Applicable to:	Potential Clinical Utility
With rapid cycling	At least four episodes in previous 12 months	Bipolar I disorder, bipolar II disorder	Specific treatment needs (e.g., less likely to respond to lithium)
With seasonal pattern	Regular temporal relationship between onset of major depressive episodes and time of year and remission at a characteristic time of the year	Bipolar I disorder, bipolar II disorder, major depressive disorder	Utility of light therapy
With interepisode recovery/without interepisode recovery	Whether or not full remission is attained between two most recent mood episodes	Bipolar I disorder, bipolar II disorder, major depressive disorder	Indicates need for interepisode treatment; more difficult to treat

Interview guides

Training and experience with diagnostic interview guides are very useful in helping clinicians become better diagnosticians by becoming familiar with efficient ways to pose questions and to focus on important differential diagnostic issues. Ideally, focused training for the specific procedure will have been obtained. The two such procedures that are most widely used are briefly described below.

Structured Clinical Interview for DSM-IV Axis I Disorders (SCID-IV)

The most commonly used clinical interview procedures are versions of the Structured Clinical Interview for DSM-IV Axis I Disorders (SCID-IV) (First *et al.* 2002). Versions of the SCID-IV include semistructured interview guides designed for use with patients or with nonpatient subjects who are being evaluated for psychopathology. The interview guides include probe questions and suggested follow-up questions, as well as skip-out instructions when a subject's symptoms do not meet a critical criterion for a diagnosis. The items to be scored are the individual diagnostic criteria for the diagnosis covered by a particular module. The diagnostic modules of the SCID-IV include Mood Episodes, Psychotic Symptoms, Psychotic Disorders Differential, Mood Disorders Differential, Substance Use, Anxiety Disorders, Somatoform Disorders, Eating Disorders, and Adjustment Disorders. The SCID-CV is the Clinician Version (First *et al.* 1996) designed to be used in nonresearch settings. The modular organization also allows a clinician to focus on particular diagnoses following an initial open diagnostic evaluation.

Mini International Neuropsychiatric Interview (MINI)

The MINI (Sheehan *et al.* 1998) is a highly structured diagnostic interview designed to provide a brief diagnostic evaluation. Each module has a series of closed-ended yes/no questions focused upon the diagnostic criteria for a specific disorder. In contrast to the SCID, each of the MINI modules is designed to be overinclusive, thus potentially allowing more false positive diagnoses. In settings where more precise diagnoses are needed, the clinician is expected to seek more clarification regarding the criteria.

Diagnostic self-report questionnaires

Self-report procedures are best used for screening rather than for a formal differential diagnostic evaluation. They are designed to be reviewed by clinicians and depending upon the patient's responses, definitive diagnoses must be verified. The Psychiatric Diagnostic Screening Questionnaire (PDSQ) (Zimmerman and Mattia, 1999) and the Patient Health Questionnaire (PHQ) (Spitzer *et al.* 1999) are the two most widely used, with the PDSQ having broader coverage than the PHQ.

Psychiatric Diagnostic Screening Questionnaire (PDSQ)

The PDSQ screens for the 13 most commonly experienced DSM-IV Axis I outpatient disorders: bulimia/binge-eating disorder, major depressive disorder, panic disorder, agoraphobia, PTSD, obsessive compulsive disorder, generalized anxiety disorder, social phobia, alcohol and drug abuse/dependence, somatization disorder, and hypochondriasis. There is also a short psychosis screen. Items are grouped by diagnosis and are in a yes/no format. An interview guide is available to aid the clinician in confirming the self-report responses or ruling out diagnoses.

Patient Health Questionnaire (PHQ)

The PHQ has questions for eight DSM-IV diagnoses (major depressive syndrome, other depressive syndrome, panic disorder, other anxiety syndrome, somatoform disorder, bulimia nervosa, binge-eating disorder, and alcohol abuse). There are algorithms for diagnoses and instructions for ruling out certain diagnoses (e.g., due to a physical disorder).

Evaluation of severity of mood disorders

There are many different procedures available for the assessment of the presence and severity of symptoms of depression and mania. While some involve clinical interviews, self-report questionnaires are more frequently used. Use of such procedures detects changes in clinical status that are very valuable in determining the potential need for changes in treatment. They are designed to be used at baseline and periodically thereafter to monitor clinical changes. Ideally, clinicians would use such scales regularly, as such use should lead to greater understanding of the meaningfulness of the scores.

Self-report measures of severity of mood episodes

There are many different self-report questionnaires designed for the assessment of the severity of depressive symptoms. The self-report versions or the IDS and the QIDS (described below) are currently considered to have the "best" coverage and to be the most sensitive to change in the severity of depression, and are now the most commonly used in clinical settings.

Inventory of Depressive Symptomatology (IDS); Quick Inventory of Depressive Symptomatology (QIDS)

Both the IDS and the QIDS were designed to cover all of the criterion symptoms of DSM-IV major depressive episode (Rush *et al.* 2000, 2003, Trivedi *et al.* 2004). There are two versions of both measures, self-rated and clinician-rated, and scores from the two versions are highly correlated. The 16 QIDS items cover the nine symptom groups used to define a major depressive episode. The IDS contains 30 items, including some for frequently associated symptoms such as anxiety, as well as items for atypical or melancholic features. The IDS also has a wider range in total score than other available procedures for assessing depression severity, whether clinician-rated or self-report, making the measure more suitable for assessing change in less severely ill patients.

Self-report measures of depression for special groups

Given the problems of evaluating severity of depression in patients with general medical conditions, several different self-report questionnaires are more

appropriate. They include the Edinburgh Postnatal Depression Scale with 10 items, the Geriatric Depression Scale with 30 items, and the Hospital Anxiety and Depression Scale with 14 items.

Self-report measure of severity of manic symptoms

Although some clinicians are skeptical regarding the usefulness of self-report measures of manic symptoms, the Altman Self-Rating Mania Scale (ASRMS)(Altman *et al.* 1997) has been found to provide reliable and valid measures of the severity of five manic symptoms. These measures have relatively high correlations with clinician ratings and have been shown to be sensitive to changes in clinical status. Unfortunately, efforts to include items for the assessment of psychotic symptoms in patients with bipolar manic disorder were unsuccessful.

Clinical interview measures of severity of mood disorders

The severity measures that involve clinical interviews depend upon the clinician's ability to establish frequency, intensity, and pervasiveness of the various symptoms prior to scoring their severity. Brief descriptions of the most frequently employed interview procedures are given below.

Inventory of Depressive Symptomatology (IDS); Quick Inventory of Depressive Symptomatology (QIDS)

The IDS and QIDS are described above. The clinician-rated versions include semistructured interview guides.

Montgomery–Asberg Depression Rating Scale (MADRS)

The MADRS (Montgomery and Asberg, 1979) has 10 items descriptive of features of major depressive disorder that were selected because they were generally sensitive to change. In addition, the items often describe cognitive features and thus are less likely to be scored in patients with general medical illnesses. The items are rated on seven-point scales with descriptive anchors for every second level. The MADRS has usually been completed without the use of a structured interview guide.

Hamilton Rating Scale for Depression (HAM-D)

The Ham-D (Hamilton, 1960) has been the most commonly used interview-based measure of the severity of depression. However, some of the Ham-D's properties have been problematic, particularly when used with outpatients or with patients who have general medical illnesses. The item content is more appropriate for use with inpatients that have relatively severe major depressive disorder. The items are scored on three- or four-point severity scales with defined levels that at times involve more than one clinical feature. There are now many different versions of the Ham-D ranging from 17 to over 30 items. The ratings are often made on the basis of unstructured clinical interviews, although several interview guides are now available and these have been shown to improve the reliability of the scores.

Clinician-Administered Rating Scale For Mania (CARS-M)

The CARS-M (Altman *et al.* 1994) was developed to evaluate both the features of the manic syndrome (10 items) as well as psychotic symptoms (five items) with all but one rated on six-point scales with defined levels of severity. Questions are available to aid the clinician and, in addition, clinicians are encouraged to use all other sources of information (e.g., family reports).

Young Mania Rating Scale (YMRS)

The YMRS (Young *et al.* 1978) has 11 items designed to assess both mild and severe symptoms of mania. Some items are scored on five-point scales, others on nine-point scales with defined levels of severity. No interview guide is available.

DSM-5

The next edition of the *Diagnostic and Statistical Manual of Mental Disorders*, DSM-5, is expected to be published in May 2013. Compared to other sections of the manual, changes to the Mood Disorders section are relatively modest. On an organizational level, one change is to split the mood disorders grouping into two separate groupings: bipolar and related disorders, and depressive disorders. The bipolar and related disorders section will essentially contain the same disorders as in DSM-IV: bipolar I disorder, bipolar II disorder, cyclothymic disorder, substance-induced bipolar disorder, and bipolar disorder attributed to another medical condition. Regarding changes to the disorders themselves, the criteria for a manic and hypomanic episode now require both a mood disturbance (i.e., elevated, euphoric, or irritable mood) *and* an increase in activity or energy. Manic or hypomanic episodes triggered by somatic treatment of depression (e.g., antidepressant medication, light therapy, ECT) and that persist beyond the physiological effect of that treatment are considered to be bona fide manic or hypomanic episodes in DSM-5; in DSM-IV they were classified as substance-induced mood episodes and would not count towards a diagnosis of bipolar I or bipolar II disorder. The construct of a "mixed episode" as a variety of manic episode has been dropped in DSM-5. Instead, depressive symptoms that occur nearly every day during a manic episode justify use of the specifier "with mixed features."

More significant changes have been made to the depressive disorders section. Dysthymic disorder is being renamed "persistent depressive disorder" and can now be given regardless of the co-occurrence or history of any major depressive episodes. Two new depressive disorders will be included in DSM-5; premenstrual dysphoric disorder and disruptive mood dysregulation disorder. Premenstrual dysphoric disorder is for presentations of dysphoric mood and other symptoms that occur in the week prior to menses and that improve within a few days after menses, and has been in the DSM research appendix in some form since 1987. Disruptive mood dysregulation disorder, newly included in DSM-5, is for presentations with persistently irritable mood occurring nearly every day punctuated by severe recurrent temper outbursts in response to common stressors that occur at least three or more times per week for at least 12 months. It is being included with the hope that it will reduce the inappropriate application of the bipolar label to children.

References

Akiskal, H.S. and McKinney, W.T., Jr. (1975). Overview of recent research in depression. Integration of ten conceptual models into a comprehensive clinical frame. *Archives of General Psychiatry*, 32, 285–305.

Altman, E.G., Hedeker, D., Peterson, J.L., and Davis, J.M. (1997). The Altman Self-Rating Mania Scale. *Biological Psychiatry*, 42, 948–955.

Altman, E.G., Hedeker, D.R., Janicak, P.G., Peterson, J.L., and Davis, J.M. (1994). The Altman Self-Rating Mania Scale. *Biological Psychiatry*, 36, 124–134.

American Psychiatric Association (1980). *Diagnostic and Statistical Manual of Mental Disorders, Third Edition*. Washington, DC: American Psychiatric Association.

American Psychiatric Association (2000). *Diagnostic and Statistical Manual of Mental Disorders, Fourth Edition, Text Revision*. Washington, DC: American Psychiatric Association.

Angst, J., Azorin, J.M., Bowden, C.L. *et al.* (2011). Prevalence and characteristics of undiagnosed bipolar disorders in patients with a major depressive episode: The BRIDGE study. *Archives of General Psychiatry*, 68, 791–798.

Clayton, P.J., Halikes, J.A., and Maurice, W.L. (1971). The bereavement of the widowed. *Diseases of the Nervous System*, 32, 597–604.

Feighner, J.P., Robins, E., Guze, S.B. *et al.* (1972). Diagnostic criteria for use in psychiatric research. *Archives of General Psychiatry*, 26, 57–63.

First, M.B., Spitzer, R.L., Gibbon, M., and Williams, J.B.W. (1996). *Structured Clinical Interview for DSM-IV Axis I Disorders, Clinician Version (SCID-CV)*. Washington, DC: American Psychiatric Press, Inc.

First, M.B., Spitzer, R.L., Gibbon, M., and Williams, J.B.W. (2002). *Structured Clinical Interview for DSM-IV-TR Axis I Disorders Research Version, Patient Edition (SCID-I/P)*. New York: Biometrics Research, New York State Psychiatric Institute.

Hamilton, M. (1960). A rating scale for depression. *Journal of Neurology, Neurosurgery and Psychiatry*, 23, 56–62.

Kendell, R.E. (1989). Clinical validity. *Psychological Medicine*, 19, 45–55.

Kendler, K.S., Myers, J., and Zisook, S. (2008). Does bereavement-related major depression differ from major depression associated with other stressful life events? *American Journal of Psychiatry*, 165, 1449–1455.

Lamb, K., Pies, R., and Zisook, S. (2010). The bereavement exclusion for the diagnosis of major depression: To be or not to be. *Psychiatry*, 7, 19–25.

Mojtabai, R. (2011). Bereavement-related depressive episodes: Characteristics, 3-year course and implications for the DSM-5. *Archives of General Psychiatry*, 68, 920–928.

Montgomery, S.A. and Asberg, M. (1979). A new depression scale designed to be sensitive to change. *British Journal of Psychiatry*, 23, 56–62.

Reed, G.M., Correia, J.M., Esparza, P., Saxena, S., and Maj, M. (2011). The WPA-WHO Global Survey of Psychiatrists' Attitudes Towards Mental Disorders Classification. *World Psychiatry*, 10, 118–131.

Rush, A.J., Carmody, T.J., and Reimitz, P.E. (2000). The Inventory of Depressive Symptomatology (IDS): clinician (IDS-C) and self-report (IDS-SR) ratings of depressive symptoms. *International Journal of Methods in Psychiatric Research*, 9, 45–49.

Rush, A., First, M., and Blacker, D. (2008). *Handbook of Psychiatric Measures Second Edition*. Arlington, VA: American Psychiatric Publishing, Inc.

Rush, A.J., Trivedi, M.H., Ibrahim, H.M. *et al.* (2003). The 16-item Quick Inventory of Depressive Symptomatology (QIDS), clinician rating (QIDS-C), and self-report (QIDS-SR): A psychometric evaluation in patients with chronic major depression. *Biological Psychiatry*, 54, 573–583.

Sato, T., Bottlender, R., Schröter, A., and Möller, H.J. (2003). Frequency of manic symptoms during a depressive episode and unipolar "depressive mixed state" as bipolar spectrum. *Acta Psychiatrica Scandinavica*, 107, 268–274.

Sheehan, D.V., Lecrubier, Y., K., H.-S., Amorim, P. *et al.* (1998). The Mini-International Neuropsychiatric Interview (M.I.N.I.): The development and validation of a structured diagnostic psychiatric interview for DSM-IV and ICD-10. *Journal of Clinical Psychiatry*, 59, 22–33.

Spitzer, R.L., Kroenke, K., and Williams, J.B.W. (1999). Validation and utility of a self-report version of PRIME-MD: The PHQ primary care study. Primary Care Evaluation of Mental Disorders. Patient Health Questionnaire. *Journal of the American Medical Association*, 282, 1737–1744.

The APA Task Force on Laboratory Tests in Psychiatry (1987). The dexamethasone suppression test: an overview of its current status in psychiatry. *American Journal of Psychiatry*, 144, 1253–1263.

Trivedi, M.H., Rush, A.J., Ibrahim, H.M. *et al.* (2004). The Inventory of Depressive Symptomatology, Clinician Rating (IDS-C) and Self-Report (IDS-SR), and the Quick Inventory of Depressive Symptomatology, Clinician Rating (QIDS-C) and Self-Report (QIDS-SR). *Psychological Medicine*, 34, 73–82.

Wakefield, J.C. and First, M.B. (2012). Validity of the bereavement exclusion to major depression: Does the empirical evidence support the proposal to eliminate the exclusion in DSM-5? *World Psychiatry*, 11, 3–10.

Wakefield, J.C. and Schmitz, M.F. (2012). Recurrence of bereavement-related depression: Evidence for the validity of the DSM-IV bereavement exclusion from the Epidemiological Catchment Area Study. *Journal of Nervous and Mental Diseases*, 200, 480–485.

Wakefield, J., Schmitz, M., First, M., and Horwitz, A. (2007). Extending the bereavement exclusion for major depression to other losses: Evidence from the National Comorbidity Survey. *Archives of General Psychiatry*, 64, 433–440.

World Health Organization (1992). *The ICD-10 Classification of Mental and Behavioral Disorders: Clinical Descriptions and Diagnostic Guidelines Tenth Edition*. Geneva: World Health Organization.

Young, R.C., Biggs, J.T., Ziegler, V.E., and Meyer, D.A. (1978). A rating scale for mania: Reliability, validity and sensitivity. *British Journal of Psychiatry*, 133, 429–435.

Zimmerman, M. and Mattia, J.I. (1999). The reliability and validity of a screening questionnaire for 13 DSM-IV Axis I disorders (the Psychiatric Diagnostic Screening Questionnaire) in psychiatric outpatients. *Journal of Clinical Psychiatry*, 60, 677–683.

Zisook, S., Shear, K., and Kendler, K. (2007). Validity of the bereavement exclusion criterion for the diagnosis of major depressive episode. *World Psychiatry*, 6, 102–107.

Chapter

3

Dysthymia and chronic depression

David J. Hellerstein and Jordan W. Eipper

Introduction

Clinical case vignette

Mr. S is a 35-year-old single, unemployed white male who describes life-long depression that has worsened since he lost his job 3 months ago. He feels depressed most of the day, nearly every day, without diurnal variation. Over the past 3 months his sleep, which has always been irregular, has worsened. He feels pessimistic and guilty, but denies extreme fatigue or leaden paralysis. His appetite, concentration, and motor activity are normal. However, feeling "immobilized," he rarely leaves his apartment and lacks motivation to find a new job, despite worsening financial problems.

Mr. S's depression began when he was 12 years old, and he reports feeling depressed approximately 80% of the time since then. In college, after he broke up with a girlfriend, his depression became "more serious" for several months, but it is unclear whether he met criteria for a major depressive episode (MDE). Following an 8-month period of euthymia at age 24, Mr. S's depression gradually returned. His symptoms have worsened in recent months following the afore-mentioned job loss. There is no evidence for ADHD or anxiety disorders, and no history of hypomania or mania. Mr. S was briefly prescribed sertraline (50 mg/day) in high school, which he stopped taking after a few months because of "jitters," and bupropion (up to 200 mg/day) 2 years ago. Bupropion offered some relief, but Mr. S discontinued it following a change in insurance coverage. Mr. S has been in group therapy for the past 10 years, which has helped alleviate his isolation, but has not improved his mood.

Stress stemming from multiple family moves during childhood caused Mr. S to lose friends and to struggle academically. Following college, he held jobs in broadcast entertainment until being downsized 6 years ago. Since then, he has gotten temporary jobs. He feels that depression interferes with work performance: he has trouble staying motivated and engaged, and often cannot finish projects on time. He also has difficulties in workplace relationships, feeling withdrawn and lacking confidence when interacting with co-workers. Mr. S is involved with a girlfriend of 7 years, although they currently do not live together. She complains that he is too negative and becomes "too dependent" on her. Mr. S's mother, brother, and paternal grandmother have been treated for depression, and a maternal cousin has bipolar I disorder. Mr. S denies a family history of suicide, schizophrenia, or substance abuse.

He is unshaven and appears slightly overweight. His thoughts are coherent and goal-directed. He is pre-occupied with pessimistic ideas, e.g., that there is no purpose to life and that he will never get another job. He denies current suicidal ideation, but acknowledges occasionally wondering "what's the point of living?"

Mr. S was diagnosed with dysthymic disorder (DD), early onset. Although his symptoms have worsened recently, he does not meet criteria for major depression. Mr. S was started on an SNRI antidepressant medication, and after 6 weeks his HAM-D score (Hamilton, 1960) dropped from 22 to 6. After his depression remitted, Mr. S began treatment with behavioral activation therapy (Erickson and Hellerstein, 2011), an activity-focused psychotherapy, in order to address residual affective, interpersonal, and vocational issues.

Clinical Handbook for the Management of Mood Disorders, ed. J. John Mann, Patrick J. McGrath, and Steven P. Roose.
Published by Cambridge University Press. © Cambridge University Press 2013.

Background

Though traditionally viewed as an episodic and periodically remitting disorder, in the last several decades, it has become clear that depression often has a chronic course, and is associated with high personal and socioeconomic costs (Weissman and Klerman, 1977, Akiskal, 1980, Kessler *et al.* 1994, Klein *et al.* 2000).

Concurrently, the psychiatric nosology has evolved in attempts to characterize the varied presentations of chronic depression. The 1980 DSM-III relabeled "neurotic depression" as "dysthymia" and classified it among the affective disorders. DSM-III-R differentiated between chronic major depression, a more severe form of chronic depression, and the milder condition of dysthymia (McCullough, 2000). DSM-IV complicated the picture by describing other sub-types of chronic depression, including: recurrent major depression with incomplete interepisode recovery, concurrent dysthymia and major depression ("double depression," Keller and Shapiro, 1982), and major depression in incomplete remission.

Yet it has become clear that there are few meaningful differences among these sub-types, which exhibit few differences in clinically relevant variables such as longitudinal course, treatment response, symptomatology, psychosocial functioning, co-morbidity, family history, or demographics (DSM-5 Work Group, McCullough *et al.* 2000, 2003). In contrast, numerous variables differentiate chronic from acute depression: higher rates of suicidality (Klein *et al.* 2000), greater functional impairment (Klein *et al.* 1988), more Axis I and Axis II co-morbidity (Markowitz *et al.* 1992, Pepper *et al.* 1995), stronger family history (Klein *et al.* 1988, 1995), higher rates of childhood adversity (Lizardi *et al.* 1995), a lower rate of treatment response (Kocsis, 2003), and earlier age of onset (Garvey *et al.* 1986, Yang and Dunner, 2001, Klein *et al.* 2004). Thus, the chronic depressions, while at times differing in terms of cross-sectional severity, are at once highly similar and distinct from episodic major depression.

Consequently, the DSM-5 Mood Disorder Work Group recently proposed draft criteria in which the category of dysthymic disorder will be replaced by a new diagnosis, chronic depressive disorder (CDD) (DSM-5 Work Group), which will subsume various forms of chronic depression under a single category. The new category will no longer require clinicians to differentiate between disorders, such as residual major depression and DD, which require retrospective distinctions that often have questionable reliability. While varying in pattern of onset and cross-sectional severity, these conditions are all characterized, by definition, by chronicity. Hence, DSM-5 will emphasize that chronicity (≥ 2 years) of depression has a major impact on presentation and outcome. (There have been differences of opinion regarding the length of time needed to define chronicity; some investigators consider 1 year of consistent symptoms sufficient to mark a chronic episode) (Brown and Moran, 1994). More recently, however, DSM-5 draft criteria were revised to retain a separation between dysthymic disorder and chronic MDD, with the following justification: "We believe it important to distinguish from dysthymic disorder the relatively high illness severity implicit in the DSM-IV definition of chronic MDD, a definition that requires the continuous presence of the full major depressive syndrome over a two-year period." Thus, currently the only changes in DSM-5 draft criteria for dysthymic disorder are in criteria D and E, removing language excluding individuals with major depression in the first 2 years of the disorder and those with prior cyclothymia diagnoses. The major consequence will be that among patients currently meeting criteria for dysthymia (but without current MDD), clinicians will no longer need to attempt to distinguish between dysthymic disorder and residual major depression.

Epidemiology and burden

Epidemiological studies have confirmed clinical findings that chronic depression is both common and disabling. Early research found rates of dysthymia ranging from 2.3 to 4.8% in women and 1.3 to 2.3% in men, with a mean lifetime prevalence of 3.1% across five nationwide sites (Weissman *et al.* 1988). Subsequent reports have found values between 2.5% (Kessler *et al.* 2005) and 6.4% (Kessler *et al.* 1994). Similar to episodic depression, rates of dysthymia are nearly twice as high in females as in males. Perhaps 12 to 20% of major depressive episodes take a chronic course (Weissman and Klerman 1977, Scott 1988, Gilmer *et al.* 2005). Since the lifetime prevalence of major depression has been estimated to be from 4.9 to 17.1% (Weissman *et al.* 1991, Kessler *et al.* 1994), it is clear that chronic depressions make up a substantial portion of the illness's burden in the community. In clinical settings, chronic depression is more prevalent than in the general community, with dysthymia reported in 5 (Brown *et al.* 1999) to 9% (site range = 5–15%, Spitzer *et al.* 1994) of primary care patients and 22 (Klein *et al.* 1989) to 36% (Markowitz *et al.* 1992) of psychiatric outpatients.

The morbidity of chronic depression is often overlooked, especially when it does not reach the severity of major depression. Given a longitudinal outlook, however, a sizeable literature demonstrates a considerable disease burden. Wells *et al.* (1989) found that in a mixed sample (both MDD and dysthymia) depression was correlated with poorer social functioning than medical conditions such as diabetes and coronary artery disease. Other research has found dysthymia to be associated with greater physical, emotional, and social impairment over a 2-year period than several chronic medical conditions, as well as episodic major depression (Hays *et al.* 1995). Compared to individuals with episodic major depression and the general population, chronically depressed individuals are more likely to be in poor physical health and to use medical services (Howland 1993, Angst *et al.* 2009, Satyanarayana *et al.* 2009), and they exhibit more depressive symptoms in any given time period during a 2-year follow-up than individuals with episodic major depression (Wells *et al.* 1992). At 5- and 10-year follow-up, Klein *et al.* (2000) found that dysthymic patients – with or without superimposed MDD –were significantly more depressed than episodic major depressives, and had significantly more suicide attempts and psychiatric hospitalizations.

Chronic depression, regardless of severity, is associated with psychosocial impairment, in both clinical and epidemiological samples. Dysthymic disorder, double depression, and MDD chronic type are associated with greater impairment than episodic MDD (Leader and Klein, 1996). In a clinical sample, Klein *et al.* (1988) concluded that individuals with early-onset DD experience more social impairment than patients with episodic MDD, with significantly higher levels of self-criticism, lower levels of extraversion and social support, and higher levels of chronic strain and perceived stress. Early-onset dysthymic patients exhibited significantly greater depression and poorer social and global functioning over a 6-month follow-up than those with late-onset dysthymia, suggesting an insidious effect of greater chronicity. DeLisio and colleagues (1986) also found greater dysfunction in the domains

of work, family, and primary relationships in a dysthymic sample than in MDD. Yang and Dunner (2001) even found that patients with dysthymic disorder had greater functional impairment than patients with both chronic and nonchronic major depression. When compared with healthy controls, individuals with dysthymia have been shown to have less stable work histories, greater incidence of significant work problems, and more than twice as much workplace productivity loss (Stewart *et al.* 2003, Adler *et al.* 2004). Baune and colleagues' (2009) cross-sectional study among 4181 German subjects similarly found a large work disability burden among individuals with DD compared to MDD. Our recent report from the large epidemiological NESARC study demonstrated that individuals with DD (N = 328) were significantly less likely to work full time than individuals with episodic MDD (N = 712) (36.2% vs. 44%; OR = 0.70, CI = 0.54,0.92), and more likely to be receiving Social Security disability income (SSI) (13.9% vs. 4.5%; OR = 3.4, CI = 2.0,5.9) and Medicaid (20.2% vs. 13%; OR = 1.7, CI = 1.1,2.6). Individuals with DD were also more likely to receive SSI (13.9% vs. 2.9%; OR = 4.6, CI = 3.4,6.2) and Medicaid (20.2% vs. 5.9%; OR = 2.9, CI = 2.0,4.1) when compared to the NESARC community sample (N = 42 052) (Hellerstein and Agosti *et al.* 2010). Angst's epidemiological sample demonstrated that individuals with chronic depression are more likely to be unemployed and to receive Social Security benefits in comparison to those with episodic depression; they are also more often unmarried (Angst *et al.* 2009).

While results (McCullough *et al.* 1994, Evans *et al.* 1996, Adler *et al.* 2004) have sometimes been mixed, the literature provides a clear and not necessarily intuitive picture: although often less severe on a cross-sectional basis than episodic MDD, dysthymia and other forms of chronic depression are generally associated with greater long-term impairment. When a major depressive episode is superimposed on an underlying dysthymia, the impact is usually more marked. These results suggest that clinical findings generalize to the community setting, and that disability among chronically depressed individuals constitutes a significant public health burden.

Course [see Figure 3.1]

Chronic depression can persist over decades. Shelton *et al.* (1997) found a mean duration of illness

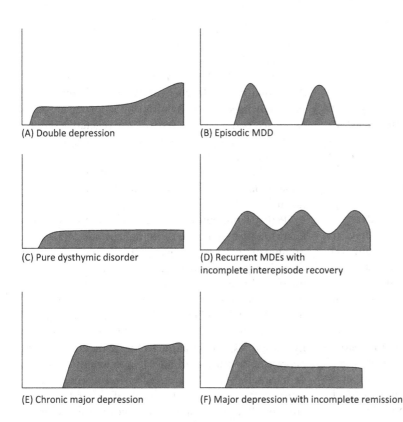

Figure 3.1 Various causes of chronic depression

(A) Double depression

(B) Episodic MDD

(C) Pure dysthymic disorder

(D) Recurrent MDEs with incomplete interepisode recovery

(E) Chronic major depression

(F) Major depression with incomplete remission

approaching 30 years in their dysthymic sample. In a psychiatrically treated sample, Klein and colleagues (Klein *et al.* 2006) found that only 52.9% and 69.5% of dysthymic patients experienced recovery at 5 years and 10 years, respectively. Over half of these (54.7%) relapsed to chronic depression (Klein *et al.* 2006). Doubly depressed patients (i.e., dysthymia with a superimposed MDE) were significantly more likely to re-experience a major depressive episode than individuals with episodic major depression.

Longitudinal studies have revealed the evolving presentation of chronic depression. Among children with an index episode of dysthymic disorder and no history of major depression, Kovacs *et al.* (1994) found an 81% cumulative probability of developing an initial major depressive episode over 9 years of follow-up. Half of the patients followed by Wells *et al.* (1992) who were dysthymic at baseline – with or without a superimposed major depressive episode – had an MDE during the 2-year follow-up period. In a sample of 190 dysthymic patients, Keller and colleagues found lifetime rates of major depression approaching 80%

(Keller *et al.* 1995). In a primary-care sample of 222 dysthymic patients, Brown *et al.* (1999) found the 12-month prevalence of co-occuring major depression to be 28.8%. Klein and colleagues have done the most extensive longitudinal evaluation comparing chronically and episodically depressed patients, though with relatively small sample size. Klein's dysthymic sample (N = 87) contained patients both with and without a superimposed major depressive episode. Of those in the dysthymia group, the majority (77.9%) had had a major depressive episode at some point, whether current or past. Of those with no history of MDD, 73.7% developed an MDE at some point during the 5-year follow-up, at which point 94.2% of the dysthymia group had experienced a lifetime MDE. Thus, while studies vary, it appears that nearly all individuals with dysthymia will experience at least one major depressive episode at some point. As Klein and colleagues sensibly conclude, double depression and dysthymic disorder are likely the same condition seen at different points in a naturally fluctuating course.

Diagnostic evaluation

Clinical diagnostic features of chronic depression

What are the main symptoms of chronic depression, and do they differ from the most common symptoms of MDD? The DSM-IV distinguishes between dysthymia and major depressive disorder based on the number and chronicity of symptoms in a shared group. Several authors (Keller *et al.* 1995, Gwirtsman *et al.* 1997) have noted the shortcomings of a diagnostic system that largely ignores symptom differences between episodic and chronic depression. Clinicians treating dysthymic patients will quickly encounter the paradox that the DSM-IV definition of the disorder may not reflect many of the most common, and most troubling symptoms presented by patients seeking treatment, since DSM-IV criteria include primarily vegetative symptoms. In addition to the required depressed mood, they must include two of the following: poor appetite or overeating, insomnia or hypersomnia, low energy or fatigue, low self-esteem, poor concentration or difficulty making decisions, and feelings of hopelessness. The DSM-IV Mood Disorders Field Trial (Keller, 1995) found that cognitive, interpersonal, and emotional symptoms were more common than vegetative symptoms among the dysthymic cohort. Among the most common symptoms found in patients with dysthymia are pessimism, feelings of inadequacy, social withdrawal, and decreased work productivity. The Field Trials authors argued that the content validity of dysthymic disorder criteria could be improved by including more cognitive/affective symptoms, and by decreasing emphasis on vegetative symptoms, and we agree.

Cognitive/affective symptoms, however, do not themselves distinguish dysthymic disorder from major depression. In the DSM-IV Field Trials sample, this class of symptoms was also heavily endorsed in the major depressive cohort. Whereas major depression is commonly marked by the presence of both somatic/vegetative and cognitive/affective symptoms, dysthymic disorder is notable in its frequency of cognitive/affective symptoms, but a relative lack of somatic/vegetative symptoms (Han *et al.* 1995). The DSM-IV-TR Appendix includes an alternative list (Alternative Research Criterion B) that shifts the focus to cognitive/affective symptoms (DSM-IV-TR). Barzega *et al.* (2001) assessed a dysthymic sample

using this list, finding that Alternative Criterion B symptoms were in fact highly prevalent in the group. They also found that the somatic/vegetative symptoms present in the DSM-IV main text criteria for dysthymia were infrequent in their dysthymic sample. Clinicians should be aware that for chronically depressed patients, resolution of any vegetative symptoms may falsely signal the remission of illness. Given the relative weight of cognitive and affective symptoms in the dysthymic profile, significant burden may remain once sleep and appetite have returned to normal.

Patients presenting with chronic depression are likely to differ from those with nonchronic MDD in a number of significant categories (Klein, 2008): they are more likely to exhibit suicidality, functional impairment, and neuroticism, more likely to have an early onset of depression, and to have familial loading of mood disorders and family history of chronic depression. Note, however, that a family history may be easily missed: especially among older patients, chronic depression is often attributed to personality disorder or "character" and therefore rarely results in diagnosis or treatment. Finally, chronically depressed patients are more likely to exhibit a number of other complicating features, including greater Axis I and Axis II co-morbidity (see Complicating diagnostic and clinical factors).

In general, the evaluating clinician should be aware that clinical presentations of chronic depression may be heterogeneous. Some patients present during a major depressive episode superimposed on long-standing dysthymia, or with an MDE that is itself of chronic duration; others present with low-grade depression, or so-called "pure" dysthymia, which may be overlooked among other presenting problems. Patients with early age of onset may never have known euthymic mood, and thus may not consider their depression something that is treatable (Klein and Santiago, 2003).

Diagnostic tools (laboratory) and standardized assessments

Clinicians should obtain a medical history or work-up to rule out medical conditions as potential sources of depression. Laboratory tests generally include a comprehensive serum metabolic profile, complete blood count, urinalysis, urine toxicology, and serum tests for thyroid function and folate/vitamin B12 levels (homocysteine and methylmalonic acid levels may be more useful in the detection of folate/B12-related depression than vitamin levels themselves) (Klee, 2000).

Various clinical tools can aid clinicians in diagnosing and sub-typing mood disorders. The Structured Clinical Interview for DSM-IV-TR Axis I Disorders (First *et al.* 1995) provides an organized framework for Axis I assessment and diagnosis under the current DSM-IV-TR nosology, though it is likely too cumbersome for routine use in clinical settings. A clinician form of the SCID (SCID-CV, First *et al.* 1997) may be useful, but lacks specifiers for some types of chronic depression (e.g., the SCID-CV does not differentiate between early- and late-onset DD). A number of clinician-administered instruments aid in the assessment of depression severity, though none is diagnostic. The gold standard Hamilton Depression Rating Scale (Hamilton, 1960) is intended for use in major depression, and was developed in an inpatient context. As a result, it emphasizes vegetative symptoms more likely to typify major depression than DD. The 17-item HAM-D may not be sufficiently sensitive to pick up the more subtle cognitive and affective symptoms that predominate in dysthymia. Longer versions of the HAM-D, with 21, 24, 27, 29, and 31 items can be more useful in that regard; or, alternatively, scales such as the Cornell Dysthymia Rating Scale (CDRS, Mason *et al.* 1993), a 20-item scale developed specifically for DD. In a study (Hellerstein, 2002) of 110 patients with DD, we found that CDRS was a much more sensitive measure of patients' symptomatology than the HAM-D.

Self-report measures are also an important means of evaluating depression. Commonly used instruments include the Quick Inventory of Depressive Symptomatology – Self Report (QIDS-SR16, Rush *et al.* 2003), the PHQ-9 (Kroenke *et al.* 2001), and the Beck Depression Inventory (BDI, Beck, 1961). Since these are completed independently, they serve as useful tools to complement clinicians' assessment of depressive symptoms.

Ancillary

Information from past medical records, family members, and other treating clinicians can aid in the assessment and diagnosis of chronic depression. In addition to course of illness, precipitants, and co-morbidities, clinicians should seek information on psychopharmacological history, including medications, doses, durations, and response to treatment. Both clinician-rated (Antidepressant Treatment History Form, Sackeim, 2001) and patient-rated (MGH – Antidepressant Treatment Response Questionnaire, Chandler *et al.* 2010) measures can be useful. In assessing psychotherapy, clinicians should evaluate response to depression-focused therapies such as interpersonal psychotherapy (IPT), cognitive behavior therapy (CBT), and behavioral activation therapy. Information gathered from an array of sources can be useful, as a patient's current mental state may distort self-reporting of depression history. Collateral information may also aid the clinician in ruling out other potential causes of depression such as general medical conditions, bipolar disorder, and substance abuse; past hypomania and substance abuse are often under-reported.

Complicating diagnostic and clinical factors

Anxiety disorders: Nearly half of individuals meeting lifetime criteria for major depression also meet criteria for a co-morbid anxiety disorder (Regier *et al.* 1998), particularly generalized anxiety disorder and social anxiety disorder. Chronic depression and dysthymia are even more likely to co-exist with anxiety disorders (Klein *et al.* 2004, Gilmer *et al.* 2005); indeed, some authors argue that dysthymic disorder is less common in a "pure" form than in a mixed depression–anxiety co-morbidity, for which the term "cothymia" has been proposed (Tyrer *et al.* 2001). Anxiety disorder co-morbidity in DD is associated with greater impairment (Tyrer *et al.* 2001) and lower likelihood of recovery (Hayden and Klein, 2001). Anxiety disorders may be distinguished from depressive disorders by autonomic, cardiovascular, or respiratory hyperarousal, muscle tension, subjective reports of anxiety and worry, and threat-related cognitions (Clark *et al.* 1994). Generalized anxiety disorder is a common childhood antecedent of mood disorders. In co-morbid adults, distinguishing whether depression or anxiety is more troubling may be difficult.

Substance-use disorders: Rates of substance-use disorders in major depressive and dysthymic populations have been found to range from 18 to 30% (Regier *et al.* 1990, Grant *et al.* 2004). It is unclear whether DD is associated with substance abuse to a higher degree than is MDD, with studies yielding mixed results (Regier *et al.* 1990, Kessler *et al.* 1997, Compton *et al.* 2000, Klein *et al.* 2000, Grant *et al.* 2004). The prognostic impact of co-occurring substance-abuse disorders has not been adequately studied in chronic depression, although active alcohol abuse predicts a significantly lower likelihood of recovery from major depression (Mueller *et al.* 1994). In assessing co-morbid mood and anxiety disorders, it is important to differentiate independent mood symptoms from those that occur as a direct result of substance intoxication or withdrawal. Substance-abuse disorders and depressive disorders have various inter-relationships: depression can arise as a result of substance abuse, substance abuse can develop in an attempt to self-medicate depression, life events resulting from one condition can serve a causal role in bringing about the other, or both conditions can exist simultaneously and independently, possibly sharing common etiological factors.

The DSM-IV stipulates that a mood disorder can be deemed independent of a co-occurring substance-use disorder when it either has onset before the substance-use disorder, or persists for at least 4 weeks following cessation of substance abuse or withdrawal. Applying these criteria in an epidemiological sample, Grant and colleagues (2004) found that mood disorders existing concurrently with substance-abuse disorders are mostly independent, that is, not substance-induced. Earlier studies, however, arrived at different conclusions (see Swendson and Merikangas, 2000). In co-morbid individuals, Compton *et al.* (2000) found that depression and dysthymia are equally as likely to precede the onset of substance abuse as they are to follow it.

To assess this issue, the evaluating clinician should determine whether substance abuse preceded the onset of a mood disorder or vice versa. Clinicians should also pay attention to instances in which substance abuse or depression remits, noting whether the remission has any impact on the co-morbid disorder. Such careful assessment can aid the clinician in uncovering the causal relationship, if any, between a patient's co-morbid substance abuse and depression.

Attention deficit disorders: Attention deficit hyperactivity disorder (ADHD) is an under-recognized problem in adults and is a common complicating factor in depression. The National Comorbidity Survey Replication (Kessler *et al.* 2006) reported a 4.4% prevalence of ADHD in the adult US population, and found a striking co-morbidity with depression: 9.4% of those with MDD and 22.6% of those with dysthymia have ADHD. ADHD's prevalence in the dysthymic cohort was the highest among all DSM-IV disorders examined, with the exception of drug dependence. That ADHD and dysthymia often present concurrently

makes clinical sense, since the functional and behavioral impairments caused by ADHD can lead to stress, anxiety, and depression; also, poor concentration and attention are common symptoms of depression. There may be more fundamental links between the two conditions, as multiple studies have found support for family linkages of ADHD and depression in first-degree relatives (Biederman *et al.* 1987, 1991). As both chronic depression and ADHD are underdiagnosed in adults, clinicians may under-recognize their concomitant presentation. Differential diagnosis is made more difficult by symptoms shared by ADHD and DD, such as inattention, memory difficulties, motivational problems/procrastination, irritability, and restlessness (Thakkar and Adler, 2006). Wender and colleagues described patients with ADHD and long-standing but intermittent depression marked by "ups and downs." Such patients, often classified under DSM-II nosology as "neurotically" or "secondarily" depressed, apparently exhibited better response to stimulant therapy than to tricyclic antidepressants (Wender *et al.* 1981), though to our knowledge this has not been tested with modern antidepressants. For ADHD patients in whom depressive symptoms fluctuate, stimulant treatment may be a logical first choice.

Personality disorders: There is a growing literature on the relation between Axis I disorders, such as dysthymia, and Axis II disorders, and between mood disorders and temperament. While a full review of these areas is beyond the scope of this chapter, it is worth pointing out that the relation between mood disorders and "personality" is complex. In individuals with an early-onset dysthymic disorder, it may be unclear what their underlying "personality" is. There are broader issues as well: in many dysthymics, apparent Axis II traits may be part of a mood disorder; alternatively, apparent mood symptoms may be part of a personality disorder. Despite these complex inter-relationships, it is important to distinguish between the two conditions. As previously discussed, a now outdated view holds that all low-severity depressions are based in character or personality, and that such "characterological" depressions are not amenable to medication treatment. To the contrary, research findings support the contention that dysthymia belongs to the family of affective disorders, and numerous studies demonstrate the effectiveness of antidepressant medication in treating DD (see Efficacy of psychopharmacology).

Individuals with chronic depression frequently have impairment in personality functioning, where personality is defined as a "complex hierarchic system that can be naturally decomposed into distinct psychobiological dimensions of temperament and character" (Cloninger, 1987). Frank and Thase state, "The mood disorders themselves may alter or "scar" personality development; conversely, people who have problems with excessive dependence on others, shyness or avoidance of emotionally charged circumstances may be more likely to develop a syndromal episode of depression" (Frank and Thase, 1999).

People with depression have more Axis II disorders (most commonly dependent, avoidant, histrionic, or borderline personality disorder) than the general population (Klein and Santiago, 2003). Individuals with chronic depression have more co-morbid Axis II disorders than do individuals with episodic major depression. Individuals with Axis II disorders are also at greater risk for developing depression than the general population. People with both depression *and* Axis II disorders have worse outcomes than those with single diagnoses. An Axis II diagnosis may even "go away" when depression remits – not because of a dramatic change in personality but because the individual may no longer meet a sufficient number of Axis II criteria to merit a diagnosis (Black, 1997). DD also predisposes to nonremission of personality disorders (PDs) (Hellerstein *et al.* 2010b). Of note is the category of "depressive personality disorder" (DPD), which appears in Appendix B of DSM-IV-TR. DPD is typified by life-long depressive traits, dispositions, and cognitions, but not by persistent depressed mood and vegetative symptoms required for diagnoses of major depression and dysthymia (Klein, 1998). While DPD is related to dysthymia, the correlation is modest: fewer than one half of the individuals in one diagnostic category tend to meet criteria for the other (Laptook, 2006). Interestingly, DPD diagnosis predicts a slower rate of improvement among individuals with a concomitant diagnosis of dysthymic disorder (Laptook, 2006).

Temperamental and cognitive factors: Studies have found that dysthymic patients exhibit elevated levels of harm avoidance and negative emotionality and low levels of reward dependence (on Cloninger's Tridimensional Personality Questionnaire) (Hellerstein *et al.* 2000) and positive emotionality (Klein and Santiago, 2003). Chronically depressed patients also exhibit impaired autonomy and more dysfunctional attitudes (Riso *et al.* 2003). Even in the absence of a personality disorder, chronically depressed patients often suffer impairment in social functioning and in core

views of self-worth and agency (Friedman, 1993). Such cognitive and temperamental abnormalities are clinically relevant in DD. Social impairment and low social support, for example, both increase the risk of developing a depressive episode and predict a lower likelihood of recovery (Brugha *et al.* 1990, Hays *et al.* 1997, Lara *et al.* 1997, Joiner, 2000).

In summary, the interplay between depression, personality, temperament, and cognitive style is complex and multi-directional. Many patients with chronic depression live a constricted life, with few close relationships and poor vocational functioning. In patients with chronic depression, prolonged illness may have left "scars" on personality and functioning. Conversely, personality impairment may serve as a "substrate" for depression. In other words, characterological traits can predispose to recurrent depressive episodes.

Other relevant considerations in the evaluation of chronic depression

Age of onset – childhood, mid-life, or geriatric – may be an important factor in the course of chronic depression. Early-onset chronic depression may be the most severe. It is associated with increased rates of Cluster B and C Axis II diagnoses (Garyfallos, 1999) and more likelihood of double depression. Early onset is also more highly correlated with childhood adversity and higher rates of mood disorders in family members (Klein and Santiago, 2003). In chronic major depression, early onset is associated with longer episodes, higher rates of substance abuse, more depressive personality traits, and psychiatric hospitalization (Klein *et al.* 1999). DD in some patients (especially mid-life onset) has been hypothesized to be related to gonadal hypofunction. Seidman *et al.*'s (2009) study with testosterone replacement showed benefit in DD patients. A recent study (Markianos *et al.* 2007) of mid-life onset DD showed reduced levels of DHEAS in both males and females, and low serum testosterone levels in younger (<50 years) rather than older patients. In older patients, chronic depression is associated with less history of MDD, lower incidence of Axis II co-morbidity, and differential treatment response, with less response to SSRI medication (Devanand, 1994, 2000). Geriatric-onset chronic depression is more likely to attend major losses and health issues (Klein and Santiago, 2003), and a growing body of research suggests that many cases of late-life depression are attributable to cerebrovascular disease. Cerebrovascular etiology may be especially likely in patients presenting with executive dysfunction and psychomotor retardation, but lacking psychosocial stressors and family history of depressive illness (Kales *et al.* 2005).

In the STAR*D sample (Gilmer *et al.* 2005), a number of variables were associated with chronic episodes of major depression. Medical co-morbidity and co-occurring generalized anxiety disorder were associated with chronic episodes, as were unemployment, less education, Hispanic ethnicity, African American race, and nonexistent or public health insurance. Hays *et al.* (1997) found diminished social support and physical impairment were correlated with chronicity of depression. Length of depression before initiation of treatment and low income (Keller *et al.* 1984) as well as multiple deaths of family members, disabled spouses, co-morbid medical illness, and sedative, hypnotic, and alcohol abuse (Akiskal 1982, Mueller *et al.* 1994) have also been associated with chronicity of major depression. Hayden and Klein (2001) found that chronic stress, greater familial loading of chronic depression, poor parental relationships, childhood abuse, higher levels of neuroticism, depressive personality traits, and histories of personality, anxiety, and eating disorders were all associated with higher levels of depression at 5-year follow-up. In short, psychosocial stressors, psychiatric and medical co-morbidities, and socioeconomic constraints are frequently seen in the presence of chronic depression and may predict a prolonged course.

Clinical pearls of diagnostic wisdom

There are a number of special considerations that the clinician should keep in mind when assessing chronic depression:

- Assessment of Axis I co-morbidity can be complex. Bipolar II disorder may be difficult to ascertain in a brief psychiatric evaluation or even a structured clinical interview (Dunner and Tay, 1993, Benazzi, 2003). Current or past substance abuse, which may factor strongly in diagnostic decision-making, may not be volunteered by chronically depressed patients.
- Similarly, personality factors which bear on etiology and outcome may be difficult to determine at initial assessment. Confirming an Axis II diagnosis often requires extended evaluation.

- While severe chronic depression – chronic MDD or double depression – is likely to be noticed, clinicians may overlook the apparently less severe dysthymic disorder. It is not uncommon for patients to receive many years of psychiatric treatment, particularly psychotherapy, before a diagnosis of DD is made.
- Patients with DD may have become acclimated to a basal level of depression, and may be highly skeptical as to the potential for improvement through treatment.
- Even in very chronic depression, response can be remarkable. Antidepressant medication or depression-focused psychotherapy often allows patients to achieve a level of well-being greater than any they can remember.
- After medication response, such individuals may suffer from residual functional impairment – including avoidant behaviors, procrastination, decreased willingness to try new activities, and cognitive symptoms such as pessimism and ruminations. These may require additional modalities of treatment, as discussed below.

Treatment

Efficacy of psychopharmacology

A wide range of medications have been shown to be effective for dysthymic disorder, although none currently has an FDA-approved indication for this condition. Recent controversial reports (e.g., Kirsch *et al.* 2008, Fournier *et al.* 2010) claim that antidepressants are only effective in more severe depressions, and imply that mild depression responds to antidepressant medication no more than to placebo. To the contrary, psychopharmacology studies of dysthymic disorder, which presents with mild severity in cross-section, almost invariably separate active medication from placebo. The placebo response rate is low in DD (Levkovitz *et al.* 2011), and the medication response rate, though perhaps lower than seen in MDD, is reproducibly higher than placebo response. Medication has been found to be significantly more effective than placebo in nearly all double-blind controlled studies of dysthymia in the world literature.

A recently updated Cochrane Review (Silva de Lima *et al.* 2009) of the literature reported that there are at least 17 randomized, double-blind, placebo-controlled studies of dysthymic disorder. Seven of these investigated "pure dysthymia," or patients whose disorder did not currently meet criteria for an episode of major depression. (The importance of such studies is that they can test whether the disorder of dysthymia itself responds to medication treatment, whereas in double depression it may be difficult to determine whether the acute or the chronic depression is responding to treatment). Ranging in duration from 4 to 12 weeks, these studies included a total of 1964 patients, and evaluated medications including tricyclic antidepressants (TCAs), monoamine oxidase inhibitors (MAOIs), selective serotonin reuptake inhibitors (SSRIs), and medications not currently available in the United States (the reversible MAOI meclobemide and the antipsychotics amisulpride and ritanserin, as well as the atypical tricyclic amineptine). Similar results were found for TCAs, SRIs, MAOIs, and these other drugs in terms of overall efficacy. The "number needed to treat" ranged from 2.9 (MAOIs) to 4.3 (TCAs) to 5.0 (SSRIs). Using full remission as a more stringent criterion for improvement, the Cochrane reviewers found the same results. In another review, Griffiths *et al.* (2000) listed 19 double-blind studies, 17 of which demonstrated that active medication was superior to placebo.

A recent meta-analysis of dysthymia studies (Levkovitz *et al.* 2011) included 17 randomized double-blind, placebo-controlled studies of dysthmic disorder, and determined that antidepressant therapy was significantly more effective than placebo in dysthymic disorder. These 17 trials with DD were compared to 177 with MDD. Meta-regression analyses suggested "a statistically significant difference in the RR of responding to antidepressants vs. placebo" when comparing studies of DD to MDD, which suggested a greater RR for response with dysthymia than MDD (co-efficient of -0.113, $p = 0.007$). The number needed to treat (NNT) for dysthymic disorder was 4.4 compared to 6.1 for MDD, which was not significantly different. In treatment of DD, the risk ratio was 1.75, and 95% CI was 1.49–2.04, with $p < 0.0001$. In addition, placebo response rates in dysthymic disorder were significantly lower than those found for MDD: 29.9% vs. 37.9%, $p = 0.042$.

In short, despite a relative paucity of studies, RCTs demonstrate that dysthymic disorder responds well to treatment with antidepressants. Moreover, initial medication responses appear to continue in long-term treatment (Vanelle *et al.* 1997). Limited evidence suggests that those who do not respond to

an initial medication trial may experience benefit at an increased dose (Vanelle *et al.* 1997). Medication selection, supplementation, and dosing strategies in DD and other forms of chronic depression, in the almost complete absence of data specific to these disorders, should generally follow the conventions used in other forms of unipolar depression.

Psychotherapy of dysthymic disorder

The persistent social dysfunction of patients with dysthymia, as well as the preference of many people for nonpharmacological treatments, raises the question of the efficacy of psychotherapy. In the DSM-II era, chronically depressed people were believed to suffer from "neurotic depression" and were generally treated with psychodynamic psychotherapy. Even after the DSM-III reclassification of dysthymia as a mood disorder, this practice persists, and many psychotherapists have caseloads of patients who might meet criteria for dysthymia and yet who are not considered for medication treatment. The efficacy (or lack of efficacy) of psychodynamic therapy for dysthymia has not been determined. In a 1994 review of psychotherapy of dysthymia (Markowitz, 1994), Markowitz noted, "Although long-term psychodynamic psychotherapy continues to be frequently prescribed for dysthymic patients, there is no evidence that either short- or long-term psychodynamic treatment benefits such patients."

Studies of psychotherapy (Markowitz, 1994) in dysthymia tend to be "small, usually uncontrolled studies with varying methods and limited follow-up." In a summary of cognitive behavior therapy (CBT), Markowitz noted an approximate response rate of 41%. Interpersonal therapy (IPT) (Klerman *et al.* 1984) is a treatment modality designed by Klerman and Weissman; a series of IPT cases noted in this review had a 64% response rate. More recently, Arnow and Constantino (2003) reviewed the literature on psychotherapy vs. medication in dysthymia and chronic major depression. In chronic major depression, combined psychotherapy and medication were found to be more effective than either therapy alone in the treatment of both depressive symptoms and secondary co-morbidities. For dysthymia, the authors concluded that medication has a clear advantage over psychotherapy in achieving remission of depression. While evidence for the superiority of a combined treatment approach is limited, the authors suggest that combined therapy may be superior to medication alone when considering a broader range of outcome measures.

Many studies of combined medication and psychotherapy have somewhat divergent findings, and it is difficult to generalize from their results. Small sample size may lead to an inability to show true differences between treatments (Ravindran *et al.* 1999). Different psychotherapies have been studied, such as the cognitive behavioral analysis system of psychotherapy (CBASP, McCullough 1991, Kocsis 2009), cognitive behavior therapy (CBT, Dunner *et al.* 1996, Ravindran *et al.* 1999), interpersonal psychotherapy (IPT, deMello *et al.* 2001, Markowitz *et al.* 2005), brief supportive psychotherapy (BSP, Markowitz *et al.* 2005, Kocsis *et al.* 2009), cognitive-interpersonal group psychotherapy for chronic depression (CIGP-CD, Hellerstein *et al.* 2001), and problem-solving treatment in primary care (PST-PC, Williams *et al.* 2000). Although many treatments share some features (such as cognitive therapy techniques), differences between therapies may account for varying results. Study samples also have had different characteristics, with more severely depressed patients in some (Keller *et al.* 2000) and geriatric dysthymics in others (Williams *et al.* 2000).

A few general conclusions, however, can be drawn. Medication appears to be more effective than psychotherapy in achieving remission of acute depressive symptoms. Psychotherapy likely takes longer to achieve an effect in chronic depression (Imel *et al.* 2008), but may play a valuable role in sustaining remission. The value of psychotherapy may be especially apparent in patients exhibiting impairment in the domains of social and occupational functioning: while there is evidence that successful depression treatment can have beneficial effects in these domains (Kocsis *et al.* 1997), considerable morbidity often remains once euthymia has been achieved (Kocsis *et al.* 1988, Stewart *et al.* 1988, Friedman *et al.* 1995, 1999). Thus, the recommendation of combined treatment might take into account a number of factors, such as patient preference, Axis II co-morbidities, psychosocial impairment, behavioral patterns, and residual depressive symptoms. Lastly, it is clear that some studies have found similar levels of effectiveness for medication and depression-oriented (i.e., nonpsychodynamic) psychotherapies (e.g., Keller *et al.* 2000, Kocsis *et al.* 2009). Thus, antidepression-focused psychotherapy (CBT, IPT, behavioral activation therapy) remains a clinically reasonable first-line treatment

in chronic depression. Alternative therapies such as exercise (Martinsen, 2008) and mindfulness meditation (Butler *et al.* 2008, Barnhofer *et al.* 2009) have also been shown to have a beneficial effect in chronic depression. Clinicians must recognize that all patients presenting with chronic depression warrant some form of therapeutic trial, whether medication, psychotherapy, or combined treatment. Treatment should proceed with careful attention to symptom response, with a goal of achieving prolonged remission (HAM-D < 7), and ineffective therapies should be discontinued or augmented until the end-goal of persistent remission of depressive pathology has been achieved.

Future directions

Neuroscience is likely to bring sweeping changes in the assessment, treatment, and understanding of chronic depression. Various lines of research demonstrate that depression is associated with neurobiological abnormalities, including chronic stress activation of neurohormonal and immunological systems and changes in brain anatomy, function, and connectivity, consistent with neurotoxic effects of chronic stress. Drevets *et al.* (2008) describe how neural networks that moderate aspects of normal emotional behavior "have been implicated in the pathophysiology of mood disorders by converging evidence from neuroimaging, neuropathological and imaging studies." Key depression-related brain areas include the medial prefrontal cortex and the medial and caudolateral orbital cortex as well as the amygdala, hippocampus, and ventromedial portions of the basal ganglia.

Furthermore, studies suggest that chronic depression is associated with more severe abnormalities than acute depression. Frodl *et al.* (2008) showed that negative neuroplastic changes were greater in nonremitted individuals with MDD over 3 years prospective assessment in comparison to remitted patients and healthy controls, suggesting an association with stress-related changes in areas of the brain including hippocampus, dorsomedial prefrontal cortex, dorsolateral prefrontal cortex, and anterior cingulate.

In dysthymic disorder, Ravindran *et al.* (2009, 2010) found that unmedicated patients had reduced activation in the dorsolateral prefrontal cortex, and increased amygdala activation compared to age-, sex-, and education-matched controls. This suggests that the brain circuitry involved with dysthymia may involve altered activation of the PFC, anterior cingulate, amygdala, and insula, which is similar to MDD, but may show some differences that are distinct to DD. Ravindran *et al.*'s (2010) repeat fMRI scans following SSRI treatment showed changes suggesting that paroxetine normalizes the activity of such areas as the middle frontal gyrus, cingulate gyrus, and insula in response to emotional stimuli.

Some studies demonstrate neurobiological commonalities between DD and MDD: for example, Bruder *et al.*'s (2012) EEG study demonstrated that DD and MDD share a common abnormality of hemispheric asymmetry for dichotic listening. Other avenues of research have found additional biological features in DD, such as lower rates of HPA disturbance and higher levels of interleukin 1-beta (Anisman *et al.* 1999, Schlatter *et al.* 2001) that may distinguish chronic from episodic depression. The likelihood of a biological substrate for many individuals with chronic depression is also supported by the findings of familial aggregation of chronic depression (Klein *et al.* 1995, Mondimore *et al.* 2006), although the result has not been supported elsewhere (Lyons *et al.* 1998). Future research will elucidate the etiological role of chronic depression's complex biological correlates and should aid in the development of more effective treatments.

Conclusions

Chronic depression, regardless of severity level, is associated with considerable functional impairment and morbidity. Chronic low-grade depression causes significant impairment and suffering. Dysthymia can be conceptualized as a prodromal disorder, since nearly all individuals with DD will at some point experience a full-blown major depressive episode. Clinicians should focus on early identification of chronic depression and dysthymia, with the goals of preventing the progression of DD to MDD and reversing a trajectory of chronic social and vocational dysfunction. While current treatments are imperfect, it is frequently possible to achieve sustained remission of chronic depression and significant psychosocial rehabilitation. The ideal interventions vary from patient to patient, and often include both pharmacological and psychotherapeutic approaches. Future research will expand the range and efficacy of treatments and explore novel therapeutic pathways.

References

Adler, D.A., Irish, J., Mclaughlin, T.J. *et al.* (2004). The work impact of dysthymia in a primary care population. *General Hospital Psychiatry*, 26, 269–276.

Akiskal, H.S. (1982). Factors associated with incomplete recovery in primary depressive illness. *Journal of Clinical Psychiatry*, 43, 266–271.

Akiskal, H.S., Rosenthal, T., Haykal, R. *et al.* (1980). Characterological depressions: Clinican and sleep EEG findings separating subaffective dysthymias from character spectrum disorders. *Archives of General Psychiatry*, 37, 777–783.

American Psychiatric Association (1980). *Diagnostic and Statistical Manual of Mental Disorders, Third Edition*. Washington, DC: American Psychiatric Association.

American Psychiatric Association (1987). *Diagnostic and Statistical Manual of Mental Disorders, Third Edition, Revised*. Washington, DC: American Psychiatric Association.

American Psychiatric Association (1994). *Diagnostic and Statistical Manual of Mental Disorders, Fourth Edition*. Washington, DC: American Psychiatric Association.

American Psychiatric Association (2000). *Diagnostic and Statistical Manual of Mental Disorders, Fourth Edition, Text Revision*. Washington, DC: American Psychiatric Association.

American Psychiatric Association DSM 5 Development (2010). *D03 Chronic Depressive Disorder (Dysthymia)* [Online]. Available: http://www.dsm5.org/ProposedRevisions/Pages/proposedrevision.aspx?rid=46 (accessed September 2012).

Angst, J., Gamma, A., Roessler, W., Ajdacic, V., and Klein, D.N. (2009). Long-term depression versus episodic major depression: Results from the prospective Zurich study of a community sample. *Journal of Affective Disorders*, 115, 112–121.

Anisman, H., Ravindran, A.V., Griffiths, J., and Merali, Z. (1999). Endocrine and cytokine correlates of major depression and dysthymia with typical or atypical features. *Molecular Psychiatry*, 4, 182–188.

Arnow, B.A. and Constantino, M.J. (2003). Effectiveness of psychotherapy and combination treatment for chronic depression. *Journal of Clinical Psychology*, 59, 893–905.

Barnhofer, T., Crane, C., Hargus, E. *et al.* (2009). Mindfulness-based cognitive therapy as a treatment for chronic depression: A preliminary study. *Behaviour Research and Therapy*, 47, 366–373.

Barzega, G., Maina, G., Venturello, S., and Bogetto, F. (2001). Dysthymic disorder: Clinical characteristics in relation to age at onset. *Journal of Affective Disorders*, 66, 39–46.

Baune, B.T., Caniato, R.N., Arolt, V., and Berger, K. (2009). The effects of dysthymic disorder on health-related quality of life and disability days in persons with comorbid medical conditions in the general population. *Psychotherapy and Psychosomatics*, 78, 161–166.

Beck, A.T., Erbaugh, J., Ward, C.H., Mock, J., and Mendelsohn, M. (1961). An inventory for measuring depression. *Archives of General Psychiatry*, 4, 561–571.

Benazzi, F. (2003). Diagnosis of bipolar II disorder: a comparison of structured versus semistructured interviews. *Progress in Neuro-Psychopharmacology and Biological Psychiatry*, 27, 985–991.

Biederman, J., Faraone, S.V., Keenan, K., and Tsuang, M.T. (1991). Evidence of familial association between attention-deficit disorder and major affective disorders. *Archives of General Psychiatry*, 48, 633–642.

Biederman, J., Munir, K., Knee, D. *et al.* (1987). High rate of affective disorders in probands with attention-deficit disorder and in their relatives: A controlled family study. *American Journal of Psychiatry*, 144, 330–333.

Black, K.J. and Sheline, Y.I. (1997). Personality disorder scores improve with effective pharmacotherapy of depression. *Journal of Affective Disorders*, 43, 11–18.

Brown, G.W. and Moran, P. (1994). Clinical and psychosocial origins of chronic depressive episodes. I: A community survey. *British Journal of Psychiatry*, 165, 447–456.

Browne, G., Steiner, M., Roberts, J. *et al.* (1999). Prevalence of dysthymic disorder in primary care. *Journal of Affective Disorders*, 54, 303–308.

Bruder, G.E., Stewart, J.W., Hellerstein, D. *et al.* (2012). Abnormal functional brain asymmetry in depression: Evidence of biologic commonality between major depression and dysthymia. *Psychiatry Research*, 196, 250–254.

Brugha, T.S., Bebbington, P.E., Maccarthy, B. *et al.* (1990). Gender, social support and recovery from depressive disorders: A prospective clinical study. *Psychological Medicine*, 20, 147–156.

Butler, L., Waelde, L., Hastl, T. *et al.* (2008). Meditation with yoga, group therapy with hypnosis, and psychoeducation for long-term depressed mood: A randomized pilot trial. *Journal of Clinical Psychology*, 64, 806–820.

Chandler, G.M., Iosifescu, D.V., Pollack, M.H., Targum, S.D., and Fava, M. (2010). Validation of the Massachusetts General Hospital Antidepressant Treatment History Questionnaire (ATRQ). *CNS Neuroscience and Therapeutics*, 16, 322–325.

Clark, D.A., Beck, A.T., and Beck, J.S. (1994). Symptom differences in major depression, dysthymia, panic disorder, and generalized anxiety disorder. *American Journal of Psychiatry*, 151, 205–209.

Cloninger, C.R. (1987). A systematic method for clinical description and classification of personality variants: A proposal. *Archives of General Psychiatry*, 44, 573–588.

Compton, W.M., Cottler, L.B., Phelps, D.L., Ben Abdallah, A., and Spitznagel, E.L. (2000). Psychiatric disorders among drug dependent subjects: Are they primary or secondary? *American Journal on Addictions*, 9, 126–134.

Delisio, G., Maremmani, I.P., Perugi, G. *et al.* (1986). Impairment of work and leisure in depressed outpatients: A preliminary communication. *Journal of Affective Disorders*, 10, 79–84.

De Mello, M.F., Myczcowisk, L.M., and Menezes, P.R. (2001). A randomized controlled trial comparing moclobemide and moclobemide plus interpersonal psychotherapy in the treatment of dysthymic disorder. *The Journal of Psychotherapy Practice and Research*, 10, 117–123.

Devanand, D.P., Nobler, M.S., Singer, T. *et al.* (1994). Is dysthymia a different disorder in the elderly? *American Journal of Psychiatry*, 151, 1592–1599.

Devanand, D.P., Turret, N., Moody, B.J. *et al.* (2000). Personality disorders in elderly patients with dysthymic disorder. *American Journal of Geriatric Psychiatry*, 8, 188–195.

Drevets, W.C., Price, J.L., and Furey, M.L. (2008). Brain structural and functional abnormalities in mood disorders: implications for neurocircuitry models of depression. *Brain Structure and Function*, 213, 93–118.

Dunner, D.L. and Tay, L.K. (1993). Diagnostic reliability of the history of hypomania in bipolar-II patients and patients with major depression. *Comprehensive Psychiatry*, 34, 303–307.

Dunner, D.L., Schmaling, K.B., Hendrickson, H. *et al.* (1996). Cognitive therapy versus fluoxetine in the treatment of dysthymic disorder. *Depression*, 4, 34–41.

Erickson, G. and Hellerstein, D. (2011). Behavioral activation therapy for remediating persistent social deficits in medication-responsive chronic depression. *Journal of Psychiatric Practice*, 17, 161–169.

Evans, S., Cloitre, M., Kocsis, J. *et al.* (1996). Social-vocational adjustment in unipolar mood disorders: Results of the DSM IV field trial. *Journal of Affective Disorders*, 38, 73–80.

First, M., Spitzer, R., Gibbon, M., and Williams, J. (1997). *Structured Clinical Interview for DSM-IV Axis I Disorders – Clinician Version*. Washington, DC: American Psychiatric Press.

First, M.B., Spitzer, R.L., Williams, J.B.W., and Gibbon, M. (1995). *Structured Clinical Interview for DSM-IV (SCID)*. Washington, DC: American Psychiatric Association.

Fournier, J.C., Derubeis, R.J., Hollon, S.D. *et al.* (2010). Antidepressant drug effects and depression severity: A patient-level meta-analysis. *Journal of the American Medical Association*, 303, 47–53.

Frank, E. and Thase, M.E. (1999). Natural history and preventative treatment of recurrent mood disorders. *Annual Review of Medicine*, 50, 453–468.

Friedman, R.A. (1993). Social impairment in dysthymia. *Psychiatric Annals*, 23, 632–637.

Friedman, R.A., Markowitz, J.C., Parides, M., and Kocsis, J.H. (1995). Acute response of social functioning in dysthymic patients with desipramine. *Journal of Affective Disorders*, 34, 85–88.

Friedman, R.A., Markowitz, J.C., Parides, M., Gniwesch, L., and Kocsis, J.H. (1999). Six months of desipramine for dysthymia: Can dysthymic patients achieve normal social functioning? *Journal of Affective Disorders*, 54, 283–286.

Frodl, T.S., Koutsouleris, N., Bottlender, R. *et al.* (2008). Depression-related variation in brain morphology over 3 years: Effects of stress? *Archives of General Psychiatry*, 65, 1156–1165.

Garvey, M.J., Tollefson, G.D., and Tuason, V.B. (1986). Is chronic primary major depression a distinct depression subtype? *Comprehensive Psychiatry*, 27, 446–448.

Garyfallos, G., Adamopoulou, A., Karastergiou, A. *et al.* (1999). Personality disorders in dysthymia and major depression. *Acta Psychiatrica Scandinavica*, 99, 332–340.

Gilmer, W., Trivedi, M., Rush, A. *et al.* (2005). Factors associated with chronic depressive episodes: A preliminary report from the STAR-D project. *Acta Psychiatrica Scandinavica*, 112, 425–433.

Grant, B.F., Stinson, F.S., Dawson, D.A. *et al.* (2004). Prevalence and co-occurrence of substance use disorders and independent mood and anxiety disorders: Results from the national epidemiologic survey on alcohol and related conditions. *Archives of General Psychiatry*, 61, 807–816.

Griffiths, J., Ravindran, A., Merali, Z., and Anisman, H. (2000). Dysthymia: A review of pharmacological and behavioral factors. *Molecular Psychiatry*, 5, 242–261.

Gwirtsman, H., Blehar, M., McCullough, J., Kocsis, J., and Prien, R. (1997). Standardized assessment of dysthymia: report of a National Institute of Mental Health conference. *Psychopharmacology Bulletin*, 33, 3–11.

Hamilton, M. (1960). A rating scale for depression. *Journal of Neurology, Neurosurgery and Psychiatry*, 23, 56–62.

Han, L., Schmaling, K., and Dunner, D. (1995). Descriptive validity and stability of diagnostic criteria for dysthymic disorder. *Comprehensive Psychiatry*, 36, 338–343.

Hayden, E.P. and Klein, D.N. (2001). Outcome of dysthymic disorder at 5-year follow-up: The effect of familial psychopathology, early adversity, personality, comorbidity, and chronic stress. *American Journal of Psychiatry*, 158, 1864–1870.

Hays, J.C., Krishnan, K.R.R., George, L.K. *et al.* (1997). Psychosocial and physical correlates of chronic depression. *Psychiatry Research*, 72, 149–159.

Hays, R., Wells, K., Sherbourne, C., Rogers, W., and Spritzer, K. (1995). Functioning and well-being outcomes of patients with depression compared with chronic general medical illnesses. *Archives of General Psychiatry*, 52, 11–19.

Hellerstein, D., Little, S., Samstag, L. *et al.* (2001). Combined medication and group psychotherapy in dysthymia: A randomized prospective outcome study. *Journal of Psychotherapy Practice and Research*, 10, 93–103.

Hellerstein, D., Skodol, A., Petkova, E. *et al.* (2010a). The impact of comorbid dysthymic disorder on outcome in personality disorders. *Comprehensive Psychiatry*, 51, 449–457.

Hellerstein, D.J., Batchelder, S.T., Lee, A., and Borisovskaya, M. (2002). Rating dysthymia: an assessment of the construct and content validity of the Cornell Dysthymia Rating Scale. *Journal of Affective Disorders*, 71, 85–96.

Hellerstein, D.J., Agosti, V., Bosi, M., and Black, S.R. (2010b). Impairment in psychosocial functioning associated with dysthymic disorder in the NESARC study. *Journal of Affective Disorders*, 127, 84–88.

Hellerstein, D.J., Kocsis, J.H., Chapman, D., Stewart, J.W., and Harrison, W. (2000). Double-blind comparison of sertraline, imipramine, and placebo in the treatment of dysthymia: Effects on personality. *American Journal of Psychiatry*, 157, 1436–1444.

Howland, R.H. (1993). General health, health-care utilization, and medical comorbidity in dysthymia. *International Journal of Psychiatry in Medicine*, 23, 211–238.

Imel, Z.E., Malterer, M.B., McKay, K.M., and Wampold, B.E. (2008). A meta-analysis of psychotherapy and medication in unipolar depression and dysthymia. *Journal of Affective Disorders*, 110, 197–206.

Joiner, T.E. (2000). Depression's vicious scree: self-propagating and erosive processes in depression chronicity. *Clinical Psychology – Science and Practice*, 7, 203–218.

Kales, H.C., Maixner, D.F., and Mellow, A.M. (2005). Cerebrovascular disease and late-life depression. *American Journal of Geriatric Psychiatry*, 13, 88–98.

Keller, M.B. and Shapiro, R.W. (1982). Double depression – superimposition of acute depressive episodes on chronic depressive disorders. *American Journal of Psychiatry*, 139, 438–442.

Keller, M.B., Klerman, G.L., Lavori, P.W. *et al.* (1984). Long-term outcome of episodes of major depression:

clinical and public-health significance. *Journal of the American Medical Association*, 252, 788–792.

Keller, M.B., Klein, D.N., Hirschfeld, R.M.A. *et al.* (1995). Results of the DSM-IV Mood Disorders Field Trial. *American Journal of Psychiatry*, 152, 843–849.

Keller, M.B., McCullough, J.P., Klein, D.N. *et al.* (2000). A comparison of nefazodone, the cognitive behavioral-analysis system of psychotherapy, and their combination for the treatment of chronic depression. *New England Journal of Medicine*, 342, 1462–1470.

Kessler, R., Chiu, W., Demler, O., Merikangas, K., and Walters, E. (2005). Prevalence, severity, and comorbidity of 12-month DSM-IV disorders in the National Comorbidity Survey Replication. *Archives of General Psychiatry*, 62, 709.

Kessler, R.C., McGonagle, K., Zhao, S. *et al.* (1994). Lifetime and 12 month prevalence of DSM-III-R psychiatric disorders in the United States: Results from the National Comorbidity Survey. *Archives of General Psychiatry*, 51, 8–19.

Kessler, R.C., Crum, R.M., Warner, L.A. *et al.* (1997). Lifetime co-occurrence of DSM-III-R alcohol abuse and dependence with other psychiatric disorders in the National Comorbidity Survey. *Archives of General Psychiatry*, 54, 313–321.

Kessler, R.C., Adler, L., Barkley, R. *et al.* (2006). The prevalence and correlates of adult ADHD in the United States: results from the National Comorbidity Survey Replication. *American Journal of Psychiatry*, 163, 716–723.

Kirsch, I., Deacon, B.J., Huedo-Medina, T.B. *et al.* (2008). Initial severity and antidepressant benefits: A meta-analysis of data submitted to the food and drug administration. *PLOS Medicine*, 5, 260–268.

Klee, G. (2000). Cobalamin and folate evaluation: measurement of methylmalonic acid and homocysteine vs vitamin B-12 and folate. *Clinical Chemistry*, 46, 1277–1283.

Klein, D. (2008). Classification of depressive disorders in the DSM-V: Proposal for a two-dimension system. *Journal of Abnormal Psychology*, 117, 552–560.

Klein, D. and Santiago, N. (2003). Dysthymia and chronic depression: Introduction, classification, risk factors, and course. *Journal of Clinical Psychology*, 59, 807–816.

Klein, D., Shankman, S., and Rose, S. (2006). Ten-year prospective follow-up study of the naturalistic course of dysthymic disorder and double depression. *American Journal of Psychiatry*, 163, 872–880.

Klein, D., Taylor, E., Dickstein, S., and Harding, K. (1988). Primary early-onset dysthymia: Comparison with primary non-bipolar non-chronic major depression on demographic, clinical, familial, personality, and socioenvironmental characteristics and short-term outcome. *Journal of Abnormal Psychology*, 97, 387–398.

Klein, D., Dickstein, S., Taylor, E., and Harding, K. (1989). Identifying chronic affective disorders in outpatients: Validation of the General Behavior Inventory. *Journal of Consulting and Clinical Psychology*, 57, 106–111.

Klein, D., Schwartz, J., Rose, S., and Leader, J. (2000). Five-year course and outcome of dysthymic disorder: A prospective, naturalistic follow-up study. *American Journal of Psychiatry*, 157, 931–939.

Klein, D., Shankman, S., Lewinsohn, P., Rohde, P., and Seeley, J. (2004). Family study of chronic depression in a community sample of young adults. *American Journal of Psychiatry*, 161, 646–653.

Klein, D.N. and Shih, J.H. (1998). Depressive personality: Associations with DSM-III-R mood and personality disorders and negative and positive affectivity, 30-month stability, and prediction of course of Axis I depressive disorders. *Journal of Abnormal Psychology*, 107, 319–327.

Klein, D.N., Riso, L.P., Donaldson, S.K. *et al.* (1995). Family study of early-onset dysthymia: Mood and personality disorders in relatives of outpatients with dysthymia and episodic major depression and normal controls. *Archives of General Psychiatry*, 52, 487–496.

Klein, D.N., Schatzberg, A.F., McCullough, J.P. *et al.* (1999). Age of onset in chronic major depression: Relation to demographic and clinical variables, family history, and treatment response. *Journal of Affective Disorders*, 55, 149–157.

Klerman, G., Weissman, M., Rounsaville, B., and Chevron, E. (1984). *Interpersonal Psychotherapy of Depression*. New York: Basic Books.

Kocsis, J.H. (2003). Pharmacotherapy for chronic depression. *Journal of Clinical Psychology*, 59, 885–892.

Kocsis, J.H., Frances, A.J., Voss, C. *et al.* (1988). Imipramine and social-vocational adjustment in chronic depression. *American Journal of Psychiatry*, 145, 997–999.

Kocsis, J.H., Zisook, S., Davidson, J. *et al.* (1997). Double-blind comparison of sertraline, imipramine, and placebo in the treatment of dysthymia: Psychosocial outcomes. *American Journal of Psychiatry*, 154, 390–395.

Kocsis, J.H., Gelenberg, A.J., Rothbaum, B.O. *et al.* (2009). Cognitive Behavioral Analysis System of Psychotherapy and Brief Supportive Psychotherapy for augmentation of antidepressant nonresponse in chronic depression. *Archives of General Psychiatry*, 66, 1178–1188.

Kovacs, M., Akiskal, H., Gatsonis, C., and Parrone, P. (1994). Childhood onset dysthymic disorder: Clinical features and prospective naturalistic outcome. *Archives of General Psychiatry*, 51, 365–374.

Kroenke, K., Spitzer, R.L., and Williams, J.B.W. (2001). The PHQ-9: Validity of a brief depression severity measure. *Journal of General Internal Medicine*, 16, 606–613.

Laptook, R., Klein, D., and Dougherty, L. (2006). Ten-year stability of depressive personality disorder in depressed outpatients. *American Journal of Psychiatry*, 163, 865–871.

Lara, M.E., Leader, J., and Klein, D.N. (1997). The association between social support and course of depression: is it confounded with personality? *Journal of Abnormal Psychology*, 106, 478–482.

Leader, J. and Klein, D. (1996). Social adjustment in dysthymia, double depression and episodic major depression. *Journal of Affective Disorders*, 37, 91–101.

Levkovitz, Y., Tedeschini, E., and Papakostas, G.I. (2011). Efficacy of antidepressants for dysthymia: A meta-analysis of placebo-controlled randomized trials. *Journal of Clinical Psychiatry*, 72, 509–514.

Lizardi, H., Klein, D.N., Ouimette, P.C. et al. (1995). Reports of the childhood home environment in early-onset dysthymia and episodic major depression. *Journal of Abnormal Psychology*, 104, 132–139.

Lyons, M.J., Eisen, S.A., Goldberg, J. et al. (1998). A registry-based twin study of depression in men. *Archives of General Psychiatry*, 55, 468–472.

Markianos, M., Tripodianakis, J., Sarantidis, D., and Hatzimanolis, J. (2007). Plasma testosterone and dehydroepiandrosterone sulfate in male and female patients with dysthymic disorder. *Journal of Affective Disorders*, 101, 255–258.

Markowitz, J., Moran, M., Kocsis, J., and Frances, A. (1992). Prevalence and comorbidity of dysthymic disorder among psychiatric outpatients. *Journal of Affective Disorders*, 24, 63–71.

Markowitz, J.C. (1994). Psychotherapy of dysthymia. *American Journal of Psychiatry*, 151, 1114–1121.

Markowitz, J.C., Kocsis, J.H., Bleiberg, K.L., Christos, P.J., and Sacks, M. (2005). A comparative trial of psychotherapy and pharmacotherapy for "pure" dysthymic patients. *Journal of Affective Disorders*, 89, 167–175.

Martinsen, E. (2008). Physical activity in the prevention and treatment of anxiety and depression. *Nordic Journal of Psychiatry*, 62, 25–29.

Mason, B.J., Kocsis, J.H., Leon, A.C. et al. (1993). Measurement of severity and treatment response in dysthymia. *Psychiatric Annals*, 23, 625–631.

McCullough, J., Klein, D., Keller, M. et al. (2000). Comparison of DSM-III-R chronic major depression and major depression superimposed on dysthymia (double depression): Validity of the distinction. *Journal of Abnormal Psychology*, 109, 419–427.

McCullough, J., Klein, D., Borian, F. et al. (2003). Group comparisons of DSM-IV subtypes of chronic depression: Validity of the distinctions, part 2. *Journal of Abnormal Psychology*, 112, 614–622.

McCullough, J.P. (1991). Psychotherapy for dysthymia: A naturalistic study of 10 patients. *Journal of Nervous and Mental Disease*, 179, 734–740.

McCullough, J.P. (1994). Social adjustment, coping style, and clinical course among DSM-III-R community unipolar depressives. *Depression*, 2, 36.

Mondimore, F.M., Zandi, P.P., Mackinnon, D.F. et al. (2006). Familial aggregation of illness chronicity in recurrent, early-onset major depression pedigrees. *American Journal of Psychiatry*, 163, 1554–1560.

Mueller, T.I., Lavori, P.W., Keller, M.B. et al. (1994). Prognostic effect of the variable course of alcoholism on the 10-year course of depression. *American Journal of Psychiatry*, 151, 701–706.

Pepper, C.M., Klein, D.N., Anderson, R.L. et al. (1995). DSM-III-R Axis II comorbidity in dysthymia and major depression. *American Journal of Psychiatry*, 152, 239–247.

Ravindran, A., Smith, A., Georgescu, T. et al. (2010). Effect of antidepressant treatment on the neural circuitry in dysthymia: A functional magnetic resonance imaging study. *European Neuropsychopharmacology*, 20, S301–S302.

Ravindran, A.V., Anisman, H., Merali, Z. et al. (1999). Treatment of primary dysthymia with group cognitive therapy and pharmacotherapy: Clinical symptoms and functional impairments. *American Journal of Psychiatry*, 156, 1608–1617.

Ravindran, A.V., Smith, A., Cameron, C. et al. (2009). Toward a functional neuroanatomy of dysthymia: A functional magnetic resonance imaging study. *Journal of Affective Disorders*, 119, 9–15.

Regier, D.A., Rae, D.S., Narrow, W.E., Kaelber, C.T., and Schatzberg, A.F. (1998). Prevalence of anxiety disorders and their comorbidity with mood and addictive disorders. *British Journal of Psychiatry*, 173, 24–28.

Regier, D.A., Farmer, M.E., Rae, D.S. et al. (1990). Comorbidity of mental disorders with alcohol and other drug abuse: Results from the Epidemiologic Catchment Area (ECA) study. *Journal of the American Medical Association*, 264, 2511–2518.

Riso, L.P., Du Toit, P.L., Blandino, J.A. et al. (2003). Cognitive aspects of chronic depression. *Journal of Abnormal Psychology*, 112, 72–80.

Rush, A.J., Trivedi, M.H., Ibrahim, H.M. et al. (2003). The 16-item Quick Inventory of Depressive Symptomatology

(QIDS), clinician rating (QIDS-C), and self-report (QIDS-SR): A psychometric evaluation in patients with chronic major depression. *Biological Psychiatry*, 54, 573–583.

Sackeim, H.A. (2001). The definition and meaning of treatment-resistant depression. *The Journal of Clinical Psychiatry*, 62 Suppl 16, 10–17.

Satyanarayana, S., Enns, M.W., Cox, B.J., and Sareen, J. (2009). Prevalence and correlates of chronic depression in the Canadian Community Health Survey: Mental health and well-being. *Canadian Journal of Psychiatry – Revue Canadienne De Psychiatrie*, 54, 389–398.

Schlatter, J., Ortuno, F., and Cervera-Enguix, S. (2001). Differences in interleukins' patterns between dysthymia and major depression. *European Psychiatry*, 16, 317–319.

Scott, J. (1988). Chronic depression. *British Journal of Psychiatry*, 153, 287–297.

Seidman, S., Orr, G., Raviv, G. *et al.* (2009). Effects of testosterone replacement in middle-aged men with dysthymia: A randomized, placebo-controlled clinical trial. *Journal of Clinical Psychopharmacology*, 29, 216–221.

Shelton, R., Davidson, J., Yonkers, K. *et al.* (1997). The undertreatment of dysthymia. *Journal of Clinical Psychiatry*, 58, 59–65.

Silva De Lima, M., Moncrieff, J., and Soares, B. (2009). Drugs versus placebo for dysthymia. *Cochrane Database of Systematic Reviews*.

Spitzer, R., Williams, J., Kroenke, K. *et al.* (1994). Utility of a new procedure for diagnosing mental disorders in primary care: The PRIME-MD 1000 Study. *Journal of the American Medical Association*, 272, 1749–1756.

Stewart, J.W., Quitkin, F.M., McGrath, P.J. *et al.* (1988). Social functioning in chronic depression – effect of 6 weeks of antidepressant treatment. *Psychiatry Research*, 25, 213–222.

Stewart, W.F., Ricci, J.A., Chee, E., Hahn, S.R., and Morganstein, D. (2003). Cost of lost productive work time among US workers with depression. *Journal of the American Medical Association*, 289, 3135–3144.

Swendsen, J.D. and Merikangas, K.R. (2000). The comorbidity of depression and substance use disorders. *Clinical Psychology Review*, 20, 173–189.

Thakkar, V. and Adler, L. ( ). *Depression and ADHD: What You Need to Know* [Online]. MedScape. Available: http://www.medscape.org/viewarticle/549018 (accessed September 2012).

Tyrer, P., Seivewright, H., Simmonds, S., and Johnson, T. (2001). Prospective studies of cothymia (mixed anxiety-depression): How do they inform clinical practice? *European Archives of Psychiatry and Clinical Neuroscience*, 251, 53–56.

Vanelle, J.M., Attarlevy, D., Poirier, M.F. *et al.* (1997). Controlled efficacy study of fluoxetine in dysthymia. *British Journal of Psychiatry*, 170, 345–350.

Weissman, M. and Klerman, G. (1977). The chronic depressive in the community: Unrecognized and poorly treated. *Comprehensive Psychiatry*, 18, 523–532.

Weissman, M., Leaf, P., Bruce, M., and Florio, L. (1988). The epidemiology of dysthymia in 5 communities: Rates, risks, comorbidity, and treatment. *American Journal of Psychiatry*, 145, 815–819.

Weissman, M.M., Bruce, M.L., Leaf, P.J., Florio, L.P., and Holzer, C.I. (1991). Affective disorders. In Robins, L.N. and Regier, D.A., eds. *Psychiatric Disorders in America: The Epidemiologic Catchment Area Study*. New York: The Free Press, 53–80.

Wells, K., Burnam, M., Rogers, W., Hays, R., and Camp, P. (1992). The course of depression in adult outpatients: Results from the medical outcomes study. *Archives of General Psychiatry*, 49, 788–794.

Wells, K., Stewart, A., Hays, R. *et al.* (1989). The functioning and well-being of depressed patients: Results from the Medical Outcomes Study. *Journal of the American Medical Association*, 262, 914–919.

Wender, P.H., Reimherr, F.W., and Wood, D.R. (1981). Attention deficit disorder (minimal brain-dysfunction) in adults. *Archives of General Psychiatry*, 38, 449–456.

Williams, J.W., Barrett, J., Oxman, T. *et al.* (2000). Treatment of dysthymia and minor depression in primary care: A randomized controlled trial in older adults. *Journal of the American Medical Association*, 284, 1519–1526.

Yang, T. and Dunner, D. (2001). Differential subtyping of depression. *Depression and Anxiety*, 13, 11–17.

Chapter

4

Management of adult major depressive disorder

J. John Mann, Steven P. Roose, and Patrick J. McGrath

Introduction

Major depressive disorder (MDD) is a common, recurrent, or chronic illness, and a major cause of death and disability. In Western nations, most psychological autopsy studies find that mood disorders are present in about 60% of all suicides. In the United States that means about 20 000 suicides per year in individuals with mood disorders. Worldwide, MDD is projected to account for 78.7 million disability-adjusted life years (DALYs) lost, second amongst all diseases by the year 2020 (Murray *et al*. 1997). The prevalence of MDD in the USA is 5.4–8.9% (Narrow *et al*. 2002). Major depression is common in medical outpatient clinics (5–13%) and in primary care practice, where it often presents with somatic complaints (Katon *et al*. 1992, Coyne *et al*. 1994, Kroenke *et al*. 1994). The somatic symptoms can include anorexia and weight loss, hyperphagia and weight gain, constipation, disturbed sleep, anergia, loss of libido, aches and pains, and memory and concentration deficiencies. Unless the clinician asks specifically about depression, guilt, anxiety, and hopelessness, the diagnosis of depression may be missed. Prominent somatic symptoms, or accepting atribution to life stressors, are some reasons depression may be undiagnosed and therefore untreated (Hirschfeld *et al*. 1997, Goldman *et al*. 1999). Treatment is received in the United States by only about two-thirds of persons with major depression, and in only half of those is treatment of adequate intensity and duration. Treatment duration should be at least 6 months for a single episode, but is often shorter. Maintenance treatment is indicated in highly recurrent cases. Clinicians often do not continue to adjust treatment to achieve remission in partial responders, as a result, MDD is often undertreated even when correctly diagnosed (Goldman *et al*. 1999).

Suicidal ideation and suicide attempts are a risk in moderately as well as the most severely depressed, and should be part of the routine evaluation of such patients. That risk is most strongly associated with a personal or family history of a suicide attempt, and further increased by co-morbid substance-use disorder, borderline personality disorder, and antisocial personality disorder (Mann *et al*. 2006b, 2007). The short-term risk is best estimated by severity of suicial ideation and specifically having a current plan for a specific method for a suicide attempt or attempt to suicide. Psychological studies show that most depressed patients are untreated at the time of suicide, and also the risk of a suicide attempt is greater during an episode of major depression compared to between episodes. Psychotic symptoms may complicate major depression, such as delusions of guilt and somatic disease, especially postpartum, and these are further risk factors for suicide. This subtype of depression is the subject of Chapter 6. Depressive episodes in bipolar disorder are similar to MDD and, together with mixed states, are addressed in the chapters on bipolar disorder (Chapters 7–8). It is not always easy to make the differential diagnosis of bipolar disorder, and particularly difficult when the patient presents initially in a depressive episode (Bebbington *et al*. 1995). Interviewing a collateral informant is often critical in establishing the presence of bipolar disorder.

Approximately 75–85% of patients presenting with one major depressive episode will have future episodes (Keller *et al*. 1986, Mueller *et al*. 1999). This chapter will address episodic recurrent depression; chronic major depression, double depression, and dysthymia have separate chapters devoted to them (see Chapters 3 and 10).

Clinical Handbook for the Management of Mood Disorders, ed. J. John Mann, Patrick J. McGrath, and Steven P. Roose.
Published by Cambridge University Press. © Cambridge University Press 2013.

Pathophysiology of depression

The clinical picture of depression varies enormously from episode to episode within the same depressed patient (Oquendo *et al.* 2004). This pleomorphic clinical picture, because it is seen within individuals, indicates that MDD is really a single superfamily of mood disorders that despite its many clinical pictures may potentially have a common pathology. We find the manifestation of this variable psychopathology as assessed by relative regional brain activity, appears to vary from episode to episode in terms of affected brain regions, even within the same patient, and is in contrast to the more static picture or trait-like character of abnormal neurotransmitter systems (Milak *et al.* 2005, Miller *et al.* 2009a). That neurotransmitter-based trait pathology is more likely to be part of a disease process common to perhaps a larger sub-set of depression, makes it detectable in a modest sample of patients under study.

Specific neurotransmitter system abnormalities in MDD fall into two broad categories. The first category includes hypothesized deficiencies in neurotransmitter levels or signal transduction, that include serotonin, norepinephrine, dopamine, GABA, and some peptidergic transmitters, as well as trophic factors such as BDNF, somatostatin and thyroid-related hormones (see Mann *et al.* 2005). The second category of peptides and neurotransmitter system abnormalities are thought to involve overactivation and include acetylcholine, glutamate corticotrophin-releasing factor, and substance P (Mann *et al.* 2005). How these neurotransmitter abnormalities are related to each other, and whether different neurotransmitters are involved in the MDD of different patients, is not known.

We know less about the etiology of major depression compared to its pathophysiology. MDD is moderately heritable (Kendler and Karkowski-Shuman 1997, Kendler *et al.* 2006) and reported childhood adversity such as reported physical or sexual abuse is associated with increased risk of major depression in adolescence and adulthood (Risch *et al.* 2009). However, the specific genes remain to be identified (Sullivan *et al.* 2000, Major Depressive Disorder Working Group of the Psychiatric GWAS Consortium 2012) and it is minimally understood how genes and early life experience mold the brain developmentally to create the predisposition for major depressive disorder (see Mann *et al.* 2006a for a summary). It has been proposed on the basis of animal studies that familial transmission of psychopathology such as major depression may result from either genetic factors or transmission of epigenetic modifications resulting from early life experience.

Genes and stress during earlier periods of life affect stress response systems in the brain and their components outside the brain such as the hypothalamic pituitary adrenal axis (HPA axis), and the noradrenergic system. Early childhood stress in animal models of maternal deprivation sensitize these two major stress response systems and that super-sensitive response persists into adulthood, as shown when the adult animal is stressed (Kaufman *et al.* 2000, Heim and Nemeroff, 2001). Cross-sectional studies in depressed patients reporting physical or sexual abuse suggest such hyperactive stress responses may be found in depressed patients (Heim *et al.* 2001). Other aspects of altered pathophysiology include altered neuroplasticity, diminished cellular resilience, and neurogenesis (see Charney *et al.* 2004 for a review and Boldrini *et al.* 2009). In rodent models stress and glucocorticoids reduce neurogenesis, and this effect can be reversed or prevented by antidepressant medication administration. In postmortem studies of depressed suicides, reported childhood adversity is associated with increased DNA methylation in key parts of the regulatory region of the glucocorticoid receptor gene and that in turn can explain the observed lower gene expression, and contribute to HPA axis hyper-responsiveness to stress (McGowan *et al.* 2009). How that in turn may affect neurogenesis remains to be determined. Persistently elevated cortisol levels in rodents leads to hippocampal atrophy and both elevated corticosteroids and smaller hippocampus characterize some moderate to severe depressions. Therefore enhanced cortisol release in MDD may explain smaller hippocampal volume which has been reported to be proportional to duration of untreated depression lifetime (Sheline *et al.* 2002), and which progresses with lack of remission of depression (MacQueen *et al.* 2008).

More recently, gene–environment interactions have been observed that help to explain why childhood adversity can have a negative long-term outcome in some people and not others. The best known example is the report that children exposed to childhood adversity and who carry lower expressing gene variants of the promotor or regulatory region of the serotonin transporter gene (the target of SSRIs) have an elevated risk of major depression when exposed to stress in their mid-twenties (Caspi *et al.* 2003). Although there is debate over this finding (Risch *et al.* 2009), the same gene variant favors hyper-responsiveness of the amygdala on functional magnetic resonance imaging when matching frightened faces. A hyperactive amygdala is also reported in major depression and its overactivity may facilitate encoding of painful memories leading to stress sensitivity in adulthood and greater likelihood of depression when stressed (Hariri *et al.* 2005). In nonhuman primates these gene variants are associated with reduction of serotonin function in response to maternal deprivation, an effect that persists into adulthood (Ichise *et al.* 2006) and may explain part of the biologic impact of childhood adversity in genetically susceptible individuals who are more prone to depression in adulthood (Brent *et al.* 2004). We found that patients with MDD who report childhood adversity, also have lower serotonin transporter binding on PET scanning (Miller *et al.* 2009b). Maternal deprivation may remodel the serotonin system changes in the genetically vulnerable person and this may be a biological phenotype associated with a vulnerability to stress-induced MDD in adulthood. Mice that have the serotonin transporter blocked for a few days in infancy through short-term administration of an SSRI, grow up to manifest a depressive behavioral phenotype (Gingrich *et al.* 2001). Since the SSRI given after infancy has an antidepressant effect, the vulnerability to less serotonin transporter is confined to a critical period of only a few days after birth in the rodent. That transient short-term effect in infancy appears to be sufficient to alter the developing brain downstream to produce the vulnerability to depression. Several clinical studies have shown that the carriers of the lower-expressing alleles and those with major depression, have altered brain connectivity between the amygdala and the anterior cingulate, two brain regions known to be involved in the pathophysiology of MDD (Pezawas *et al.* 2005). Such potential effect on brain circuitry and connectivity are one hypothesized way in which the low-expressing alleles of the serotonin transporter gene interact with early childhood experience to remodel the brain to produce the diathesis for MDD. In general, a research approach looking at gene–environment interactions may help to provide a more complete picture of the pathogenesis of MDD. Although some promising clinical and animal studies suggest a role for the serotonin transporter gene, a gene–environment approach needs to include a broader range of genes involved in risk and resilience for MDD.

Alterations in structure and/or activity in a number of brain regions in major depression have been identified by brain imaging. Greater brain activity is reported in ventral brain structures, including limbic structures and hypoactivity in dorsal and lateral prefrontal cortex. Recovery from an episode of major depression is associated with reversal of much of this picture with changes in brain activity in the direction of that found in healthy volunteers (Mayberg, 1997, Milak *et al.* 2005). Structural changes in the brain in MDD are much smaller than the functional changes (Soares *et al.* 1997a, 1997b). The disordered neurocircuitry of major depression more specifically includes hypoactivity in the ventral, medial, and dorsolateral prefrontal cortex, the anterior insula, the ventral striatum, the posterior cingulate gyrus, and hippocampus, and hyperactivity in the anterior cingulate cortex (ACC), medial thalamus, amygdale, and brainstem (for a review see Milak *et al.* 2005). These brain areas regulate emotional, cognitive, autonomic, sleep, and stress response behaviours, which are impaired in MDD.

MDD is so pleomorphic from episode to episode even within a single patient, making it less probable that a different etiology underlies all the different clinical manifestations of MDD. The answer to this puzzle may have important treatment implications in terms of choosing the optimal pharmacological medication or perhaps the use of a psychotherapy for each patient and for each of their episodes of MDD. We predict that the current nosology, which is entirely based on clinical features will be complemented by an orthogonal, biological classification system based on measurable biosignatures that will improve prognostication and help in treatment selection.

Diagnosis of major depression

Diagnosis of major depressive disorder is entirely clinical at present, and based on criteria such as DSM-IV (1994) which is mostly used within the US, or ICD-10 which is the international standard. The details can be found in Chapter 2. The DSM-IV diagnosis requires the presence nearly every day for at least 2 weeks of depressed mood or loss of interest or diminished sense of pleasure, plus four of seven other features that include: weight change of at least 5% in one month or persistent appetite change, insomnia or hypersomnia most days, changes in psychomotor state, fatigue, feelings of guilt and worthlessness, diminished concentration and decisiveness, and suicidal ideation or an attempt. These features should constitute a change from normal function and episodes generally last an average of 3 months, although they can persist for years. Planning treatment with respect to hospitalization requires estimation of suicide risk by inquiring about previous suicide attempts, current suicidal ideation, including a plan or intent for suicide, level of agitation, and the presence of delusions. Some patients are so depressed they cannot eat or drink adequately, manage personal hygiene, or co-operate with taking medication. Inpatient treatment can therefore be required.

Children and adolescents may initially manifest an anxiety disorder that then evolves into a mood disorder (Brent et al. 2002, Weissman 2006). Early episodes often have milder symptomatology and are shorter and therefore may not meet diagnostic criteria for MDD. On the other hand, earlier onset mood disorders can have a more severe course (Zisook et al. 2004). Each episode has the potential to extract a toll in terms of broken relationships, education failure, and loss of employment, and therefore early diagnosis and treatment may mitigate such adverse effects. Serious physical illnesses such as pancreatic cancer, lung cancer, anterior strokes, demyelinating diseases, epilepsy, or marked anemia may trigger a depression that clinically looks like a primary mood disorder and can respond to antidepressants somewhat independently of how well the medical illness responds to treatment (Bauer et al. 2002). MDD, like bipolar disorder, is moderately heritable (Kendler et al. 1997, 2006). A family history of bipolar disorder may indicate a higher probability of the ultimate diagnosis being a bipolar disorder, particularly where bipolar disorder presents with a depressive episode, although there are many examples of MDD and bipolar disorder being found in the same families. As a general rule, a spouse or friend may clarify the diagnosis, because some patients with bipolar disorder may deny manic symptoms, regarding them not as a sign of illness but of wellbeing.

Classes of medications

Antidepressants

Reported response rates to antidepressants, and improve with time and with successive courses of antidepressants, and are estimated at 47% to a course of an SSRI in an outpatient population of major depression (Trivedi et al. 2006). Some argue that this response rate is rather modest, namely that only about half the patients with moderate to severe depression will respond to a first-line antidepressant. It is notable that response rates to antihypertensive medications in patients with stage I or II hypertension are much better. Response rates based on meta-analysis of study-level data have been modest for antidepressants in comparison to placebo, but a patient-level meta-analysis of published and unpublished studies of the efficacy of fluoxetine and venlafaxine found that medication response relative to placebo to be quite robust (Gibbons et al. 2012). A debate has also been underway about the impact of illness severity on antidepressant response (Mulrow, 1999). Some large-scale studies have not found severity of depression to predict antidepressant medication outcome (Walsh et al. 2002, Gibbons et al. 2012). While it had been suggested that less severity of depression predicts better response to psychotherapies like cognitive therapy (Elkin et al. 1995), more recent studies did not confirm this finding (DeRubeis et al. 2005).

Another factor that may be related to antidepressant medication response is the pharmacologic class of antidepressant. Classes of antidepressant agents are defined by mechanism of action. Most effective antidepressants amplify signaling by inhibiting serotonin or norepinephrine reuptake at the synaptic cleft. These drugs include selective serotonin reuptake inhibitors (SSRIs), selective norepinephrine reuptake inhibitors (NRIs), and dual-action agents that inhibit uptake of serotonin and norepinephrine (SNRIs and an older class of antidepressants such as tricyclic antidepressants (TCAs)). Monoamine oxidase inhibitors (MAOIs) inhibit monoamine degradation by monoamine oxidase A or B (Westenberg, 1999). Other antidepressants are alpha-2-adrenergic autoreceptor antagonists and thereby *enhance* norepinephrine firing, and/or $5-HT_{2A}$ receptor antagonists, including many atypical antipsychotics that are used as augmenting or adjunctive treatments for depression (Westenberg, 1999). Efficacy of individual agents generally appears comparable both between and within classes of antidepressants (Mulrow 1999, Rush 2007).

Then there are antidepressants that act on different neurotransmitter systems like the NMDA antagonist, ketamine, lamotrigine, which acts on the GABAergic system and affects glutamate release, and lithium, which has many pharmacologic effects; the ones related to its antidepressant and antidepressant augmentation benefit are uncertain. Of note, electroconvulsive treatment raises seizure threshold, which is also a consequence of many antiepileptic drugs that are now used as mood stabilizers and some of which may have antidepressant effects such as valproate and lamotrigine.

Selective serotonin reuptake inhibitors (SSRIs)

SSRI treatment has become the standard first-line medication for the initial pharmacotherapy of MDD because of better tolerability, lower cardiovascular risk, and lower risk of mortality in overdose compared to first-generation antidepressants (Mulrow, 1999). Since their introduction in 1989, SSRIs have transformed the therapy of MDD, as well as of other psychiatric disorders such as anxiety disorders. For example, there were 2.5 million prescriptions for fluoxetine in 1988 and 33.3 million prescriptions in 2002 in the USA. Meta-analyses generally find no difference in efficacy or tolerability between SSRIs (Mulrow, 1999, Stahl, 2000, Kroenke et al. 2001), or between SSRIs and other classes of antidepressants (Simon et al. 1996, Mulrow, 1999, Anderson, 2000, Geddes et al. 2000, MacGillivray et al. 2003), but there are some specific differences. An exception is escitalopram that has been reported to be very modestly superior to other SSRIs and comparable to venlafaxine (Kennedy et al. 2006). Fluoxetine and its active metabolite have a longer half-life than other SSRIs which reduces the impact of missed doses, allows for once a day dosing or even less frequently, and mitigates the discontinuation syndrome (Rosenbaumy 1998). Paroxetine and sertraline have shorter half-lives and are more prone to the discontinuation syndrome, and some report that in higher doses these drugs may block dopamine reuptake, although not to the degree that it seems likely to contribute to their antidepressant action (Mulrow, 1999, Anderson, 2000, Peretti et al. 2000, MacGillivray et al. 2003, Nemeroff et al. 2004). For patients presenting with predominantly physical symptoms and/or pain, SSRIs appear to be less effective than TCAs and NRIs (Briley, 2004). The SSRI fluoxetine is the only antidepressant shown by most studies to be effective in youth (March et al. 2004) and SSRIs may be superior to NRIs in younger adults (18 24) (Mulder et al. 2003). Finally, (Grunebaum et al. 2012) found an SSRI to be more effective than bupropion for major depression, and also for suicidal ideation,

independently of antidepressant benefit, with the advantage being greater in those who reported more severe suicidal ideation prior to the clinical treatment trial. This was only a pilot study and the results need to be replicated because, if confirmed, they have great implications for treatment selection in depressed patients with suicidal ideation.

Older dual-action reuptake inhibitors

A sub-set of tricyclic antidepressants (imipramine, amitriptyline) inhibit both serotonin and norepinephrine reuptake. A newer nontricyclic set of antidepressants, such as duloxetine and venlafaxine, also inhibit reuptake of both NE and 5-HT. Some studies report no difference in overall efficacy between TCAs, SSRIs, and MAOIs, (Anderson, 2000, MacGillivray et al. 2003) however, other studies find the dual-action drugs have more benefit and fewer side effects (Tran et al. 2003). The type of depression has been suggested as an explanation for the different study outcomes, for example, TCAs are reported to have superior efficacy as compared to SSRIs in hospitalized patients and in people with severe MDD or depression with melancholic features (Boyce et al. 1999, Geddes, 1999, Anderson, 2000). In bipolar depression, tricyclics may be associated with higher rates of mania or hypomania, or rapid cycling compared with SSRIs (Peet 1994, Gijsman et al. 2004). Since many bipolar patients present initially with an episode of depression, this risk can be difficult to predict.

Newer dual-action antidepressants

New-generation serotonin–norepinephrine reuptake inhibitors (SNRIs) such as duloxetine or venlafaxine block both monoamine transporters, but differ from tricyclics by having much less affinity for cholinergic, histaminergic, or alpha-adrenergic receptors (Hirschfeld et al. 2004). Superior efficacy and higher rates of remission for SNRIs compared to SSRIs are not found consistently across this class of antidepressants, although they are reported to be more effective than SSRIs in several studies (Anderson, 2001, Olver et al. 2001, Thase et al. 2001, Rudolph, 2002, Smith et al. 2002, Stahl et al. 2002, Tran et al. 2003). On the other hand, duloxetine was reported to have comparable efficacy to the SSRI paroxetine (Detke et al. 2004). Venlafaxine is effective in treatment of chronic pain (Rowbotham et al. 2004) and duloxetine in co-morbid pain and depression (Goldstein et al. 2004, Brannan et al. 2005), an advantage for patients presenting with depression in the context of physical illness, somatic symptoms, and pain.

Bupropion inhibits norepinephrine, and to a modest and probably clinically insignificant degree, dopamine reuptake, but has no direct action on the serotonin system. It has comparable efficacy to TCAs (Mulrow, 1999) and SSRIs (Nieuwstraten et al. 2001). It is associated with less nausea, diarrhea, somnolence, and sexual dysfunction compared with SSRIs (Nieuwstraten and Dolovich 2001). It may be an alternative, or adjunctive therapy, for SSRI nonresponders (DeBattista et al. 2003, Fava et al. 2003). On the other hand, in a preliminary and as yet unreplicated study, buproprion appears to be less effective than the SSRI, paroxetine, for both major depression and suicidal ideation in depressed patients presenting with more severe suicidal ideation (Grunebaum et al. 2012).

Norepinephrine reuptake inhibitors (NRIs)

Some tricyclic and tetracyclic drugs, such as nortriptyline, maprotiline, and desipramine, are relatively selective norepinephrine reuptake inhibitors, and are marketed in many countries including the USA, but have antihistaminic and anticholinergic effects, as well as cardiotoxicity on overdose. Tricyclics can also suppress ventricular ectopics, which could be theraputic in some patients, yet other patients are potentially endangered in terms of heart block, such as those with pre-existing conduction defects, even at doses in the therapeutic range. Reboxetine is a selective norepinephrine reuptake inhibitor, with debatable effectiveness compared to TCAs and SSRIs (Mulrow, 1999) because it failed in efficacy trials for the FDA and consequently it is not available in the USA.

Monoamine oxidase inhibitors

Although MAOIs generally appear to have comparable antidepressant efficacy to each other and to TCAs (Thase et al. 1995), they may be superior to TCAs for atypical depression (Quitkin et al. 1993) and sometimes work in TCA, SSRI, and SNRI nonresponders (Thase et al. 1992a, Thase et al. 1992b, Nolen et al. 1993, McGrath et al. 2006). More detailed discussion of MAOI pharmacotherapy can be found in Chapter 5, which discusses atypical depression, where MAOIs are effective.

Other antidepressants and new novel treatments

Mirtazapine blocks alpha-2-adrenergic autoreceptors, serotonin 5-HT$_{2A}$, 5-HT$_3$, and histamine H$_1$ receptors. The blockade of the alpha-2-adrenergic autoreceptors enhances norepinephrine transmission by increasing firing rate and NE release. Blocking H$_1$ receptors produces sedation, making the drug more tolerable when given in the evening or at bedtime. It has comparable efficacy to TCAs and SSRIs (Benkert et al. 2002), although perhaps not for severe depression, (Kasper, 1997, Hirschfeld, 1999) and has been shown in controlled studies to augment SSRI antidepressants (Blier et al. 2009, 2010). Mirtazapine is reported to have fewer sexual side effects than the SSRI, paroxetine (Montejo et al. 2001), and less sleep disturbance than the SNRI, venlafaxine (Guelfi et al. 2001). The propensity of mirtazapine to cause sedation and weight gain makes it an appealing choice for patients with typical melancholic depression characterized by pronounced insomnia, and/or weight loss. Nefazodone blocks the 5-HT$_{2A}$ serotonin receptor, and to a lesser degree than mirtazapine it also blocks the alpha-1-adrenergic receptor. It also is reported to have comparable antidepressant efficacy to SSRIs with fewer sexual and sleep-related side effects, although a US FDA "Black Box" warning concerning hepatotoxicity has limited its use (Feiger et al. 1996, Rush et al. 1998). Trazadone, related to both these drugs, is a proven antidepressant (Mann et al. 1981), but so sedating that it has found a place as an adjunctive medication in the treatment of depression when given at bedtime to help sleep. Atypical antipsychotics also block the 5-HT$_{2A}$ receptor and some are reported to have antidepressant effects (see below).

New treatments that are in the process of evaluation include: ketamine, in sub-anesthetic doses sufficient to block the NMDA receptor, which produces a rapid antidepressant effect that is manifested in about 4 hours. This medication has been evaluated in about nine studies with positive results, and works in treatment-resistant depression, and has a striking effect on suicidal ideation (see Chapter 27 for details). The benefit persists for about 5 days. Research into the best approach for sustaining this rapid benefit is underway. It is noteworthy that this rapid clinical action is accompanied by an equally rapid increase in dendritic spines on cortical neurons that may be related to the antidepressant action (Duman et al. 2012).

The observations of hyperactive hypothalamic pituitry adrenal axis function in major depression, especially delusional and more severe forms of depression, led to the evaluation of mifepristone, a glucocorticoid antagonist, for the treatment of delusional depression where it has proven to be at best modestly effective (Stahl *et al.* 2003). A disappointing new antidepressant drug target involved the use of substance P antagonists for depression, where several drugs all proved ineffective (Stahl and Grady, 2003).

Augmenting and adjunctive medications

These medications are used in conjunction with other antidepressants to either augment antidepressant effect or target a different component of psychopathology, such as delusions, or prevent a switch into mania.

Mood stabilizers

Lithium, an antimanic agent, is used for maintenance treatment of bipolar disease to prevent episodes of mania and depression (see Chapters 7 and 8 for details), and in major depressive disorder for the prevention of recurrence of depressive episodes. Lithium may be superior to placebo for bipolar depression (Zornberg *et al.* 1993), and although its efficacy as an antidepressant for MDD is debated, it is an effective augmenting agent for patients whose depression did not respond to a single antidepressant (de Montigny 1994, Bauer *et al.* 2003). Lamotrigine, an antiepileptic drug, reduces glutamatergic activity perhaps via GABA enhancement, but its efficacy for bipolar depression is debatable and its efficacy as an augmenting treatment in MDD is also unlcear (Normann *et al.* 2002, Barbosa *et al.* 2003).

Antipsychotic drugs

Typical antipsychotic agents (chlorpromazine, haloperidol) mostly block the D_2 dopamine receptor, and "atypical" antipsychotic agents (e.g., olanzapine, risperidone, quetiapine, ziprasidone, aripiprazole) target additional neurotransmitter systems, such as serotonin via $5-HT_{2A}$ blockade (Sanger, 2004). Antipsychotic drugs are combined with antidepressants for depression with psychotic features because antidepressant monotherapy is less effective compared with a combination of an antidepressant and antipsychotic. The alternative to medication for psychotic

depression is electroconvulsive therapy (Masan 2004, Rothschild *et al.* 2004). In addition to psychotic depression, treatment-resistant major depression can also respond to augmentation with most atypical antipsychotics (Yatham *et al.* 2003, Baldassano *et al.* 2004, Papakostas *et al.* 2008).

Atypical antipsychotic drugs have a more favorable side-effect profile in terms of parkinsonism, akathisia, and tardive dyskinesia, better tolerability, and have comparable or better antidepressant efficacy compared with typical antipsychotic agents. Thus, they are the preferred choice over typical antipsychotics in mood disorders. However, atypical antipsychotics have more risk of drug-induced arrhythmia, diabetes, including a hyperosmolar ketotic crisis, weight gain, and hyperlipidemia, the latter three features are known as metabolic syndrome. Risk of diabetes-related side effects is lower for risperidone and quetiapine (Cohen, 2004). Patients being considered for atypical antipsychotics should be screened for diabetes, hyperlipidemias, and cardiac abnormalities. Because of these risks, these medications are not first-line antidepressants.

Thyroid supplements

The addition of synthroid or T4, and less commonly T3, is used to augment antidepressant medications, particularly when the TSH is elevated (Bauer *et al.* 1990). These hormonal supplements appear to accelerate antidepressant response and enhance response in treatment-resistant depression treated with first-generation antidepressants, and also with SSRIs (Agid *et al.* 2003). How they work remains unclear.

Overall therapeutic strategy

Successful treatment of major depression may require a multi-modal approach including pharmacotherapy, education, and psychotherapy (Figure 4.1). Diagnosis may require seeing a family member in addition to the patient, and reassessment is indicated if mania, suicidal ideation or behavior, or psychotic features emerge in the course of treatment. Reviewing past medical records may offer valuable clues as to what were the therapeutic and side effects of previously used medications in specific doses. Treatment with medication requires monitoring side effects, clinical response, and especially suicidal ideation or behavior. The patient and their family must be educated about the course of

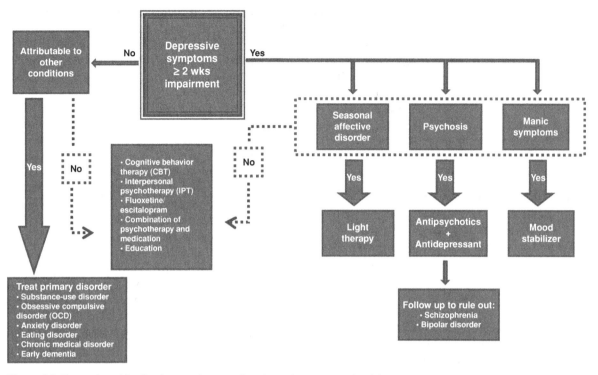

Figure 4.1 Diagnostic and first-line therapeutic approach to depressive symptoms in adults

illness so that they can understand that the initial clinical response can take a couple of months to become fully manifest, although recent data indicate that the onset of antidepressant action compared to placebo begins to appear within the first week (Walsh *et al.* 2002). It may require longer, up to several weeks, for the improvement to be clearly detectable by patient and family. Figure 4.2 summarizes the acute treatment of major depression. The family and patient must also understand the basis for the need for adherence to therapy, given that the median duration of treatment of an episode of depression in a general population is about 3 months, although potentially longer in hospital clinic populations (Spijker *et al.* 2002). It has been shown that shorter courses of treatment result in higher relapse rates (Melfi *et al.* 1998, Geddes *et al.* 2003).

A treatment plan takes into account previous treatment outcomes because such a history gives an indication of both the class of medication that might work and the dose. Mood disorder sub-type will affect choice of medication type, such as use of an atypical antipsychotic or medication to help associated psychotic features or an SSRI for panic attacks or obsessive compulsive symptoms, or a light box for

a seasonal component (Figure 4.3). SSRIs may be more effective for major depression characterized by prominent suicidal ideation (Grunebaum *et al.* 2012). A personal or family history of suicidal behavior or current ideation with a specific suicide plan or intent, including evidence the patient has begun preparations for suicide such as acquiring the means or preparing their will or insurance papers, are indications favoring management as an inpatient because they signify greater risk of suicide (Figure 4.2). Current severity of depression is a consideration because certain treatments may work better for more severe depression like tricyclics and dual-action antidepressants known as SNRIs that include venlafaxine and duloxetine (Figure 4.2). Co-morbid psychiatric and somatic conditions such as pain favor use of an SNRI. Nonpsychiatric medications may interfere with the use of some antidepressants because of drug interactions or summation of side effects. For example, the use of diuretics or antihypertensive medications which block alpha-1-adrenergic receptors may result in an excessive drop in blood pressure if combined with a TCA or an atypical antipsychotic antidepressant which also blocks alpha-1-adrenergic receptors. Psychological stressors such as relationship

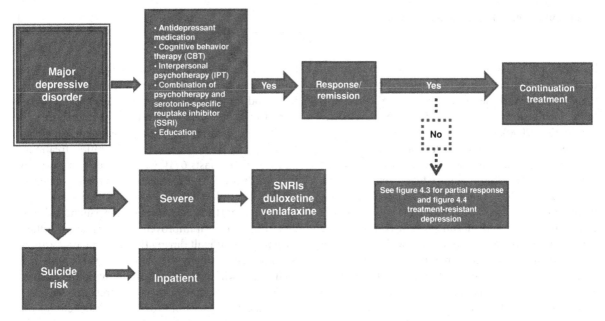

Figure 4.2 Acute treatment of major depression

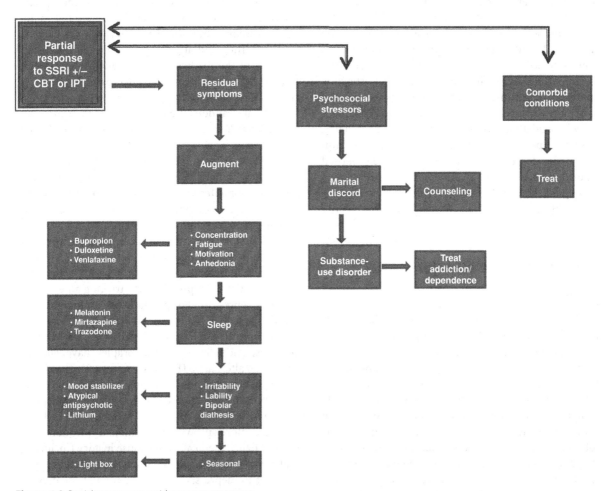

Figure 4.3 Partial response to antidepressant treatment

breakup or job loss may lead the patient to abandon treatment in the belief that their depression is due to their situation and therefore is not going to respond to a medication approach (American Psychiatric Association, 2000).

Treatment for major depression involves three phases: acute, which lasts about 2 months and where the goal is complete or almost total (remission) or moderate symptom relief (response); continuation treatment, which lasts about 6 months and where the goal is to sustain benefit and prevent relapse of the episode; and maintenance treatment which is used in those patients whose frequency or severity of recurrent major depressive episodes requires the goal of active treatment to be preventing recurrence of a new episode of major depression. Maintenance treatment, in those patients where it is required, can be lifetime or indefinite. Standard practice indicates that indefinite maintenance treatment is indicated after three episodes of MDE, and should be considered after two (American Psychiatric Association, 1993, Pence *et al.* 2012). Although most clinicians use a relative nonsystematic and intuitive approach, in fact using treatment algorithms in order to apply a systematic approach to treatment of major depressive episodes can improve outcome as compared to usual treatment (Hawley *et al.* 1998, Adli *et al.* 2002, Trivedi *et al.* 2004). Figure 4.2 presents a basic acute treatment algorithm for a major depressive episode in MDD. The proposed algorithm is based on treatment models developed from published treatment algorithm studies (Hawley *et al.* 1998, Adli *et al.* 2002, Trivedi *et al.* 2004, Mann, 2005).

Major depressive disorder

Acute phase

Antidepressant treatment in the acute phase seeks remission, namely minimal symptoms, no longer meeting criteria for a major depressive episode, and marked improvement in psychosocial functioning based on patient and family report, or if that proves difficult, then at least response which is moderate symptom relief and improvement in psychosocial function to the degree the patient can handle their job, and have rewarding experiences and relationships. Anything less than that requires ongoing revisions to the treatment in order to achieve these goals. Early treatment can potentially modify the course of illness

by reducing the time until an episode improves or remits, and because treatment earlier in an episode may produce a better outcome (Keller, 1989). Prevention of subsequent episodes is important, because successive episodes may become less treatment responsive (Kupfer *et al.* 1989). The acute medication treatment phase generally lasts 6–10 weeks. Weekly or biweekly visits with a treating physician are recommended to address clinical state, side effects, adjust doses, and provide support and education for the patient and family until substantial improvement is achieved. Adherence is often difficult during this acute phase for three main reasons. Initially the patient may lack hope that medication will work, as part of the symptomatic pessimism that characterizes major depression. Secondly, the medication does not provide much benefit for the first couple of weeks, even when it is going to work eventually. Thirdly, side effects are most pronounced when the medication is introduced and may partly improve with the passage of time, although that is not much comfort when the benefit has not yet become manifest. Thus, initially the patient has all the disadvantages of the medication and none of the benefit. Improving compliance by regular patient contact is crucial. One cause of treatment nonresponse is when the patient abandons the medication at their own initiative, and does not tell the doctor about not taking it.

In Western countries, including the USA, most depressed patients are treated by primary care physicians or internists, and not psychiatrists. These doctors are almost never trained in the specialized psychotherapies (cognitive therapy or interpersonal psychotherapy) shown in clinical trials to work for mild and perhaps moderately severe major depressive episodes. Therefore, primary care physicians and internists use antidepressants for treating all episodes of major depression. For psychiatrists, antidepressants are the first-line treatment choice for moderate to severe episodes of major depression. For milder episodes, specialized psychotherapies have efficacy and are an alternative (Figures 4.1 and 4.2). The choice of medication depends partly on a consideration of the effectiveness and side effects of available antidepressants and depressive sub-type (presence of psychotic features, more pronounced suicidal ideation, comorbid pain), medication response history (including that of first-degree relatives), medication tolerability (a sedating antidepressant for anxious or agitated depression, a nonsedating or activating antidepressant for a depression characterized by significant psychomotor retradation), and the pattern of side effects such as avoiding anticholinergic effects in a patient with pre-existing constipation or prostatic enlargement that interferes with urination. Cardiac conduction defects would lead to avoidance of tricyclics, hypertension may be worsened by SNRIs and bupropion, whereas weight gain and sexual dysfunction are potentially less problematic with bupropion compared with SSRIs. Bupropion is superior to an SSRI for migraine, which may be worsened by a serotonin-enhancing drug and not by a drug targeting the noradrenergic system. Medication choice is also influenced by the use of nonpsychiatric drugs, the cost of medication and what is covered by health insurance.

Outpatients with suicidal ideation should not be treated with antidepressant drugs that can be lethal in the event of an overdose, e.g., tricyclics or prescribed smaller quantities of safer antidepressants until they are much improved and stable. In general, at the beginning of treatment, a patient should be given prescriptions for smaller quantities of medication, not only in case of a suicide attempt by an overdose of the medication, but also because the dose and even the medication itself may need to be changed, depending on clinical response and side effects. SSRIs and other newer antidepressant drugs that have a greater safety margin on overdose, compared with tricyclic antidepressants, are currently the first-line medications for moderate–severe depression, particularly for outpatients, patients treated by primary care physicians, and for patients with cardiovascular disease (American Psychiatric Association, 2000, Bauer *et al.* 2002, Swenson *et al.* 2003). To improve compliance and make side effects more tolerable, one begins with lower doses and then increases the dose, depending on both degree of clinical response and severity of side effects. When to raise the dose, change the medication, or add another medication requires experience and judgment in gauging the trajectory of clinical response (Adli *et al.* 2005). For example, raising the dose of the SSRI paroxetine, or for that matter the norepinephrine reuptake inhibitor maprotiline, in depression that has not responded after 3 weeks of treatment, have been found to produce no more improvement than that achieved after a longer duration of treatment at the lower dose (Benkert *et al.* 1997). Although treatment guidelines such as those from the American Psychiatric Association suggest dosage increments in all patients not responding well to lower dosages, raising

the dose may sometimes produce more side effects without accelerating recovery.

Monitoring treatment response

Patient response to treatment needs systematic monitoring, not only to improve compliance, but to make sound decisions about the need to raise the dose to achieve an optimal antidepressant effect and to monitor side effects (Rush, 2007). The goal of treatment should be remisson and the STAR*D study demonstrated that the use of "measurement-based care," whereby clinicians used rating scales to quantify clinical response and made treatment decisions based on degree of quantified improvement instead of clinical impression (Trivedi *et al.* 2006), was probably the reason that treatment outcomes for primary care physicians were comparable to those obtained by psychiatrists (Rush, 2007). Another way of thinking about this approach is that it leaves less to guesswork by requiring criteria like 50% improvement to qualify as clinical response, and less improvement than that requiring a treatment decision like increase the dose, add another medication, switch medication class, or continue the current medication for longer. Less than that level of improvement is associated with less functionality and quality of life, and with higher risk of relapse. Pessimism is a symptom of depression and patients are easily discouraged when antidepressant medication does not work within days. Frequent initial contact can help compliance substantially, as well as providing better treatment. Physicians often settle for insufficient improvement, especially nonpsychiatrists who are less experienced in gauging the degree of improvement and how close the patient is to their baseline state of wellness, which is mitigated by use of standard instruments for monitoring treatment response.

Here is a quantifiable set of response criteria. Nonresponse is a decrease in baseline severity of 25% or less, partial response, a 26–49% decrease in baseline severity, partial remission or clinical response is a 50% or greater decrease in baseline severity (residual symptoms), and absence of symptoms, or minimal symptoms, is remission (Bauer *et al.* 2002). Remission is defined in STAR*D as a 17-item Hamilton Depression Rating Scale score of 7 or less. We believe that remission should be the goal of treatment, and the results of STAR*D support this view because the results of continuation treatment were better for those entering such treatment when already in remission. Persisting with treatment modification continues to achieve the benefit associated with remission because after level 1 treatment 37% remitted, after level 2, 31% remitted, after level 3, 14%, and after level 4, 13% remitted. By level 3 and 4 the complexity of the treatments in terms of multiple medications and making choices of alternative medications means that such treatment should be carried out by psychiatrists and so the measurement also provides an objective threshold for patient referral (Trivedi *et al.* 2006). In addition to remission having a better prognosis, less than remission, such as clinical response, still leaves significant residual symptoms with impaired social relationships, impaired work performance, and increased risk of suicide.

The best clinical predictors of outcome are improvement in anhedonia or loss of pleasure, and less psychomotor retardation (Charney *et al.* 1998). Sometimes the family will notice early improvement before the patient is aware of it. It is therefore necessary to both enquire about other domains of depression beyond "depressed mood," including the above, and to ask the family whether they have noticed any change in the patient. Suicidal ideation or risk for suicidal acts, diurnal variation, pessimism, guilt, and other cognitions may take longer to improve than vegetative symptoms, such as sleep or appetite (Greco *et al.* 2004). Changing medication dose, or switching medications or adding additional medications, are considered if initial treatment response does not progress to remission, or if side effects prevent the medication being used in adequate doses. Note that the presence of side effects often means the dose is adequate. Reducing the dose if side effect interfere with compliance may be indicated. Almost half the patients will have a good response or remission on a first-line treatment. Therefore, 30–50% of patients have substantial residual symptoms defined as clinical nonresponse, even after adequate doses of a first-line treatment (Amsterdam *et al.* 1994). No improvement after 4 weeks of a given drug at an adequate dose predicts an inadequate ultimate response to that medication (Bauer *et al.* 2002). Partial response after 4–6 weeks requires careful monitoring of the trajectory of response, because it signifies a greater likelihood of a full clinical response after a total of 8–12 weeks of treatment (Rush *et al.* 2001).

The factors determining the dose required to produce a remission in depression in a patient are only partly understood. One factor is blood level of medication. That bears a distant relationship to oral dose.

A 10- to 20-fold range in blood levels, and therefore potentially side effects, is seen in a group of patients receiving the same oral dose of a given drug, because of individual variations in drug metabolism due to genetic differences and drug clearance by the kidney or liver, drug effects on liver enzymes, or the effects of aging resulting in a combination of pharmacokinetic and pharmacodynamic effects. While blood levels have been shown to be associated with response to first-generation antidepressant medictions, multiple studies have failed to show such a relationship with second-generation medications, including SSRIs and SNRIs. In terms of the response of the pathophysiology of depression to medication that is not related to drug level and termed pharmacodynamic effects, even less is known. Studies have shown that patients with more impaired serotonin function have a poorer response to SSRIs (Parsey *et al.* 2006, Miller *et al.* 2008), and yet there are no pronounced clinical differences. Thus, the biology of the depression appears to be different in antidepressant responders compared with nonresponders, despite little clinical difference, and this finding has major implications in terms of predicting clinical remission on an antidepressant using a laboratory test (see Chapter 28 for details). Given that the clinician at present relies solely on clinical picture, there is a need to develop better laboratory predictors of clinical outcome.

Before switching medication, or raising the dose, there should be a reappraisal of the diagnosis and reassessment of adequacy of dose and patient adherence. Nonadherence is frequently the reason for nonresponse, and unless asked about, will often not be revealed by the patient. Co-existing medical conditions, alcoholism, substance-use disorder, or nonpsychiatric medication such as beta-blockers and corticosteroids, may also contribute to medication nonresponse.

Once nonresponse to a particular drug is observed, despite an adequate dose and duration of treatment, alternative therapeutic strategies should be considered (see Figures 4.3 and 4.4). The simplest is to switch to an antidepressant from a different pharmacological class. This approach avoids polypharmacy, and thereby reduces the risk of adverse drug–drug interactions and potential summation of side effects that can occur with combinations of similar drugs (Benkert *et al.* 1997, Adli *et al.* 2005, Trivedi *et al.* 2006, Rush, 2007). Generally, prescribing fewer medications enhance adherence. The challenge of switching from one kind

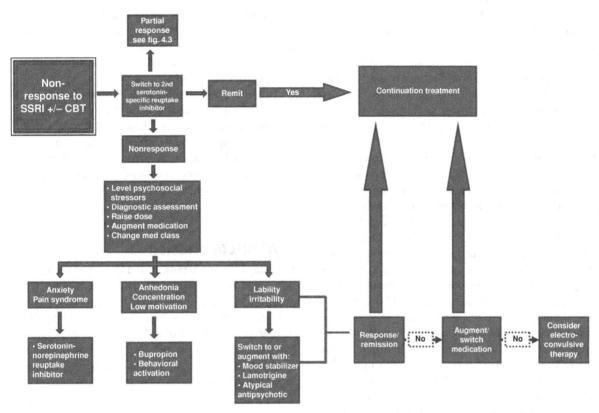

Figure 4.4 Treatment-resistant depression

of medication to another is having to deal with loss of possible partial response achieved with the initial drug, the delay in onset of antidepressant action from the second medication, and finally, for short-acting SSRIs and related medications, unlike fluoxetine, there is a requirement for tapering to avoid symptoms from rapid discontinuation (such as nausea, headache, and sensory changes), which may increase the risk of clinical deterioration unless one starts the new medication before the taper of the previous medication is complete. Drug–drug interactions are a consideration when switching from irreversible MAOIs to most other agents, and that switch requires a minimum 2-week period off the MAOI to allow enough new MAO to be synthesized. Perhaps surprisingly, even switching to another antidepressant from the same pharmacological class is an option, because nonresponders to one SSRI have a 40–70% chance of responding to a second SSRI (Thase *et al.* 1997).

A third option is to combine two antidepressants from different classes with complementary mechanisms of action (Blier *et al.* 2010), and the remission

rate on fluoxetine alone (25% in this study) was about half that observed on a combination of fluoxetine with mirtazapine (52%), or venlafaxine with mirtazapine (58%), or buproprion and mirtazapine (46%). Combinations of medications have been compared in few studies, but these results make the case for further evaluation and the STAR*D study found patients were willing to choose such combinations in the hope of better clinical outcomes (Rush, 2007). Combinations of medications require more vigilance regarding drug–drug interactions and new side effects, and mean higher medication cost. Irreversible MAOIs should not be combined with most antidepressants, but when used in combinations require careful monitoring to avoid drug–drug interactions such as a serotonin syndrome or a hypertensive reaction.

Adjunctive and augmenting treatment

Adjunctive treatment is an additional treatment for some specific symptom or component of symptoms such as medication for insomnia or anxiety. An augmenting treatment is an additional treatment for the core depression, including accelerating response to antidepressants.

Adjunctive treatment may improve compliance with treatment and is most commonly used to control anxiety or treat insomnia. For anxiety the short-term use of benzodiazepines or the use of antidepressants with an antianxiety effect can be helpful. Benzodiazepines should be restricted to the short-term treatment of free-floating or generalized anxiety, relief of severe panic attacks, and co-morbid PTSD. SSRIs are the first-line treatment for anxiety related to panic attacks, PTSD, or obsessive complusive symptoms, which can be part of the depressive picture, but they take time to work. Short-term use of benzodiazepines can be used for rapid symptom relief from distressing anxiety, panic attacks, or PTSD until such time as SSRIs begin to work. Other options for anxious depression are antiepileptic drugs that have debatable antidepressant effect, like lamotrigine, but in general there is little good evidence for efficacy for either the anxiety or the depression. For insomnia, a good choice is trazodone in a dose of 50–300 mg. It has some antidepressant effect, but is quite sedating. At the same time it has a short half-life of about 3–4 hours so many patients sleep well without lingering fatigue or sedation in the morning. It also promotes sleep with less disruption to the sleep architecture and is not prone to tolerance or dependency. Other options are new-generation hypnotics used for a short course until the insomnia improves as the depression remits. Note that benzodiazepines lack antidepressant efficacy, and are an adjunctive treatment option for insomnia. They are probably overused because 30–60% of depressed patients receive tranquillizers concomitantly with antidepressant agents (Furukawa *et al.* 2001) for anxiety, agitation, and insomnia. Nevertheless, it is reported that combination antidepressant–benzodiazepine treatment may improve response and reduces treatment discontinuation when compared with antidepressant alone (Furukawa *et al.* 2001). Benzodiazepines have disadvantages because they cause psychomotor slowing, memory impairment, and carry the risk of dependence. There is an increased risk of falls, fractures, traffic accidents, and mortality in the elderly (Hemmelgarn *et al.* 1997, Vinkers *et al.* 2003). In addition, some clinicians believe that chronic use of high-dose benzodiazepines may result in treatment-resistant depression. A history of current alcohol or drug abuse/dependency is a contraindication to the use of benzodiazepines. Modafinil, like other stimulants, can alleviate residual sleepiness and fatigue, though controlled trials have not shown an augmented antidepressant response on mood (Fava *et al.* 2003, Demyttenaere *et al.* 2005).

Patients with sub-clinical hypothyroidism should receive thyroxine, but otherwise the use of thyroxine is of uncertain value. See Chapter 18 for the role of nutritional supplements such as fish oil as a source of omega-3 fatty acids with possible antidepressant properties, but in general vitamin B12, folic acid, iron, etc. work only when there is some evidence of a deficiency.

Psychotic depression

See Chapter 6 for details. Mood disorders with delusions and/or hallucinations require treatment with an antidepressant–antipsychotic combination rather than either class of medication alone, or with ECT (Spiker *et al.* 1985, Rothschild *et al.* 1993). Treatment of this more severe form of depression that carries an elevated risk of suicide, generally requires inpatient care and some will require electroconvulsive therapy.

Continuation treatment phase

The continuation phase of treatment generally lasts 6–9 months and is the time to eliminate residual symptoms, restore prior levels of occupational and social functioning, and prevent recurrence or early relapse. Residual symptoms indicate partial remission and predict recurrence or early relapse (Paykel *et al.* 1995) or a more chronic course (Judd *et al.* 2000). Treatment should continue to be adjusted until remission is achieved or all options exhausted. A history of episodes lasting more than 6 months require longer continuation treatment of up to 12 months, and generally continuation treatment will be longer for psychotic depression (Rush and Kupfer, 2001). The medications and doses used to achieve relief in the acute phase should be continued in the continuation phase of therapy (Thase, 1999, American Psychiatric Association, 2000). There is no evidence that supports tapering the dose of antidepressants in the transition from the acute treatment phase to the continuation treatment phase. The rule of thumb is that whatever got the patient better is what is needed to keep them better.

Treatment discontinuation

If there is no recurrence or relapse during continuation therapy, gradual medication discontinuation may be undertaken after at least 6 months of treatment. Earlier discontinuation is associated with a 77% higher risk of relapse compared with continuation treatment (Melfi *et al.* 1998). At that point in time a medication taper over a couple of weeks permits detection of emerging or returning symptoms. A return of symptoms should lead to reinstitution of a full medication dose for another 3–6 months (Bauer *et al.* 2002). A medication taper minimizes a discontinuation syndrome that otherwise may last days or longer, involving physical symptoms of imbalance, gastrointestinal and flu-like symptoms, sensory and sleep disturbances, and psychological symptoms such as anxiety and/or agitation, crying spells, and irritability (Schatzberg *et al.* 1997). The discontinuation syndrome is sometimes called a withdrawal syndrome, erroneously implying drug dependence.

Maintenance treatment phase

The goal of maintenance therapy is to prevent future episodes of depression. Maintenance treatment for 12–36 months reduces risk of recurrence by two-thirds (Geddes *et al.* 2003). It is indicated for patients who have a high risk of recurrence such as episodes occurring roughly yearly, patients who have impairment due to sub-syndromal residual symptoms, chronicity of major depression or dysthymia, and so without treatment remain symptomatic and impaired, or patients whose episodes are extremely severe and have high risk of suicide (Keller *et al.* 1986, American Psychiatric Association, 2000, Judd *et al.* 2000, Bauer *et al.* 2002). Duration of such maintenance treatment may be indefinite, given that the natural history of the illness does not lead to remission with aging, and if anything depressive episodes that last longer.

The maintenance phase begins with continuing the antidepressant or combination of mediations used in the continuation phase (American Psychiatric Association, 2000). While adjunctive medications such as for sleep may be discontinued once remission or a good response is attained, in general the medications that have worked during the continuation phase are used in the same doses in the maintenance phase. Sometimes patients will relapse during maintenance treatment and the cause may be that the dose was too low, or they have started a drug that counteracts the antidepressant such as a beta-blocker. Others have developed a medical illness that affects the brain or interferes with drug action, are abusing alcohol, or have another drug–drug interaction that affects availability of the antidepressant. Sometimes recurrences are caused by seasonal effects and require raising the dose or adding a light box to the treatment plan during fall and winter. Some patients are sensitive to time-zone changes and consistently relapse after long flights. Treatment of such patients requires careful attention to the specifics of their biological clock vulnerabilities, discussed in more detail by Terman in Chapter 26.

In terms of medication choice for maintenance treatment, the first requirement is to use a medication or combination that has worked for that patient in acute treatment. The second requirement is to optimize acceptability of the treatment by minimizing side effects and frequency of dosing so that taking the medication is as simple and tolerable as possible. Side effects that may be acceptable to the patient in the short term because they are so pleased that the depression is improved, become intolerable when the depression is absent. An example are the sexual side effects of SSRIs. The longer the patient is feeling well the less acceptable it is to have sexual dysfunction. Switching to or augmenting with buproprion or a phosphodiesterase inhibitor like sildenafil, dose reduction, and brief drug breaks, for example for an occasional weekend, may relieve sexual dysfuncion (Rothschild, 2000). In terms of medication options for maintenance treatment, lithium has no advantage over antidepressants in prophylaxis (De Souza *et al.* 1991), but may reduce suicide risk independently of its effect on mood (Thies-Flechtner *et al.* 1996). TCAs, SSRIs, MAOIs, bupropion, and the newer antidepressants, nefazadone, mirtazapine, and venlafaxine, all prevent recurrence (De Souza *et al.* 1991, Thies-Flechtner *et al.* 1996, Montgomery *et al.* 1998, Bauer *et al.* 2002, Simon *et al.* 2004). Doctor visits during the maintenance phase should take place at 3–6 month intervals in stable patients. As in other phases, adherence should be monitored and breakthrough symptoms detected early. Patient and family education reduces treatment attrition and improves outcome (Rush, 1999).

Summary

Antidepressant and adjunctive pharmacological agents allow successful acute treatment and prevention of future episodes of major depression in most patients (Serretti *et al.* 2004). There is a need for new treatments which may work faster and one day remove the need for continuation and maintenance treatment. Until that time, the clinician must optimize the clinical response during both the acute and continuation phases of treatment, the goal being remission, and then minimize side effects and sustain remission in the sub-group of patients who require maintenance treatment.

References

Adli, M., Baethge, C., Heinz, A., Langlitz, N., and Bauer, M. (2005). Is dose escalation of antidepressants a rational strategy after a medium-dose treatment has failed? A systematic review. *European Archives of Psychiatry and Clinical Neuroscience*, 255, 387–400.

Adli, M., Berghofer, A., Linden, M. *et al.* (2002). Effectiveness and feasibility of a standardized stepwise drug treatment regimen algorithm for inpatients with depressive disorders: Results of a 2-year observational algorithm study. *Journal of Clinical Psychiatry*, 63, 782–790.

Agid, O. and Lerer, B. (2003). Algorithm-based treatment of major depression in an outpatient clinic: Clinical correlates of response to a specific serotonin reuptake inhibitor and to triiodothyronine augmentation. *International Journal of Neuropsychopharmacology*, 6, 41–49.

American Psychiatric Association (1993). *Practice Guideline for Major Depressive Disorder in Adults, First Edition*. Washington, DC: American Psychiatric Association.

American Psychiatric Association (1994). *Diagnostic and Statistical Manual for Mental Disorders, DSM-IV, Fourth Edition*. Washington, DC: American Psychiatric Association.

American Psychiatric Association (2000). Practice guideline for the treatment of patients with major depressive disorder (revision). *American Journal of Psychiatry*, 157 Suppl, 1–45.

Amsterdam, J.D., Maislin, G., and Potter, L. (1994). Fluoxetine efficacy in treatment resistant depression. *Progress In Neuropsychopharmacology and Biological Psychiatry*, 18, 243–261.

Anderson, I.M. (2000). Selective serotonin reuptake inhibitors versus tricyclic antidepressants: A meta-analysis of efficacy and tolerability. *Journal of Affective Disorders*, 58, 19–36.

Anderson, I.M. (2001). Meta-analytical studies on new antidepressants. *British Medical Bulletin*, 57, 161–178.

Baldassano, C.F., Ballas, C.A., and O'Reardon, J.P. (2004). Rethinking the treatment paradigm for bipolar depression: the importance of long-term management. *CNS Spectrums*, 9 Suppl 9, 11–18.

Barbosa, L., Berk, M., and Vorster, M. (2003). A double-blind, randomized, placebo-controlled trial of augmentation with lamotrigine or placebo in patients concomitantly treated with fluoxetine for resistant major depressive episodes. *Journal of Clinical Psychiatry*, 64, 403–407.

Bauer, M., Whybrow, P.C., Angst, J., Versiani, M., and Moller, H.J. (2002). World Federation of Societies of Biological Psychiatry (WFSBP) Guidelines for Biological Treatment of Unipolar Depressive Disorders, Part 1: Acute and continuation treatment of major depressive disorder. *World Journal of Biological Psychiatry*, 3, 5–43.

Bauer, M., Forsthoff, A., Baethge, C. *et al.* (2003). Lithium augmentation therapy in refractory depression-update 2002. *European Archives of Psychiatry and Clinical Neuroscience*, 253, 132–139.

Bauer, M.S. and Whybrow, P.C. (1990). Rapid cycling bipolar affective disorder. II. Treatment of refractory rapid cycling with high-dose levothyroxine: A preliminary study. *Archives of General Psychiatry*, 47, 435–440.

Bebbington, P. and Ramana, R. (1995). The epidemiology of bipolar affective disorder. *Social Psychiatry and Psychiatric Epidemiology*, 30, 279–292.

Benkert, O., Muller, M., and Szegedi, A. (2002). An overview of the clinical efficacy of mirtazapine. *Human Psychopharmacology*, 17 Suppl 1, S23–S26.

Benkert, O., Szegedi, A., Wetzel, H. *et al.* (1997). Dose escalation vs. continued doses of paroxetine and maprotiline: A prospective study in depressed out-patients with inadequate treatment response. *Acta Psychiatrica Scandinavica*, 95, 288–296.

Blier, P., Gobbi, G., Turcotte, J.E. *et al.* (2009). Mirtazapine and paroxetine in major depression: A comparison of monotherapy versus their combination from treatment initiation. *European Neuropsychopharmacology*, 19, 457–465.

Blier, P., Ward, H.E., Tremblay, P. *et al.* (2010). Combination of antidepressant medications from treatment initiation for major depressive disorder: A double-blind randomized study. *American Journal of Psychiatry*, 167, 281–288.

Boldrini, M., Underwood, M.D., Hen, R. *et al.* (2009). Antidepressants increase neural progenitor cells in the human hippocampus. *Neuropsychopharmacology*, 34, 2376–2389.

Boyce, P. and Judd, F. (1999). The place for the tricyclic antidepressants in the treatment of depression. *Australian and New Zealand Journal of Psychiatry*, 33, 323–327.

Brannan, S.K., Mallinckrodt, C.H., Brown, E.B. *et al.* (2005). Duloxetine 60 mg once-daily in the treatment of painful physical symptoms in patients with major depressive disorder. *Journal of Psychiatric Research*, 39, 43–53.

Brent, D.A., Oquendo, M.A., Birmaher, B. *et al.* (2002). Familial pathways to early-onset suicide attempt: Risk for suicidal behavior in offspring of mood-disordered suicide attempters. *Archives of General Psychiatry*, 59, 801–807.

Brent, D.A., Oquendo, M., Birmaher, B. *et al.* (2004). Familial transmission of mood disorders: Convergence and divergence with transmission of suicidal behavior. *Journal of the American Academy of Child and Adolescent Psychiatry*, 43, 1259–1266.

Briley, M. (2004). Clinical experience with dual action antidepressants in different chronic pain syndromes. *Human Psychopharmacology*, 19 Suppl 1, S21–S25.

Caspi, A., Sugden, K., Moffitt, T.E. *et al.* (2003). Influence of life stress on depression: Moderation by a polymorphism in the 5-HTT gene. *Science*, 301, 386–389.

Charney, D.S. and Manji, H.K. (2004). Life stress, genes, and depression: Multiple pathways lead to increased risk and new opportunities for intervention. *Science's STKE.*, 2004, no. 225, re5.

Charney, D.S., Berman, R., and Miller, H.L. (1998). Treatment of depression. In Schatzberg, A.F. and Nemeroff, C.B., eds., *Textbook of Psycopharmacology*. Washington, DC: American Psychiatric Press, 705–731.

Cohen, D. (2004). Atypical antipsychotics and new onset diabetes mellitus: An overview of the literature. *Pharmacopsychiatry*, 37, 1–11.

Coyne, J.C., Fechner-Bates, S., and Schwenk, T.L. (1994). Prevalence, nature, and comorbidity of depressive disorders in primary care. *General Hospital Psychiatry*, 16, 267–276.

DeBattista, C., Solvason, H.B., Poirier, J., Kendrick, E., and Schatzberg, A.F. (2003). A prospective trial of bupropion SR augmentation of partial and non-responders to serotonergic antidepressants. *Journal of Clinical Psychopharmacology*, 23, 27–30.

de Montigny, C. (1994). Lithium addition in treatment-resistant depression. *International Clinical Psychopharmacology*, 9 Suppl 2, 31–35.

Demyttenaere, K., De, F.J., and Stahl, S.M. (2005). The many faces of fatigue in major depressive disorder. *International Journal of Neuropsychopharmacology*, 8, 93–105.

DeRubeis, R.J., Hollon, S.D., Amsterdam, J.D. *et al.* (2005). Cognitive therapy vs medications in the treatment of moderate to severe depression. *Archives of General Psychiatry*, 62, 409–416.

De Souza, E.B., Zaczek, R., Culp, S., Appel, N.M., and Contrera, J.F. (1991). Comparison of the effects of repeated oral versus subcutaneous fenfluramine administration on rat brain monoamine neurons: Pharmacokinetic and dose-response data. *Pharmacology, Biochemistry and Behavior*, 39, 963–969.

Detke, M.J., Wiltse, C.G., Mallinckrodt, C.H. *et al.* (2004). Duloxetine in the acute and long-term treatment of major depressive disorder: A placebo- and paroxetine-controlled trial. *European Neuropsychopharmacology*, 14, 457–470.

Duman, R.S., Li, N., Liu, R.J., Duric, V., and Aghajanian, G. (2012). Signaling pathways underlying the rapid antidepressant actions of ketamine. *Neuropharmacology*, 62, 35–41.

Elkin, I., Gibbons, R.D., Shea, M.T. *et al.* (1995). Initial severity and differential treatment outcome in the National Institute of Mental Health Treatment of Depression Collaborative Research Program. *Journal of Consulting and Clinical Psychology*, 63, 841–847.

Fava, M., Papakostas, G.I., Petersen, T. *et al.* (2003). Switching to bupropion in fluoxetine-resistant major depressive disorder. *Annals of Clinical Psychiatry*, 15, 17–22.

Feiger, A., Kiev, A., Shrivastava, R.K., Wisselink, P.G., and Wilcox, C.S. (1996). Nefazodone versus sertraline in outpatients with major depression: Focus on efficacy, tolerability, and effects on sexual function and satisfaction. *Journal of Clinical Psychiatry*, 57 Suppl 2, 53–62.

Furukawa, T.A., Streiner, D.L., and Young, L.T. (2001). Is antidepressant-benzodiazepine combination therapy clinically more useful? A meta-analytic study. *Journal of Affective Disorders*, 65, 173–177.

Geddes, J. (1999). Suicide and homicide by people with mental illness. *British Medical Journal*, 318, 1225–1226.

Geddes, J.R., Freemantle, N., Mason, J., Eccles, M.P., and Boynton, J. (2000). SSRIs versus other antidepressants for depressive disorder. *Cochrane Database of Systematic Reviews*, 2, CD001851.

Geddes, J.R., Carney, S.M., Davies, C. *et al.* (2003). Relapse prevention with antidepressant drug treatment in depressive disorders: A systematic review. *Lancet*, 361, 653–661.

Gibbons, R.D., Hur, K., Brown, C.H., Davis, J.M., and Mann, J.J. (2012). Benefits from antidepressants: synthesis of 6-week patient-level outcomes from double-blind placebo-controlled randomized trials of fluoxetine and venlafaxine. *Archives of General Psychiatry*, 69, 572–579.

Gijsman, H.J., Geddes, J.R., Rendell, J.M., Nolen, W.A., and Goodwin, G.M. (2004). Antidepressants for bipolar depression: a systematic review of randomized, controlled trials. *American Journal of Psychiatry*, 161, 1537–1547.

Gingrich, J.A. and Hen, R. (2001). Dissecting the role of the serotonin system in neuropsychiatric disorders using knockout mice. *Psychopharmacology (Berlin)*, 155, 1–10.

Goldman, L.S., Nielsen, N.H., and Champion, H.C. (1999). Awareness, diagnosis, and treatment of depression. *Journal of General Internal Medicine*, 14, 569–580.

Goldstein, D.J., Lu, Y., Detke, M.J. *et al.* (2004). Duloxetine in the treatment of depression: A double-blind placebo-controlled comparison with paroxetine. *Journal of Clinical Psychopharmacology*, 24, 389–399.

Greco, T., Eckert, G., and Kroenke, K. (2004). The outcome of physical symptoms with treatment of depression. *Journal of General Internal Medicine*, 19, 813–818.

Grunebaum, M.F., Ellis, S.P., Duan, N. *et al.* (2012). Pilot randomized clinical trial of an SSRI vs bupropion: Effects on suicidal behavior, ideation, and mood in major depression. *Neuropsychopharmacology*, 37, 697–706.

Guelfi, J.D., Ansseau, M., Timmerman, L., and Korsgaard, S. (2001). Mirtazapine versus venlafaxine in hospitalized severely depressed patients with melancholic features. *Journal of Clinical Psychopharmacology*, 21, 425–431.

Hariri, A.R., Drabant, E.M., Munoz, K.E. *et al.* (2005). A susceptibility gene for affective disorders and the response of the human amygdale. *Archives of General Psychiatry*, 62, 146–152.

Hawley, C.J., Pattinson, H.A., Quick, S.J. *et al.* (1998). A protocol for the pharmacologic treatment of major depression: A field test of a potential prototype. *Journal of Affective Disorders*, 47, 87–96.

Heim, C. and Nemeroff, C.B. (2001). The role of childhood trauma in the neurobiology of mood and anxiety disorders: Preclinical and clinical studies. *Biological Psychiatry*, 49 (12) 1023–1039.

Heim, C., Newport, D.J., Bonsall, R., Miller, A.H., and Nemeroff, C.B. (2001). Altered pituitary-adrenal axis responses to provocative challenge tests in adult survivors of childhood abuse. *American Journal of Psychiatry*, 158, 575–581.

Hemmelgarn, B., Suissa, S., Huang, A., Boivin, J.F., and Pinard, G. (1997). Benzodiazepine use and the risk of motor vehicle crash in the elderly. *Journal of the American Medical Association*, 278, 27–31.

Hirschfeld, R.M. (1999). Efficacy of SSRIs and newer antidepressants in severe depression: Comparison with TCAs. *Journal of Clinical Psychiatry*, 60, 326–335.

Hirschfeld, R.M. and Vornik, L.A. (2004). Newer antidepressants: Review of efficacy and safety of escitalopram and duloxetine. *Journal of Clinical Psychiatry*, 65 Suppl 4, 46–52.

Hirschfeld, R.M.A., Keller, M., Panico, S. *et al.* (1997). The national depressive and manic-depressive association consensus statement on the undertreatment of depression. *Journal of the American Medical Association*, 277, 333–340.

Ichise, M., Vines, D.C., Gura, T. *et al.* (2006). Effects of early life stress on [11C]DASB positron emission tomography imaging of serotonin transporters in adolescent peer- and mother-reared rhesus monkeys. *Journal of Neuroscience*, 26, 4638–4643.

Judd, L.L., Paulus, M.J., Schettler, P.J. *et al.* (2000). Does incomplete recovery from first lifetime major depressive episode herald a chronic course of illness? *American Journal of Psychiatry*, 157, 1501–1504.

Kasper, S. (1997). Efficacy of antidepressants in the treatment of severe depression: The place of mirtazapine. *Journal of Clinical Psychopharmacology*, 17 Suppl 1, 19S–28S.

Katon, W., Von, K.M., Lin, E., Bush, T., and Ormel, J. (1992). Adequacy and duration of antidepressant treatment in primary care. *Medical Care*, 30, 67–76.

Kaufman, J., Plotsky, P.M., Nemeroff, C.B., and Charney, D.S. (2000). Effects of early adverse experiences on brain structure and function: Clinical implications. *Biological Psychiatry*, 48, 778–790.

Keller, M.B. (1989). Current concepts in affective disorders. *Journal of Clinical Psychiatry*, 50, 157–162.

Keller, M.B., Lavori, P.W., Rice, J., Coryell, W., and Hirschfeld, R.M. (1986). The persistent risk of chronicity in recurrent episodes of nonbipolar major depressive disorder: A prospective follow-up. *American Journal of Psychiatry*, 143, 24–28.

Kendler, K.S. and Karkowski-Shuman, L. (1997). Stressful life events and genetic liability to major depression: Genetic control of exposure to the environment? *Psychological Medicine*, 27, 539–547.

Kendler, K.S., Davis, C.G., and Kessler, R.C. (1997). The familial aggregation of common psychiatric and substance use disorders in the National Comorbidity Survey: A family history study. *British Journal of Psychiatry*, 170, 541–548.

Kendler, K.S., Gatz, M., Gardner, C.O., and Pedersen, N.L. (2006). A Swedish national twin study of lifetime major depression. *American Journal of Psychiatry*, 163, 109–114.

Kennedy, S.H., Andersen, H.F., and Lam, R.W. (2006). Efficacy of escitalopram in the treatment of major depressive disorder compared with conventional selective serotonin reuptake inhibitors and venlafaxine

XR: a meta-analysis. *Journal of Psychiatry and Neuroscience*, 31, 122–131.

Kroenke, K., Spitzer, R.L., Williams, J.B. *et al.* (1994). Physical symptoms in primary care: Predictors of psychiatric disorders and functional impairment. *Archives of Family Medicine*, 3, 774–779.

Kroenke, K., West, S.L., Swindle, R. *et al.* (2001). Similar effectiveness of paroxetine, fluoxetine, and sertraline in primary care: a randomized trial. *Journal of the American Medical Association*, 286, 2947–2955.

Kupfer, D.J., Frank, E., and Perel, J.M. (1989). The advantage of early treatment intervention in recurrent depression. *Archives of General Psychiatry*, 46, 771–775.

MacGillivray, S., Arroll, B., Hatcher, S. *et al.* (2003). Efficacy and tolerability of selective serotonin reuptake inhibitors compared with tricyclic antidepressants in depression treated in primary care: systematic review and meta-analysis. *BMJ*, 326, 1014.

MacQueen, G.M., Yucel, K., Taylor, V.H., Macdonald, K., and Joffe, R. (2008). Posterior hippocampal volumes are associated with remission rates in patients with major depressive disorder. *Biological Psychiatry*, 64, 880–883.

Major Depressive Disorder Working Group of the Psychiatric GWAS Consortium (2012). A mega-analysis of genome-wide association studies for major depressive disorder. *Molecuar Psychiatry*, e-pub ahead of print, doi: 10.1038/mp.2012.21.

Mann, J.J. (2005). The medical management of depression. *New England Journal of Medicine*, 353, 1819–1834.

Mann, J.J. and Currier, D. (2006a). Effects of genes and stress on the neurobiology of depression. *International Review of Neurobiology*, 73, 153–189.

Mann, J.J. and Currier, D. (2006b). Understanding and preventing suicide. In Stein, D.J., Kupfer, D.J., and Schatzberg, A.F., eds., *Amercan Psychiatric Publishing Textbook of Mood Disorders, First Edition*, Arlington, VA: American Psychiatric Publishing, 485–496.

Mann, J.J. and Currier, D. (2007). Prevention of suicide. *Psychiatric Annals*, 35, 331–339.

Mann, J.J., Georgotas, A., Newton, R., and Gershon, S. (1981). A controlled study of trazodone, imipramine, and placebo in outpatients with endogenous depression. *Journal of Clinical Psychopharmacology*, 1, 75–80.

Mann, J.J., Currier, D., Quiroz, J., and Manji, H.K. (2005). Neurobiology of severe mood and anxiety disorders. In Siegel, G.J., Albers, R.W., Brady, S., and Price, D., eds., *Basic Neurochemistry, Seventh Edition*. San Diego, CA: Elsevier.

March, J., Silva, S., Petrycki, S. *et al.* (2004). Fluoxetine, cognitive-behavioral therapy, and their combination for adolescents with depression: Treatment for Adolescents With Depression Study (TADS) randomized controlled

trial. *Journal of the American Medical Association*, 292, 807–820.

Masan, P.S. (2004). Atypical antipsychotics in the treatment of affective symptoms: A review. *Annals of Clinical Psychiatry*, 16, 3–13.

Mayberg, H.S. (1997). Limbic-cortical dysregulation: A proposed model of depression. *Joural of Neuropsychiatry and Clinical Neuroscience*, 9, 471–481.

McGowan, P.O., Sasaki, A., D'Alessio, A.C. *et al.* (2009). Epigenetic regulation of the glucocorticoid receptor in human brain associates with childhood abuse. *Nature Neuroscience*, 12, 342–348.

McGrath, P.J., Stewart, J.W., Fava, M. *et al.* (2006). Tranylcypromine versus venlafaxine plus mirtazapine following three failed antidepressant medication trials for depression: A STAR*D report. *American Journal of Psychiatry*, 163, 1531–1541.

Melfi, C.A., Chawla, A.J., Croghan, T.W. *et al.* (1998). The effects of adherence to antidepressant treatment guidelines on relapse and recurrence of depression. *Archives of General Psychiatry*, 55, 1128–1132.

Milak, M.S., Parsey, R.V., Keilp, J. *et al.* (2005). Neuroanatomic correlates of psychopathologic components of major depressive disorder. *Archives of General Psychiatry*, 62, 397–408.

Miller, J.M., Oquendo, M.A., Ogden, R.T., Mann, J.J., and Parsey, R.V. (2008). Serotonin transporter binding as a possible predictor of one-year remission in major depressive disorder. *Journal of Psychiatric Research*, 42, 1137–1144.

Miller, J.M., Brennan, K.G., Ogden, T.R. *et al.* (2009a). Elevated serotonin 1A binding in remitted major depressive disorder: Evidence for a trait biological abnormality. *Neuropsychopharmacology*, 34, 2275–2284.

Miller, J.M., Kinnally, E.L., Ogden, R.T. *et al.* (2009b). Reported childhood abuse is associated with low serotonin transporter binding in vivo in major depressive disorder. *Synapse*, 63, 565–573.

Montejo, A.L., Llorca, G., Izquierdo, J. A., and Rico-Villademoros, F. (2001). Incidence of sexual dysfunction associated with antidepressant agents: A prospective multicenter study of 1022 outpatients. Spanish Working Group for the Study of Psychotropic-Related Sexual Dysfunction. *Journal of Clinical Psychiatry*, 62 Suppl 3, 10–21.

Montgomery, S.A., Reimitz, P.E., and Zivkov, M. (1998). Mirtazapine versus amitriptyline in the long-term treatment of depression: A double-blind placebo-controlled study. *International Clinical Psychopharmacology*, 13, 63–73.

Mueller, T.I., Leon, A.C., Keller, M.B. *et al.* (1999). Recurrence after recovery from major depressive disorder during 15 years of observational follow-up. *American Journal of Psychiatry*, 156, 1000–1006.

Mulder, R.T., Watkins, W.G., Joyce, P.R., and Luty, S.E. (2003). Age may affect response to antidepressants with serotonergic and noradrenergic actions. *Journal of Affective Disorders*, 76, 143–149.

Mulrow, C.D. (1999). *Treatment of Depression: Newer Pharmacotherapies*. Rockville, MD: Agency for Health Care Policy and Research.

Murray, C.J. and Lopez, A.D. (1997). Global mortality, disability, and the contribution of risk factors: Global Burden of Disease Study. *Lancet*, 349, 1436–1442.

Narrow, W.E., Rae, D.S., Robins, L.N., and Regier, D.A. (2002). Revised prevalence estimates of mental disorders in the United States: Using a clinical significance criterion to reconcile 2 surveys' estimates. *Archives of General Psychiatry*, 59, 115–123.

Nemeroff, C.B. and Owens, M.J. (2004). Pharmacologic differences among the SSRIs: Focus on monoamine transporters and the HPA axis. *CNS Spectrums*, 9 Suppl 4, 23–31.

Nieuwstraten, C.E. and Dolovich, L.R. (2001). Bupropion versus selective serotonin-reuptake inhibitors for treatment of depression. *Annals of Pharmacotherapy*, 35, 1608–1613.

Nolen, W.A., Haffmans, P.M., Bouvy, P.F., and Duivenvoorden, H.J. (1993). Monoamine oxidase inhibitors in resistant major depression: A double-blind comparison of brofaromine and tranylcypromine in patients resistant to tricyclic antidepressants. *Journal of Affective Disorders*, 28, 189–197.

Normann, C., Hummel, B., Scharer, L.O. *et al.* (2002). Lamotrigine as adjunct to paroxetine in acute depression: A placebo-controlled, double-blind study. *Journal of Clinical Psychiatry*, 63, 337–344.

Olver, J.S., Burrows, G.D., and Norman, T.R. (2001). Third-generation antidepressants: Do they offer advantages over the SSRIs? *CNS Drugs*, 15, 941–954.

Oquendo, M.A., Barrera, A., Ellis, S.P. *et al.* (2004). Instability of symptoms in recurrent major depression: A prospective study. *American Journal of Psychiatry*, 161, 255–261.

Papakostas, G.I., Fava, M., and Thase, M.E. (2008). Treatment of SSRI-resistant depression: A meta-analysis comparing within- versus across-class switches. *Biological Psychiatry*, 63, 699–704.

Parsey, R.V., Hastings, R.S., Oquendo, M.A. *et al.* (2006). Lower serotonin transporter binding potential in the human brain during major depressive episodes. *American Journal of Psychiatry*, 163, 52–58.

Paykel, E.S., Ramana, R., Cooper, Z. *et al.* (1995). Residual symptoms after partial remission: An important outcome in depression. *Psychological Medicine*, 25, 1171–1180.

Peet, M. (1994). Induction of mania with selective serotonin re-uptake inhibitors and tricyclic antidepressants. *British Journal of Psychiatry*, 164, 549–550.

Pence, B.W., O'Donnell, J.K., and Gaynes, B.N. (2012). The depression treatment cascade in primary care: A public health perspective. *Current Psychiatry Reports*, 14, 328–335.

Peretti, S., Judge, R., and Hindmarch, I. (2000). Safety and tolerability considerations: Tricyclic antidepressants vs. selective serotonin reuptake inhibitors. *Acta Psychiatrica Scandinavica Supplementum*, 403, 17–25.

Pezawas, L., Meyer-Lindenberg, A., Drabant, E.M. *et al.* (2005). 5-HTTLPR polymorphism impacts human cingulate-amygdala interactions: A genetic susceptibility mechanism for depression. *Nature Neuroscience*, 8, 828–834.

Quitkin, F.M., Stewart, J.W., McGrath, P.J. *et al.* (1993). Columbia atypical depression: A subgroup of depressives with better response to MAOI than to tricyclic antidepressants or placebo. *British Journal of Psychiatry Supplement*, 21, 30–34.

Risch, N., Herrell, R., Lehner, T. *et al.* (2009). Interaction between the serotonin transporter gene (5-HTTLPR), stressful life events, and risk of depression: A meta-analysis. *Journal of the American Medical Association*, 301, 2462–2471.

Rosenbaum, J.F. (1998). Depression and its subtypes: A treatment update. Conclusion. *Journal of Clinical Psychiatry*, 59 Suppl 18, 37–38.

Rothschild, A.J. (2000). Sexual side effects of antidepressants. *Journal of Clinical Psychiatry*, 61 Suppl 11, 28–36.

Rothschild, A.J., Samson, J.A., Bessette, M.P., and Carter-Campbell, J.T. (1993). Efficacy of the combination of fluoxetine and perphenazine in the treatment of psychotic depression. *Journal of Clinical Psychiatry*, 54, 338–342.

Rothschild, A.J., Williamson, D.J., Tohen, M.F. *et al.* (2004). A double-blind, randomized study of olanzapine and olanzapine/fluoxetine combination for major depression with psychotic features. *Journal of Clinical Psychopharmacology*, 24, 365–373.

Rowbotham, M.C., Goli, V., Kunz, N.R., and Lei, D. (2004). Venlafaxine extended release in the treatment of painful diabetic neuropathy: A double-blind, placebo-controlled study. *Pain*, 110, 697–706.

Rudolph, R.L. (2002). Achieving remission from depression with venlafaxine and venlafaxine extended release: A literature review of comparative studies with selective serotonin reuptake inhibitors. *Acta Psychiatrica Scandinavica Supplementum*, 415, 24–30.

Rush, A.J. (1999). Strategies and tactics in the management of maintenance treatment for depressed patients. *Journal of Clinical Psychiatry*, 60 Suppl 14, 21–26.

Rush, A.J. (2007). STAR*D: What have we learned? *American Journal of Psychiatry*, 164, 201–204.

Rush, A.J. and Kupfer, D.J. (2001). Strategies and tactics in the treatment of depression. In Gabbard, G.O., ed., *Treatment of Psychiatric Disorders*. Washington, DC: American Psychiatric Publishing, 1417–1439.

Rush, A.J., Armitage, R., Gillin, J.C. *et al.* (1998). Comparative effects of nefazodone and fluoxetine on sleep in outpatients with major depressive disorder. *Biological Psychiatry*, 44, 3–14.

Sanger, D.J. (2004). The search for novel antipsychotics: Pharmacological and molecular targets. *Expert Opinion on Therapeutic Targets*, 8, 631–641.

Schatzberg, A.F., Haddad, P., Kaplan, E.M. *et al.* (1997). Serotonin reuptake inhibitor discontinuation syndrome: A hypothetical definition. *Journal of Clinical Psychiatry*, 58 Suppl 7, 5–10.

Serretti, A., Cusin, C., Rossini, D. *et al.* (2004). Further evidence of a combined effect of SERTPR and TPH on SSRIs response in mood disorders. *American Journal of Medical Genetics: B Neuropsychiatric Genetics*, 129B, 36–40.

Sheline, Y.I., Mittler, B.L., and Mintun, M.A. (2002). The hippocampus and depression. *European Psychiatry*, 17 Suppl 3, 300–305.

Simon, G.E., VonKorff, M., Heiligenstein, J.H. *et al.* (1996). Initial antidepressant choice in primary care: Effectiveness and cost of fluoxetine vs tricyclic antidepressants. *Journal of the American Medical Association*, 275, 1897–1902.

Simon, J.S., Aguiar, L.M., Kunz, N.R., and Lei, D. (2004). Extended-release venlafaxine in relapse prevention for patients with major depressive disorder. *Journal of Psychiatric Research*, 38, 249–257.

Smith, D., Dempster, C., Glanville, J., Freemantle, N., and Anderson, I. (2002). Efficacy and tolerability of venlafaxine compared with selective serotonin reuptake inhibitors and other antidepressants: A meta-analysis. *British Journal of Psychiatry*, 180, 396–404.

Soares, J.C. and Mann, J.J. (1997a). The anatomy of mood disorders: Review of structural neuroimaging studies. *Biological Psychiatry*, 41, 86–106.

Soares, J.C. and Mann, J.J. (1997b). The functional neuroanatomy of mood disorders. *Journal of Psychiatric Research*, 31, 393–432.

Spijker, J., de, G.R., Bijl, R.V., Beekman, A.T., Ormel, J., and Nolen, W.A. (2002). Duration of major depressive episodes in the general population: results from The Netherlands Mental Health Survey and Incidence Study (NEMESIS). *British Journal of Psychiatry*, 181, 208–213.

Spiker, D.G., Weiss, J.C., Dealy, R.S. *et al.* (1985). The pharmacological treatment of delusional depression. *American Journal of Psychiatry*, 142, 430–436.

Stahl, S.M. (2000). Placebo-controlled comparison of the selective serotonin reuptake inhibitors citalopram and sertraline. *Biological Psychiatry*, 48, 894–901.

Stahl, S.M. and Grady, M.M. (2003). Differences in mechanism of action between current and future antidepressants. *Journal of Clinical Psychiatry*, 64 Suppl 13, 13–17.

Stahl, S.M., Entsuah, R., and Rudolph, R.L. (2002). Comparative efficacy between venlafaxine and SSRIs: A pooled analysis of patients with depression. *Biological Psychiatry*, 52, 1166–1174.

Sullivan, P.F., Neale, M.C., and Kendler, K.S. (2000). Genetic epidemiology of major depression: Review and meta-analysis. *American Journal of Psychiatry*, 157, 1552–1562.

Swenson, J.R., O'Connor, C.M., Barton, D. *et al.* (2003). Influence of depression and effect of treatment with sertraline on quality of life after hospitalization for acute coronary syndrome. *American Journal of Cardiology*, 92, 1271–1276.

Thase, M.E. (1999). Redefining antidepressant efficacy toward long-term recovery. *Journal of Clinical Psychiatry*, 60 Suppl 6, 15–19.

Thase, M.E. and Rush, A.J. (1997). When at first you don't succeed: Sequential strategies for antidepressant nonresponders. *Journal of Clinical Psychiatry*, 58 Suppl 13, 23–29.

Thase, M.E., Trivedi, M.H., and Rush, A.J. (1995). MAOIs in the contemporary treatment of depression. *Neuropsychopharmacology*, 12, 185–219.

Thase, M.E., Entsuah, A.R., and Rudolph, R.L. (2001). Remission rates during treatment with venlafaxine or selective serotonin reuptake inhibitors. *British Journal of Psychiatry*, 178, 234–241.

Thase, M.E., Mallinger, A.G., McKnight, D., and Himmelhoch, J.M. (1992). Treatment of imipramine-resistant recurrent depression, IV: A double-blind crossover study of tranylcypromine for anergic bipolar depression. *American Journal of Psychiatry*, 149, 195–198.

Thies-Flechtner, K., Muller-Oerlinghausen, B., Seibert, W., Walther, A., and Greil, W. (1996). Effect of prophylactic treatment on suicide risk in patients with major affective disorders: Data from a randomized prospective trial. *Pharmacopsychiatry*, 29, 103–107.

Tran, P.V., Bymaster, F.P., McNamara, R.K., and Potter, W.Z. (2003). Dual monoamine modulation for improved treatment of major depressive disorder. *Journal of Clinical Psychopharmacology*, 23, 78–86.

Trivedi, M.H., Rush, A.J., Crismon, M.L. *et al.* (2004). Clinical results for patients with major depressive disorder in the Texas Medication Algorithm Project. *Archives of General Psychiatry*, 61, 669–680.

Trivedi, M.H., Rush, A.J., Wisniewski, S.R. *et al.* (2006). Evaluation of outcomes with citalopram for depression using measurement-based care in STAR*D: Implications for clinical practice. *American Journal of Psychiatry*, 163, 28–40.

Vinkers, D.J., Gussekloo, J., Van der Mast, R.C., Zitman, F.G., and Westendorp, R.G. (2003). Benzodiazepine use and risk of mortality in individuals aged 85 years or older. *Journal of the American Medical Association*, 290, 2942–2943.

Walsh, B.T., Seidman, S.N., Sysko, R., and Gould, M. (2002). Placebo response in studies of major depression: Variable, substantial, and growing. *Journal of the American Medical Association*, 287, 1840–1847.

Weissman, M.M. (2006). Recent advances in depression across the generations. *Epidemiologia e Psichiatria Sociale*, 15, 16–19.

Westenberg, H.G. (1999). Pharmacology of antidepressants: Selectivity or multiplicity? *Journal of Clinical Psychiatry*, 60 Suppl 17, 4–8.

Yatham, L.N., Calabrese, J.R., and Kusumakar, V. (2003). Bipolar depression: Criteria for treatment selection, definition of refractoriness, and treatment options. *Bipolar Disorders*, 5, 85–97.

Zisook, S., Rush, A.J., Albala, A. *et al.* (2004). Factors that differentiate early vs. later onset of major depression disorder. *Psychiatry Research*, 129, 127–140.

Zornberg, G.L. and Pope, H.G., Jr. (1993). Treatment of depression in bipolar disorder: New directions for research. *Journal of Clinical Psychopharmacology*, 13, 397–408.

Chapter 5

Atypical depression

Jonathan W. Stewart

Introduction

Depression with atypical features was added to the DSM-IV as a mood disorder specifier based on studies documenting its distinction from depression with melancholic features (Rabkin *et al.* 1996). In addition to the presence of a mood disorder (major depression, bipolar depression, or dysthymic disorder), DSM-IV criteria for "depression with atypical features" (see Table 5.1) require significant mood reactivity accompanied by two of four associated features, including significant degrees of hyperphagia or weight gain, hypersomnia, leaden paralysis, and pathologic rejection sensitivity. In addition, the patient cannot also meet criteria for melancholic or catatonic features.

Depression with atypical features is common, occurring in 0.7–2.7% of the general population (Horwath *et al.* 1992, Angst *et al.* 2002) and 17–36% of depressed outpatients (McGinn *et al.* 1996, Nierenberg *et al.* 1998, Posternak and Zimmerman, 2001, Novick *et al.* 2005). Most studies show it often has an early onset (Horwath *et al.* 1992, Stewart *et al.* 1993, Benazzi, 1999, Angst *et al.* 2002, Matza *et al.* 2003), and a chronic course (Stewart *et al.* 1993, McGinn *et al.* 1996, Benazzi, 1999, Angst *et al.* 2002). It is disabling, depressed patients with atypical features being more often unmarried and not working than those having other depressive presentations (Agosti *et al.* 2001, Matza *et al.* 2003, Novick *et al.* 2005). Depression with atypical features therefore presents a significant clinical challenge for practicing mental health clinicians.

Problems exist, however, in defining depression with atypical features, and the validity of the DSM-IV atypical features specifier has been challenged. At a minimum, important questions remain unanswered. This chapter reviews the literature on the validity of the

Table 5.1 DSM-IV criteria for atypical features specifier (of major depressive disorder, major depressive episode of bipolar disorder, or dysthymic disorder)

A. Mood reactivity (i.e., mood brightens in response to actual or potential positive events)

B. Two (or more) of the following features:

   (1) significant weight gain or increase in appetite
   (2) hypersomnia
   (3) leaden paralysis (i.e., heavy, leaden feelings in arms or legs)
   (4) long-standing pattern of interpersonal rejection sensitivity (not limited to episodes of mood disturbance) that results in significant social or occupational impairment

C. Criteria are not met for With Melancholic Features or With Catatonic Features during the same episode.

entity defined by DSM-IV and its treatment. A suggested algorithm is presented for treating depressed patients who have atypical features, a clinical vignette is described, and clinical pearls are presented.

Defining atypical depression

West and Dally (1959) first suggested the existence of a depressive sub-type characterized by increased response to monoamine oxidase inhibitors (MAOI) relative to tricyclic antidepressants (TCA), and electroconvulsive therapy (ECT). Such patients did not present with "typical" endogenous features, such as early morning wakening and weight loss, leading these authors and their colleagues at London's St. Thomas Hospital to use the term "atypical" to describe their depressive illness. The St. Thomas group wrote several papers describing the characteristics of patients with "atypical depression," but did not propose specific criteria (West and Dally, 1959, Sargant, 1960, Dally and Rohde, 1961). West and Dally (1959) characterized

Clinical Handbook for the Management of Mood Disorders, ed. J. John Mann, Patrick J. McGrath, and Steven P. Roose.
Published by Cambridge University Press. © Cambridge University Press 2013.

such patients as having hysterical, over-reactive personalities, prominent phobic and somatic anxiety, and marked fatigue. They lacked the terminal insomnia and diurnal morning worsening characteristic of patients with endogenous depression, an earlier term used to describe melancholia, and had been ill "for years."

Davidson *et al.* (1982) codified these characteristics. Not only did patients with atypical depression not have the vegetative features of melancholia; instead, some reported reverse vegetative symptoms, such as hypersomnia and hyperphagia. Some such patients seemed more anxious than depressed, such that Davidson considered their depressive symptoms to be "masked by phobic anxiety." In addition to prominent anxiety, patients with atypical depression were "over-reactive" and "hysterical," fatigue was prominent, and if insomnia was present it was initial rather than being characterized by early morning wakening. Self-reproach was common and if there was diurnal variation in mood, evenings were their worst time of day, rather than mornings, as in melancholia. Davidson suggested there are "A" (anxious) and "V" (vegetative) sub-types, but did not define criteria. Nor, to our knowledge, have Davidson's A and V sub-types of atypical depression been prospectively tested using validating principles, so their existence remains hypothetical.

A group at Columbia University sought to test the St. Thomas' group's suggestion that depressed patients exist who respond specifically to MAOIs relative to TCAs. Preliminary to their studies, they established "the Columbia criteria" for atypical depression requiring significant mood reactivity plus two of four additional symptoms (hyperphagia, hypersomnia, leaden paralysis, and pathologic rejection sensitivity). Two separate studies confirmed superior MAOI response relative to TCA in patients meeting these criteria (Liebowitz *et al.* 1988, Quitkin *et al.* 1990). Stewart *et al.* (1993) showed that, relative to patients with melancholia, patients meeting the Columbia criteria had an earlier age onset of depressive illness, a more chronic course of illness, less severely but more chronically depressed first-degree relatives, and failed to show the pattern of abnormal biological testing documented in patients with melancholia. These studies validated the inclusion of "atypical features" as a specifier of depressive disorders in DSM-IV (Rabkin *et al.* 1996), which incorporated the Columbia criteria (see Table 5.1).

While some studies have partially validated DSM-IV depression with atypical features (Lam and Stewart, 1996, Sotsky and Simmens, 1999, Posternak and Zimmerman, 2002), others have questioned the concept's legitimacy. Finding mood reactivity more associated with severity of illness than with the other atypical features, some have suggested removing this requirement (Angst, 2002, Thase, 2007). An extension of this argument is that the five elements (mood reactivity, hyperphagia, hypersomnia, leaden paralysis, and rejection sensitivity) correlate relatively poorly (Angst, 2002, Parker, 2002, Posternak, 2002) or do not demonstrate the internal consistency expected if they define a disease entity (Parker, 2002). These arguments have resulted in suggested alternatives. Angst (2002), for example, recommends using any three of the five DSM-IV items. Parker (2002) suggests considering atypical depression a "character trait" whose defining feature is rejection sensitivity. Benazzi (2000) and Perugi (2003) consider atypical depression to belong to a broadly defined "bipolar spectrum." It is possible that these suggestions will eventually be shown to identify legitimate psychiatric disorders. What is unclear is whether such reconceptualizations improve on DSM-IV's criteria or define different disorders. That is, are the patients defined by the Angst, Parker, or Benazzi criteria the same as those West and Dally, the Columbia group, and DSM-IV were attempting to identify (i.e., patients specifically responsive to MAOI relative to TCA); or alternatively, do these suggested reconceptualizations define different disorders that are phenomenologically similar?

One problem with the DSM-IV definition of depression with atypical features stems from its origin in West and Dally's observation that these are TCA-unresponsive patients. Contrary to this expectation, Stewart *et al.* (2002) noted that the Columbia group's validating studies demonstrated TCA to be superior to placebo for patients meeting their criteria for atypical depression (Liebowitz *et al.* 1988, Quitkin *et al.* 1990). Stewart *et al.* (2002) argued that if failure to respond to TCA is a characteristic of depression with atypical features, then the DSM-IV criteria must include some patients who actually have a different disorder. That is, those responding to TCA may have the same phenomenology, but not the same illness. These authors demonstrated that within patients meeting DSM-IV criteria for depression with atypical features, lack of TCA responsivity was limited to those who had both early onset (prior to age 20) and very chronic illness (no 2-month period of spontaneous well-being post-onset); in contrast, depressed patients with atypical features who report either illness onset after age 20 or at least one spontaneous remission had a robust imipramine response (Stewart *et al.* 2002). These findings were replicated in a second group of depressed patients having "probable atypical features" (Stewart *et al.* 2002), and validated in two biologic studies (Stewart *et al.* 2003, 2005) and a family study (Stewart *et al.* 2007). Because within DSM-IV depression with atypical features, those having the early onset of a very chronic disorder differ across multiple domains from those with either later onset or a less chronic illness, several criteria for validating psychiatric disorders (Robins and Guze, 1970, Kendall, 1989, Klein, 1989) indicate these are separate disorders, rather than variants of the same entity. Other proposed suggestions to change the DSM-IV criteria, such as those of Angst *et al.* and Parker *et al.* do not have supporting evidence from independent datasets; nor do they compare the suggested group with the residual group or validate their suggested criteria across multiple domains, as was done by Stewart and colleagues (summarized by Stewart *et al.* 2007). None of the suggested alternative definitions has been shown to have preferential response to MAOIs relative to TCAs; until these validating studies are done, it will remain unclear whether suggested alternatives define the illness West and Dally described.

Relationship between depression with atypical features and other disorders

Bipolar depression

Several authors have suggested a relationship exists between bipolar disorder and depression with atypical features. Indeed, DSM-IV includes bipolar disorder as one of three affective disorders (along with major depression, and dysthymic disorder) for which atypical features are to be assessed. Angst *et al.* (2002) followed virtually all Zurich 18-year-olds for 25 years. While exact atypical features were not explicitly assessed, depression with atypical features was approximated from the assessment battery. Based on these assessments, Angst *et al.* reported increased rates of bipolar II disorder, as well as a more broadly defined "bipolar spectrum" in those having depression with atypical features relative to other depressed subjects.

Based on similar findings in clinical populations, Benazzi (1997, 1999, 2000) and Perugi *et al.* (1998) suggested atypical depression may be a variant of bipolar disorder. Using a "loose" definition of hypomania allowing a diagnosis to be made if hypomanic-like symptoms last two or more days, Benazzi (1999) reported increased rates of bipolar disorder in depressed patients with atypical features relative to those without atypical features. These authors argued that the mood lability seen in depression with atypical features is a variant on the mood swings of bipolar disorder. Descriptions of bipolar mood swings, however, usually indicate that at least some are spontaneous, while those of depression with atypical features are described as reactive, perhaps an important distinction. The Stewart *et al.* (2007) reconceptualization of depression with atypical features as presenting with a relentlessly chronic course of depressive illness seems antithetical to the recurrent episodic nature of bipolar illness, suggesting that bipolar disorder with atypical-like features may be a "look-alike" having similar phenomenology, but a different underlying etiology. Nevertheless, the relationship, if any, between atypical depression and bipolar disorder is unresolved.

Himmelhoch *et al.* (1991), defined "anergic bipolar depression" (i.e., major depression plus fatigue or volitional inhibition, predominant psychomotor retardation, and either hypersomnia or >5 lb weight gain, plus a history of mania or hypomania), randomizing 56 patients meeting these criteria to 6 weeks' treatment with imipramine (to 300 mg/d) or tranylcypromine (to 60 mg/d). Significantly greater response was observed in those treated with the MAOI (81%) than with the TCA (48%; $\chi^2 = 4.2$, df = 1, p < 0.02). Thase *et al.* (1992) treated 12 imipramine nonresponders from the above study with tranylcypromine, reporting that 9 (75%) responded, while only 1 of 4 (25%) tranylcypromine nonresponders benefited when given imipramine, supporting their conclusion that anergic bipolar depression is preferentially responsive to MAOIs relative to TCAs. A major difference between the Columbia group's patients and those of Himmelhoch and Thase is that all the Thase and Himmelhoch patients had bipolar disorder, while only 11% of the Columbia patients were diagnosed with bipolar disorder. And neither Thase *et al.* nor Himmelhoch *et al.* report on other features, such as mood reactivity, rejection sensitivity, and course of illness, which the Columbia group found to distinguish patients with atypical depression

61

from other depressive conditions. As with bipolar disorder in general, it is unclear whether anergic bipolar depression is akin to depression with atypical features or represents a bipolar "look-alike." Of note, however, this is the only group offering alternative definitions to that of the Columbia group to have tested and demonstrated increased MAOI vs. TCA responsivity, the original West and Dally benchmark considered crucial to pharmacologic dissection (Klein, 1989).

Personality disorders

Pathologic rejection sensitivity is the most common feature of depression with atypical features (McGrath *et al.* 1992, Posternak and Zimmerman, 2001). The criteria used by the Columbia group (Stewart *et al.* 1993) make clear that rejection sensitivity is a life-long pattern rather than a cross-sectional symptom, as are the other atypical features, assessment of which is limited to the past 3 months or current episode, whichever is shorter. Instead, rejection sensitivity is rated during any 2-year period. Unstated in the criteria is the expectation that whatever is captured during that period will be characteristic of the individual during their lifetime. Parker (2007) has argued that such a pathological personality trait is better captured on Axis II than as an Axis I symptom. While an interesting philosophical argument, Parker does not provide independent validity evidence, such as that within patients meeting DSM-IV criteria for atypical depression. Relative to those without rejection sensitivity, those with rejection sensitivity have different family histories, biology, or treatment response.

If conceptualized as a disorder of excessive mood reactivity resulting in difficulties maintaining relationships, depression with atypical features includes characteristics of borderline personality, including affective instability and unstable interpersonal relationships. The Stewart *et al.* (2007) reconceptualization of depression with atypical features highlights the early onset and chronic nature of the illness, further likening it to a personality disorder. Little literature addresses this possible relationship, however. Parsons *et al.* (1989) demonstrated particularly robust MAOI response coupled with lack of TCA response in the sub-set of patients with atypical depression who also had borderline personality disorder. Other validating features comparing atypical depression with and without borderline personality disorder, such as family history and biological testing, have

not been reported. We are also unaware of studies evaluating differences between depressed patients having borderline personality and depressed patients with atypical features but not borderline personality. Thus, the relationship, if any, between depression with atypical features and borderline personality disorder remains largely theoretical.

Treatment studies

MAOIs

Following up on West and Dally's 1959 observations, Liebowitz *et al.* (1984, 1988) published the first papers testing the hypothesis that operationally defined patients with atypical depression would preferentially respond to MAOIs relative to TCAs or placebo. Using the "Columbia criteria," two randomized studies (Liebowitz *et al.* 1988, Quitkin *et al.* 1990) showed similar results, namely that improvement was significantly more likely in patients treated with a representative MAOI, phenelzine (71 and 83% responded, respectively), than in those treated with the TCA, imipramine, (50% responded in each study), or placebo (28 and 19% responded, respectively). Similar results were shown in patients having "probable" atypical depression (significant mood reactivity plus one of the four DSM-IV associated symptoms; 71, 47, and 29% responded, respectively, to phenelzine, imipramine, and placebo), but this was a smaller (N = 60) and unreplicated study (Quitkin *et al.* 1988). Sixty patients with mood reactivity but none of the DSM-IV associated ("B") symptoms did not demonstrate superiority of phenelzine (75% responded) relative to imipramine (74% responded) (Quitkin *et al.* 1989), suggesting specificity existed rather than that phenelzine is a better antidepressant than imipramine for all depressed patients.

Selegiline, though not the transdermal formulation, has been studied in depressed patients with atypical features. It was hoped that because at low dose selegiline has negligible inhibition of MAO-A, the enzyme that metabolizes tyramine, a tyramine-free diet would not be required. Quitkin *et al.* (1984) reported on 17 patients having depression with atypical features treated openly with selegiline (then called l-deprenyl), reporting significant improvement in nine (53%) patients, though eight required doses above 20 mg/d, the apparent threshold for selegiline's MAO-B selectivity. As this study was not placebo-controlled, at best it suggests efficacy. Mann *et al.* (1989) treated 44 depressed patients including 13 with atypical features using doses of selegiline up to 30 mg/d, reporting both overall efficacy, and efficacy within those with atypical features, relative to placebo. McGrath *et al.* (1989) compared the sub-set from a larger study randomly assigned to treatment with selegiline (to 40 mg/d) or placebo for 6 weeks, reporting increased response to active selegiline (50%) relative to placebo (28%). McGrath *et al.*, however, did not compare selegiline response to phenelzine or imipramine, the other two drugs included in the study. We are unaware of reports of the efficacy of the selegiline patch as treatment for depression with atypical features. While it seems reasonable to assume delivery by the patch ought to be effective if oral delivery is, it is unclear what the patch equivalent to 30 or 40 mg/d is, rendering it unclear whether to anticipate efficacy similar to those reported by Mann *et al.* and McGrath *et al.* at selegiline's marketed dosing.

The reversible MAOI, moclobemide, has been studied. Larsen *et al.* (1991), for example, compared moclobemide to clomipramine (a TCA) and isocarboxazid (an irreversible MAOI) in a randomized study of 167 outpatients with atypical depression, finding equivalent response rates, although the numerically lower moclobemide response rate (46 vs. 64% remission on the other two agents) suggests a larger study might demonstrate clomipramine or isocarboxazid is the superior agent; two pluses of this study are the prospective determination of diagnosis and random assignment; three limitations are low doses of all three medications, lack of a control group, and small sample size. Of note, 130 subjects would be needed in each treatment group to have an 80% chance of detecting the difference between 46 and 64%, nearly 200 patients more than Larsen studied, while Larsen's sample size provided approximately a 40% chance of demonstrating a significant between-group difference in response rates. Lonnqvist *et al.* (1994) randomly assigned 209 depressed patients, including 53 with atypical features to moclobemide up to 450 mg/d or fluoxetine up to 40 mg/d for 6 weeks. While they assert moclobemide may be superior to fluoxetine in the sub-group with atypical depression (60% responded to moclobemide, 48% to fluoxetine), they do not show any statistical analysis to back up this assertion. Søgaard *et al.* (1999) randomly assigned 197 patients having atypical depression to treatment with moclobemide (to 450 mg/d) or sertraline (to 100 mg/d), reporting a trend for superior outcome with the sertraline (77.5% responded vs. 67.5% to moclobemide; p = 0.052). We found no placebo-controlled studies of moclobemide in atypical depression, so at best, conclusions are tentative. Overall, these three studies are suggestive that moclobemide might be about as effective as irreversible MAOIs or SSRIs in treating atypical depression, but more definitive studies are needed.

SSRIs (selective serotonin reuptake inhibitors)

While MAOI studies suggested that MAOIs might be useful first-line agents in treatment of depression with atypical features, dietary restrictions, high rates of side effects, such as weight gain and sexual dysfunction, and significant drug–drug interactions make MAOIs less attractive in practice. Hence, the advent of the more user-friendly selective serotonin reuptake inhibitors (SSRIs) had significant appeal. Ideally, studies would demonstrate both noninferiority of SSRIs relative to MAOIs and superiority of SSRIs relative to TCAs. Indeed, in a double-blind randomized study limited to patients having depression with atypical features, Pande *et al.* (1996) reported similarly high response rates to phenelzine and fluoxetine (about 80% responded to each treatment). However, there was no placebo control group, and the sample size was too small (20 in each group) to detect any but large differences between the treatments. As noted above, Lonnqvist *et al.* (1994) and Søgaard *et al.* (1999) did not find significant differences between the reversible MAOI, moclobemide, and an SSRI. Reimherr *et al.* (1984) randomly assigned patients to fluoxetine, imipramine, or placebo, including 28 patients having atypical depression who were randomized to an active drug; significantly more patients responded to fluoxetine (65%) than imipramine (13%). However, Reimherr did not report placebo response of patients with atypical depression and sample size was small. McGrath *et al.* (2000) randomly assigned 154 depressed patients with atypical features to fluoxetine (to maximum dose 60 mg/d), imipramine (to maximum dose 300 mg/d), or placebo (to maximum six pills daily), reporting both active medications to have increased efficacy relative to placebo (response rates: fluoxetine 51%, imipramine 53%, placebo 23%), but the two drugs did not differ from each other. Stratta *et al.* (1991) also compared fluoxetine to imipramine, reporting no difference in efficacy, but this was an underpowered study (N = 14 on each treatment) and did not include a placebo group. Thus, three underpowered studies suggest SSRIs' noninferiority to MAOIs, and two underpowered studies did not demonstrate SSRIs' superiority vs. TCAs, leading us to conclude that SSRIs' place relative to MAOI and TCA is unclear. Nevertheless, we conclude that SSRIs should be considered a first-line medication.

CBT (cognitive behavior therapy)

Mercier *et al.* (1992) first suggested cognitive behavior therapy (CBT) might be an effective treatment for atypical depression, but did not have a control group. Jarrett *et al.* (1999) randomly assigned depressed patients with atypical features phenelzine to CBT and placebo. Phenelzine and CBT were comparably effective and both were superior to placebo. The main problem with this study was there was a high dropout rate on placebo (64%), raising questions about the blind and the appropriateness of statistical comparisons between the other treatments and placebo. Acceptably low attrition on the active treatments (phenelzine: 25%; CBT: 14%), however, suggests comparisons between the active treatments may be valid. Therefore, CBT may be a reasonable alternative to phenelzine in the treatment of depression with atypical features.

Stewart *et al.* (1998) reanalyzed data from the National Institute of Mental Health Treatment of Depression Collaborative Research Program (Elkin *et al.* 1989), a study that randomized patients with major depression to interpersonal psychotherapy, cognitive behavior therapy, imipramine, or placebo. The Stewart *et al.* reanalysis showed imipramine to be significantly more effective in depressed patients without than in those with atypical features, corroborating earlier findings. The two psychotherapies were numerically but not statistically superior to placebo in both sub-types, although the sample size limited the power to detect between-group differences. The strength of this study is its inclusion of a placebo control group, while two drawbacks are atypical depression was determined post-hoc by algorithm, and the modest sample size of patients with atypical depression (13–22 per group) limited the likelihood of detecting differences between treatments. We do not consider these studies of psychotherapy for treating depression with

atypical features definitive, but they are suggestive that psychotherapy may be a reasonable alternative for atypically depressed patients who cannot take or prefer not to use antidepressant medications.

Bupropion

Goodnick and Extein (1989) gave open-label bupropion or fluoxetine to 57 depressed patients, reporting bupropion to be more effective for those having bipolar or atypical depression, while the SSRI was more effective for those having "typical" depression. Goodnick *et al.* (1998) gave 41 depressed patients open-label bupropion, also reporting a better response in those having atypical features or bipolar depression, than in other depressed subjects. These open-label, non-randomized reports require substantiation using formal randomized, double-blind studies before accepting their suggestion that bupropion is an effective treatment for depression with atypical features.

SNRI (serotonin–norepinephrine reuptake inhibitor)

Roose *et al.* (2004) gave open-label venlafaxine to 17 elderly depressed patients with atypical features, reporting 65% remitted. Most, however, had onset after age 50, suggesting it may be tenuous to generalize this to the patients included in the DSM-IV validation studies and in particular the early-onset patients Stewart *et al.* proposed as representing a reconceptualized definition of depression with atypical features. Therefore, at best this open-label study implies possible venlafaxine efficacy for elderly patients having late-onset illness.

Stewart reported 50% of depressed younger adults (aged 18–65) with atypical features responded to open-label duloxetine dosed to a maximum of 120 mg/d. This study did not report on possible differential efficacy between study patients with and without early onset and very chronic depressive illness. The open-label nature of the study suggests caution in generalizing from this report.

Other antidepressant medications

We did not find other studies and in particular RTCs of the efficacy of other marketed antidepressants in depression with atypical features, such as mirtazapine, trazodone, and velazodone. McGrath *et al.* (1994) reported significant efficacy for the unmarketed drug, gepirone, but as this agent is unavailable, it can play no role in the current treatment of this disorder.

Chromium

Case reports suggested chromium might be helpful for depressed patients who had carbohydrate craving and/or excessive appetite, perhaps because of chromium's facilitation of insulin action (McLeod *et al.* 2000). A small (N = 15) double-blind, placebo-controlled study testing this observation confirmed chromium's efficacy in such patients (Davidson *et al.* 2003). However, a larger double-blind study of 113 patients having atypical depression failed to demonstrate an overall benefit for chromium, although carbohydrate craving was markedly reduced in chromium-treated patients presenting with cravings (Docherty *et al.* 2005). While the literature is mixed on whether chromium is an effective treatment for depression with atypical features, the Docherty *et al.* suggestion that it may reduce carbohydrate craving and overeating is consistent with chromium's proposed action as an insulin facilitator (Anderson *et al.* 1998).

ECT (electroconvulsive therapy)

Although remarked upon as relatively ineffective for patients with atypical depression since West and Dally's initial report (1959), there is little supportive literature. Husain *et al.* (2008) reported that 80% of 36 ECT-treated depressed patients with atypical features remitted. While an impressive remission rate, it is based on a small group of inpatients, limiting its generalizability. Nevertheless, ECT should always be considered, especially for highly treatment-refractory patients.

Treatment algorithm

The literature is clear that phenelzine is a superior choice over imipramine for the treatment of depression with atypical features, particularly if onset is early and the course is very chronic. Although some randomized controlled trials suggest the efficacy of SSRIs and CBT for the treatment of atypical depression, the literature is not clear as to the order in which such treatments ought to be used. Therefore, our algorithm is based more on practicality than strong evidence.

Our first-line treatment is CBT, as it has a modest demonstration of efficacy, perhaps is comparable to MAOIs, and does not entail dietary restrictions, medication side effects, or drug–drug interactions. We also find it acceptable to most treatment-naïve patients. CBT should provide 20 sessions over 12–16 weeks, but if marked improvement does not occur in this time frame, medication should be instituted.

Our first-line medication is an SSRI, for example, fluoxetine. While flaws exist in the few existing comparison studies, none suggested inferiority of SSRIs relative to MAOIs. Any SSRI is started at the lowest marketed dose (e.g., 10 mg for fluoxetine) giving the first dose with food, as this minimizes excessive gastrointestinal stimulation. After 1–4 weeks, the dose is increased iteratively if tolerated to maximal PDR dose (80 mg/d for fluoxetine). If the patient remits, we continue the same medication at least an additional 6 months before considering a trial off the medication. If there is no benefit after 4 weeks on maximally tolerated dose, the SSRI should be tapered and discontinued.

Our second-line medication is bupropion for patients without increased seizure risk, such as in the presence of anorexia and/or bulimia, or concomitant use of another medication that lowers the seizure threshold. We use bupropion XL, as it can be given safely once daily, starting at 150 mg/d and, if tolerated and the patient's depressive symptoms have not remitted, the dose should be pushed to the PDR maximum (450 mg/d) for 4 weeks.

If bupropion is not effective, mirtazapine or an atypical antipsychotic may be added as adjunctive treatment, or an SNRI may be tried instead, such as venlafaxine, desvenlafaxine, or duloxetine. At some point, however, one should consider a trial with a TCA or an MAOI. Our choice between these original antidepressants rests on the patient's history. The early onset of a very chronic depressive illness would favor use of an MAOI, while onset after age 20 or periods of spontaneous remission would favor use of a TCA. Our TCA choice is nortriptyline because it appears to be the best tolerated of the medication class. Prior to starting a TCA, we obtain an electrocardiogram to rule out evidence of a cardiac conduction defect, as TCAs may increase the QT_C interval; if the baseline QT_C is greater than 500 ms, TCA should probably be avoided. We give TCA all as a single dose at bedtime, starting nortriptyline at 25 mg and increasing by 25 mg every 3 days to 75 mg q hs, if tolerated, then obtain a blood level and electrocardiogram 5–7 days later. While laboratories commonly list 50–150 ng/ml as the target blood level, we find best results in patients with blood levels between 125–150 ng/ml. The repeated electrocardiograms are to determine whether the QT_C has increased and we do not increase the dose further if the QT_C approaches 500 ms.

If a TCA is skipped or ineffective, we then treat with an MAOI. Accepted practice is to taper and discontinue the TCA and any SRI, then wait 2 weeks before starting the MAOI. We are not aware of studies comparing any of the MAOIs marketed in the USA. Not surprisingly, then, the author of this chapter and the editors of this book disagree on which MAOI should be used. Some prefer starting with selegiline, based on its presumed increased tolerability. Others prefer tranylcypromine based on its presumed increased efficacy and the need to taper and wait 2 weeks between MAOIs should selegiline prove ineffective. We note, however, that neither the selegiline patch nor tranylcypromine has randomized, controlled study data supporting its use in depression with atypical features. Dosing of selegiline begins with a 6 mg/24 hour patch, noting that the tyramine-free diet does not have to be followed at this dose, and that the location of the patch should be changed every day. After 4 weeks, if tolerated and insufficient benefit has been achieved, the patch should be changed to the 9 mg/24 hour dosing and the tyramine-free diet must be started. If response remains insufficient after 4 weeks the patch should be increased to 12 mg/24 hours for 4 weeks.

Whether selegiline is used or skipped, the next treatment should be an oral MAOI, such as tranylcypromine, following a 2-week wait after the last dose of the prior medication. Dosing of tranylcypromine starts at 10 mg/d with twice weekly dose increases to 40 mg/d, then increasing by weekly 10 mg increments to a maximum of 60 mg/d, if tolerated, waiting longer or stopping dose increases should side effects become intolerable, and not instituting dose increases if remission has occurred. Doses above 30 mg/d should be given in divided doses because single doses above 30 mg/d can increase the blood pressure. We keep patients on the highest tolerated dose up to 60 mg/d for 4 weeks before making a change. If they tolerate 60 mg/d and have not remitted after 4 weeks, we consider increasing the dose further, recognizing this is beyond the PDR limits. One problem with increasing the dose above 60 mg/d is one either has to take it more than twice a day, creating adherence problems, or carefully measure the blood pressure, instituting antihypertensive treatment should the blood pressure increase. Our protocol is to have the patient come

to the office without having taken their second dose of tranylcypromine. After we obtain their blood pressure, they take the increased dose and we take their blood pressure every half hour for 90 minutes. If the blood pressure increases by 30 mm Hg systolic or 20 mm Hg diastolic, we have them take an antihypertensive, such as nifedipine 10 mg/d, and repeat the blood pressure testing after they have begun taking nifedipine. This procedure is repeated each time the afternoon dose is increased, that is, every other dose increase. If tolerated and not remitted, we continue weekly 10 mg dose raises to 120 mg/d (i.e., 60 mg bid or 40 mg tid).

MAOI (tyramine-free) diet

Prior to starting an MAOI, the patient must be educated about the content of and rationale for the tyramine-free diet and dangerous medications, such as SSRIs and meperidine. Because tyramine is a strong pressor agent, its presence in sufficient concentration can raise the blood pressure, potentially to hypertensive crisis levels, necessitating emergency intervention to prevent a bleed. In the worst-case scenario, a hemorrhagic stroke results. As tyramine is mainly metabolized by MAO-A, in the presence of an inhibitor of MAO-A, one must carefully avoid tyramine-containing foods to prevent a sudden rise in blood pressure. These foods include aged meats (such as salami and sausage), aged cheeses (such as blue cheese and cheddar), and a few other foods, including broad beans (such as fava beans) and tap beer. A relatively simple avoidance diet accompanies the package insert of the selegiline patch. Concomitant over-the-counter decongestants can also cause a hypertensive crisis, while mixing MAOIs and SSRIs can result in a serotonin syndrome, so these combinations must be avoided.

Partial remission

The algorithm above and shown in Figure 5.1 is best applied to patients who do not benefit at each step. There are no studies suggesting the next best treatment for depressed patients with atypical features who improve without remitting at each step. Therefore, one must generalize from more general studies. Even for depression in general, the data are not clear however. For example, most treatment-refractory studies do not separate out patients who had not improved from those who had a partial response. Also, very few

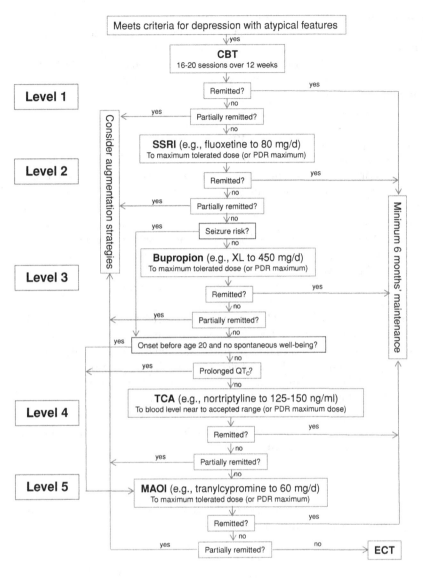

Figure 5.1 Treatment algorithm for depression with atypical features

- **Combination strategies: add a 2nd antidepressant**
  - Bupropion
  - Mirtazapine
  - Tricyclic antidepressant
  - Trazodone
  - Psychotherapy (CBT or IPT)
- **Augmentation strategies: add a nonantidepressant**
  - Lithium
  - Thyroid (triiodothyronine)
  - Antipsychotic
  - Buspirone

studies compared multiple possible options. The one exception is the NIMH-sponsored Sequenced Treatment Alternatives to Relieve Depression (STAR*D) study, but subsequent treatments (Fava *et al.* 2006, McGrath *et al.* 2006, Nierenberg *et al.* 2006, Rush *et al.* 2006, Trivedi *et al.* 2006, Thase *et al.* 2007) were equivalent, so the results do not direct an algorithm. Also, because STAR*D allowed equipoise randomization, in which patients and their physicians could choose among the alternatives (Rush *et al.* 2004), it was not possible to compare a "switch" strategy to an "augment" strategy. Therefore, we recommend a "switch" strategy for patients who do not benefit from current treatment (i.e., stop current treatment and then switch to a different treatment) and an "augment" strategy for patients who benefit, but insufficiently.

Because the literature is largely unhelpful in choosing among augmentation strategies, we recommend the least troublesome be added first, the likely most troublesome last. As psychotherapy is unlikely to cause adverse events, this should be tried first, unless already unsuccessful. Nevertheless, a different psychotherapeutic approach may be effective (e.g., interpersonal psychotherapy when CBT was ineffective initially). Our next choice is to add an antidepressant, considered by some "combination therapy" rather than "augmentation" (i.e., the addition of a medication not thought to have intrinsic antidepressant properties). When combining antidepressants, we add one presumed not to produce drug–drug interactions while offering a different mechanism of action. Thus, we would add bupropion to an SSRI, but would not add a second SSRI or an SNRI. If we wanted to add an NRI to an SSRI, we would either add a TCA or switch to an SNRI, not add the latter. If combining antidepressants is ineffective, we either move to the next step of the algorithm (i.e., "switch") or augment. Augmenters include lithium, thyroid, buspirone, and the antipsychotic medications. We avoid the latter if possible due to their poor tolerability, but also recognize their demonstrated effectiveness.

Managing side effects

SSRIs

Two initial problems are nausea and agitation. Nausea is minimized by taking the initial dose with a meal, so we instruct patients to take the first dose of any SRI with food. Fortunately, nausea usually subsides quickly, typically after the first ingestion or a few subsequent doses. Agitation may be related to the suicidality that prompted the FDA to issue a warning. Agitation is discomfiting and requires lowering of the dose or discontinuation of the medication. We find it important to warn patients about this possibility and instruct them to call to discuss how to ameliorate it should it occur. Sexual dysfunction and weight gain are later problems for patients taking SRI medications. Most commonly, sexual dysfunction consists of anorgasmia or difficulty reaching orgasm. We find skipping a dose the best way to handle the sexual dysfunction of SSRIs. That is, the patient is instructed to skip their SSRI dose on the morning of the day when

sexual activity will occur, then take the medication afterwards. Occasionally, two doses must be skipped. Weight gain is usually small, but problematic when more than a few pounds. We have not found simple solutions beyond urging healthy eating and regular exercise.

Bupropion

Bupropion can induce irritability. While many adverse events wane with continued use of antidepressant medications, the irritability resulting from bupropion seems to continue as long as the drug is continued at the same dose. Therefore, we warn patients about increased irritability and lower the dose should it arise, discontinuing and switching treatments should a lower dose be ineffective. Insomnia can be problematic if the patient takes it too late in the day, so we recommend it be taken first thing in the morning. Patients must be warned about the risk for seizures and should not take bupropion if they have increased seizure risk, for example if they have a diagnosis of anorexia, bulimia, or alcohol abuse/dependence, or they are taking other medications known to lower the seizure threshold. In addition, at 450 mg/d some patients' blood pressure increases so we obtain blood pressure readings before treatment and if we raise the dose to 450 mg/d.

TCAs

TCAs commonly cause dry mouth, constipation, daytime sleepiness, urinary retention, and weight gain. Sucking on a lemon drop (sugar-free) helps with a dry mouth, while heavy doses of stool softeners allay constipation (e.g., two tablespoons Metamucil or 100 mg Colace with each meal). If a patient has trouble waking or feels "drugged" in the morning, taking the drug earlier often helps. We ask the patient what time their brain finally wakes up, then instruct them to take the medication that much earlier. If this makes them too sleepy in the evening, we have them take some of the medication earlier and the rest at bedtime. Bethanechol 5 or 10 mg three or four times a day helps urinary retention. We deal with weight gain as with SSRIs. Because TCAs can prolong the QT_C, we obtain an electrocardiogram prior to TCA use and after reaching a stable dose, skipping this medication class if the baseline QT_C is >500 ms, and do not increase the dose further if the QT_C approaches 500 ms.

MAOIs

The selegiline patch has the side effects of other MAOIs, but they tend to be milder and less frequent, plus a rash can occur at the site of application. The latter can be reduced by moving the patch locations and use of a local antihistamine gel. Phenelzine and isocarboxazid cause weight gain, sleep disturbance, fluid retention, and sexual dysfunction. While these problems can occur with tranylcypromine, we find them less problematic, except for the sleep disturbance and orthostasis, which can be more severe with tranylcypromine than the other MAOIs. The sleep disturbance of phenelzine tends to be displaced sleep (e.g., the patient cannot sleep at night, but cannot stay awake during the day) or hypersomnia, although night-time insomnia can also occur. Phenelzine also causes sudden daytime sleepiness, typically in the late afternoon, mimicking narcolepsy, and can be dangerous if driving when this occurs, so patients must be warned. With tranylcypromine, total sleep time decreases, and some patients have trouble functioning due to marked sleep deprivation. We find trazodone 50–200 mg at hs helpful for night-time insomnia. The daytime sleepiness of phenelzine is helped by alerting medications such as modafinil.

Clinical pearls

These represent our clinical observations and reflect our clinical experience rather than evidence from clinical trials.

Mirtazapine is a "dirty" drug, in that it affects many neurotransmitter systems. As its highest affinity is for the histamine receptor, its effects at lowest doses are those of antihistamines – sleep inducing and appetite stimulation. While these effects may be desired in some patients, for example, those with melancholia, they are undesired in others, including patients with atypical depression. As mirtazapine's dose is increased, other actions begin to be seen, including antagonism of several serotonin and norepinephrine receptors. As these effects may counteract mirtazapine's antihistaminic actions, some patients tolerate this drug better at higher doses than the usual starting dose of 15 mg/d. Because of this observation, some practitioners begin mirtazapine at 30 or 45 mg/d rather than the suggested starting dose of 15 mg/d. As poor sleep and appetite are common problems in the elderly, some geriatricians make use of mirtazapine's ameliorative effects on these symptoms.

TCAs often cause dry mouth and constipation. As dry mouth results from decreased saliva flow rather than representing dehydration, drinking liquids is relatively ineffective, as the mouth is immediately dry again once the liquid is swallowed. Instead, we recommend stimulation of saliva by lemon drops; these must be sugar-free, as saliva is the first defense against tooth decay and coating the teeth with sugar in a saliva-deficient mouth invites bacterial growth. Because constipation is so common with TCAs, we prophylactically have patients increase roughage, while watching for a hardening of their stool. Should hardening occur, we immediately have them begin large quantities of stool softeners, such as two tablespoons Metamucil three times a day or 100 mg Colace three times a day.

MAOIs: Phenelzine causes narcolepsy, so patients must be warned to watch for this and not to drive at times it occurs, usually 3–5 in the afternoon. Although stimulants are thought to be contraindicated with MAOIs, we find them to be safe and to counteract the narcoleptic effect of phenelzine. All MAOIs can interfere with sleep. For MAOI-induced insomnia, we find trazodone 50–200 mg hs useful. For sleep phase shifts, bright lights are more effective than sleep-inducing medications. Tranylcypromine at single doses above 30 mg at a time can directly increase the blood pressure; therefore, we obtain blood pressure 45–60 minutes after each dose increase above 30 mg and treat with standard antihypertensive medications should the systolic blood pressure increase more than 15 mm Hg or diastolic increase more than 10 mm Hg.

Stimulants and MAOIs: This combination has long been thought to be contraindicated. We assume this is from extension from indirect sympathomimetic drugs, such as ephedrine and pseudoephedrine, which clearly can produce a hypertensive crisis if taken by someone on an MAOI. We and others (Feighner *et al.* 1985, Satel and Nelson, 1989, Stewart *et al.* pers. comm.) have not found direct-acting sympathomimetics to produce significant blood pressure increases when given to patients already taking MAOIs, so consider them safe in this regard. While some patients do well for many years on combined stimulant plus MAOI, we have also had patients who have achieved remarkable improvement only when stimulants and MAOIs were combined but who eventually developed psychotic symptoms. We have had patients report parasitosis, frank paranoia, and other forms of psychosis, which seem to respond poorly to the introduction of antipsychotic medication, but slowly resolve with discontinuation of the offending medications.

Sexual dysfunction: Many drugs used by psychiatrists affect sexual functioning, including libido, arousal, and orgasm. We are unaware of suggested treatments for decreased libido. Sildenafil and similar agents improve erectile dysfunction. Multiple agents have been suggested for prolonged time to orgasm and anorgasmia, including yohimbine (Price and Greenhouse, 1990), bupropion (Masand *et al.* 2001), buspirone (Norden, 1994) amantadine (Balogh *et al.* 1992), and cyproheptidine (Lauerma, 1996). Only the bupropion study was an RTC, but failed to find a difference between low-dose bupropion (150 mg/d) and placebo. We are unaware of definitive RTCs demonstrating efficacy of any of these agents and have rarely found them useful in practice. Instead, we use "mini drug holidays." That is, a dose or two of the drug is skipped, then given once sexual activity is completed. This works well with shorter half-life drugs, such as venlafaxine and paroxetine, less well with long half-life drugs such as fluoxetine. One caution is induction of withdrawal symptoms, particularly with short half-life drugs.

Orthostatic hypotension: Dizziness on standing is often a problem with TCAs and MAOIs. We first caution patients to watch for dizziness on standing, especially after lying for long periods, such as following a night's sleep, or after a long, hot soak in the tub. Our first method of counteracting such orthostatic dizziness is to have the patient rise more slowly, for example, sitting on the edge of the bed first thing in the morning before standing or sitting on the edge of the tub before rising. Second, is lowering the dose if it is unclear that the orthostatis-inducing dose is not required. Third, is increased salt; increasing salt intake, such as by eating pickles or adding extra salt is simple, but there are also salt pills available in pharmacies. Fourth, is surgical support stockings. If all else fails, we prescribe the mineralocorticoid, fludrocortisone, 0.1–0.2 mg/d.

Vignette

Ms. A reported "I was born depressed." She brought in a picture in which she was about five with a frown on her face, while her sister, 2 years her senior, had a winning smile. She was currently about 100 lb overweight with a history of chronic weight problems and rollercoaster dieting, losing considerable weight when she would go on a "crash" diet, and regaining it when she would succumb to her cravings for sweets. She could be temporarily cheered by good news, but "then I would look for something to bring me down again" and her mood would plummet when she subsequently noted some way she was being put down. At such times, her carbohydrate cravings would escalate, she would retreat to bed and feel physically unable to move, she felt so weighed down. She had received good trials with multiple antidepressants, experiencing only side effects, felt "I understood myself better" after dynamic psychotherapy "but my mood did not change." On phenelzine 60 mg/d, her sleep had nearly normalized and mood was much improved, though still mildly depressed half the time; she remained too sensitive to the way she was treated, but less so. On 90 mg/d, her mood completely lifted, and she was able to withstand interactions she had previously considered as evidence she was being rejected. She experienced persistent euthymia for the first time in her life.

Future directions

Despite considerable controversy as to how to define atypical depression, all seem to recognize some such entity exists. The major issue is which criteria best define it. Our view is that the existing data support adding early onset and extreme chronicity to the DSM-IV criteria, recognizing, however, that demurral exists. It seems critical for those espousing alternative definitions to demonstrate that their suggested alternative definition better identifies atypical depression than the Stewart *et al.* (2007) criteria. As the original conceptualization of atypical depression was that it was a syndrome preferentially responsive to MAOIs relative to TCA, it seems this ought to be demonstrated by any proposed alternative definition. Without meeting this requirement, a similar phenomenological presentation (anergic bipolar depression?) might be defined that nevertheless represents a different entity. A candidate "look-alike" of depression with atypical features is bipolar depression which frequently presents with atypical features, as is recognized by DSM-IV. If Stewart *et al.* are correct that the "true" atypical depression is a life-long illness unpunctuated by spontaneous periods of undepressed mood, the fluctuating episodicity of bipolar illness cannot be the same illness, despite dysphoric periods of hypersomnia and hyperphagia. Alternatively, should particularly biologic data demonstrate similar biosignature and family history, then anergic bipolar depression is the "real McCoy," not a "look-alike" and Stewart *et al.* are wrong.

In determining whether alternative criteria are superior to, say, Stewart *et al.* or DSM-IV, it is important to compare groups that meet one set of criteria, but not the other. That is, for example, patients who meet the Stewart *et al.* criteria but not those of Angst are compared to those who meet Angst but not Stewart. The question is, which group is closer to those who meet both criteria in terms of such validating criteria as course of illness, treatment outcome, family history, or biology? Stewart *et al.* (2007) have partially performed such comparisons, while we are not aware of such a strategy having been applied to other alternatives to DSM-IV.

Determining the underlying biology of whatever best defines atypical depression seems the next order of business, as this will ultimately lead to the best understanding of its etiology and treatment. Once the biology and etiology are understood, better treatments ought to eminate. Until that time, we are limited to our current trial-and-error approach, hoping to find an alternative to MAOIs for each individual patient before finally turning to these agents.

References

Agosti, V. and Stewart, J.W. (2001). Atypical and non-atypical subtypes of depression: Comparison of social functioning, symptoms, course of illness, co-morbidity and demographic features. *Journal of Affective Disorders*, 65, 75–79.

Anderson, R.A. (1998). Chromium, glucose intolerance and diabetes. *Journal of the American College of Nutrition*, 17, 548–555.

Angst, J., Gamma, A., Sellaro, R., Zhang, H., and Merikangas, K. (2002). Toward validation of atypical depression in the community: Results of the Zurich cohort study. *Journal of Affective Disorders*, 72, 125–138.

Balogh, S., Hendricks, S.E., and Kang, J. (1992). Treatment of fluoxetine-induced anorgasmia with amantadine. *Journal of Clinical Psychiatry*, 53, 212–213.

Benazzi, F. (1997). Prevalence of bipolar II disorder in outpatient depression: A 203-case study in private practice. *Journal of Affective Disorders*, 43,163–166.

Benazzi, F. (1999). Prevalence and clinical features of atypical depression in depressed outpatients: A 467-case study. *Psychiatry Research*, 86, 259–265.

Benazzi, F. (2000). Depression with DSM-IV atypical features: A marker for bipolar II disorder. *European Archives of Psychiatry*, 250, 53–55.

Dally, P.J. and Rohde, P. (1961). Comparison of antidepressant drugs in depressive illnesses. *Lancet*, 1, 18–20.

Davidson, J.R.T., Miller, R.D., Turnbull, C.D., and Sullivan, J.L. (1982). Atypical depression. *Archives of General Psychiatry*, 39, 527–534.

Davidson, J.R.T., Abraham, K., Connor, K.M., and McLeod, M.N. (2003). Effectiveness of chromium in atypical depression: A placebo-controlled study. *Biological Psychiatry*, 53, 261–264.

Docherty, J.P., Sack, D.A., Roffman, M., Finch, M., and Komorowski, J.R. (2005). A double-blind, placebo-controlled, exploratory trial of chromium picolinate in atypical depresssion: Effect on carbohydrate craving. *Journal of Psychiatric Practice*, 11, 302–314.

Elkin, I., Shea, T., Watkins, J.T. *et al.* (1989). National Institute of Mental Health Treatment of Depression Collaborative Research Program: General effectiveness of treatments. *Archives of General Psychiatry*, 46, 971–982.

Fava, M., Rush, A.J., Wisniewski, S.R. *et al.* (2006). STAR*D Study Team: A comparison of mirtazapine and nortriptyline following two consecutive failed mediation treatments for depressed outpatients: A STAR*D Report. *American Journal of Psychiatry*, 163, 1161–1172.

Feighner, J.P., Herbstein, J., and Damlouji, N. (1985). Combined MAOI, TCA and direct stimulant therapy of treatment-resistant depression. *Journal of Clinical Psychiatry*, 46, 206–209.

Goodnick, P.J. and Extein, I.L. (1989). Bupropion and fluoxetine in depressive subtypes. *Annals of Clinical Psychiatry*, 1, 119–122.

Goodnick, P.J., Dominguez, R.A., DeVane, C.L., and Bowden, C.L. (1998). Bupropion slow-release response in depression: Diagnosis and biochemistry. *Biological Psychiatry*, 44, 629–631.

Himmelhoch, J.M., Thase, M.E., Mallinger, A.G., and Houck, P. (1991). Tranylcypromine versus imipramine in anergic bipolar depression. *American Journal of Psychiatry*, 148, 910–916.

Horwath, E., Johnson, J., Weissman, M.M., and Hornig, C.D. (1992). The validity of major depression with atypical features based on a community study. *Journal of Affective Disorders*, 26, 117–125.

Husain, M.M., McClintock, S.M., Rush, A.J. *et al.* (2008). The efficacy of acute electroconvulsive therapy in atypical depression. *Journal of Clinical Psychiatry*, 69, 406–411.

Jarrett, R.B., Schaffer, M., McIntire, D. *et al.* (1999). Treatment of atypical depression with cognitive therapy or phenelzine: A double-blind, placebo-controlled trial. *Archives of General Psychiatry*, 56, 431–437.

Kendell, R.E. (1989). Clinical validity. *Psychological Medicine*, 19, 45–55.

Klein, D.F. (1989). The pharmacological validation of psychiatric diagnosis. In Robins, L. and Barrett, J., eds., *Validity of Psychiatric Diagnosis*. New York: Raven, 203–216.

Lam, R.W. and Stewart, J.N. (1996). The validity of atypical depression in DSM-IV. *Comprehensive Psychiatry*, 37, 375–383.

Larsen, J.K., Gjerris, A., Holm, P. *et al.* (1991). Moclobemide in depression: A randomized multicentre trial against isocarboxazide and clomipramine emphasizing atypical depression. *Acta Psychiatrica Scandanavica*, 84, 564–570.

Lauerma, H. (1996). Successful treatment of citalopram-induced anorgasmia by cyproheptadine. *Acta Psychiatrica Scandinavica*, 93, 69–70.

Liebowitz, M.R., Quitkin, F.M., Stewart, J.W. *et al.* (1984). Phenelzine v imipramine in atypical depression: A preliminary report. *Archives of General Psychiatry*, 41, 669–677.

Liebowitz, M.R., Quitkin, F.M., Stewart, J.W. *et al.* (1988). Antidepressant specificity in atypical depression. *Archives of General Psychiatry*, 45, 129–137.

Lonnqvist, J., Sihvo, S., Syvälahti, E., and Kiviruusu, O. (1994). Moclobemide and fluoxetine in atypical depression: A double-blind trial. *Journal of Affective Disorders*, 32 169–177.

Mann, J.J., Aarons, S.F., Wilner, P.J. *et al.* (1989). A controlled study of the antidepressant efficacy and side effects of (-)-deprenyl: A selective monoamine oxidase inhibitor. *Archives of General Psychiatry*, 46, 45–50.

Masand, P.S., Ashton, A.K., Gupta, S., and Franks, B. (2001). Sustained-release bupropion for selective serotonin reuptake inhibitor-induced sexual dysfunction: A randomized, double-blind, placebo-controlled, parallel-group study. *Ameican Journal of Psychiatry*, 158, 805–807.

Matza, L.S., Revicki, D.A., Davidson, J.R., and Stewart, J.W. (2003). Depression with atypical features in the National Comorbidity Survey: Classification, description, and consequences. *Archives of General Psychiatry*, 60, 817–826.

McGinn, L.K., Asnis, G.M., and Rubinson, E. (1996). Biological and clinical validation of atypical depression. *Psychiatry Research*, 60, 191–198.

McGrath, P.J., Stewart, J.W., Harrison, W. *et al.* (1989). A placebo-controlled trial of L-deprenyl in atypical depression. *Psychopharmacology Bulletin*, 25, 63–67.

McGrath, P.J., Stewart, J.W., Harrison, W.M. *et al.* (1992). Predictive value of symptoms of atypical depression for differential drug treatment outcome. *Journal of Clinical Psychopharmacology*, 12, 197–202.

McGrath, P.J., Stewart, J.W., Nunes, E.V. *et al.* (1993). A double-blind cross-over trial of imipramine and phenelzine for outpatients with treatment-refractory depression. *American Journal of Psychiatry*, 150, 118–123.

McGrath, P.J., Stewart, J.W., Quitkin, F.M. *et al.* (1994). Gepirone treatment of atypical depression: Preliminary evidence of serotonergic involvement. *Journal of Clinical Psychopharmacology*, 14, 347–352.

McGrath, P.J., Stewart, J.W., Janal, M.N. *et al.* (2000). A placebo-controlled study of fluoxetine versus imipramine in the acute treatment of atypical depression. *American Journal of Psychiatry*, 157, 344–350.

McGrath, P.J., Stewart, J.W., Fava, M. *et al.* (2006). STAR*D Study Team: tranylcypromine versus venlafaxine plus mirtazapine following three failed antidepressant medication trials for depression: A STAR*D report. *American Journal of Psychiatry*, 163, 1531–1541.

McLeod, M.N. and Golden, R.N. (2000). Chromium treatment of depression. *International Journal of Neuropsychopharmacology*, 3, 311–314.

Mercier, M.A., Stewart, J.W., and Quitkin, F.M. (1992). A pilot sequential study of cognitive therapy and pharmacotherapy of atypical depression. *Journal of Clinical Psychiatry*, 53, 166–170.

Nierenberg, A.A., Fava, M., Trivedi, M.H. *et al.* (2006). STAR*D Study Team: A comparison of lithium and T3 augmentation following two failed medication treatments for depression: A STAR*D report. *American Journal of Psychiatry*, 163, 1519–1530.

Nierenberg, A.A., Alpert, J.E., Pava, J., Rosenbaum, J.F., and Fava, M. (1998). Course and treatment of atypical depression. *Journal of Clinical Psychiatry*, 59 Suppl 18, 5–9.

Norden, M.J. (1994). Buspirone treatment of sexual dysfunction associated with selective serotonin re-uptake inhibitors. *Depression*, 2, 109–112.

Novick, J.S., Stewart, J.W., Wisniewski, S.R. *et al.* (2005). Clinical and demographic features of atypical depression in outpatients with major depressive disorder: Preliminary findings from STAR*D. *Journal of Clinical Psychiatry*, 66, 1002–1011.

Pande, A.C., Birkett, M., Fechner-Batesa, S., Haskett, B.S., and Greden, J.F. (1996). Fluoxetine versus phenelzine in atypical depression. *Biological Psychiatry*, 40, 1017–1020.

Parker, G., Roy, K., Mitchell, P. *et al.* (2002). Atypical depression: A reappraisal. *American Journal of Psychiatry*, 159, 1470–1479.

Parker, G.B. (2007). Atypical depression: A valid subtype? *Journal of Clinical Psychiatry*, 68 Suppl 3, 18–22.

Parsons, B., Quitkin, F.M., McGrath, P.J. *et al.* (1989). Phenelzine, imipramine, and placebo in borderline patients meeting criteria for atypical depression. *Psychopharmacology Bulletin*, 25, 524–534.

Perugi, G., Toni, C., Travierso, M.C., and Akiskal, H.S. (2003). The role of cyclothymia in atypical depression: toward a data-based reconceptualization of the borderline-bipolar II connection. *Journal of Affective Disorders*, 73, 87–98.

Perugi, G., Akiskal, H.S., Lattanxi, L. *et al.* (1998). The high prevalence of "soft" bipolar (II) features in atypical depression *Comprehensive Psychiatry*, 39, 63–71.

Posternak, M.A. and Zimmerman, M. (2001). Symptoms of atypical depression. *Psychiatry Research*, 104, 175–181.

Posternak, M.A. and Zimmerman, M. (2002). Partial validation of atypical features subtype of major depressive disorder. *Archives of General Psychiatry*, 59, 70–76.

Price, J. and Grunhaus, L.J. (1990). Treatment of clomipramine-induced anorgasmia with yohimbine: A case report. *Journal of Clinical Psychiatry*, 51, 32–33.

Quitkin, F.M., Liebowitz, M.R., Stewart, J.W. *et al.* (1984). L-deprenyl in atypical depressives. *Archives of General Psychiatry*, 41, 777–781.

Quitkin, F.M., Stewart, J.W., McGrath, P.J. *et al.* (1988). Phenelzine versus imipramine in the treatment of probable atypical depression: Defining syndrome boundaries of selective MAOI responders. *American Journal of Psychiatry*, 145, 306–311.

Quitkin, F.M., McGrath, P.J., Stewart, J.W. *et al.* (1989). Phenelzine and imipramine in mood reactive depressives: Further delineation of the syndrome of atypical depression. *Archives of General Psychiatry*, 46, 787–793.

Quitkin, F.M., McGrath, P.J., Stewart, J.W. *et al.* (1990). Atypical depression, panic attacks, and response to imipramine and phenelzine: A replication. *Archives of General Psychiatry*, 47, 935–941.

Rabkin, J.G., Stewart, J.W., Quitkin, F.M. *et al.* (1996). Should atypical depression be included in DSM-IV? In Widiger, T.A., Frances, A.J., Pincus, H.A. *et al.*, eds, *DSM-IV Sourcebook*, 2. Washington, DC: American Psychiatric Association, 239–260.

Reimherr, F.W., Wood, D.R., Byerley, B., Brainard, J., and Grosser, B.I. (1984). Characteristics of responders to fluoxetine. *Psychopharmacology Bulletin*, 20, 70–72.

Robertson, H.A., Lam, R.W., Stewart, J.N. *et al.* (1996). Atypical depressive symptoms and clusters in unipolar and bipolar depression. *Acta Psychiatrica Scandanavica*, 94, 421–427.

Robins, E. and Guze, S.B. (1970). Establishment of diagnostic validity in psychiatric illness: Its application to schizophrenia. *American Journal of Psychiatry*, 126, 983–987.

Roose, S.P., Miyazaki, M., Devanand, D. *et al.* (2004). An open trial of venlafaxine for the treatment of late-life atypical depression. *International Journal of Geriatric Psychiatry*, 10, 989–994.

Rush, A.J., Fava, M., Wisniewski, S.R. *et al.* (2004). STAR*D Investigators Group: Sequenced treatment alternatives to relieve depression (STAR*D): rationale and design. *Controlled Clinial Trials*, 25, 119–142.

Rush, A.J., Trivedi, M.H., Wisniewski, S.R. *et al.* (2006). STAR*D Study Team. *New England Journal of Medicine*, 354, 1231–1242.

Sargant, W. (1960). Drugs in the treatment of depression. *British Medical Journal*, 1, 14–17.

Satel, S.L. and Nelson, J.C. (1989). Stimulants in the treatment of depression: A critical overview. *Journal of Clinical Psychiatry*, 50, 241–249.

Søgaard, J., Lane, R., Latimer, P. *et al.* (1999). A 12-week study comparing moclobemide and sertraline in the treatment of outpatients with atypical depression. *Journal of Psychopharmacology*, 13, 406–414.

Sotsky, S.M. and Simmens, S.J. (1999). Pharmacotherapy response and diagnostic validity in atypical depression. *Journal of Affective Disorders*, 54, 237–247.

Stewart, J.W. (2007). Treating depression with atypical features. *Journal of Clinical Psychiatry*, 68 Suppl 3, 25–29.

Stewart, J.W., McGrath, P.J., and Quitkin, F.M. (2002). Do age of onset and course of illness predict different treatment outcome among DSM IV depressive disorders with atypical features? *Neuropsychopharmacology*, 26, 237–245.

Stewart, J.W., McGrath, P.J., Rabkin, J.G., and Quitkin, F.M. (1993). Atypical depression: A valid clinical entity? *Psychiatric Clinics of North America*, 16, 479–495.

Stewart, J.W., Bruder, G.E., McGrath, P.J., and Quitkin, F.M. (2003). Do age of onset and course of illness define biologically distinct groups within atypical depression? *Journal of Abnormal Psychology*, 112, 253–262.

Stewart, J.W., Quitkin, F.M., McGrath, P.J., and Klien, D.F. (2005). Defining the boundaries of atypical depression: Evidence from the HPA axis supports course of illness distinctions. *Journal of Affective Disorders*, 86, 161–167.

Stewart, J.W., Garfinkel, R., Nunes, E.V., Donovan, S., and Klein, D.F. (1998). Atypical features and treatment response in the National Institute of Mental Health Treatment of Depression Collaborative Research Program. *Journal of Clinical Psychopharmacology*, 18, 429–434.

Stratta, P., Bolino, F., Cupillari, M., and Casacchia, M. (1991). A double-blind parallel study comparing fluoxetine with imipramine in the treatment of atypical depression. *International Clinical Psychopharmacology*, 6, 193–196.

Thase, M.E. (2007). New directions in the treatment of atypical depression. *Journal of Clinical Psychiatry*, 68 Suppl 3, 25–29.

Thase, M.E., Malinger, A.G., McKnight, D., and Himmelhoch, J.M. (1992). Treatment of imipramine-resistant recurrent depression: IV. A double-blind crossover study of tranylcypromine for anergic bipolar depression. *American Journal of Psychiatry*, 149, 195–198.

Thase, M.E., Friedman, E.S., Biggs, M.M. *et al.* (2007). Cognitive therapy versus medication in augmentation and switch strategies as second-step treatments: A STAR*D Report. *American Journal of Psychiatry*, 164, 739–752.

Trivedi, M.H., Fava, M., Wisniewski, S.R. *et al.* (2006). Medication augmentation after the failure of SSRIs for depression. *New England Journal of Medicine*, 354, 1243–1252.

West, E.D. and Dalley, P.J. (1959). Effects of iproniazid in depressive syndromes. *British Journal of Medicine*, 1, 1491–1494.

Psychotic depression

Barnett S. Meyers and Jimmy N. Avari

Introduction

Definition

The diagnosis of psychotic major depression (MDpsy) requires that a delusion or hallucination has developed in association with an episode of major depression (MDD) (American Psychiatric Association, 2000). Because MDpsy is a relatively recent addition to psychiatric nomenclature, this chapter begins with a discussion of the historical evolution of MDpsy in relationship to advances in psychopharmacology. A discussion of the public health and prognostic significance of MDpsy follows. The section on Management emphasizes diagnostic and treatment considerations.

Psychotic major depression (MDPsy) consists of an episode of major depression accompanied by delusions, and/or hallucinations. Because MDpsy associated with hallucinations without delusions is rare (Coryell *et al.* 1998), MDpsy is considered equivalent to delusional depression.

Historical background and evolution of the diagnosis

Psychiatric texts from the early twentieth century recognized that delusions and hallucinations occurred in severe cases of depressive illness. Kraepelin (1907) classified patients with both a mood disorder and delusions or hallucinations as suffering from manic depressive illness, whether or not episodes of mania had occurred. Kraepelin and others (Hoch and MacCurdy, 1922, Lewis, 1934) who reported on case series from the pre-electroconvulsive therapy (ECT) era, recognized that the presence of delusions was associated with a poorer prognosis, but did not specify delusional depression as a specific sub-type of illness.

DSM-III (American Psychiatric Association, 1980) formally recognized MDpsy as a distinct sub-type of affective disorder if delusions, hallucinations, or grossly bizarre behavior indicative of impaired reality testing were present. Interest in the syndrome of delusional depression developed following publication of early tricyclic antidepressant (TCA) trials (Friedman *et al.* 1961, Hordern *et al.* 1963) demonstrating that depressions with delusions were associated with poor response rates. The classic report by Glassman *et al.* (1977) demonstrating that high concentrations of imipramine were associated with remission in 95% of patients with nondelusional melancholic depression, in contrast to a 33% remission rate in delusional patients underscored the impact of delusions on treatment response.

The next phase in the diagnostic evolution of MDpsy considered the diagnostic import of the content of delusions and hallucinations. Research Diagnostic criteria (RDC) (Spitzer *et al.* 1975) assigned diagnostic significance to whether the content of psychotic phenomena (delusions and hallucinations) were "nonaffective" and considered specific psychotic phenomena, such as delusions of control and thought insertion or control, as exclusion criteria for MDD. However, a subsequent review demonstrated that delusional content did not distinguish affective psychoses from schizophrenia on either prognosis or treatment response (Pope and Lipinski, 1978). Similarly, Kendler (1991) subsequently reported that the characteristics of delusional phenomena, including their congruence or the presence of "first-rank symptoms" typical of schizophrenia (Schneider 1959), did not have diagnostic or prognostic significance. Thus, the diagnosis of MDpsy does not depend on the content of delusions (American Psychiatric Association, 2000).

Clinical Handbook for the Management of Mood Disorders, ed. J. John Mann, Patrick J. McGrath, and Steven P. Roose.
Published by Cambridge University Press. © Cambridge University Press 2013.

Comparisons between delusional and nondelusional depression

Relationship to bipolar disorder

Multiple studies have demonstrated that MDpsy occurs more frequently in bipolar than in unipolar depression (Guze *et al.* 1975, Endicott *et al.* 1985, Goes *et al.* 2007), although conflicting reports exist (Serretti *et al.* 1999). Longitudinal studies have demonstrated 20% switch rates from unipolar MDpsy to bipolar I disorder (Akiskal *et al.* 1983), with a first affective episode of MDpsy leading to a bipolar course in 37.5% of one cohort of patients (Goes *et al.* 2007). Similarly, a high switch rate occurs among young adults and adolescents with an initial unipolar MDpsy (Strober and Carlson, 1982). In contrast, patients with MDpsy have comparable frequencies of having a unipolar or a bipolar II course (Goes *et al.* 2007).

Although higher rates of bipolar I disorder in the relatives of probands with unipolar MDpsy have been reported (Weissman *et al.* 1984a, Maj *et al.* 2007), evidence for this association is inconsistent (Goes *et al.* 2007).

Relationship of delusions to severity of depressive symptoms

A long-standing controversy exists regarding whether MDpsy represents a more severe variant of unipolar MDD (Frances *et al.* 1981, Koscis *et al.* 1990, Maj *et al.* 1990) or a biologically distinct clinical syndrome (Schatzberg and Rothschild, 1992). Forty *et al.* (2009) addressed this question by comparing the severity of mood symptoms reported during depressive episodes among individuals with recurrent nondelusional depression to symptom severity among individuals who had experienced MDpsy. The within-group comparison demonstrated that more severe depressive symptoms occurred during MDpsy episodes in individuals MDpsy. A comparison between MDpsy and consistently nondelusional patients failed to find between-group differences in severity. These findings parallel the earlier NIMH Collaborative Longitudinal Study's finding that the delusional episodes of MDpsy patients are more severe and last longer than nondelusional episodes (Coryell *et al.* 1996). Also, patients with one MDpsy episode are more likely to have additional psychotic episodes than individuals with

an index nondelusional MDD (Charney and Nelson, 1981a, Lykouras *et al.* 1986). Despite the recent report of high switch rates to other diagnoses over 10 years among individuals with one or more MDpsy episodes, 31.7% of subjects retained the diagnosis of MDpsy at all four assessments, and 54.8% of individuals with an index MDpsy retained the diagnosis of either unipolar or bipolar depression at year 10 (Ruggerio *et al.* 2011). These data are consistent with considering the psychotic features of MDpsy as occurring in individuals who have a vulnerability to developing psychotic symptoms.

Scope of the problem and public health significance

Epidemiology

The community prevalence of MDpsy has been estimated at 0.4%, comprising 20% of individuals meeting criteria for current MDD (Ohayon and Schatzberg, 2002). Rates in psychiatric inpatient settings are higher with a rate of 18.5 to 25% reported in mixed-age inpatients (Guze *et al.* 1975, Coryell *et al.* 1996), which increases to 45% in geriatric psychiatry inpatients (Meyers and Greenberg, 1986).

Costs

Most MDpsy patients receive acute treatment on inpatient services (Gaudiano *et al.* 2009). In the recently completed Study of the Pharmacotherapy of Psychotic Depression (STOP PD-I) (Meyers *et al.* 2009), 69% of the 259 participants began the study as inpatients. Among Medicaid recipients, the annual health care cost per case of depression alone is $5505 compared to $18 318 for each case of MDpsy (Garis *et al.* 2002). The threefold higher costs are attributable to a greater frequency of hospitalizations, longer lengths of stay, and greater use of outpatient mental health specialists by MDpsy patients (Garis *et al.* 2002). MDD is the most common cause of psychiatric admission for Medicare patients (Ettner and Hermann, 1998). Initiation of ECT 5 days or longer after admission and being $\geq$ 65 years of age are associated with more costly and longer hospital stays (Olfson *et al.* 1998), a finding consistent with MDpsy contributing disproportionately to the Medicare costs for inpatient psychiatric care.

Course of illness

Following an initial remission, the risks for relapse and recurrence are high. Observational studies have shown a 17 to 50% relapse rate over 12 months and recurrence rates ranging from 43 to 85%, 4 to 6 years after an initial remission (Spiker *et al.* 1985, Aronson *et al.* 1988, Baldwin 1988, Coryell *et al.* 1996, Naz *et al.* 2007).

Follow-up studies have demonstrated that MDpsy is associated with more residual symptoms and greater functional impairment than nondelusional depression (Johnson *et al.* 1991, Coryell 1998, Maj *et al.* 2007). Among community residents, an index MDspy predicts poorer occupational, marital, and financial status, and an increased likelihood of receiving public assistance 1 year later (Johnson *et al.* 1991).

MDpsy and suicide

High rates of both current episode suicide attempts (18.5%) and lifetime attempts (34%) have been reported (Meyers *et al.* 2009). These data are consistent with previous reports of more frequent suicide attempts in MDpsy than in nonpsychotic depression (Thakur *et al.* 1999, Maj *et al.* 2007, Goes *et al.* 2007). Rates of actual suicide were significantly higher following an initial suicide attempt in MDpsy nonpsychotic MDD during a 4-year follow-up (Suominen *et al.* 2009) and a 25-year follow-up reporting a five times greater risk for suicide after an index MDpsy than after an index nonpsychotic MDD (Roose *et al.* 1983). The poor long-term prognosis is also demonstrated by reports of a twofold greater mortality than in nondelusional MDD over 15 years after controlling for suicides (Vythilingam *et al.* 2003).

Management

Differential diagnosis

Management begins with establishing the diagnosis. DSM-IV (American Psychiatric Association, 2000) recognizes that depression may occur during the prodromal, active, and residual phases of schizophrenia, and limits MDpsy to patients whose episodes of psychosis occur exclusively during episodes of MDD. In contrast to MDpsy, the mood symptoms of schizophrenia are brief in relation to the duration of the psychotic disorder. A diagnosis of schizoaffective disorder is made if psychotic symptoms have persisted for at least 2 weeks without an associated mood disturbance and the patient does not meet the full criteria for schizophrenia. Reliance on historical information about the existence and duration of previous psychotic symptoms complicate the differentiation of schizoaffective disorder from MDpsy (Coryll, 1998) and underscore the importance of obtaining a careful history. Differential diagnosis must also consider nonschizophrenic disorders, such as obsessive compulsive and body dysmorphic disorders, that can be associated with both MDD and psychotic symptoms.

Identification of delusions

Depressive, anxious, and suspicious thought content that might be present must be identified and characterized. Specific attention is given to determine whether preoccupations that developed during the MDD are resistant to the laws of logic and affect behavior. Although the disturbed mood of MDD generally influences thought content, patients with unwavering conviction about the validity of their depressive or frightening concerns are susceptible to giving up hope, acting irrationally, and being nonadherent to prescribed treatments. The belief that a condition is hopeless is inconsistent with taking prescribed medications. Suicide may result from fixed beliefs of deserved punishment, impending financial ruin, or hopelessness. Establishing whether delusions are present and whether these ideas are likely to affect behavior is critical to deciding whether patients require inpatient treatment.

We have previously demonstrated that conviction about depressive ruminations can be reliably assessed in MDpsy patients by evaluating the patient's "subjective sense of certainty" and establishing whether the patient can "accommodate" to the interviewer's use of confrontation. Accommodation includes assessing the patient's ability to consider evidence that the idea might result from the current state of depression and might not be a valid concern (Meyers *et al.* 2006). After training of interviewers, inter-rater reliability for a factor of "conviction" was 0.77, with conviction most strongly reflecting the patient's "subjective sense of certainty" and ability to "accommodate" to the interviewer's offer of alternative explanations. Therefore, clinicians can reliably identify the presence of delusional ideas when historical information is integrated with a careful assessment of current concerns.

Obstacles to diagnosis

The emphasis on high volume clinical practice that is endemic to modern emergency rooms and short-length-of-stay inpatient psychiatric units militates against careful clinical assessment. Data from participants in STOP PD I demonstrated that the present of psychotic features was commonly "missed" among patients admitted to academic medical centers (Rothschild *et al.* 2008). A review of the charts of study participants, all of whom had a well-defined delusion based on a research interview, found that a diagnosis of psychotic depression was not listed, including as a rule-out, in 39% of subjects' emergency room charts and missed in >20% of inpatient charts. Missing the diagnosis of MDpsy was associated with failures to identify either delusions or hallucinations (Rothschild *et al.* 2008).

Choice of treatment setting

Assessment of delusions must consider the "impact" of irrational beliefs that may be present. Impact refers specifically to the extent to which patients with MDpsy are distressed by and initiate actions based on their delusions (Meyers *et al.* 2006). Clinicians easily recognize the distress that ruminations about ideas of guilt, financial ruin, persecution, and disease cause their patients, but too infrequently consider the possible consequences of this distress. Acting on a belief is a corollary of conviction. Thus, patients with somatic delusions will make frequent visits to specialists, and patients with paranoid delusions will commonly ask for police assistance. Patients with more focused depressive delusions of guilt, impending financial disaster, or hopelessness, will consider ways to protect loved ones from being harmed by their problems. These patients frequently consider suicide to both relieve their own pain and protect family. Friends, family members, and previous caregivers are generally aware of the patient's depressive ideas and actions that have been based on them. Having expressed suicidal thoughts or making a will indicate the patient is at high risk for suicide. If suicidal ideation is denied in the presence of delusions of hopelessness or deserved punishment, the clinician should inquire about reasons why suicide was not considered in light of these firmly held pessimistic beliefs. A patient's denial of having suicidal ideation should not be accepted as an absence of risk. Both MDpsy patients and their family members, when practical, should be involved in a discussion of suicide to minimize both the short- and longer-term risks.

Determining a patient's imminent risk for suicide is critical for determining whether hospital treatment is required. Although the infrequency of suicide undermines the systematic investigation of risk factors, a strong family history of suicide, having made previous suicide attempts, and the presence of delusions all increase suicidal risk. Even if these risk factors are not present, clinicians should be particularly vigilant about suicide risk in patients who are preoccupied with delusions of guilt or hopelessness that could logically justify a suicidal act.

Acute treatment

An appropriate goal of acute treatment is to achieve both the remission of major depression and the resolution of delusional ideas. Empirical data on the time course of recovery from these domains of psychopathology are not available, nor do we know the extent to which full remission is associated with the insight that a previously held delusional idea was irrational.

The number of randomized placebo-controlled trials (RCTs) for the treatment of MDpsy is limited. Early evidence that placebo is ineffective (Glassman and Roose, 1981, Spiker and Kupfer, 1988), concerns about the severity of illness in trial participants, and reliance on inpatient services have limited the use of placebo arms in RCTs. As a result, nearly all RCTs for MDpsy use active comparators with the result that participants know they will receive a treatment that might be effective. Furthermore, investigators have used different methods for establishing the presence of delusions without a consistent measurement of delusional resolution.

Combination pharmacotherapy: antidepressants plus an antipsychotic

Spiker *et al.* (1986) reported results from the first NIMH-supported controlled trial of pharmacotherapy for MDpsy. High doses (approximately 50 mg/d) of perphenazine, a phenothiazine-type antipsychotic, combined with serum-level-controlled treatment with the tricyclic antidepressant amitriptyline was associated with a 78% remission rate, compared to a 41% frequency with an average of 217 mg/d of amitriptyline. Additional support for combination therapy was provided in reviews of comparison studies (Kroessler *et al.* 1985, Chan *et al.* 1987), a retrospective analysis of the dose–response relationship to combination therapy (Nelson *et al.* 1986), and a comprehensive meta-analysis that demonstrated numerical but not statistical superiority for combination treatment (Parker *et al.* 1992). These results and the evidence from studies of electroconvulsive therapy (ECT) described below led to the recommendation of combination antipsychotic and antidepressant treatment or ECT for MDpsy in the American Association Practice Guidelines of 2000 and 2010 (American Psychiatric Association, 2000, American Psychiatric Aassociation, 2010).

Nevertheless, the dearth of comparisons between combination treatment and monotherapy prevents drawing a firm conclusion. Thus, a recent meta-analysis concluded that "there is no evidence for the clinical belief that an antidepressant alone is ineffective for the treatment of psychotic depression" (Wijkstra *et al.* 2006). By pooling the data from three comparisons of combination treatment to antipsychotic monotherapy, Wijkstra *et al.* (2006) demonstrated the superiority of combination therapy; however, pooling data from the two combination therapies versus TCA comparison trials available at that time, Spiker *et al.* 1985 and Mulsant *et al.* 2001 did not demonstrate superiority for combination treatment.

Of interest, positive antidepressant monotherapy studies in the Wijkstra *et al.* meta-analysis (2006) were conducted using therapeutic concentrations of imipramine in subjects with mood-congruent delusions. A post-hoc analysis of pooled data from previously published RCTs (Birkenhager *et al.* 2008), found that the 40 subjects with mood-congruent delusions randomized to imipramine had significantly higher response rates than nondelusional subjects treated with imipramine. The sample was limited to subjects with delusions of guilt/sin, paranoia, somaticism, nihilism, and poverty, with two participants reporting hallucinations. Nondelusional subjects had numerically longer-duration episodes and had failed prior pharmacotherapy more frequently, factors that would contribute to the superiority of imipramine in the mood-congruent MDpsy subjects. Also, pooled data from RCTs comparing TCAs to other antidepressants demonstrated significantly higher response rates to imipramine in mood congruent MDpsy subjects than to non-TCA antidepressants (mirtazapine and fluvoxamine) (Bruijn *et al.* 1996, Van den Broek *et al.* 2004). A recent trial demonstrated that high

doses of venlafaxine (target of 375 mg/d) combined with 600 mg of quetiapine had greater efficacy than monotherapy with either venlafaxine or imipramine. Most participants had mood-congruent delusions and none had only mood-incongruent. Therefore, despite some studies demonstrating that mood-congruent MDpsy may respond to therapeutic concentrations of imipramine, the accumulated literature is consistent with practice guidelines endorsing the use of combination treatment and not antidepressant monotherapy as an acute pharmacological treatment of MDpsy (American Psychiatric Association, 2000).

One of two parallel trials that compared fixed ratios of combined olanzapine and fluoxetine to olanzapine monotherapy and placebo also demonstrated the superiority of combination treatment (Rothschild *et al.* 2004). Although the explanation for the unusually high placebo response rates in both trials is uncertain, the use of 23 sites in these industry-sponsored studies and the requirement that participants begin as inpatients until a pre-specified level of improvement was achieved may have contributed to rapid early improvement. Results from the four-site NIMH-supported STOP PD trial provide the strongest evidence for the efficacy of combination therapy (Meyers *et al.* 2009). Of 259 MDpsy subjects with mood-congruent and/or -incongruent delusions, the remission rate of 41.9% associated with combined olanzapine plus sertraline was comparable to remission rates reported in RCTs of nondelusional depression and was significantly higher than the 23.9% remission rate associated with olanzapine plus placebo. Also, STOP PD was the first study to demonstrate the efficacy of combination therapy in geriatric MDpsy. Efficacy in the 142 older subjects with an average age of 71.2 was numerically superior and statistically comparable to that in younger adults.

ECT

The effectiveness of ECT for psychotic major depression observed during the first half of the twentieth century (Lewis, 1934) received empirical support by the report that only 40% of these patients responded to high doses of imipramine compared to an 83% response rate to ECT (Avery and Lubrano, 1979). A subsequent British RCT of ECT demonstrated a clear efficacy of real compared to sham ECT among patients with delusional MDD, a difference that was not observed in nondelusional MDD (Buchan *et al.* 1992). Additional support for greater efficacy of ECT in MDpsy comes from the CORE study in which 96% of MDpsy participants achieved remission compared to 83% in subjects with nonpsychotic MDD (Petrides *et al.* 2001).

Novel approaches: mifepristone and the glucocorticoid hypothesis

Episodes of MDpsy have been associated with dysregulation of the hypothalamic pituitary axis with hypercortisolemia (Schatzberg *et al.* 1985, Nelson and Davis, 1997, Duval *et al.* 2006). Mifepristone, a potent central glucocorticoid receptor antagonist, has been studied as a potential treatment. Early small-sample-size studies demonstrated rapid early improvement in psychotic symptoms but not depression without persistence of benefits (Belanoff 2001, 2002, DeBattista *et al.* 2006). A recent placebo-controlled trial failed to demonstrate efficacy overall (Blasey, 2011), but demonstrated a rapid and sustained benefit in association with mifepristone among subjects who achieved pre-specified high plasma levels. The potential benefits of using mifepristone to modulate the excess central glucocorticoid activity hypothesized to stimulate the psychotic features of MDpsy remains under investigation.

Maintenance and continuation treatment

Remarkably little systematic data is available to guide continuation treatment to prevent relapses in the 4–6 months following remission and no studies are available on the prevention of recurrences after 6 months. Follow-up studies in both young adults (Robinson and Spiker, 1985) and geriatric patients (Flint and Rifat, 1998) have demonstrated greater chronicity and higher relapse rates in MDpsy than in patients with nondelusional depression when medications associated with the initial remission were continued. Nevertheless, the specific contribution of continuing antipsychotic medications was not assessed. In an open trial, Rothschild and Duval (2003) demonstrated that discontinuation of the antipsychotic medication in MDpsy patients who had remained in remission during 4 months of continuation combination therapy was associated with a 27% relapse rate over the next 8 months. The finding of low relapse rates and gradually increasing remission during 4 months of continuing the treatment associated with remission

(Wijkstra *et al.* 2010a) argues against discontinuing a medication associated with an initial response.

Deciding about continuation and maintenance treatment following ECT is also hindered by limited systematic data. Spiker *et al.* (1985) demonstrated a 50% relapse rate among delusional depression patients after successful ECT, which included a 75% rate of rehospitalization following relapse. Sackheim's post-ECT RCT of continuation pharmacotherapy (Sackeim *et al.* 2001) found higher relapse rates among initially nondelusional subjects than those with MDpsy, but initial treatment resistance, which was a significant predictor of early relapse, was more common among nondelusional subjects. The CORE study (Kellner *et al.* 2006) found that continuation ECT and pharmacotherapy using combined lithium plus nortriptyline were associated with comparable 6-month relapse rates of 37.1% and 31.6% respectively. As in Sackeim's study, MDpsy was associated with lower relapse rates, but the contribution of initial treatment resistance to relapse rates was not assessed. Relapse within 1 week of the last ECT occurred in 5.9% of remitters in the Sackeim study (2001) and in 20.5% of remitters in the Kellner *et al.* trial (2006), underscoring the importance of rapidly initiating continuation treatment. The only RCT comparing continuation combination treatment to TCA monotherapy following remission with ECT found a 27% overall relapse rate over 6 months without an effect for treatment assignment (Meyers *et al.* 2001). The relapse rate in this geriatric sample was comparable to the 27% overall rate reported by Kellner *et al.* (2006) in mixed-age adults.

A post-hoc analysis of pooled data from continuation RCTs comparing relapse rates in unipolar MDpsy to nonpsychotic depression, found lower rates in MDpsy at 1 year after controlling for both the duration of the index episode and whether post-remission assignment had been to placebo continuation (Birkenhager *et al.* 2005). Few subjects had been rated as treatment resistant initially. Only 1 of the 29 MDpsy subjects who received imipramine or imipramine plus lithium after remission relapsed in the initial 4 months and none relapsed in the subsequent 8 months of follow-up, a finding suggesting that continuation pharmacotherapy may be more effective for MDpsy than for nondelusional MDD.

Whether post-remission combination treatment is more efficacious than monotherapy for preventing relapses of unipolar MDpsy following remission with either ECT or combination treatment has not been studied. A current NIMH-supported RCT (STOP PD-II) will compare 36 weeks of continuation combination therapy with olanzapine plus sertraline, to sertraline plus placebo to assess whether continuing an atypical antipsychotic medication reduces the risk of relapse. Despite the limited empirical data to guide a best practice approach, results from acute studies and clinical experience are consistent with continuing combination treatment following remission. Gradual tapering of the antipsychotic can be considered after a minimum of 6 months, while considering side effects from the antipsychotic, the frequency and severity of previous episodes, and whether suicidality occurred during previous MDpsy episodes.

Case example

History and presenting symptoms

Ms. G, a 75-year-old widow was referred for psychiatric admission to treat symptoms of sadness, anhedonia, diminished energy, poor appetite, poor concentration, and somatic ruminations about memory loss. She had not received psychiatric treatment previously. Ms. G's present illness began 6 months earlier and was marked by increasing crying spells, social withdrawal, and repeated visits to her primary care physician and specialists for evaluation of her memory. She had voiced concerns that she had "Alzheimer's disease" or a "brain tumor" and had informed her family that her physicians were "missing something." Ms. G had repeatedly discounted her internist's reassurance that her memory was normal. She had been referred to a neurologist and then to a neuropsychologist. Both neuroimaging studies and neuropsychological testing were normal. Ms. G's admission was precipitated by repeated tearful phone calls to family members during which she expressed feelings of hopelessness.

Hospital treatment and post-hospital course

Ms. G was diagnosed as suffering from a major depression with pessimistic and somatic ruminations. Although she complained the test was too difficult, Ms. G achieved a score of 28 on her Mini Mental State Examination, despite frequently doubting her responses. A diagnosis of major depression associated with subjective complaints of memory impairment and anxiety about having an undiagnosed brain disease. Clinical assessment and functioning in the hospital did not reveal evidence of cognitive impairment.

Ms. G denied having suicidal ideation, but admitted that she would want to die if she was suffering from an incurable brain disease. She was reassured that poor concentration and a decrease in memory are commonly associated with depression and that these symptoms were normal in a depressed person of her age.

Ms. G was treated with sertraline, an SSRI, at a dose of 100 mg/d. Her mood brightened with increased engagement in activities during 2 weeks of hospital treatment and she acknowledged that her depression was "50% better." Ms. G remained concerned that she was suffering from an undiagnosed brain disease, but appeared less preoccupied with the idea that she was losing her memory. Ms. G was discharged as moderately improved and referred to a psychiatrist in her community. Shortly after discharge, Ms. G made a consultation appointment with a different neurologist. After examining Ms. G and reviewing her records, the neurologist informed her that further testing was not needed and advised Ms. G to discuss her concerns with her psychiatrist. Ms. G returned home, but took a lethal overdose of all the medicine in her cabinet that night. She left a suicide note explaining to her family that she did not wish to burden them with caring for a person with dementia.

Comment

Ms. G exemplifies a patient with MDpsy associated with a somatic delusion that was not identified or successfully treated and who had an unrecognized risk for suicide. Despite the fact that reassurance was ineffective, the possibility that Ms. G's cognitive concerns were delusional and required additional specific treatment was not recognized by the treatment staff. Her wish to die if an incurable brain disease was present was not explored. Her thoughts about dying and awareness that she did not have an incurable brain disease were not monitored as her depressed feelings improved. Careful inquiry might have determined whether Ms. G's cognitive concerns were delusional and whether additional treatment with ECT or adding an antipsychotic medication was needed. By attributing Ms. G's initially marked memory complaints and their persistence to depression and aging, treating clinicians missed the opportunity to identify and then treat a delusional belief that contributed to Ms. G's suicide. Her post-hospital course is consistent with improvement in depression and an associated increase in activity without resolution of her somatic delusion.

Conclusions

Unipolar MDpsy is a severe disorder that is highly recurrent but can be effectively treated with either combination pharmacotherapy or ECT. Based on current knowledge, antidepressant monotherapy is considered inadequate. The identification of delusions can be difficult, particularly the differentiation of depressive delusions from pessimistic ruminations that are not held with delusional conviction. The increased risk of suicide associated with MDpsy may result from patients acting as though their beliefs were valid. Suicidal acts may be more likely when guilty delusions of deserved punishment or somatic delusions associated with hopelessness are present. Also, delusional beliefs are obstacles to seeking and adhering to treatment. Therefore, inpatient treatment is generally required to both maximize patient safety and assure adherence.

The outcomes of untreated or inadequately treated MDpsy are poor, with high rates of suicide attempts, recurrences, and residual disability. Therefore, effective acute, maintainence, and continuation treatments are critical. For individuals who achieve remission with ECT, maintainence treatment should be initiated rapidly. A combination of the doses of TCAs and lithium that achieve standard therapeutic concentrations appears to prevent relapses. Among patients who remit with combination pharmacotherapy, continuing the treatment associated with remission appears to be effective, but relapse-prevention studies are needed to determine the risks vs. benefits of continuing the antipsychotic. Novel treatments designed to address the hypothesized pathophysiology of MDpsy have been promising and are ongoing.

References

Akiskal, P., Walker, V.R., Puzantian, D. *et al.* (1983). Bipolar outcome in the course of depressive illness. *Journal of Affective Disorders*, 5, 115–128.

American Psychiatric Association (1968). *Diagnostic and Statistical Manual of Mental Disorders, Second Edition (DSM II)*. Washington DC: American Psychiatric Association.

American Psychiatric Association (1980). *Diagnostic and Statistical Manual of Mental Disorders, Third Edition (DSM III)*. Washington DC: American Psychiatric Association.

American Psychiatric Association (2000). Practice guideline for the treatment of patients with major depressive disorder (revision). *American Journal of Psychiatry*, 157 Suppl 4, 1–45.

American Psychiatric Association (2010). *Practice Guideline for the Treatment of Patients with Major Depressive Disorder, Third Edition*. Washington DC: American Psychiatric Association.

Andreescu, C., Mulsant, B.H., Peasley-Miklus, C. *et al.* (2007). Persisting low use of antipsychotic the treatment of major depression with psychotic features. *Journal of Clinical Psychiatry*, 68, 194–200.

Aronson, T.A., Shukla, S., Gujavarty, K. *et al.* (1988). Relapse in delusional depression: A retrospective study of the course of treatment. *Comprehensive Psychiatry*, 29, 12–21.

Avery, D. and Lubrano, A. (1979). Depression treated with imipramine and ECT: The DeCarolis study reconsidered. *American Journal of Psychiatry*, 136, 559–562.

Baldwin, R.C. (1988). Delusional and non-delusional depression in late life: Evidence for distinct subtypes. *British Journal of Psychiatry*, 153, 39–44.

Belanoff, J.K., Flores, B.H., Kalezhan, M. *et al.* (2001). Rapid reversal of psychotic depression using mifepristone. *Journal of Clinical Psychopharmacology*, 21, 516–521.

Belanoff, J.K., Rothschild, A.J., Cassidy, F. *et al.* (2002). An open label trial of C-1073 (mifepristone) for psychotic major depression. *Biological Psychiatry*, 52, 386–392.

Birkenhager, T.K., Van den Broek, W.W., Mulder, P.G. *et al.* (2005). One year outcome of psychotic depression after ECT. *Journal of ECT*, 21, 221–226.

Birkenhager, T.K., Van den Broek, W.W., Mulder, P.G. *et al.* (2008). Efficacy of imipramine in psychotic versus nonpsychotic depression. *Journal of Clinical Psychopharmacology*, 28, 166–170.

Blasey, C.M., Block, C.M., Belanoff, J.K. *et al.* (2011). Efficacy and safety of mifepristone for the treatment of psychotic depression. *Journal of Clinical Psychopharmacology*, 31, 436–440.

Bruijn, A.J., Moleman, P., Mulder, P.G.H. *et al.* (1996). A double-blind fixed blood-level study comparing mirtazapine with imipramine in depressed in-patients. *Psychopharmacology*, 127, 231–237.

Buchanan, H., Johnstone, E., McPherson, K. *et al.* (1992). Who benefits from electroconvulsive therapy? Combined results from the Leicester and Northwick Park Trials. *British Journal of Psychiatry*, 160, 355–359.

Chan, C.H., Janicak, P.G., Davis, J.M. *et al.* (1987). Response of psychotic and nonpsychotic depressed patients to tricyclic antidepressants. *Journal of Clinical Psychiatry*, 48, 197–200.

Charney, D.S. and Nelson, J.C. (1981). Delusional and nondelusional unipolar depression: Further evidence for distinct subtypes. *American Journal of Psychiatry*, 138, 328–333.

Coryell, W. (1998). The treatment of psychotic depression. *Journal of Clinical Psychiatry*, 59 suppl 1, 22–27.

Coryell, W., Zimmerman, M., and Pfohl, B. (1986). Outcome at discharge and six months in major depression: The significance of psychotic features. *Journal of Nervous and Mental Disease*, 174, 92–96.

Coryell, W., Leon, A., Winokur, G. *et al.* (1996). Importance of psychotic symptoms to long-term course of major depression. *American Journal of Psychiatry*, 153, 483–489.

DeBattista, C., Belanoff, J., Glass, S. *et al.* (2006). Mifepristone versus placebo in the treatment of psychosis in patients with psychotic major depression. *Biological Psychiatry*, 60, 1343–1349.

Duval, F., Mokrani, M.-C., and Monreal-Ortiz, J.A. (2006). Cortisol hypersecretion in unipolar major depression with melancholic and psychotic features: Dopaminergic, noradrenergic and thyroid correlates. *Psychoneuroendocrinology*, 31, 876–888.

Endicott, J., Nee, J., Andreasen, N. *et al.* (1985). Bipolar II. Combine or keep separate? *Journal of Affective Disorders*, 8, 17–28.

Ettner, S.L. and Hermann, R.C. (1998). Inpatient psychiatric treatment of elderly Medicare beneficiaries. *Psychiatric Services*, 49, 1173–1179.

Flint, A.J. and Rifat, S.L. (1998). Two-year outcome of psychotic depression in late life. *American Journal of Psychiatry*, 155, 178–183.

Folstein, M.F., Folstein, S.E., and McHugh, P.R. (1975). Mini-Mental State: A practical method for grading the cognitive state of patients for the clinician. *Journal of Psychiatric Research*, 12, 189–198.

Forty, L., Jones, L., Jones, I. *et al.* (2009). Is depression severity the sole cause of psychotic symptoms during an episode of unipolar major depression? A study both between and within subjects. *Journal of Affective Disorders*, 114, 103–109.

Frances, A., Brown, R.P., Kocsis, J.H. *et al.* (1981). Psychotic depression: A distinct entity? *American Journal of Psychiatry*, 138, 831–833.

Friedman, C., Mowbray, M.S., and Hamilton, V.J. (1961). Imipramine (Tofranil) in depressive states. *Journal of Mental Science*, 107, 948–953.

Garis, R.I. and Farmer, K.C. (2002). Examining costs of chronic conditions in a Medicaid population. *Managed Care*, 11, 43–50.

Gaudiano, B.A., Dalrymple, K.L., and Zimmerman, M. (2009). Prevalence and clinical characteristics of psychotic versus nonpsychotic major depression in a general psychiatric outpatient clinic. *Depression and Anxiety*, 26, 54–64.

Glassman, A. and Roose, S. (1981). Delusional depression. *Archives of General Psychiatry*, 38, 424–427.

Glassman, A.H., Perel, J.M., Shostak, M., Kantor, S.J., and Fleiss, J.L. (1977). Clinical implications of imipramine plasma levels for depressive illness. *Archives of General Psychiatry*, 34, 197–204.

Goes, F.S., Sadler, B., Toolan, J. *et al.* (2007). Psychotic features in bipolar and unipolar depression. *Bipolar Disorders*, 9, 901–906.

Guze, S.B., Woodruff, R.A., and Clayton, P.J. (1975). The significance of psychotic affective disorders. *Archives of General Psychiatry*, 32, 1147–1150.

Hoch, A. and MacCurdy, J.T. (1922). The prognosis of involutionary melancholia. *Archives of Neurology and Psychiatry*, 7, 1–17.

Hordern, A., Holt, N.F., Burt, C.G. *et al.* (1963). Amitriptyline in depressive states. *British Journal of Psychiatry*, 109, 815–825.

Johnson, J., Horwath, E., and Weissman, M.M. (1991). The validity of major depression with psychotic features based on a community sample. *Archives of General Psychiatry*, 48, 1075–1081.

Kellner, C.H., Knapp, R., Petrides, G. *et al.* (2006). Continuation electroconvulsive therapy vs pharmacotherapy for relapse prevention in major depression. *Archives of General Psychiatry*, 63, 1337–1344.

Kendler, K.S. (1991). Mood-incongruent psychotic affective illness. *Archives of General Psychiatry*, 48, 362–369.

Kocsis, J.H., Croughan, J.L., Katz, M.M. *et al.* (1990). Response to treatment with antidepressants of patients with severe or moderate nonpsychotic depression and of patients with psychotic depression. *American Journal of Psychiatry*, 147, 621–624.

Kraepelin, E. (Diefendorf, A.R., trans.) (1907). *Clinical Psychiatry: A Textbook for Students and Physicians*. New York, NY: Macmillan Publishing Co. Inc.

Kroessler, D. (1985). Relative efficacy rates for therapies of delusional depression. *Convulsive Therapy*, 1, 173–182.

Lewis, A.J. (1934). Melancholia: a clinical survey of depressive states. *Journal of Medical Science*, 80, 277–378.

Lykouras, E., Malliaras, D., Christodoulou, G.N. *et al.* (1986). Delusional depression: Phenomenology and response to treatment, a prospective study. *Acta Psychiatric a Scandinavica*, 73, 324–329.

Maj, M., Pirozzi, R., and Di Caprio E. (1990). Major depression with mood-congruent psychotic features: a distinct diagnostic entity or a more severe subtype of depression? *Acta Psychiatrica Scandinavica*, 82, 439–444.

Maj, M., Pirozzi, R., and Magliano, L. (2007). Phenomenology and prognostic significance of delusions in major depressive disorder: A 10-year prospective follow-up study. *Journal of Clinical Psychiatry*, 68, 1411–1417.

Meyers, B.S. and Greenberg, R. (1986). Late-life delusional depression. *Journal of Affective Disorders*, 11, 133–137.

Meyers, B.S., Klimstra, S.A., Gabriele, M. *et al.* (2001). Continuation treatment of delusional depression in older adults. *American Journal of Geriatric Psychiatry*, 9, 415–422.

Meyers, B.S., English, J.M., Peasley-Micklus, C. *et al.* (2006). Delusion assessment scale for psychotic major depression: Reliability, validity and utility. *Biological Psychiatry*, 60, 1336–1342.

Meyers, B.S., Flint, A.J., Rothschild, A.J. *et al.* (2009). A double-blind randomized controlled trial of olanzapine plus sertraline vs. olanzapine plus placebo for psychotic depression: The Study of Pharmacotherapy of Psychotic Depression (STOP-PD). *Archives of General Psychiatry*, 66, 838–847.

Mugdha, T., Hays, J., and Krishnan, K.R.R. (1999). Clinical, demographic and social characteristics of psychotic depression. *Psychiatric Research*, 86, 99–106.

Mulsant, B.H., Sweet, R.A., Rosen, J. *et al.* (2001). A double-blind randomized comparison of nortriptyline plus perphenazine versus nortriptyline plus placebo in the treatment of psychotic depression in late life. *Journal of Clinical Psychiatry*, 62, 597–604.

Naz, B., Craig, T.J., Bromet, E.J. *et al.* (2007). Remission and relapse after the first hospital admission in psychotic depression: A 4-year naturalistic follow-up. *Psychological Medicine*, 37, 1173–1181.

Nelson, J.C. and Davis, J.M. (1997). DST studies in psychotic depression: A meta-analysis. *American Journal of Psychiatry*, 154, 1497–1503.

Nelson, J.C., Price, L.H., and Jatlow, P.I. (1986). Neuroleptic dose and desipramine concentrations during combined treatment of unipolar delusional depression. *American Journal of Psychiatry*, 143, 1151–1154.

Ohayon, M.M. and Schatzberg, A.F. (2002). Prevalence of depressive episodes with psychotic features in the general population. *American Journal of Psychiatry*, 159, 1855–1861.

Olfson, M., Marcus, S., Sackeim, H.A. *et al.* (1998). Use of ECT for the inpatient treatment of recurrent depression. *American Journal of Psychiatry*, 155, 22–29.

Parker, G., Roy, K., Hadzi-Pavlovic, D., and Pedic F. (1992). Psychotic (delusional) depression: A meta-analysis of physical treatments. *Journal of Affective Disorders*, 24, 17–24.

Parker, G., Hadzi-Pavlovic, D., Hickie, I. *et al.* (1991). Distinguishing psychotic and non-psychotic melancholia. *Journal of Affective Disorders*, 22, 135–148.

Petrides, G., Fink, M., Husain, M.M. *et al.* (2001). ECT remission rates in psychotic versus nonpsychotic depressed patients: A report from CORE. *Journal of ECT*, 17, 244–253.

Pope, H.G., Jr., and Lipinski, J.F. (1978). Diagnosis in schizophrenia and manic-depressive illness: Reassessment of the specificity of "schizophrenic" symptoms in the light of current research. *Archives of General Psychiatry*, 35, 811–828.

Robinson, D.G. and Spiker, D.G. (1985). Delusional depression: A one-year follow-up. *Journal of Affective Disorders*, 9, 79–83.

Roose, S.P., Glassman, T., Woodring, S., and Vital-Herne, J. (1983). Depression, delusions and suicide. *American Journal of Psychiatry*, 140, 1159–1162.

Rothschild, A.J. and Duval, S.E. (2003). How long should patients with psychotic depression stay on the antipsychotic medication? *Journal of Clinical Psychiatry*, 64, 390–396.

Rothschild, A.J., Williamson, D.J., Tohen, M.F. *et al.* (2004). A double-blind, randomized study of olanzapine and olanzapine/fluoxetine combination for major depression with psychotic features. *Journal of Clinical Psychopharmacology*, 24, 365–373.

Rothschild, A.J., Winer, J., Flint, A.J. *et al.* (2008). Missed diagnosis of psychotic depression at 4 academic centers. *Journal of Clinical Psychiatry*, 69, 1293–1296.

Ruggerior, C.J., Kotov, R., and Carlson, G.A. (2011). Diagnostic consistency of major depression with psychosis across 10 years. *Journal of Clinical Psychiatry*, 72, 1207–1213.

Sackeim, H.A., Haskett, R.F., Mulsant, B.H. *et al.* (2001). Continuation pharmacotherapy in the prevention of relapse following electroconvulsive therapy: A randomized controlled trial. *Journal of the American Medical Association*, 285, 1299–1307.

Serretti, A., Lattuada, E., Cusin, C. *et al.* (1999). Clinical and demographic features of psychotic and nonpsychotic depression. *Comprehensive Psychiatry*, 40, 358–362.

Schatzberg, A.F. and Rothschild, A.J. (1992). Psychotic (delusional) major depression: Should it be included as a distinct syndrome in DSM-IV? *American Journal of Psychiatry*, 149, 733–745.

Schatzberg, A.F., Rothschild, A.J., Langlais, P.J. *et al.* (1985). A corticosteroid/dopamine hypothesis for psychotic depression and related states. *Journal of Psychiatric Research*, 19, 57–64.

Schneider, K. (Hamilton, M.W., trans.) (1959). *Clinical Psychopathology*. New York, NY: Grune and Stratton Inc.

Simpson, G.M., El Sheshai, A., Rady, A. *et al.* (2003). Sertraline as monotherapy in the treatment of psychotic and nonpsychotic depression. *Journal of Clinical Psychiatry*, 64, 959–965.

Spiker, D. and Kupfer, D. (1988). Placebo response rates in psychotic and nonpsychotic depression. *Journal of Affective Disorders*, 14, 21–23.

Spiker, D.G., Stein, J., and Rich, C.L. (1985). Delusional depression and electroconvulsive therapy. One year later. *Convulsive Therapy*, 1, 167–172.

Spiker, D.G., Weiss, J.C., Dealy, R.S. *et al.* (1986). The pharmacological treatment of delusional depression. *American Journal of Psychiatry*, 142, 430–436.

Spitzer, R.L., Endicott, J., and Robins, E. (1975). *Research Diagnostic Criteria for a Selected Group of Functional Disorders, Second Edition*. New York, NY: New York State Psychiatric Institute.

Strober, M. and Carlson, G. (1982). Bipolar illness in adolescents with major depression. *Archives of General Psychiatry*, 39, 549–555.

Suominen, K., Haukka, J., Valtonen, H.M., and Lönnqvist, J. (2009). Outcome of patients with major depressive disorder after serious suicide attempt. *Journal of Clinical Psychiatry*, 70, 1372–1378.

Thakur, M., Hays, J., and Krishnan, R.R. (1999). Clinical, demographic and social characteristics of psychotic depression. *Psychiatry Research*, 86, 99–106.

Van den Broek, W.W., Birkenhager, T.K., Mulder, P.G.H. *et al.* (2004). A double-blind study of comparing imipramine with fluvoxamine in depressed inpatients. *Psychopharmacology*, 175, 481–486.

Vythilingam, M., Chen, J., Bremner, J.D. *et al.* (2003). Psychotic depression and mortality. *American Journal of Psychiatry*, 160, 574–576.

Weissman, M.M., Prusoff, B.A., and Merikangas, K.R. (1984). Is delusional depression related to bipolar disorder? *American Journal of Psychiatry*, 141, 892–893.

Wijkstra, J., Lijmer, J., Balk, F.J. *et al.* (2006). Pharmacological treatment of unipolar psychotic depression. *British Journal of Psychiatry*, 188, 410–415.

Wijkstra, J., Burger, H., Van den Broek, W.W. *et al.* (2010a). Long-term response to acute pharmacological treatment of psychotic depression. *Journal of Affective Disorders*, 123, 238–242.

Wijkstra, J., Burther, H., Van den Broek, W.W. *et al.* (2010b). Treatment of unipolar psychotic depression: A randomized, double-blind study comparing imipramine, venlafaxine and venlafaxine plus quetiapine. *Acta Psychiatrica Scandinavica*, 121, 190–200.

Pharmacologic and somatic treatments for bipolar depression

Lucas Giner, S. Aidan Kelly, and Maria A. Oquendo

Bipolar disorder is a chronic disease that generates high annual costs, estimated at about $US45 billion in 1991 (Wyatt and Henter, 1995), with higher costs expected currently (Kleinman *et al.* 2003). Depression is the most prevalent phase of bipolar disorder (Judd and Akiskal, 2003), up to three times more common than others (Kupka *et al.* 2007). The depressive phase of bipolar disorder, known as bipolar depression, causes patients disability similar to or greater than a manic phase of equivalent severity (Altshuler *et al.* 2006). Moreover, minor depression and sub-syndromal depression are more chronic and as a result can cause more psychosocial disability than hypomania and sub-syndromal hypomania (Judd *et al.* 2005). Disability also appears to increase according to the severity of depressive symptoms, both in subjects with bipolar disorder I and with bipolar disorder II (Judd *et al.* 2005). Likewise, patients with depressive symptomatology experience lower quality of life than those with symptoms of hypomania, mania, or euthymia (Vojta *et al.* 2001, Zhang *et al.* 2006). Finally and critically, the majority of suicides among bipolar patients occur during depressive or mixed states (Isometsa *et al.* 1994, Valtonen *et al.* 2007), as do most suicide attempts (Dilsaver *et al.* 1997, Valtonen *et al.* 2008).

For all these reasons, preventing and managing the depressive phase is essential. Nonetheless, the majority of research has focused on treatment of the manic phase and until recently, as indicated by Fountoulakis and Vieta (2008), there were few recommendations and no FDA-approved medications for the treatment of bipolar depression. In 2003, a combination of fluoxetine and olanzapine became the first medication approved specifically for depression in the context of adult bipolar disorder. The recommended dosage

is from 6 to 18 mg of olanzapine and 25 to 50 mg of fluoxetine (Food and Drug Administration, 2011). In 2006, quetiapine was approved for the treatment of acute depression in bipolar adults, but not in those under 18 years. Recommended dosage is 300 mg/d, with precautions for certain populations (for more information, consult the package insert). In this review, we describe medications that have been studied to assess their utility in the treatment of bipolar depression, regardless of their current FDA approval.

Lithium

The mood-altering properties of lithium have been recognized since the nineteenth century. In fact, it appears waters rich in lithium were used to treat mental disease as early as the fifth century (Marmol, 2006). Based on its effects in animal studies, lithium was first used to treat mania and prevent relapse in bipolar disorder by John Cade in 1949. In 1954, Schou *et al.* published the first RCT testing lithium's efficacy (Schou *et al.* 1954). Since receiving FDA-approval in 1970, lithium has proven to be an effective treatment for acute mania and hypomania (Suppes *et al.* 2008), and also helps prevent both the manic and depressive phases of bipolar disorder I and II (Tondo *et al.* 1998), as well as cyclothymic disorder (Peselow *et al.* 1982).

Lithium's acute effects on bipolar depression

Few recent studies have examined lithium's acute effects. However, earlier small studies with open treatment and of short duration suggested effectiveness in treating bipolar depression. Goodwin *et al.* (1969) studied six bipolar disorder I subjects and six bipolar disorder II. A response was seen in 5 of the 12 treated with therapeutic doses of lithium. The same group was

Clinical Handbook for the Management of Mood Disorders, ed. J. John Mann, Patrick J. McGrath, and Steven P. Roose.
Published by Cambridge University Press. © Cambridge University Press 2013.

later expanded to 40 patients with bipolar depression. Patients received 6 days of placebo followed by 2 weeks of lithium. Clinical response was seen in 12 patients (30%) and partial response in 20 (50%), while 8 had worsening depression and the rest remained unchanged.

Lithium has also shown effectiveness in treating acute depression in bipolar I adolescents (Patel *et al.* 2006) and in open studies without a placebo group (Suppes *et al.* 2008). While more recent studies have not confirmed that lithium treatment improves depressive symptoms more than placebo, this may be due to sampling or other methodological factors (Young *et al.* 2010).

Maintenance studies of lithium

Studies including patients with depression in the course of bipolar disorder I or II indicate lithium's effectiveness in the treatment and prevention of bipolar depression (Kane *et al.* 1982, Tondo *et al.* 1998). Tondo *et al.* (1998) examined the clinical research charts of 317 patients and compared the frequency of depressive episodes with and without lithium treatment. Depression-free periods before lithium had an average duration of 8 months compared to 35 months once receiving lithium (Wilcoxon $\chi^2 = 56.9$, df $= 1$, p < 0.0001), an observation that was stronger in the first year of treatment. Subjects with bipolar disorder II showed far greater remission periods, 5.9 times longer than among those with bipolar disorder I (Tondo *et al.* 1998). Although Tondo *et al.* found that lithium was more effective in reducing manic/hypomanic episodes (3.3-fold fewer per year and lasting 3.0-fold less time) than depressive episodes (2.1-fold fewer per year lasting 2.3-fold less time), the effect on depression was still robust. It is worth noting that the response to lithium was negatively associated with the duration of illness without lithium treatment (r = −0.44, df = 315, p < 0.0001), supporting the use of lithium early in the course of illness.

Recent studies have examined lithium's antidepressive effects in more specific populations. An RCT by Calabrese *et al.* (2001) of 173 stable bipolar I patients that assigned lamotrigine, lithium, or placebo over 76 weeks, suggested that subjects treated with lithium showed a duration between depressive episodes similar to those treated with placebo. However, lithium was more effective than placebo in the prevention of manic episodes (Calabrese *et al.* 2001).

Among middle-aged and elderly subjects (>60 years) with either bipolar or unipolar depression, lithium treatment appears to reduce the frequency of depressive episodes and related events, such as suicidal ideas and attempts (Lepkifker *et al.* 2007). Since treatment with lithium has been associated with an increase in gray matter volume in the orbito-frontal cortex, it is possible that the antidepressant effects of lithium are mediated by a more generalized trophic effect than neurogenesis, which is thought to be confined to the dentate gyrus and the olfactory cortex (Benedetti *et al.* 2011).

Thus, the bulk of the data suggest that lithium is useful for both the treatment and prevention of bipolar depression.

Antidepressants

Some controversy remains regarding the use of antidepressants in bipolar disorder due to the potential risk of provoking a "switch" to mania and the paucity of data regarding their efficacy in treating bipolar depression. Nonetheless, more than 50% of subjects with bipolar disorder in the US are treated with antidepressants, second only to stimulants (Ghaemi *et al.* 2006).

Antidepressants' acute effects

Some investigators suggest that depressive episodes which have not responded to lithium or which arise despite preventive maintenance treatment should be treated with antidepressants (Sachs *et al.* 2000, Thase and Sachs, 2000, American Psychiatric Association, 2006). Many clinicians follow this practice. However, a review of published research does not consistently support this approach. Several studies suggest that antidepressants lack efficacy, though the studies have limitations, such as use of low doses of antidepressant (Sachs *et al.* 2007, McElroy *et al.* 2010) and small samples (McElroy *et al.* 2010). For example, the Systematic Treatment Enhancement Program for Bipolar Disorder (STEP-BD) (Sachs *et al.* 2007) included 366 subjects and did not show clinical response to treatment with paroxetine (median dose = 30 mg; range 20–40 mg) or bupropion (median dose = 300 mg; range 150–375 mg), perhaps due to the modest doses used.

On the other hand, Altshuler *et al.* carried out a randomized, double-blind study examining the response to either bupropion, sertraline, or venlafaxine over 10 weeks among 83 subjects with bipolar depression. After 10 weeks, 51% responded. Because patients were eligible to enter two subsequent reran-domizations, they found that 63% responded to at least one of the antidepressants (Altshuler *et al.* 2009), sug-gesting that antidepressants are quite useful in bipolar depression and that after an initial failure to respond, alternate antidepressants should be utilized.

Meta-analyses examining antidepressant treat-ment of acute bipolar depression, though limited by the quality of the studies included, do provide modest support for use of antidepressants for bipolar depression. Gijsman *et al.* (2004) included four previous studies with a total of 662 patients and found greater recovery from depressive symptoms in those treated with antidepressants compared with placebo (RR = 1.86, 95% CI = 1.49–2.30), including after using a random effect model (RR = 2.29, 95% CI = 1.29–4.04). A response to treatment was seen in approximately 75% of subjects that received concomi-tant medication. Further, Gijsman *et al.* (2004) found that TCAs were less effective than SSRIs (RR = 0.60, 95% CI = 0.36–100; z = 1.96, p = 0.05) and MAOIs (RR = 0.48, 95% CI = 0.28–0.82; z = 2.69, p = 0.007). Of interest, Gijsman *et al.* (2004) concluded that the extent of antidepressant effect in bipolar depression is similar to that observed in unipolar depression, based on the study by Peet (1994). A more recent meta-analysis (Sidor and MacQueen, 2011) examined six studies in terms of antidepressant efficacy relative to placebo. In these studies, 68% of patients were simultaneously receiving a mood stabilizer. Clinical response could be determined in five of the six studies and indicated a slight difference in favor of the antide-pressants that did not reach statistical significance (RR = 1.18, 95% CI = 0.99–1.40). The same was true for remission (RR = 1.20, 95% CI = 0.98–1.47). Of note, in another systematic review by Vieta *et al.* (2010), imipramine was the only antidepressant to have greater clinical response than placebo. However, a recent meta-analysis examining acute treatment of bipolar depression suggested that when TCAs and other antidepressants were compared with bupropion, the rates of clinical response and remission were similar across all antidepressants considered, as was the rate of discontinuation (Sidor and MacQueen, 2011).

According to Gijsman *et al.* (2004), clinical remission was measured in two studies in which the subjects received treatment with mood stabilizer or atypical antipsychotic medication. The results noted greater clinical remission for those taking add-on antidepressants compared to add-on placebo (RR = 1.41, 95% CI = 1.11–1.80). The frequency of response was greater than that of remission, as shown by a number needed to treat (NNT) of 4.2 (95% CI = 3.2–6.4) and 8.4 (95% CI = 4.8–33), respectively. Comparing antidepressants to other medications, Sidor and MacQueen (2011) found a trend for antide-pressants to be superior in clinical response relative to lamotrigine, lithium, or divalproex (RR = 1.12, 95% CI = 0.98–1.28), and in the rate of remission relative to lamotrigine (RR = 1.17, 95% CI = 0.97–1.41), but the effect did not reach statistical significance. Clearly, more work is needed to determine the utility of adding antidepressants for patients suffering from acute bipolar depression.

Given that the risk of switching associated with antidepressant treatment appears to be lower than previously thought, their potential benefits, includ-ing reducing risk of suicide, may outweigh the risks. Nonetheless, close follow-up of depressed bipolar patients is essential, not only due to the risk of suicide, but also to monitor for emergent mania or hypomania.

Maintenance with antidepressants

A handful of studies have focused on the use of antidepressants as maintenance treatment for bipolar patients. A small study (n = 70) noted that when antidepressant treatment was maintained rather than discontinued, there was a trend towards delaying recurrence of depressive symptoms (Ghaemi *et al.* 2010). Altshuler *et al.* (2009) carried out a randomized, double-blind study. The continuation phase tracked 89 responders or partial responders over a year of monthly evaluations. In that phase, 69% showed a positive response to antidepressants and 27% responded partially ($\chi^2 = 11.5$, p < 0.001), with a remission rate of 53%.

Clinical use of antidepressants in bipolar disorder is extensive, as documented by retrospective natural-istic and pharmacoepidemiological studies. Ghaemi *et al.* (2006) observed that only one-quarter of bipo-lar patients studied were in a depressive phase, but around 40% were receiving antidepressants, presum-ably as a maintenance strategy to prevent relapse. Subsequently, Fu *et al.* (2007) focused specifically on the relationship between the prescription of second-generation antidepressants (selective serotonin reup-take inhibitors, serotonin–norepinephrine reuptake inhibitors, serotonin reuptake inhibitors, dopamine reuptake inhibitors, and noradrenergic antagonists) and the number of annual visits due to depressive symptomatology. They found that those on monotherapy with antidepressants had fewer visits (odds ratio (OR) = 0.68, 95% CI = 0.56–0.82) compared with those on combined treatment with antidepressants and mood stabilizers (OR = 0.65, 95% CI = 0.52–0.81), and compared with those on no antidepressants. Together these data suggest some utility of antidepressants in lowering bipolar depressive symptoms over time.

Switching

Long-standing concerns that antidepressant treatment of bipolar depression may induce a switch to mania, an onset of rapid cycling, or treatment resistance (Ananth *et al.* 1993, Manning *et al.* 1998, Bowden *et al.* 2000, Truman *et al.* 2007) have been somewhat mitigated. Diverse data support the safety of antidepressant use. Randomized controlled clinical trials (Sachs *et al.* 2007, Altshuler *et al.* 2009) along with naturalistic (Bauer *et al.* 2005), pharmacoepidemiologic (Fu *et al.* 2007), and meta-analytic studies (Gijsman *et al.* 2004, Sidor and MacQueen, 2011) all suggest that switching to mania is no more common among those on antidepressants compared with those on no antidepressant. It may be that second-generation antidepressants do not trigger the emergence of manic or hypomanic episodes (Fu *et al.* 2007), or at least do so at a lower rate than TCAs (Truman *et al.* 2007). In fact, in a comparison of TCAs and other antidepressants, Gijsman *et al.* (2004) found an increased rate of switching on TCAs, with a risk of 2.92 (95% CI = 1.28–6.71) and a difference of absolute risk from other antidepressants of 6.8% (95% CI = 1.7–11.9%). Comparing TCAs to SSRIs specifically, there was a trend for increased switching with TCAs (RR = 6.59, 95% CI = 0.83–52.54; z = 1.78, p = 0.08). Meanwhile, Sidor and MacQueen (2011) compared TCAs and other antidepressants with bupropion with regard to switching rates and found bupropion to be safer (RR = 0.34, 95% CI = 0.13–0.88).

In two studies of similar design, an acute phase was treated with antidepressants and some subjects subsequently entered a continuation phase (Leverich *et al.* 2006, Post *et al.* 2006). In the first study, 228 subjects entered, and 174 entered the second study for treatment of acute depression. In the first study, 159 subjects and in the second, 83 continued to the maintenance phase with antidepressant treatment (sertraline,

bupropion, or venlafaxine). Improvement was seen among 48.7% of subjects in one study and 49–51% in the other. In the first study (Leverich *et al.* 2006), 38.5% improved without any type of switching. Among those who did have switching, 4.8% had a brief hypomanic episode, 7.0% had more than one episode of hypomania, and 7.9% had a full switch to mania. In the second study, using data from the Stanley Foundation Bipolar Network (Post *et al.* 2006), Post *et al.* specified rates of switching according to the antidepressant received. Switching to mania/hypomania occurred in 10% of patients taking bupropion, 9% taking sertraline, and 29% taking venlafaxine (log rank χ^2 = 12.462, df = 2, p = 0.002). Differences were significant after controlling for lithium (log rank χ^2 = 11.99, df = 2, p < 0.01), although it is important to view these data cautiously, as with those of Leverich, since they do not represent randomized controlled trials per se and include the same subjects in various groups.

Subsequently, a randomized, double-blind study conducted by Altshuler *et al.* (2009) compared the acute and maintenance responses to three different antidepressants. In the first phase, only 42.5% responded without any switching. Episodes of brief hypomania were found in 4.6% of patients, recurrent hypomania in 13.8%, and mania in 14.9%. In the continuation phase, rates of switching to mania/hypomania were 13% and 22% (χ^2 = 1.1, p = ns) for the responders and partial responders, respectively. Naturally, maintenance phases tend to be longer than acute phases permitting more time for depressive symptoms to reappear.

Subjects with bipolar disorder I appear to have greater risk of affective switching than those with bipolar disorder II. The presence of manic or hypomanic symptoms during a depressive period is also associated with a greater risk of switching. Therefore, symptoms such as increased motor activity or speech and language–thought disorder should be assessed before initiating antidepressant treatment in bipolar patients (Peet, 1994, Kupfer *et al.* 2001, Joffe *et al.* 2002, Serretti *et al.* 2003, Frye *et al.* 2009).

Recently introduced to the market in Europe, agomelatine represents a special case among antidepressants due to its action on melatonergic receptors. A naturalistic study of the effectiveness of agomelatine on bipolar depression included 21 patients in treatment with lithium or valpromide. The results are encouraging, with a rate of response greater than 80% (Calabrese *et al.* 2007). However, further studies, including RCTs, in bipolar depression are required to confirm its utility.

Overall, the efficacy of antidepressants is far from proven, but the risk of switching fairly low. These data appear in contrast to the recommendation against antidepressant treatment during the depressive phase of bipolar disorder. Nevertheless, the best option appears to be combined therapy with a mood stabilizer and antidepressant, ideally an SSRI or bupropion.

Quetiapine

Quetiapine is one of only two medications approved by the FDA specifically for the treatment of bipolar depression and has good efficacy and tolerability (Thase, 2008, Bogart and Chavez, 2009, Janicak and Rado, 2011). However, the medication is tolerated less well by patients with bipolar depression than by those with schizophrenia or mania (Wang *et al.* 2011).

Quetiapine's acute effects

Quetiapine compared to placebo

Quetiapine was first studied in the BOLDER (BipO-Lar DEpRession) trials (Calabrese *et al.* 2005, Thase *et al.* 2006). In the first of these (Calabrese *et al.* 2005), 542 currently depressed patients with bipolar disorder I (n = 360) or bipolar disorder II (n = 182) received randomized treatment with quetiapine (300 or 600 mg/d) or placebo. Both groups receiving active treatment achieved significant improvement after the first week. After 8 weeks of treatment, the average decrease on the Montgomery–Asberg Depression Rating Scale (MADRS) was 16.7 in the 600 mg/d group and 16.4 in the 300 mg/d group, compared to 10.3 in the placebo group (p < 0.001). Similarly, the decrease in Hamilton Depression Scale scores was 13.8 and 13.4 for quetiapine (300 and 600 mg/d, respectively) compared to 8.5 for placebo. The onset of action was also greater in those receiving quetiapine (median 22 days vs. 36 days; log rank χ^2 = 33.1, df = 2, p < 0.001). No difference was found among the various groups regarding treatment-emergent mania.

Comparable results were reported in a second BOLDER study of similar design including 509 patients (Thase *et al.* 2006). From the first week to the end of the study, mean HAM-D scores were significantly lower in subjects receiving quetiapine (300 and 600 mg/d) compared with placebo (p < 0.001). Similarly, remission rates were higher with both quetiapine dosages. This second study also found a lower rate of treatment-emergent mania or hypomania in subjects treated with quetiapine (both dosages) compared to the placebo group. Post-hoc analysis of bipolar disorder II subjects from both BOLDER studies confirmed a greater response to quetiapine compared to placebo on the MADRS, HAM-D, HAM-A, and CGI (Clinical Global Impression). Of note, these studies have drop-out rates between 24% and 47%, although this rate is similar to that observed in a study of dropout rates in bipolar subjects (Moon *et al.* 2012).

Weisler *et al.* (2008) performed a combined analysis of two RCTs that administered 300 or 600 mg of quetiapine and placebo to a total of 694 bipolar depression patients. Both dosages produced a greater response than placebo at 8 weeks. Improvement was observed among most key symptoms of depression evaluated with the MADRS. In particular, difficulty concentrating and pessimistic thoughts improved significantly by the second week, suggesting that improvements were not simply related to sedation from active drug. The response rates (≥50% decrease in MADRS total score from baseline), within the first week were 17.5% and 24.1% and within the second week, the rates achieved were 36.6% and 39.5% among subjects that received 300 and 600 mg/d respectively. By the eighth week, remission (MADRS total scores ≤ 12) was achieved in 55.3% and 53.6%, respectively, for 300 and 600 mg/d. Dropout due to side effects was more common among those receiving the 600 mg dosage, with a rate of 16.8% compared to 10.3% of those receiving 300 mg/d.

There are two more recent studies examining quetiapine known as EMBOLDEN I (Young *et al.* 2010) and II (McElroy *et al.* 2010). The first study compared quetiapine treatment at 300 and 600 mg/d with both placebo and lithium, studying 805 patients over 8 weeks. Both the 600 mg/d dosage and the 300 mg/d dosage of quetiapine showed greater efficacy than placebo, as measured by the MADRS. As was true in the BOLDER study (Calabrese *et al.* 2005), differences in response to quetiapine compared to placebo were significant in bipolar disorder I subjects, but not in bipolar disorder II. Both dosages of quetiapine also demonstrated improved response compared to placebo on other scales, including the HAM-D, HAM-A, CGI, and Sheehan Disability Scale, none of which showed any difference between lithium and placebo.

However, EMBOLDEN I found different results for a certain sub-group. Among those with rapid cycling, quetiapine was not superior to placebo, although the number of such subjects (n = 40) was small, limiting power.

The second EMBOLDEN study (McElroy *et al.* 2010) examined the antidepressant efficacy of quetiapine compared to placebo and paroxetine, instead of lithium, which was used in EMBOLDEN I. The results from 740 depressed subjects (bipolar disorder I and II) showed a superior response with quetiapine (300 and 600 mg/d) compared to placebo (–16.19, p < 0.001 and –16.31, p < 0.001, respectively) as measured by the MADRS. Similar results were found using the HAM-D (quetiapine 300: –14.68, p < 0.001; quetiapine 600: –15.09, p < 0.001 compared to placebo). Both bipolar disorder I and II subjects had improved response as measured by the HAM-A and CGI-BP-S with both dosages of quetiapine compared to placebo. The incidence of treatment-emergent mania or hypomania was greater with placebo (8.9%) than with quetiapine (2.1% for quetiapine 300 mg/d and 4.1% for quetiapine 600 mg/d), though not statistically significantly so.

Quetiapine compared to active comparators

EMBOLDEN I (Young *et al.* 2010) compared quetiapine treatment at 300 and 600 mg/d to both placebo and lithium, examining 805 patients over 8 weeks. The lithium group displayed no difference relative to placebo in the improvement of depressive symptoms. The 600 mg/d dosage of quetiapine showed greater efficacy than lithium or placebo as measured by the MADRS, while the 300 mg/d dosage did not. The EMBOLDEN II study (McElroy *et al.* 2010) examined the antidepressant efficacy of quetiapine compared to placebo and paroxetine. Results from 740 depressed subjects (bipolar disorder I and II) showed a superior response with quetiapine (300 and 600 mg/d) compared to paroxetine (–2.43, p = 0.017 and –2.55, p = 0.012) as measured by the MADRS. Similar results were found using the HAM-D for quetiapine 300 (–2.15, p = 0.010) and quetiapine 600 (–2.56, p = 0.002) compared to paroxetine. In fact, paroxetine showed no difference in response compared to placebo after 8 weeks. The incidence of treatment-emergent mania or hypomania was greater with paroxetine (10.7%) than with quetiapine (2.1% for quetiapine 300 mg/d and 4.1% for quetiapine 600 mg/d), though this finding was not statistically significant.

Of interest, the most recent meta-analysis does not indicate a greater efficacy for quetiapine than for other second-generation antipsychotics such as olanzapine and aripiprazole (De Fruyt *et al.* 2012). MADRS mean change from baseline to endpoint was significantly greater with quetiapine than placebo 600 (–4.64; 95% CI = –5.82–3.46), quetiapine 300 (–4.76; 95% CI = –5.75–3.76), and olanzapine (–3.1; 95% CI = –4.57–3.76) (Tohen *et al.* 2003). The relative risk for response was 1.33 for quetiapine 300 mg/d (95% CI = 1.19–1.47), 1.36 for quetiapine 600 mg/d (95% CI = 1.23–1.49), 1.28 for olanzapine (95% CI = 1.05–1.28, and 1.05 for aripiprazole (95% CI = 0.88–1.25). Differences in response to placebo compared to aripiprazole are not significant since the confidence intervals overlap. Similarly, the remission RR was 1.39 (95% CI = 1.19–1.63) and 1.36 (95% CI = 1.18–1.57) for quetiapine 300 and 600 mg/d, respectively, while it was 1.34 (95% CI = 1.06–1.69) for olanzapine and 0.99 (95% CI = 0.78–1.25) for aripiprazole. Of note, aripiprazole did not show benefit in terms of either response or remission (confidence interval crossed 1).

Moreover, a systematic review of RCTs showed two drugs to be most effective for bipolar depression in terms of efficacy, response, and remission: quetiapine and fluoxetine/olanzapine outperformed paroxetine, lamotrigine, aripiprazole, lithium, and olanzapine alone (Vieta *et al.* 2010). Likewise, the 600 mg/d dosage and the 300 mg/d extended release dosage showed superior tolerability profiles, in terms of the number needed to harm, compared to aripiprazole and olanzapine.

Maintenance studies of quetiapine

Quetiapine's efficacy as a maintenance treatment has been seen in various studies. An open-label continuation study of 55 subjects found a decrease in both occurrence and duration of depressive symptoms in those receiving quetiapine (mean dosage: 122; SD = 149) (Suppes *et al.* 2007). More recently, an RCT continuation study examined subjects with bipolar disorder I in which the episode index could be either mania, depression, or mixed states (Weisler *et al.* 2011). A total of 1226 subjects were stabilized with quetiapine (dosage range: 300–800 mg/d) and entered the randomization phase in three groups (quetiapine, lithium, or placebo) for up to 104 weeks. Compared with placebo, the risk of suffering a depressive episode was lower in subjects taking quetiapine (HR = 0.30, 95% CI = 0.20–0.44, p < 0.0001) and lithium (HR = 0.59, 95% CI = 0.42–0.84, p < 0.004). It is also worth noting that manic episodes were similarly decreased with both active medications compared to placebo (quetiapine: HR = 0.29, 95% CI = 0.21–0.40, p < 0.0001; lithium: HR = 0.37, 95% CI = 0.27–0.53, p < 0.0001) (Weisler *et al.* 2011).

Other considerations

The quetiapine extended-release formulation appears to be similar to the regular-release formulation in terms of efficacy (Cristancho and Thase, 2010, Suppes *et al.* 2010). The antidepressant efficacy of quetiapine appears to be independent of improvement in anxiety symptoms (Weisler *et al.* 2008).

Lamotrigine

As Swartz and Thase (2011) indicate in their recent review, lamotrigine has an "exceptionally controversial status." Early research found high efficacy in monotherapy, including long term (McElroy *et al.* 2004), while later studies evaluated lamotrigine as an adjunct medication in bipolar depression.

Efficacy and meta-analyses of lamotrigine's acute effects

Lamotrigine compared to placebo

Initially, two RCTs (Calabrese *et al.* 1999, 2000) indicated good response to lamotrigine in acute depressive episodes among subjects with rapid-cycling bipolar disorder or bipolar disorder I, along with indicators of good tolerability and safety. However, a later analysis of five RCTs (two unpublished) found no difference in response between lamotrigine and placebo (Calabrese *et al.* 2008). Subsequently, another meta-analysis examined four of the five RCTs used by Calabrese *et al.* (2008) and found lamotrigine only slightly better than placebo: RR = 1.27, 95% CI = 1.09–1.47, p = 0.002 according to the Hamilton Rating Scale for Depression, and RR = 1.22, 95% CI = 1.06–1.41, p = 0.005 according to the MADRS. Of interest, these two very similar meta-analyses did identify a better relative response to lamotrigine in those subjects presenting with more severe depression (HRSD score >24), with an RR = 1.47 (95% CI = 1.16–1.87, p = 0.001) (Geddes *et al.* 2009).

Lamotrigine compared to active comparators

Recently, a naturalistic study found lithium (n = 3518) to be more clinically effective than lamotrigine (n = 730) in bipolar depression (Kessing *et al.* 2011). A previous open study comparing lamotrigine (n = 44) with lithium (n = 54) in monotherapy found similar efficacy for the treatment of acute depression in patients with bipolar disorder II. However, side effects were more frequent in the lithium group (Suppes *et al.* 2008). Adding or switching to an alternate medication (antidepressants, antipsychotics, or other anticonvulsants) produced more benefit in those receiving lithium compared with lamotrigine (HR = 2.60, 95% CI = 2.23–3.04). The risk of hospitalization was also greater with lamotrigine (HR = 1.45, 95% CI = 1.28–1.65), for both currently depressed (HR = 1.31, 95% CI = 1.01–1.70) and currently manic (HR = 1.65, 95% CI = 1.31–2.09) subjects. Yet, randomized studies comparing lithium monotherapy with lamotrigine in terms of improving depression in the course of bipolar disorder II have observed comparable response rates for both drugs, although lamotrigine showed a better tolerability profile (Suppes *et al.* 2008).

Though recent work calls into question lamotrigine's antidepressant efficacy in monotherapy, evidence suggests possible efficacy as an add-on. A recent study of 124 depressed bipolar disorder I or II patients being treated with lithium, added lamotrigine or placebo in a randomized, double-blind design (van der Loos *et al.* 2009). Results indicated a better response in the active arm, as measured by the MADRS. Other naturalistic studies have shown good response among bipolar disorder II subjects following the addition of lamotrigine in cases of partial response to mood stabilizer, or other medications (Sharma *et al.* 2008, Chang *et al.* 2010). According to an analysis of 39 naturalistic studies, 48.2% of bipolar depression subjects resistant to lamotrigine or quetiapine monotherapy achieved euthymia following the addition of quetiapine or lamotrigine, respectively (Ahn *et al.* 2011). Subsyndromal symptoms decreased from 20.5 to 15.4%, along with an overall symptomatic decrease from 79.5 to 30.8% (Sharma *et al.* 2008). Combined with a mood stabilizer, lamotrigine's efficacy in treating resistant depression has been found comparable to that of antidepressants such as citalopram (Schaffer *et al.* 2006). Of note, secondary analyses from STEP-BD in patients who had failed at least one trial of mood stabilizer plus antidepressant found that those randomized to lamotrigine added on to a mood stabilizer had a better depressive symptom response compared to inositol and risperidone add-ons (Nierenberg *et al.* 2006).

It has been proposed that lamotrigine may be effective in certain sub-groups of bipolar depression patients. Wang *et al.* (2010) studied a small group of subjects with recreational drug use and rapid cycling who showed little response to the combination of lithium and valproate. Adding lamotrigine led to greater reduction of depressive symptoms than did the addition of placebo.

Of note, some genetic polymorphisms may predict response to lamotrigine. An RCT compared the combination of olanzapine/fluoxetine with lamotrigine in bipolar depression subjects over 7 weeks and associated a better response to lamotrigine with SNPs in the HRH1, dopamine beta-hydroxylase, dopamine D2 receptor, glucororticoid receptor, and melanocortin 2 receptor genes (Perlis *et al.* 2010). Pharmacogenetics may help identify individuals who are more likely to respond to a given drug and may assist in the development of a personalized approach to psychopharmacology.

Maintenance studies of lamotrigine

Calabrese *et al.* (2001) performed a 76-week-long RCT with 173 stable bipolar I subjects. Patients were randomized into three groups: lamotrigine (100–400 mg), lithium, and placebo. Results indicated greater time to intervention for lithium and lamotrigine compared to placebo. Specifically, lamotrigine was superior to placebo in preventing the appearance of depressive episodes, but not in preventing manic episodes.

Calabrese *et al.* (2000) also carried out an RCT examining lamotrigine's efficacy over 6 months in 177 subjects (bipolar disorder I and II) with rapid cycling. There was no difference between lamotrigine and placebo regarding the rate of emergent symptoms requiring additional pharmacotherapy (50% vs. 56%; p = ns). However, the survival analysis indicated that the lamotrigine group had an average premature discontinuation rate of 14 weeks compared to 8 weeks with placebo (p = 0.036). This difference was most visible in patients with bipolar disorder II (n = 52) (17 vs. 7 weeks, p = 0.015), while for the bipolar disorder I group it did not reach statistical significance. HAM-D scores were also recorded at the time of intervention

with additional medication; lamotrigine and placebo groups had similar scores. Nonetheless, the authors noted an increased proportion of clinically stable subjects among those receiving lamotrigine relative to those receiving placebo (41% vs. 26%, p = 0.03). This difference was greatest among bipolar disorder II patients (46% vs. 18%, p = 0.04), but did not reach statistical significance for those with bipolar disorder I.

In a more recent RCT, Licht *et al.* (2010) examined 155 stable bipolar I patients for a minimum of 1 year and up to 5.8 years for some. Results indicated that those taking lamotrigine (n = 77) had an increased risk of dropout compared to those taking lithium (hazard rate ratio: HRR = 0.92, 95% CI = 0.60–1.40), particularly among those with an index episode of mania (HRR = 1.91, 95% CI: = 0.73–5.04). The HRR for time to depressive episode with lamotrigine compared to lithium was 0.69 (95% CI = 0.41–1.22). Of those receiving lamotrigine, 30% suffered a depressive episode and 17% became manic. The authors note only 2/29 patients in any group who remained on monotherapy for 5 years. Taken together, the evidence for lamotrigine as either acute or maintenance therapy is inconsistent, as outlined by Swartz and Thase (2011).

Olanzapine/fluoxetine

The combination of fluoxetine/olanzapine was the first FDA-approved treatment for bipolar depression. Studies show the combination achieves greater efficacy than either molecule individually, along with good tolerability and a risk of switching that is comparable to placebo (Deeks and Keating, 2008a, 2008b).

Olanzapine/fluoxetine's acute effects

Tohen *et al.* (2003) found olanzapine/fluoxetine superior to placebo or olanzapine alone. Another RCT found a fluoxetine/olanzapine group had a faster rate of response compared with lamotrigine (week 7) (Brown *et al.* 2006) and a better outcome in terms of suicidal behavior. However, the rate of side effects (principally somnolence, increased appetite, dry mouth, sedation, weight gain, and tremor) was also greater in the fluoxetine/olanzapine group. Since then, four post-hoc analyses of olanzapine/fluoxetine have been published with various outcome measures: function and quality of life (Shi *et al.* 2004), treatment-emergent mania (Keck, Jr. *et al.* 2005), speed of response (Dube *et al.* 2007), and response in mixed depression (Benazzi *et al.* 2009).

Quality of life, functioning and speed of response in mixed states were better in those receiving combined fluoxetine/olanzapine. Rates of switching to mania were similar to placebo, in line with previous results (Amsterdam and Shults, 2005).

Maintenance studies of olanzapine/fluoxetine

A follow-up study lasting 24 weeks included subjects that had completed a trial for an acute depressive phase in which they were randomized to either olanzapine/fluoxetine, olanzapine, or placebo. For the maintenance phase, after receiving 1 week of olanzapine, participants and their physicians could switch treatments between olanzapine/fluoxetine or olanzapine at any point, provided it occurred during a study visit. Post-hoc, the participants were divided into three groups: group 1 continued olanzapine, group 2 switched to fluoxetine/olanzapine at any of three different dosages, and group 3 switched to the other treatment. After 24 weeks, remitters after the acute trial who switched treatment olanzapine to olanzapine plus fluoxetine or the other way around (group 3) were most likely to relapse (50%). Relapse was less frequent among those who opted for olanzapine/fluoxetine (24%) and lowest among those who continued with olanzapine monotherapy (11%) (Corya et al. 2006). Whether this is due to the fact that those who were switched were likely to be the ones less responsive to medication or specific medication effects cannot be determined with this type of study design. Of note, more than 60% of subjects achieved remission at some point in the study in all three groups (group 1: 64.7%; group 2: 66.7%; and group 3: 62.5%). Subsequently, an RCT examined 410 patients after 25 weeks. Compared to the lamotrigine group, the fluoxetine/olanzapine group had greater response (week 25) (Brown et al. 2009). A 12-week continuation study also indicated maintained improvement and/or remission of depressive symptoms, but along with greater weight gain in comparison with subjects that had received olanzapine monotherapy (Tamayo et al. 2009).

Despite the evidence supporting the efficacy and tolerability of combined fluoxetine/olanzapine, there has been low clinical use. This may be due to resistance to use of combined medications or troublesome side effects related to weight gain and increased risk of developing type 2 diabetes and metabolic syndrome (Shelton, 2006). That a recent study indicates the possibility of genetics influencing the rates of response to combined fluoxetine/olanzapine may permit more personalized selection of this treatment in the future (Perlis et al. 2010).

Aripiprazole

Aripiprazole has been approved by the FDA for the treatment of acute mania; it has shown greater efficacy than placebo or haloperidol (Keck, Jr. et al. 2003, Vieta et al. 2005) and is comparable to lithium (Keck et al. 2009). Furthermore it has been shown to better prevent recurrence of affective episodes when combined with lithium or valproate than either of these drugs combined with placebo (Marcus et al. 2011). Additionally, a handful of studies have examined its effects on bipolar depression.

Aripiprazole's acute effects

Initial small, open-label studies evaluating response to aripiprazole in bipolar depression found efficacy among subjects with treatment-resistant depression (Ketter et al. 2006, Kemp et al. 2007, McElroy et al. 2007). One-third of such patients showed a response (>50% reduction in the MADRS) following the addition of aripiprazole. However, these studies also indicated a high rate (29–42%) of discontinuation due to side effects, primarily akathisia. Similarly, a small retrospective study indicated response in 7 of 10 subjects with treatment-resistant bipolar depression, along with a high incidence of akathisia (Sokolski, 2007).

Thase et al. (2008) carried out one study on the effectiveness of aripiprazole in bipolar depression. They analyzed two unpublished RCTs lasting about 2 years, including a total of 373 subjects in the active arm and 376 receiving placebo. Although aripiprazole was superior to placebo during the first 6 weeks of the trial, by the end of the study, improvement of depressive symptoms was similar to placebo (Thase et al. 2008). Another study combining the same two RCTs that Thase et al. (2008) analyzed, returned similar results regarding the predictive potential of initial response. Among 617 patients (306 assigned to aripiprazole and 311 to placebo), the rate of improvement in the first 3 weeks (reduction of ≥20% from baseline in MARDS total score) was a highly sensitive predictor of later response (MADRS reduction of total score at the end of study ≥50%; sensitivity: 81%) or remission

(MADRS total score at the end of study ≤10; sensitivity: 82.9%) of depressive symptoms with a mean aripiprazole dose at endpoints of 17.8 mg/d (Kemp *et al.* 2010).

Two more studies have examined aripriprazole, though with limited samples. In an open-label study of 20 patients, aripiprazole was added to treatment already being administered, resulting in a 44% response rate (Dunn *et al.* 2008). Another study compared the efficacy over 6 weeks of adding either aripiprazole or citalopram to a mood stabilizer. Based on data from 23 subjects hospitalized for bipolar depression, results indicated a similar response in both groups (Quante *et al.* 2010). More recently, Thase *et al.* (2012) conducted a post-hoc analysis of two RCTs in which total sample (n = 745) was split into more depressed (n = 133, Bech-6 score > 15) and less depressed (n = 612, Bech-6 score < 15) groups. The more depressed group showed fairly little change in MADRS score based on treatment (–19.4 for aripiprazole vs. –15.4 for placebo, p = 0.14). However, there was significant difference (–13.8 vs. –10.3, p = 0.07) in six specific items identified as core depressive symptoms. Overall, results regarding aripiprazole's efficacy as either a monotherapy or an add-on strategy remain unclear. Whether observed negative results are due to factors such as the high rate of response to placebo, rapid titration of aripiprazole, or use of low doses is unknown (Yatham, 2011).

Ziprasidone

Studies to date on ziprasidone treatment for bipolar depression show inconclusive results. The first was an open-label study (n = 30) of depressed patients with bipolar disorder II (bipolar I was an exclusion criterion), but results are difficult to interpret due to ambiguity in the number of responders and remitters (Liebowitz *et al.* 2009). The second began with 265 bipolar depression subjects all receiving a mood stabilizer, though only192 completed the study. Of them, 88 received add-on ziprasidone (mean dosage: 89.8 mg/d) and 104 received only the mood stabilizer plus placebo (Sachs *et al.* 2011). In terms of change in depressed mood, active treatment showed no difference compared to the placebo group. However, the active drug group had better outcomes on the GAF (Global Assessment of Functioning) and Sheehan Disability Scale. The authors note that the low dosage of ziprasidone employed may have contributed to the negative

findings and post-hoc analyses also cite inconsistencies in subject rating (Lombardo *et al.* 2012).

Risperidone

Few studies have examined efficacy of risperidone treatment for depressive symptoms in bipolar depression. None to date include risperidone monotherapy. Combined with a mood stabilizer, risperidone shows efficacy similar to placebo (Shelton and Stahl, 2004, Nierenberg *et al.* 2006).

Carbamazepine

The antidepressant effect of carbamazepine has been examined in a handful of studies. The majority of data regarding carbamazepine's antidepressive efficacy come from studies comparing it with lithium. Greil and Kleindienst (1999) published a study in which carbamazepine appeared superior to lithium in preventing affective episodes for a specific sub-group of subjects with bipolar disorder II, schizoaffective disorder, and co-morbid substance use. Moreover, the combination of carbamazepine/lithium has been suggested to be more effective at preventing affective episodes among rapid cyclers than either medication in monotherapy (Denicoff *et al.* 1997). A small, open study by Dilsaver *et al.* (1996) examined 36 bipolar depression subjects (9 with mixed symptomatology and 18 with psychotic symptoms) over 21 days. In those with psychotic symptoms, the average decrease in HDRS was 23.7 ± 10.9 (df = 26; t = 11.2, p < 0.0001) and 63% reached remission (HDRS score ≤ 8) by the end of the study. Those with psychotic symptoms had lower remission rates, although this difference was not statistically significant (55.6% vs. 72.2%; p = ns) (Dilsaver *et al.* 1996). Thus, the literature on carbamazepine is too limited to confidently state it has specific antidepressant properties.

Valproate

Studies examining the response to valproate in bipolar depression were conducted in response to observations of a positive response in open-label studies of unipolar major depression (Davis *et al.* 1996) and to RCTs focused on the manic phase, which suggested that subjects with depressive symptoms had worse responses to lithium than to valproate. A meta-analysis by Smith *et al.* (2010) analyzed four RCTs, two of which were presented as abstracts in conferences (Sachs *et al.*

2001, Davis *et al.* 2005, Ghaemi *et al.* 2007, Muzina *et al.* 2008), bringing together 142 subjects. The results of the meta-analysis indicated a significantly greater response with valproate compared to placebo (SMD – 0.35, –0.69, –0.02; p = 0.04) and an observed active treatment effect of RR 2.00 (95% CI = 1.13–3.53; p = 0.02). The results of the meta-analysis indicated an absolute risk difference of 0.22 (0.07, 0.36; p = 0.003; I2 = 0%) or 22% generating an NNT of 5. No increased risk of switching was found with valproate compared to placebo. Thus, the literature is sparse, but may suggest valproate's modest utility for bipolar depression.

Other treatments

Electroconvulsive therapy

The efficacy of electroconvulsive therapy (ECT) in major depressive disorder has been verified in numerous studies (Janicak *et al.* 1985). Fewer studies regarding bipolar depression are published. Medda *et al.* (2009) compared the response to ECT in unipolar depression (n = 17) to depression in bipolar disorder I (n = 46) and to depression in bipolar disorder II, (n = 67). In all three groups, improvement was seen from baseline scores. The rate of response (50% reduction in the HAM-D) was 88.2% in MDD, 73.1% in bipolar II, and 69.6% in bipolar I, differences that were not statistically significant. However, the rate of remission (HAM-D < 8) was significantly greater in MDD (70.6%) compared to 43.3% and 34.8% in bipolar I and II subjects, respectively. The authors noted a tendency for persistence of manic and psychotic symptoms in subjects with bipolar depression I.

Daly *et al.* (2001) compared 162 subjects with MDD to 66 subjects with bipolar depression. Bipolar depression subjects achieved lower scores on the HRSD by the final treatments (4th, 5th, 6th, 7th, and 8th). The survival analysis also indicated increased rate of response among bipolar subjects, (Peto–Peto $\chi^2(1) = 7.07$, p = 0.008). The number of treatments to response was 6.33 ± 2.82 for unipolars and 4.35 ± 1.97 for bipolars (t(133) = 4.04, p < 0.0001). Of note, the rate of response was similar in both groups and appeared to be influenced by the type of stimulus received. These data are consistent with those from Black *et al.* (1986) and Grunhaus *et al.* (2002). Black *et al.* conducted a chart review study and found rates of effectiveness (69.8% in MDD compared to 69.1% in bipolar depression subjects), with no difference in response based on whether there was bilateral or unilateral application of ECT (Black *et al.* 1986). In another chart review, Grunhaus *et al.* (2002) studied 111 unipolar depressed patients and 20 bipolar depressed patients. The response rate was 57% but there were no significant differences in either response rates or in HRSD or GAF scores in bipolar compared to unipolar patients.

Deep brain stimulation

In a recent study, DBS therapy for treatment-resistant depression in patients with major depressive disorder (n = 10) was compared with bipolar disorder II (n = 7) (Holtzheimer *et al.* 2012). Depression was deemed treatment-resistant if no response had been seen with four different antidepressants at adequate dosage and treatment duration. Electrodes were inserted bilaterally into the white matter of the subcallosal cingulate. Treatment consisted of 4 weeks of single-blind sham stimulation followed by 24 weeks of active stimulation. After 24 weeks, 41% (7/17) of patients showed good response. 18% (3/17 patients) achieved symptomatic remission (HDRS score < 8). Following 2 years of active stimulation, 58% (7/12 patients) were in remission and 92% (11/12 patients) had obtained a positive response. No switching to mania or hypomania was observed.

Transcranial magnetic stimulation

Though some promising research exists, repetitive transcranial magnetic stimulation (rTMS) has not yet been shown to be effective in treating bipolar depression, largely due to the small samples sizes in extant studies. Dolberg *et al.* (2002) carried out an RCT of 20 patients with bipolar depression. Of these, 10 were randomly assigned to receive 20 sessions of real rTMS while the remaining 10 patients received 10 sessions of sham rTMS followed by 20 sessions of real rTMS. The control group had no response to the sham rTMS sessions, while both groups responded to the real sessions. The real-sessions group improved relative to control by the second week, as measured by the Hamilton Rating Scale for Depression and Brief Psychiatric Rating Scale. However, this difference disappeared at week 4, suggesting that treatment of more than 2 weeks does not offer better results.

Another RCT (Nahas *et al.* 2003) examined 21 depressed subjects and two in mixed phase (total:

14 bipolar disorder I and 9 bipolar disorder II). All patients scored >18 on the Hamilton Ratings Scale for Depression and had an optimal period of washout for antidepressants. They were randomly distributed into two groups, a control group (n = 12) that received sham rTMS and an active group that received left prefrontal rTMS (n = 11). After 2 weeks, results were similar between both groups in terms of the mean percentage change in HDRSD (active group: 25% ± 32; control group: 25% ± 31) and the percentage of responders, (active group: 36%; control group: 33%). There was no difference in any of the other scales applied (YMRS (Young Mania Rating Scale), HAM-A, Beck Depression Scale and GAF).

Dell'Osso et al. (2009) studied 11 depressed bipolar subjects with poor response to medication given for an adequate period of time and at appropriate dosages. All 11 received right dorsolateral prefrontal cortex rTMS over a 3-week period while maintaining previous antidepressant treatment. Six of the eleven subjects achieved response (reduction ≥50% in HAM-D) and four were considered remitters (HAM-D ≤8).

A naturalistic study (Cohen et al. 2010) examined 56 depressed bipolar subjects that had been effectively treated with dorsolateral prefrontal cortex rTMS and had been in remission for more than 6 months. The number of rTMS sessions received was determined clinically by the treating physician. The authors indicated that subjects with refractory (failure to remit after two or more antidepressant or mood stabilizer trials) or severe (HDRS score >24) depression in the index episode were more likely to require more than 15 sessions.

Regarding long-term efficacy, a study by Dell'Osso et al. (2011) followed 11 patients (five bipolar I and six bipolar II) that had received rTMS treatment (six full responders, three partial responders, and two nonresponders). After a year of follow-up, only four subjects maintained euthymia (three with remission after additional rTMS treatment). This may indicate that long-term efficacy is greater among those who respond to acute treatment.

Another important concern in rTMS treatment is the possibility of switching to mania/hypomania. In a review about this issue, Xia et al. (2008) indicate a rate of switching of 0.84% compared to 0.73% in the control group (p = ns). Manic/hypomanic symptoms first appeared anywhere from the first session to a week after finishing rTMS treatment. Duration of symptoms also varied, from 2 days up to 1 month. The authors suggest maintaining patients' current mood stabilizer treatment and identifying those that could be at greater risk of switching (Harel et al. 2011).

Conclusions

Despite the remarkable morbidity and mortality associated with bipolar depression, the armamentarium for its treatment remains disappointingly limited. The most solid evidence appears to be for olanzapine/fluoxetine, quetiapine, and ECT, followed by lithium and valproate. As a secondary strategy, based on existing data, it seems reasonable to use antidepressants in combination with a mood stabilizer, with attention paid to possible emergence of manic/hypomanic symptoms. Although risk of switching is not as great as previously believed and appears to be a characteristic of the disease itself, clinicians should weigh the risk of untreated depression, including suicide risk, vs. the possibility of switching when evaluating treatment options for individual patients. Despite widespread usage, the efficacy of lamotrigine for either acute or maintenance treatment of bipolar depression remains in question.

References

Ahn, Y.M., Nam, J.Y., Culver, J.L. et al. (2011). Lamotrigine plus quetiapine combination therapy in treatment-resistant bipolar depression. *Annals of Clinical Psychiatry*, 23, 17–24.

Altshuler, L.L., Post, R.M., Black, D.O. et al. (2006). Subsyndromal depressive symptoms are associated with functional impairment in patients with bipolar disorder: Results of a large, multisite study. *Journal of Clinical Psychiatry*, 67, 1551–1560.

Altshuler, L.L., Post, R.M., Hellemann, G. et al. (2009). Impact of antidepressant continuation after acute positive or partial treatment response for bipolar depression: A blinded, randomized study. *Journal of Clinical Psychiatry*, 70, 450–457.

American Psychiatric Association (2006). *Practice Guideline for the Treatment of Patients with Bipolar Disorder*. Washington, DC: American Psychiatric Assosciation.

Amsterdam, J.D. and Shults J. (2005). Comparison of fluoxetine, olanzapine, and combined fluoxetine plus olanzapine initial therapy of bipolar type I and type II major depression – lack of manic induction. *Journal of Affective Disorders*, 87, 121–130.

Ananth, J., Wohl, M., Ranganath, V., and Beshay, M. (1993). Rapid cycling patients: Conceptual and etiological factors. *Neuropsychobiology*, 27, 193–198.

Bauer, M., Rasgon, N., Grof, P. *et al.* (2005). Mood changes related to antidepressants: A longitudinal study of patients with bipolar disorder in a naturalistic setting. *Psychiatry Research*, 133, 73–80.

Benazzi, F., Berk, M., Frye, M.A. *et al.* (2009). Olanzapine/fluoxetine combination for the treatment of mixed depression in bipolar I disorder: A post hoc analysis. *Journal of Clinical Psychiatry*, 70, 1424–1431.

Benedetti, F., Radaelli, D., Poletti, S. *et al.* (2011). Opposite effects of suicidality and lithium on gray matter volumes in bipolar depression. *Journal of Affective Disorders*, 135, 139–147.

Black, D.W., Winokur, G., and Nasrallah, A. (1986). ECT in unipolar and bipolar disorders: A naturalistic evaluation of 460 patients. *Convulsive Therapy*, 2, 231–237.

Bogart, G.T. and Chavez, B. (2009). Safety and efficacy of quetiapine in bipolar depression. *Annals of Pharmacotherapy*, 43, 1848–1856.

Bowden C.L., Lecrubier Y., Bauer M. *et al.* (2000). Maintenance therapies for classic and other forms of bipolar disorder. *Journal of Affective Disorders*, 59 Suppl 1, S57–S67.

Brown, E., Dunner, D.L., McElroy, S.L. *et al.* (2009). Olanzapine/fluoxetine combination vs. lamotrigine in the 6-month treatment of bipolar I depression. *International Journal of Neuropsychopharmacology*, 12, 773–782.

Brown, E.B., McElroy, S.L., Keck, P.E., Jr. *et al.* (2006). A 7-week, randomized, double-blind trial of olanzapine/fluoxetine combination versus lamotrigine in the treatment of bipolar I depression. *Journal of Clinical Psychiatry*, 67, 1025–1033.

Calabrese, J.R., Guelfi, J.D., and Perdrizet-Chevallier, C. (2007). Agomelatine adjunctive therapy for acute bipolar depression: preliminary open data. *Bipolar Disorders*, 9, 628–635.

Calabrese, J.R., Bowden, C.L., Sachs, G.S. *et al.* (1999). A double-blind placebo-controlled study of lamotrigine monotherapy in outpatients with bipolar I depression. Lamictal 602 Study Group. *Journal of Clinical Psychiatry*, 60, 79–88.

Calabrese, J.R., Suppes, T., Bowden, C.L. *et al.* (2000). A double-blind, placebo-controlled, prophylaxis study of lamotrigine in rapid-cycling bipolar disorder. Lamictal 614 Study Group. *Journal of Clinical Psychiatry*, 61, 841–850.

Calabrese, J.R., Bowden, C.L., Deveaugh-Geiss, A. *et al.* (2001). *Lamotrigine Demonstrates Long-term Mood Stabilization in Recently Manic Patients*. Presented at the American Psychiatric Association Meeting, New Orleans, LU, USA.

Calabrese, J.R., Keck, P.E., Jr., MacFadden, W. *et al.* (2005). A randomized, double-blind, placebo-controlled trial of quetiapine in the treatment of bipolar I or II depression. *American Journal of Psychiatry*, 162, 1351–1360.

Calabrese, J.R., Huffman, R.F., White, R.L. *et al.* (2008). Lamotrigine in the acute treatment of bipolar depression: Results of five double-blind, placebo-controlled clinical trials. *Bipolar Disorders*, 10, 323–333.

Chang, J.S., Moon, E., Cha, B., and Ha K. (2010). Adjunctive lamotrigine therapy for patients with bipolar II depression partially responsive to mood stabilizers. *Progress in Neuropsychopharmacology and Biological Psychiatry*, 34, 1322–1326.

Cohen, R.B., Brunoni, A.R., Boggio, P.S., and Fregni, F. (2010). Clinical predictors associated with duration of repetitive transcranial magnetic stimulation treatment for remission in bipolar depression: A naturalistic study. *Journal of Nervous Mental Disorders*, 198, 679–681.

Corya, S.A., Perlis, R.H., Keck, P.E., Jr. *et al.* (2006). A 24-week open-label extension study of olanzapine-fluoxetine combination and olanzapine monotherapy in the treatment of bipolar depression. *Journal of Clinical Psychiatry*, 67, 798–806.

Cristancho, M.A. and Thase, M.E. (2010). The role of quetiapine extended release in the treatment of bipolar depression. *Advances in Therapy*, 27, 774–784.

Daly, J.J., Prudic, J., Devanand, D.P. *et al.* (2001). ECT in bipolar and unipolar depression: Differences in speed of response. *Bipolar Disorders*, 3, 95–104.

Davis, L.L., Bartolucci, A., and Petty, F. (2005). Divalproex in the treatment of bipolar depression: A placebo-controlled study. *Journal of Affective Disorders*, 85, 259–266.

Davis, L.L., Kabel, D., Patel, D. *et al.* (1996). Valproate as an antidepressant in major depressive disorder. *Psychopharmacology Bulletin*, 32, 647–652.

Deeks, E.D. and Keating, G.M. (2008a). Olanzapine/fluoxetine: A review of its use in the treatment of acute bipolar depression. *Drugs*, 68, 1115–1137.

Deeks, E.D. and Keating, G.M. (2008b). Spotlight on olanzapine/fluoxetine in acute bipolar depression. *CNS Drugs*, 22, 793–795.

De Fruyt, J., Deschepper, E., Audenaert, K. *et al.* (2012). Second generation antipsychotics in the treatment of bipolar depression: A systematic review and meta-analysis. *Journal of Psychopharmacology*, 26, 603–617.

Dell'Osso, B., D'Urso, N., Castellano, F., Ciabatti, M., and Altamura, A.C. (2011). Long-term efficacy after acute augmentative repetitive transcranial magnetic stimulation in bipolar depression: A I-year follow-up study. *Journal of ECT*, 27, 141–144.

Dell'Osso, B., Mundo, E., D'Urso, N. *et al.* (2009). Augmentative repetitive navigated transcranial magnetic stimulation (rTMS) in drug-resistant bipolar depression. *Bipolar Disorders*, 11, 76–81.

Denicoff, K.D., Smith-Jackson, E.E., Disney, E.R. *et al.* (1997). Comparative prophylactic efficacy of lithium, carbamazepine, and the combination in bipolar disorder. *Journal of Clinical Psychiatry*, 58, 470–478.

Dilsaver, S.C., Swann, S.C., Chen, Y.W. *et al.* (1996). Treatment of bipolar depression with carbamazepine: results of an open study. *Biological Psychiatry*, 40, 935–937.

Dilsaver, S.C., Chen, Y.W., Swann, A.C. *et al.* (1997). Suicidality, panic disorder and psychosis in bipolar depression, depressive-mania and pure-mania. *Psychiatry Research*, 73, 47–56.

Dolberg, O.T., Dannon, P.N., Schreiber, S., and Grunhaus, L. (2002). Transcranial magnetic stimulation in patients with bipolar depression: A double blind, controlled study. *Bipolar Disorder*, 4 Suppl 1, 94–95.

Dube, S., Tollefson, G.D., Thase, M.E. *et al.* (2007). Onset of antidepressant effect of olanzapine and olanzapine/fluoxetine combination in bipolar depression. *Bipolar Disorder*, 9, 618–627.

Dunn, R.T., Stan, V.A., Chriki, L.S., Filkowski, M.M., and Ghaemi, S.N. (2008). A prospective, open-label study of aripiprazole mono- and adjunctive treatment in acute bipolar depression. *Journal of Affective Disorders*, 110, 70–74.

Food and Drug Administration (2011). *Symbyax Label Information* [online]. Available at: http://www.accessdata.fda.gov/drugsatfda_docs/label/2011/021520s33lbl.pdf (accessed June 14th 2012).

Fountoulakis, K.N. and Vieta, E. (2008). Treatment of bipolar disorder: A systematic review of available data and clinical perspectives. *International Journal of Neuropsychopharmacology*, 11, 999–1029.

Frye, M.A., Helleman, G., McElroy, S.L. *et al.* (2009). Correlates of treatment-emergent mania associated with antidepressant treatment in bipolar depression. *American Journal of Psychiatry*, 166, 164–172.

Fu, A.Z., Liu, G.G., Christensen, D.B., and Hansen, R.A. (2007). Effect of second-generation antidepressants on mania- and depression-related visits in adults with bipolar disorder: A retrospective study. *Value In Health*, 10, 128–136.

Geddes, J.R., Calabrese, J.R., and Goodwin, G.M. (2009). Lamotrigine for treatment of bipolar depression: Independent meta-analysis and meta-regression of individual patient data from five randomised trials. *British Journal of Psychiatry*, 194, 4–9.

Ghaemi, S.N., Hsu, D.J., Thase, M.E. *et al.* (2006). Pharmacological treatment patterns at study entry for the first 500 STEP-BD participants. *Psychiatric Services*, 57, 660–665.

Ghaemi, S.N., Gilmer, W.S., Goldberg, J.F. *et al.* (2007). Divalproex in the treatment of acute bipolar depression: A preliminary double-blind, randomized, placebo-controlled pilot study. *Journal of Clinical Psychiatry*, 68, 1840–1844.

Ghaemi, S.N., Ostacher, M.M., El-Mallakh, R.S. *et al.* (2010). Antidepressant discontinuation in bipolar depression: A Systematic Treatment Enhancement Program for Bipolar Disorder (STEP-BD) randomized clinical trial of long-term effectiveness and safety. *Journal of Clinical Psychiatry*, 71, 372–380.

Gijsman, H.J., Geddes, J.R., Rendell, J.M., Nolen, W.A., and Goodwin, G.M. (2004). Antidepressants for bipolar depression: A systematic review of randomized, controlled trials. *American Journal of Psychiatry*, 161, 1537–1547.

Goodwin, F.K., Murphy, D.L., and Bunney, W.E., Jr. (1969). Lithium-carbonate treatment in depression and mania: A longitudinal double-blind study. *Archives of General Psychiatry*, 21, 486–496.

Greil, W. and Kleindienst, N. (1999). The comparative prophylactic efficacy of lithium and carbamazepine in patients with bipolar I disorder. *International Clinical Psychopharmacology*, 14, 277–281.

Grunhaus, L., Schreiber, S., Dolberg, O.T., Hirshman, S., and Dannon, P.N. (2002). Response to ECT in major depression: Are there differences between unipolar and bipolar depression? *Bipolar Disorders*, 4 Suppl 1, 91–93.

Harel, E.V., Zangen, A., Roth, Y. *et al.* (2011). H-coil repetitive transcranial magnetic stimulation for the treatment of bipolar depression: An add-on, safety and feasibility study. *World Journal Biological Psychiatry*, 12, 119–126.

Holtzheimer, P.E., Kelley, M.E., Gross, R.E. *et al.* (2012). Subcallosal cingulate deep brain stimulation for treatment-resistant unipolar and bipolar depression. *Archives of General Psychiatry*, 69, 150–158.

Isometsa, E.T., Henriksson, M.M., Aro, H.M., and Lonnqvist, J.K. (1994). Suicide in bipolar disorder in Finland. *American Journal of Psychiatry*, 151, 1020–1024.

Janicak, P.G. and Rado, J.T. (2011). Quetiapine monotherapy for bipolar depression. *Expert Opinion on Pharmacotherapy*, 12, 1643–1651.

Janicak, P.G., Davis, J.M., Gibbons, R.D. *et al.* (1985). Efficacy of ECT: A meta-analysis. *American Journal of Psychiatry*, 142, 297–302.

Joffe, R.T., MacQueen, G.M., Marriott, M. *et al.* (2002). Induction of mania and cycle acceleration in bipolar disorder: Effect of different classes of antidepressant. *Acta Psychiatrica Scandanivica*, 105, 427–430.

Judd, L.L. and Akiskal, H.S. (2003). Depressive episodes and symptoms dominate the longitudinal course of bipolar disorder. *Current Psychiatry Reports*, 5, 417–418.

Judd, L.L., Akiskal, H.S., Schettler, P.J. *et al.* (2005). Psychosocial disability in the course of bipolar I and II disorders: A prospective, comparative, longitudinal study. *Archives of General Psychiatry*, 62, 1322–1330.

Kane, J.M., Quitkin, F.M., Rifkin, A. *et al.* (1982). Lithium carbonate and imipramine in the prophylaxis of unipolar and bipolar II illness: A prospective, placebo-controlled comparison. *Archives of General Psychiatry*, 39, 1065–1069.

Keck, P.E., Jr., Marcus, R., Tourkodimitris, S. *et al.* (2003). A placebo-controlled, double-blind study of the efficacy and safety of aripiprazole in patients with acute bipolar mania. *American Journal of Psychiatry*, 160, 1651–1658.

Keck, P.E., Jr., Corya, S.A., Altshuler, L.L. *et al.* (2005). Analyses of treatment-emergent mania with olanzapine/fluoxetine combination in the treatment of bipolar depression. *Journal of Clinical Psychiatry*, 66, 611–616.

Keck, P.E., Orsulak, P.J., Cutler, A.J. *et al.* (2009). Aripiprazole monotherapy in the treatment of acute bipolar I mania: A randomized, double-blind, placebo- and lithium-controlled study. *Journal of Affective Disorders*, 112, 36–49.

Kemp, D.E., Gilmer, W.S., Fleck, J. *et al.* (2007). Aripiprazole augmentation in treatment-resistant bipolar depression: Early response and development of akathisia. *Progress in Neuropsychopharmacology and Biological Psychiatry*, 31, 574–577.

Kemp, D.E., Calabrese, J.R., Eudicone, J.M. *et al.* (2010). Predictive value of early improvement in bipolar depression trials: A post-hoc pooled analysis of two 8-week aripiprazole studies. *Psychopharmacology Bulletins*, 43, 5–27.

Kessing, L.V., Hellmund, G., and Andersen, P.K. (2011). An observational nationwide register based cohort study on lamotrigine versus lithium in bipolar disorder. *Journal of Psychopharmacology*, 26, 644–652.

Ketter, T.A., Wang, P.W., Chandler, R.A., Culver, J.L., and Alarcon, A.M. (2006). Adjunctive aripiprazole in treatment-resistant bipolar depression. *Annals of Clinical Psychiatry*, 18, 169–172.

Kleinman, L., Lowin, A., Flood, E. *et al.* (2003). Costs of bipolar disorder. *Pharmacoeconomics*, 21, 601–622.

Kupfer, D.J., Chengappa, K.N., Gelenberg, A.J. *et al.* (2001). Citalopram as adjunctive therapy in bipolar depression. *Journal of Clinical Psychiatry*, 62, 985–990.

Kupka, R.W., Altshuler, L.L., Nolen, W.A. *et al.* (2007). Three times more days depressed than manic or hypomanic in both bipolar I and bipolar II disorder. *Bipolar Disorders*, 9, 531–535.

Lepkifker, E., Iancu, I., Horesh, N., Strous, R.D., and Kotler, M. (2007). Lithium therapy for unipolar and bipolar depression among the middle-aged and older adult patient subpopulation. *Depression and Anxiety*, 24, 571–576.

Leverich, G.S., Altshuler, L.L., Frye, M.A. *et al.* (2006). Risk of switch in mood polarity to hypomania or mania in patients with bipolar depression during acute and continuation trials of venlafaxine, sertraline, and bupropion as adjuncts to mood stabilizers. *American Journal of Psychiatry*, 163, 232–239.

Licht, R.W., Nielsen, J.N., Gram, L.F., Vestergaard, P., and Bendz, H. (2010). Lamotrigine versus lithium as maintenance treatment in bipolar I disorder: An open, randomized effectiveness study mimicking clinical practice. The 6th trial of the Danish University Antidepressant Group (DUAG-6). *Bipolar Disorders*, 12, 483–493.

Liebowitz, M.R., Salman, E., Mech, A. *et al.* (2009). Ziprasidone monotherapy in bipolar II depression: An open trial. *Journal of Affective Disorders*, 118, 205–208.

Lombardo, I., Sachs, G., Kolluri, S., Kremer, C., and Yang, R. (2012). Two 6-week, randomized, double-blind, placebo-controlled studies of ziprasidone in outpatients with bipolar I depression: Did baseline characteristics impact trial outcome? *Journal of Clinical Psychopharmacology*, 32, 470–478.

Manning, J.S., Connor, P.D., and Sahai, A. (1998). The bipolar spectrum: A review of current concepts and implications for the management of depression in primary care. *Archives of Family Medicine*, 7, 63–71.

Marcus, R., Khan, A., Rollin, L. *et al.* (2011). Efficacy of aripiprazole adjunctive to lithium or valproate in the long-term treatment of patients with bipolar I disorder with an inadequate response to lithium or valproate monotherapy: A multicenter, double-blind, randomized study. *Bipolar Disorders*, 13, 133–144.

Marmol, F. (2006). 55 años de historia en el tratamiento del trastorno bipolar. *Medicina Clinica (Barcelona)*, 127, 189–195.

McElroy, S.L., Zarate, C.A., Cookson, J. *et al.* (2004). A 52-week, open-label continuation study of lamotrigine in the treatment of bipolar depression. *Journal of Clinical Psychiatry*, 65, 204–210.

McElroy, S.L., Suppes, T., Frye, M.A. *et al.* (2007). Open-label aripiprazole in the treatment of acute bipolar depression: A prospective pilot trial. *Journal of Affective Disorders*, 101, 275–281.

McElroy, S.L., Weisler, R.H., Chang, W. *et al.* (2010). A double-blind, placebo-controlled study of quetiapine and paroxetine as monotherapy in adults with bipolar depression (EMBOLDEN II). *Journal of Clinical Psychiatry*, 71, 163–174.

Medda, P., Perugi, G., Zanello, S., Ciuffa, M., and Cassano, G.B. (2009). Response to ECT in bipolar I, bipolar II and unipolar depression. *Journal of Affective Disorders*, 118, 55–59.

Moon, E., Chang, J.S., Kim, M.Y. *et al.* (2012). Dropout rate and associated factors in patients with bipolar disorders. *Journal of Affective Disorders*, 141, 47–54.

Muzina, D., Ganocy, S., Khalife, S. *et al.* (2008). *A Double-blind, Placebo-controlled Study of Divalproex Extended-release in Newly Diagnosed Mood Stabiliser Naive Patients with Acute Bipolar I or II Depression.* Presented at the 48th New Clinical Drug Evaluation Unit Meeting: New Approaches for Mental Health Interventions, Phoenix, AZ, USA.

Nahas, Z., Kozel, F.A., Li, X., Anderson, B., and George, M.S. (2003). Left prefrontal transcranial magnetic stimulation (TMS) treatment of depression in bipolar affective disorder: A pilot study of acute safety and efficacy. *Bipolar Disorders*, 5, 40–47.

Nierenberg, A.A., Ostacher, M.J., Calabrese, J.R. *et al.* (2006). Treatment-resistant bipolar depression: A STEP-BD equipoise randomized effectiveness trial of antidepressant augmentation with lamotrigine, inositol, or risperidone. *American Journal Psychiatry*, 163, 210–216.

Patel, N.C., Delbello, M.P., Bryan, H.S. *et al.* (2006). Open-label lithium for the treatment of adolescents with bipolar depression. *Journal of the American Academy of Child and Adolescent Psychiatry*, 45, 289–297.

Peet, M. (1994). Induction of mania with selective serotonin re-uptake inhibitors and tricyclic antidepressants. *British Journal of Psychiatry*, 164, 549–550.

Perlis, R.H., Adams, D.H., Fijal, B. *et al.* (2010). Genetic association study of treatment response with olanzapine/fluoxetine combination or lamotrigine in bipolar I depression. *Journal of Clinical Psychiatry*, 71, 599–605.

Peselow, E.D., Dunner, D.L., Fieve, R.R., and Lautin, A. (1982). Lithium prophylaxis of depression in unipolar, bipolar II, and cyclothymic patients. *American Journal of Psychiatry*, 139, 747–752.

Post, R.M., Altshuler, L.L., Leverich, G.S. *et al.* (2006). Mood switch in bipolar depression: Comparison of adjunctive venlafaxine, bupropion and sertraline. *British Journal of Psychiatry*, 189, 124–131.

Quante, A., Zeugmann, S., Luborzewski, A. *et al.* (2010). Aripiprazole as adjunct to a mood stabilizer and citalopram in bipolar depression: A randomized placebo-controlled pilot study. *Human Psychopharmacology*, 25, 126–132.

Sachs, G., Altshuler, L., Ketter, T.A. *et al.* (2001). *Divalproex versus Placebo for the Treatment of Bipolar Depression.* Presented at the 40th Annual Meeting of the American College of Neuropsychopharmacology 2001, San Juan, Puerto Rico.

Sachs, G.S., Koslow, C.L., and Ghaemi, S.N. (2000). The treatment of bipolar depression. *Bipolar Disorders*, 2, 256–260.

Sachs, G.S., Nierenberg, A.A., Calabrese, J.R. *et al.* (2007). Effectiveness of adjunctive antidepressant treatment for bipolar depression. *New England Journal of Medicine*, 356, 1711–1722.

Sachs, G.S., Ice, K.S., Chappell, P.B. *et al.* (2011). Efficacy and safety of adjunctive oral ziprasidone for acute treatment of depression in patients with bipolar I disorder: A randomized, double-blind, placebo-controlled trial. *Journal of Clinical Psychiatry*, 72, 1413–1422.

Schaffer, A., Zuker, P., and Levitt, A. (2006). Randomized, double-blind pilot trial comparing lamotrigine versus citalopram for the treatment of bipolar depression. *Journal of Affective Disorders*, 96, 95–99.

Schou, M., Juel-Nielsen, N., Stromgren, E., and Voldby, H. (1954). The treatment of manic psychoses by the administration of lithium salts. *Journal of Neurology, Neurosurgery and Psychiatry*, 17, 250–260.

Serretti, A., Artioli, P., Zanardi, R., and Rossini, D. (2003). Clinical features of antidepressant associated manic and hypomanic switches in bipolar disorder. *Progress in Neuropsychopharmacology and Biological Psychiatry*, 27, 751–757.

Sharma, V., Khan, M., and Corpse, C. (2008). Role of lamotrigine in the management of treatment-resistant bipolar II depression: A chart review. *Journal of Affective Disorders*, 111, 100–105.

Shelton, R.C. (2006). Olanzapine/fluoxetine combination for bipolar depression. *Expert Reviews of Neurotherapeutics*, 6, 33–39.

Shelton, R.C. and Stahl, S.M. (2004). Risperidone and paroxetine given singly and in combination for bipolar depression. *Journal of Clinical Psychiatry*, 65, 1715–1719.

Shi, L., Namjoshi, M.A., Swindle, R. *et al.* (2004). Effects of olanzapine alone and olanzapine/fluoxetine combination on health-related quality of life in patients with bipolar depression: Secondary analyses of a double-blind, placebo-controlled, randomized clinical trial. *Clinical Therapy*, 26, 125–134.

Sidor, M.M. and MacQueen, G.M. (2011). Antidepressants for the acute treatment of bipolar depression: A systematic review and meta-analysis. *Journal of Clinical Psychiatry*, 72, 156–167.

Smith, L.A., Cornelius, V.R., Azorin, J.M. *et al.* (2010). Valproate for the treatment of acute bipolar depression: Systematic review and meta-analysis. *Journal of Affective Disorders*, 122, 1–9.

Sokolski, K.N. (2007). Adjunctive aripiprazole in bipolar I depression. *Annals of Pharmacotherapy*, 41, 35–40.

Suppes, T., Kelly, D.I., Keck, P.E., Jr. *et al.* (2007). Quetiapine for the continuation treatment of bipolar depression: Naturalistic prospective case series from the Stanley Bipolar Treatment Network. *International Clinical Psychopharmacology*, 22, 376–381.

Suppes, T., Marangell, L.B., Bernstein, I.H. *et al.* (2008). A single blind comparison of lithium and lamotrigine for the treatment of bipolar II depression. *Journal of Affective Disorders*, 111, 334–343.

Suppes, T., Datto, C., Minkwitz, M. *et al.* (2010). Effectiveness of the extended release formulation of quetiapine as monotherapy for the treatment of acute bipolar depression. *Journal of Affective Disorders*, 121, 106–115.

Swartz, H.A. and Thase, M.E. (2011). Pharmacotherapy for the treatment of acute bipolar II depression: Current evidence. *Journal of Clinical Psychiatry*, 72, 356–366.

Tamayo, J.M., Sutton, V.K., Mattei, M.A. *et al.* (2009). Effectiveness and safety of the combination of fluoxetine and olanzapine in outpatients with bipolar depression: An open-label, randomized, flexible-dose study in Puerto Rico. *Journal of Clinical Psychopharmacology*, 29, 358–361.

Thase, M.E. (2008). Quetiapine monotherapy for bipolar depression. *Neuropsychiatric Disease and Treatment*, 4, 11–21.

Thase, M.E. and Sachs, G.S. (2000). Bipolar depression: pharmacotherapy and related therapeutic strategies. *Biological Psychiatry*, 48, 558–572.

Thase, M.E., MacFadden, W., Weisler, R.H. *et al.* (2006). Efficacy of quetiapine monotherapy in bipolar I and II depression: A double-blind, placebo-controlled study (the BOLDER II study). *Journal of Clinical Psychopharmacology*, 26, 600–609.

Thase, M.E., Jonas, A., Khan, A. *et al.* (2008). Aripiprazole monotherapy in nonpsychotic bipolar I depression: Results of 2 randomized, placebo-controlled studies. *Journal Clinical Psychopharmacology*, 28, 13–20.

Thase, M.E., Bowden, C.L., Nashat, M. *et al.* (2012). Aripiprazole in bipolar depression: A pooled, post-hoc analysis by severity of core depressive symptoms. *International Journal of Psychiatry in Clinical Practice*, 16, 121–131.

Tohen, M., Vieta, E., Calabrese, J. *et al.* (2003). Efficacy of olanzapine and olanzapine-fluoxetine combination in the treatment of bipolar I depression. *Archives of General Psychiatry*, 60, 1079–1088.

Tondo, L., Baldessarini, R.J., Hennen, J., and Floris, G. (1998). Lithium maintenance treatment of depression and mania in bipolar I and bipolar II disorders. *American Journal of Psychiatry*, 155, 638–645.

Truman, C.J., Goldberg, J.F., Ghaemi, S.N. *et al.* (2007). Self-reported history of manic/hypomanic switch associated with antidepressant use: Data from the Systematic Treatment Enhancement Program for Bipolar Disorder (STEP-BD). *Journal of Clinical Psychiatry*, 68, 1472–1479.

Valtonen, H.M., Suominen, K., Mantere, O. *et al.* (2007). Suicidal behaviour during different phases of bipolar disorder. *Journal of Affective Disorders*, 97, 101–107.

Valtonen, H.M., Suominen, K., Haukka, J. *et al.* (2008). Differences in incidence of suicide attempts during phases of bipolar I and II disorders. *Bipolar Disorders*, 10, 588–596.

Van der Loos, M.L., Mulder, P.G., Hartong, E.G. *et al.* (2009). Efficacy and safety of lamotrigine as add-on treatment to lithium in bipolar depression: A multicenter, double-blind, placebo-controlled trial. *Journal of Clinical Psychiatry*, 70, 223–231.

Vieta, E., Bourin, M., Sanchez, R. *et al.* (2005). Effectiveness of aripiprazole v. haloperidol in acute bipolar mania: Double-blind, randomised, comparative 12-week trial. *British Journal of Psychiatry*, 187, 235–242.

Vieta, E., Locklear, J., Gunther, O. *et al.* (2010). Treatment options for bipolar depression: A systematic review of randomized, controlled trials. *Journal of Clinical Psychopharmacology*, 30, 579–590.

Vojta, C., Kinosian, B., Glick, H., Altshuler, L., and Bauer, M.S. (2001). Self-reported quality of life across mood states in bipolar disorder. *Comprehensive Psychiatry*, 42, 190–195.

Wang, Z., Gao, K., Kemp, D.E. *et al.* (2010). Lamotrigine adjunctive therapy to lithium and divalproex in depressed patients with rapid cycling bipolar disorder and a recent substance use disorder: A 12-week, double-blind, placebo-controlled pilot study. *Psychopharmacology Bulletins*, 43, 5–21.

Wang, Z., Kemp, D.E., Chan, P.K. *et al.* (2011). Comparisons of the tolerability and sensitivity of quetiapine-XR in the acute treatment of schizophrenia, bipolar mania, bipolar depression, major depressive disorder, and generalized anxiety disorder. *International Journal of Neuropsychopharmacology*, 14, 131–142.

Weisler, R.H., Nolen, W.A., Neijber, A., Hellqvist, A., and Paulsson, B. (2011). Continuation of quetiapine versus switching to placebo or lithium for maintenance treatment of bipolar I disorder (trial 144: A randomized controlled study). *Journal of Clinical Psychiatry*, 72, 1452–1464.

Weisler, R.H., Calabrese, J.R., Thase, M.E. *et al.* (2008). Efficacy of quetiapine monotherapy for the treatment of depressive episodes in bipolar I disorder: A post hoc analysis of combined results from 2 double-blind, randomized, placebo-controlled studies. *Journal of Clinical Psychiatry*, 69, 769–782.

Wyatt, R.J. and Henter, I. (1995). An economic evaluation of manic-depressive illness–1991. *Social Psychiatry and Psychiatric Epidemiology*, 30, 213–219.

Xia, G., Gajwani, P., Muzina, D.J. *et al.* (2008). Treatment-emergent mania in unipolar and bipolar depression: Focus on repetitive transcranial magnetic stimulation. *International Journal of Neuropsychopharmacology*, 11, 119–130.

Yatham, L.N. (2011). A clinical review of aripiprazole in bipolar depression and maintenance therapy of bipolar disorder. *Journal of Affective Disorders*, 128 Suppl 1, S21–S28.

Young, A.H., McElroy, S.L., Bauer, M. *et al.* (2010). A double-blind, placebo-controlled study of quetiapine and lithium monotherapy in adults in the acute phase of bipolar depression (EMBOLDEN I). *Journal of Clinical Psychiatry*, 71, 150–162.

Zhang, H., Wisniewski, S.R., Bauer, M.S., Sachs, G.S., and Thase, M.E. (2006). Comparisons of perceived quality of life across clinical states in bipolar disorder: Data from the first 2000 Systematic Treatment Enhancement Program for Bipolar Disorder (STEP-BD) participants. *Comprehensive Psychiatry*, 47, 161–168.

Medication treatment of mania: Acute and preventive

David A. Kahn

Introduction

Mania, the defining feature of bipolar I disorder, is a state of elevated or irritable mood accompanied by impulsivity, high energy, lack of insight, and, when severe, psychosis and dangerous behavior. Episodes of major depression are almost always part of the long-term course and often the initial presentation; treatment with antidepressants in a person with unrecognized or as yet unmanifested bipolar disorder may lead to florid unmasking of the condition. Depressive symptoms may occur during mania (often called dysphoric mania), and frank mixed states meeting criteria for both mania and depression are not uncommon. Bipolar II disorder is characterized by episodes of hypomania and depression. Nearly all patients who have had a manic or hypomanic episode will have multiple recurrences.

This review will focus on acute and preventive treatment of mania using medication in general adult populations. This topic is inextricably linked to prevention of bipolar depression, covered in more depth in Chapter 7. Psychosocial treatment, as well attention to co-morbid conditions, particularly substance-use disorders, often crucial, are reviewed in Chapter 14 and Chapter 17. Special considerations for pediatric, geriatric, and pregnant patients are also covered elsewhere in Chapter 9, Chapter 11, Chapter 12, Chapter 15, and Chapter 16.

Over a dozen medications are effective for acute episodes of mania. Hypomania has been less a target of clinical research, but is similarly responsive. Preventing recurrence, the aim of long-term management, is more difficult to achieve than acute remission. Many individuals experience residual symptoms, which increase the risk of recurrence (Tohen *et al.* 2006). Prolonged or even chronic depression is not uncommon, especially in bipolar II disorder (Mantere *et al.* 2008). Rapid cycling poses further challenges. It is not surprising that the majority of long-term bipolar patients take three or more medications (Frye *et al.* 2000).

After reviewing the evidence for various treatments, practical clinical pathways will be presented, informed by published guidelines that have blended evidence with clinical consensus.

Overview

Time course

Treatment of mania occurs in three phases with fluid boundaries (Goodwin *et al.* 2007):

- *Acute phase* is the period from the start of an episode until a stable clinical response, ideally to the point of remission when syndromal criteria are no longer met. Once treatment starts, this lasts approximately 6 to 12 weeks.

- *Continuation phase* is the ongoing period of close monitoring until the natural course of the episode would be expected to end, usually 3 to 6 months. Resolution of mania may be complicated by cycling into depression. During continuation, high acute medication doses are often reduced for greater safety and tolerability, new preventive drugs may be added, and polypharmacy is refined for simpler, safer, long-term maintenance.

- *Maintenance phase*, also called prophylaxis, aims to prevent future episodes of mania and depression, or at least reduce their severity and frequency. Given the highly recurrent nature of bipolar illness, ongoing medication maintenance may last for years and often a lifetime. Long-term efficacy, tolerability, and safety of medications

Clinical Handbook for the Management of Mood Disorders, ed. J. John Mann, Patrick J. McGrath, and Steven P. Roose.
Published by Cambridge University Press. © Cambridge University Press 2013.

must be carefully balanced to minimize mood symptoms, while maximizing functional recovery and overall health across the lifecycle.

Return of mania during continuation is considered a *relapse*, implying the patient is still within the original episode, distinct from a *recurrence*, which is a new episode during maintenance. For simplicity, the term recurrence will be used in describing any breakthrough of mania in a previously stabilized patient.

A perspective on terminology: mood stabilizers

Lithium, valproate, and carbamazepine are traditionally called mood stabilizers, a term with no official definition. The phrase first applied to lithium because of its initially unique ability to moderate both highs and lows. It later grew to include the two anticonvulsants, distinguishing them from first-generation antipsychotics (FGAs), once the main antimanic alternatives. As second-generation antipsychotics (SGAs) came into widespread use they, too, have often been called mood stabilizers, e.g., in marketing materials.

Thoughtful researchers have tried to sharpen the definition. In a strict sense, an ideal mood stabilizer would be equally effective to treat *and* prevent both depression *and* mania (Bauer and Mitchner, 2004). Of established treatments, only lithium and electroconvulsive therapy (ECT) are seen as coming close. In a less strict definition, a mood stabilizer improves either phase, while not worsening the opposite phase (Ketter and Calabrese, 2002). In this broader conceptualization, mood stabilizers may be divided into those that are relatively more potent against mania, working "from above" baseline, contrasted with those that treat depression, "from below." While lithium and ECT are more or less bimodal, valproate, carbamazepine, and most SGAs are mood stabilizers "from above," that is, effective primarily against mania. Quetiapine among the SGAs may in fact prove to be bimodal (Weisler *et al.* 2011). Lamotrigine is distinctly a mood stabilizer "from below," effective in preventing and perhaps acutely treating bipolar depression, without exacerbating mania.

First-generation antipsychotics (FGAs) increase relapse of bipolar depression (Tohen *et al.* 2003), so while they are potent antimanic agents they are not considered mood stabilizers; antidepressants are destabilizing if used alone.

First-line medications for acute and maintenance treatment of mania

Eleven drugs are approved by the US Food and Drug Administration (FDA) for acute mania, most for mixed states as well (Table 8.1). Six are SGAs: aripiprazole, asenapine, olanzapine, quetiapine, risperidone, and ziprasidone. Paliperidone (the major active metabolite of risperidone), is indicated for add-on treatment with a mood stabilizer or antidepressant in schizoaffective disorder. While chlorpromazine is the only first-generation antipsychotic (FGA) approved for mania, other FGAs, especially haloperidol, are still in use. Along with antipsychotics, the other three drugs approved for acute mania are the traditional mood stabilizers: lithium, valproate (including divalproex, in both immediate and extended-release forms, and valproic acid), and carbamazepine. Oxcarbazepine, though not approved in mood disorders, is sometimes used as an alternative to carbamazepine, to which it is structurally related.

For bipolar maintenance, only lithium, aripiprazole, olanzapine, lamotrigine, and adjunctive quetiapine are FDA approved. In practice however, all of the acutely effective medications are used (Yatham *et al.* 2005, Grunze *et al.* 2009). Lamotrigine is beneficial only for preventing depressive relapse, despite its approved label for prevention of mania as well, a regulatory anomaly contradicted both by published and unpublished data (Cipriani *et al.* 2011).

Research evidence

Understanding research methods

The gold standard of evidence is the placebo-controlled, randomized clinical trial (RCT). RCTs in mania, heroically difficult to conduct, have two major limitations. First, subjects need to be capable of informed consent and not of immediate danger, which may select for less severely ill patients than seen in many clinical settings (Grunze *et al.* 2009). It also may be harder to show that medications work in less severely ill patients due to more improvement on placebo. Second is the problem of referral bias: patients doing well with established treatments will not enroll in a study of new medication, and those not doing well may bias outcomes against older treatments used as comparators. Further, the reporting of study results in bipolar disorder has been

Table 8.1 Approved or frequently used medications for acute mania and maintenance treatment

	Acute mania	Mixed episode	Adjunctive acutely to lithium or divalproex	Maintenance	Typical acute dose range for monotherapy, mg/day±
Antipsychotics					
Aripiprazole	+	+	+	+	15–30
Asenapine	+	+	+		10–20
Chlorpromazine	+				300–1000
Haloperidol[a]					5–20
Olanzapine	+	+	+	+	10–30
Paliperidone[b]			+		3–12
Quetiapine[c]	+	+	+	+[d]	400–800
Risperidone	+	+	+		2–6
Ziprasidone	+	+	+		80–160
Non antipsychotics					
Carbamazepine	+	+			600–1200 (serum level 4–15 mg/l)
Lamotrigine[e]				+	50–200
Lithium	+			+	600–1200 (serum level 0.8–1.3 mg/l)
Oxcarbazepine					900–1800
Valproate	+				1250–3000 (loading dose 20–30 mg/kg body weight; serum level 75–100 mg/l)

Adapted from (Grunze *et al.* 2009)

[a] Not approved by the US Food and Drug Administration for mania
[b] Approved only as adjunctive therapy to antidepressants or mood stabilizers in schizoaffective disorder
[c] Also approved for acute treatment of bipolar depressive episodes
[d] Approved only as adjunctive to lithium or valproate in maintenance
[e] Although approved to prevent mania and depression, in practice used only for depression

critiqued for omission of: (1) important details of randomization methods, a flaw which could favor active treatments, and (2) calculation of effect sizes and number needed to treat, which assess the impact of a medication in clinical practice (Strech *et al.* 2011). Most importantly perhaps, acute phase RCTs are designed to show that individual drugs work safely, and not to guide the "real-world" task of how best to navigate the panoply of medications through strategies such as optimal sequencing, combined initial treatment, and even "polypharmacy" such as two antipsychotics.

RCTs in maintenance can take two broad forms. In the first, prophylaxis, patients who have been stable for some time on any treatment are randomized into study conditions (drug vs. placebo and/or active comparator). In the second, relapse prevention, patients who responded during an acute phase to a particular medication are randomized to continue on that medication or an alternative. The latter is sometimes called

an "enriched" sample in that patients are selected for having done well initially on the drug being tested. In both, there is a hazard to withdrawing a successful treatment, which may itself artificially provoke a relapse and skew the data. In both types, the direction of the most recent episode – depression or mania – may also affect outcomes.

Maintenance trials can be difficult to compare. Study designs may differ in duration, definition of relapse (e.g., sufficient to warrant change in medication vs. meeting full syndromal criteria), or endpoint (e.g., percentage of patients episode-free at study end, average time until relapse, severity over time, including sub-syndromal symptoms, stopping medication, functional status, etc.).

The upshot, as elsewhere in medicine, is that respected professional organizations have developed treatment guidelines that blend data from individual RCTs, meta-analyses, and expert consensus to distill good advice. We will turn to these later.

Standard medications for acute mania

Monotherapy

FGAs, particularly chlorpromazine and haloperidol, have been used for mania since the 1960s. Chlorpromazine, though never evaluated against placebo, is the only FGA approved by the FDA for mania.

Lithium, the first medication compared to placebo in RCTs of mania, was approved in 1970. Lithium may appear more effective in earlier than more recent studies, perhaps reflecting the difficulty of recruiting treatment-naïve, nonrefractory patients once it became widely used. Since 1980, numerous drugs have been found to be effective. The evidence comes from industry-funded, placebo-controlled RCTs, well summarized in recent reviews and guidelines (Goodwin, 2009, Yatham *et al*. 2009, Grunze *et al*. 2010, Sachs *et al*. 2011). Some of these studies have also included active comparators such as lithium and haloperidol, providing valuable new data on the older medications. Most are conducted in hospitals with moderately to severely ill patients, allowing rescue benzodiazepines to varying degrees, and lasting 3 to 4 weeks. Response is defined as a 50% reduction in the Young Mania Rating Scale (YMRS; Young *et al*. 1978), although the absolute scores after 3 weeks often still exceeded the minimum required to gain entry into the studies, showing that the average patient is still quite symptomatic (Sachs *et al*. 2011). Mean reduction in YMRS on medication is usually around 50 to 75% compared to placebo reductions of around 25 to 40%. Typically about twice as many subjects on active medication meet categorical response criteria compared with placebo.

Two meta-analyses of monotherapy trials differ in their conclusions about whether there are meaningful differences between antimanic drugs. The first (Smith *et al*. 2007b) combined data from 13 studies involving 3089 subjects, selecting only comparisons of monotherapy to placebo for medications approved in the US or UK. Data were examined for carbamazepine, haloperidol, lithium, olanzapine, quetiapine, risperidone, valproate, and aripiprazole. The pooled response rate for antipsychotics showed that 74% more subjects responded to medication than placebo, and for the nonantipsychotics 101% more; the difference between different types of medication was not significant. Withdrawal for any reason – lack of efficacy and adverse events – was less common with drug than placebo, except with lithium, aripiprazole, and carbamazepine. Discontinuation for adverse events compared with placebo was significant only for carbamazepine, at double the rate, while extrapyramidal events were more common with risperidone and aripiprazole. The result of this study was that aside from high rates of adverse-event withdrawals with carbamazepine, little difference between agents could be discerned.

The second meta-analysis (Cipriani *et al*. 2011) evaluated a much larger set of data from 68 RCTs with over 16 000 participants. It included both unapproved drugs and unpublished data. In order of descending advantage haloperidol (often the comparator), risperidone, olanzapine, lithium, quetiapine, aripiprazole, carbamazepine, asenapine, valproate, and ziprasidone were significantly more effective than placebo, while gabapentin, lamotrigine, and topiramate were not. Among effective drugs, haloperidol was more effective than all except risperidone and olanzapine; and risperidone and olanzapine were more effective than valproate and ziprasidone. Olanzapine and risperidone were discontinued significantly less often than lithium and placebo. The study concluded that antipsychotics were significantly more effective than non-antipsychotic mood stabilizers, and that risperidone, olanzapine, and haloperidol were the most effective of all. In clinical practice, it is often desirable to sedate patients rapidly in the early portion of treatment, giving credence to the short-term preference for antipsychotics. Anecdotal preference for risperidone and olanzapine had earlier been expressed in a survey of expert clinicians (Keck *et al*. 2004), further squaring the new findings with real-life experience. An important negative result in this study is confirmation that lamotrigine, despite its product label, and gabapentin and topiramate, sometimes used off-label, are not effective in mania.

There is no reliable way to predict response to individual medications based on clusters of clinical features, though some pointers are often cited. (Yatham *et al*. 2005, Grunze *et al*. 2009). Lithium may be less effective than valproate, carbamazepine, or second-generation antipsychotics in mixed states, dysphoric mania (presence of depressive symptoms), recent rapid cycling, or more severe mania. Positive predictors of response to lithium include prior response, euphoric or "classic" mania, absence of psychosis or substance abuse, and positive family history of bipolar illness. Clinicians need not pay undue attention to these predictors as they are mainly from open studies, retrospective analysis, or unreplicated series of case reports.

Combined therapy

The few RCTs that exist of SGAs combined with other mood stabilizers have included only patients with insufficient response to initial monotherapy. One meta-analysis of eight studies included 1124 subjects with inadequate responses to lithium or valproate after 3 weeks. Antipsychotics or placebo were added for another 3 to 6 weeks. Addition of haloperidol, olanzapine, risperidone, and quetiapine, but not ziprasidone resulted in a significantly greater number of responders, in the aggregate 50% more than with placebo. Withdrawals due to weight gain on olanzapine were a significant disadvantage, but for the others, overall withdrawal rates did not differ from placebo. A second meta-analysis looked at 24 RCTs that compared SGA monotherapy to placebo, mood stabilizers (lithium or valproate), or haloperidol, and included studies of adding-on to mood stabilizers (Scherk *et al.* 2007). SGA monotherapy was comparable to haloperidol and minimally better than mood stabilizers. However, combination therapy was superior to monotherapy, albeit at the cost of more somnolence and weight gain. The comparisons were striking enough for the author to conclude that combined therapy at the outset of treatment was advisable in severe mania, even though the data involved only add-on therapy.

Aripiprazole also has been shown to be superior to placebo added to lithium or valproate in nonresponders, though with higher rates of dropout for akathisia (Vieta *et al.* 2008). Asenapine is approved for acute mania and mixed states, as well as add-on therapy. In two RCTs it was superior to placebo, but less effective than olanzapine, and caused moderate weight gain (McIntyre, 2011). Paliperidone, approved as add-on therapy in schizoaffective disorder, diminishes manic symptoms when combined with lithium or valproate (Canuso *et al.* 2010), but is not yet proven effective as monotherapy (Berwaerts *et al.* 2012).

Combinations of SGAs with carbamazepine are problematic, in part because of higher metabolism of the antipsychotics. For example, adding risperidone in patients insufficiently responsive to carbamazepine provided no advantage, whereas adding it to lithium or valproate (Tohen *et al.* 2008) improved response (Yatham *et al.* 2003). The difference correlated with markedly lower risperidone blood levels in the carbamazepine group. Carbamazepine alone or with olanzapine was compared in a double-blind 6-week trial (Tohen *et al.* 2008). There was no advantage

to the combination; in both groups about two-thirds of patients responded. However, with the combination weight gain and triglycerides were greater; and olanzapine doses had to be doubled to achieve expected serum levels due to increased metabolism.

Combined lithium and valproate has not been rigorously evaluated. However, case series have lent support, and to a lesser extent for combinations with carbamazepine (Suppes *et al.* 2005, Yatham *et al.* 2005).

Standard medications for maintenance

Lithium

Since the 1970s lithium has been known to reduce the frequency of episodes of mania and depression. An early review (Prien *et al.* 1974) showed relapse rates for up to 2 years of 20 to 50% with lithium, compared to around 90% with placebo, with similar protection against both recurrent mania and depression. Lithium monotherapy was more effective in patients who were recently manic, and less effective when the most recent episode was depression – giving rise to the notion of "mania-prone" individuals versus "depression-prone" individuals, the latter benefiting from combining lithium with the antidepressant imipramine (Shapiro *et al.* 1989). More recent studies comparing lithium, lamotrigine, and placebo showed that lithium was significantly better than placebo in preventing mania, nearly halving the risk of recurrence, but only trending toward efficacy against depressive recurrence. Early studies have been faulted for rapid discontinuation of lithium, now known to magnify relapse rates in stable patients (Yazici *et al.* 2004). The later studies may have underestimated its antidepressant effects by enriching the sample for lamotrigine responders. Another modern-era study, intended to evaluate valproate, found no difference between lithium, valproate, and placebo for 12 months following a manic episode (Bowden *et al.* 2000). This study showed an unexpectedly low rate of relapse on placebo, and the lack of difference for both lithium and valproate has been attributed to the enrollment of mildly ill patients less prone to recurrence, perhaps a consequence of having to include a placebo group (Macritchie *et al.* 2001).

Valproate

As just discussed, valproate, though clearly effective in acute mania, was not statistically better than placebo in a 12-month maintenance trial. It did, however, prolong significantly the time to a depressive relapse, and may have been more effective than placebo in a subgroup of severely ill patients (Bowden *et al.* 2000). In other RCTs divalproex was equivalent to lithium in a 20-month trial in rapid cyclers (Calabrese *et al.* 2005) and olanzapine in a 47-week trial. Relapse rates in both studies, for all three drugs, were around 50%. The difficulty proving the long-term preventive benefit of valproate has been largely discounted by every authoritative practice guideline, which uniformly recommend it as a first-line option for maintenance (American Psychiatric Association, 2002, Yatham *et al.* 2005, Goodwin 2009, Grunze *et al.* 2009).

Carbamazepine

RCTs without placebo comparing lithium and carbamazepine show comparable preventive effects, though with better tolerability for lithium (Ceron-Litvoc *et al.* 2009). Some practice guidelines consider it to be an acceptable second-line option (American Psychiatric Association, 2002, Yatham *et al.* 2005, Goodwin, 2009). There is little evidence supporting oxcarbazepine (Vasudev *et al.* 2008), though these same published guidelines suggest it as a third-line alternative to carbamazepine with few drug interactions.

SGAs

Placebo-controlled RCTs lasting at least 12 months have shown that olanzapine, quetiapine, aripiprazole, and risperidone long-acting injectable (LAI) are effective as monotherapies in preventing recurrence of mania (Yatham *et al.* 2009). All but aripiprazole are somewhat effective for depressive recurrence. Quetiapine may be more effective than the others, and twice as effective as lithium, in preventing depression (Weisler *et al.* 2011). In a 2-year RCT of quetiapine versus placebo added to lithium or valproate in over 600 patients, the active combinations reduced overall relapse rates from 52 to 20% (Suppes *et al.* 2009), with equivalent effects on mania and depression. Significantly more patients on quetiapine stopped due to adverse events, including sedation, weight gain, and elevated glucose. Risperidone LAI added to a mood stabilizer also showed a halving of relapse rates compared to placebo injection in a 2-year RCT (Macfadden *et al.* 2009) with a relatively low discontinuation rate. Adjunctive ziprasidone with lithium or valproate was similarly effective and well tolerated in a 6-month RCT (Bowden *et al.* 2010). A critique of these adjunctive maintenance trials is that they often were drawn from enriched samples of patients who did not respond acutely to lithium or valproate, improved when the SGA was added, and then were randomized to continue or withdraw the SGA. This would bias the results, and not necessarily inform the decision to continue two-drug therapy (Bowden, 2011), since the SGA alone might be all that was needed.

Other established acute and maintenance treatments

Benzodiazepines

Widely used as adjuncts to promote sleep and sedation in mania, benzodiazepines have no specific or lasting benefits when used by themselves. A meta-analysis evaluated seven studies in which clonazepam or lorazepam were compared to placebo, to each other, to lithium, or to haloperidol for days to weeks in acute mania (Curtin and Schulz, 2004). Clonazepam, but not lorazepam, at doses up to 16 mg/d was better than placebo and lithium, but inferior to haloperidol. The results are questionable in the light of variable study designs and rating tools, and often brief time frames in which lithium's delayed action placed it at a disadvantage. The safest conclusion from these is that initial sedative effects may buy time. However, these effects are short lived as tolerance develops: an initial study of clonazepam as maintenance monotherapy was terminated for rapid relapse within weeks (Aronson *et al.* 1989).

Electroconvulsive therapy (ECT)

ECT (see Chapter 24 for more detailed discussion) is considered to be effective in mania even though there are only a handful of actual clinical trials, none optimally designed given the difficulty of providing a sham condition and obtaining informed consent (Fink, 2006). Accumulated experience suggests response rates of about 80%, higher than with medications and successful when medications have failed (Mukherjee *et al.* 1994). In a comparison trial, it was more rapidly effective than lithium, especially in mixed or severe mania (Small *et al.* 1988), although outcomes at 8 weeks were ultimately similar. Results may be superior when combined with medications, including chlorpromazine (Sikdar *et al.* 1994). Moreover it can be effective even while continuing to administer valproate or carbamazepine (Zarate *et al.* 1997). Maintenance

ECT, generally combined with medication, appears to reduce hospitalizations (Vaidya *et al.* 2003).

Clozapine

While there are no RCTs of clozapine in mania, its reputation for superiority to other SGAs in schizophrenia (Asenjo Lobos *et al.* 2010) makes it of great interest for treatment-resistant bipolar illness. An uncontrolled study in 1977 reported a rapid response within 1 or 2 days, and shortened hospital stay, in half of 52 manic patients (Muller and Heipertz, 1977). Zarate *et al.* (1995) reported marked improvement in 65% of 17 manic or mixed patients refractory to standard treatments. Green *et al.* (2000) reported over 50% reductions in mania ratings in a group of 22 treatment-refractory patients. Barbini and colleagues found a more rapid response with clozapine, compared to chlorpromazine, when added to lithium in acute mania (Barbini *et al.* 1997). An open, randomized, 1-year study comparing adjunctive clozapine to treatment as usual in 38 treatment-resistant patients showed significant reductions in mania, general measures of psychopathology, use of other medications, and side-effect burden, but not depression.

Experimental antimanic treatments

Based on a proposed role for protein kinase C in mania, investigation of the aromatase inhibitor tamoxifen has yielded promising results in pilot studies (Zarate *et al.* 2007, Yildiz *et al.* 2008). Calcium channel antagonists have been explored in mania for decades due to the resemblance between ionic calcium and lithium. Some data suggest an acute antimanic role for verapamil adjunctive to lithium, but not as monotherapy (Mallinger *et al.* 2008), and for nimodipine, especially in rapid cycling (Goodnick, 2000). Chronobiological approaches seek to regulate mood through normalization of circadian rhythm. Sleep deprivation can treat depression as well as trigger hypomania (Colombo *et al.* 1999). As a corollary, amber eyeglasses that screen out blue wavelengths have been proposed for use in hypomania (Phelps, 2008).

Many anticonvulsants have been investigated in mania and cycling. Positive anecdotal reports were not replicated in controlled trials of gabapentin, levetiracetam, phenytoin, topiramate, and zonisamide. They are therefore not recommended for routine mood stabilization, though idiosyncratic, individual patient responses may conceivably occur.

There are insufficient data to recommend unregulated supplements such as omega-3 fatty acids and *N*-acetylcysteine, though clinicians turn to them in treatment-refractory patients since they appear harmless.

Differentiating medications based on safety and side-effect concerns

All of the medications reviewed have potentially serious adverse consequences that obligate careful pretreatment and ongoing monitoring, and that call for personalized treatment selection. A few major side effects differentiate them; clinicians must also consider nonspecific side effects such as sedation and cognitive problems at higher doses.

SGAs often cause weight gain progressing to a metabolic syndrome, including hyperlipidemia and impaired glucose tolerance. This is most serious with olanzapine and quetiapine, intermediate for risperidone, and least for ziprasidone and aripiprazole (Meyer *et al.* 2008). Compared with FGAs, they have fewer acute extrapyramidal side effects, and at the time of their introduction were assumed to convey less risk of tardive dyskinesia (TD) (Keck *et al.* 2000). However, prospective studies in schizophrenia have found relative TD rates compared to FGAs ranging from 50% (Correll and Schenk, 2008) to equivalency (Woods *et al.* 2010). Given evidence that FGAs caused TD at higher rates in patients with bipolar disorder than with schizophrenia (Keck *et al.* 2000), the potential risk of TD from SGAs may be underappreciated.

Lithium causes a host of side effects, including hypothyroidism, acne, and tremor, all reversible with medication antidotes, as well as more problematic weight gain. There is a serious risk of acute or chronic neurotoxicity at blood levels barely exceeding the therapeutic range. Blood levels should be monitored frequently at the beginning of treatment, every 3 to 6 months once stable, and whenever a change in level is suspected based on side effects or anticipated due to dehydration or medical problems (American Psychiatric Association, 2002). Of greatest concern in long-term treatment is the possibility of permanent kidney damage, often heralded by polyuria (reflecting antagonism of antidiuretic hormone and potential interstitial nephritis), rising serum creatinine, and proteinuria. End-stage kidney disease leading to renal replacement therapy such as dialysis is estimated to occur at up to a sixfold rate compared to the general population. Monitoring of serum kidney functions is advised every 3 to 6 months, with measurement of 24 h urine volume and creatinine clearance when deterioration is suspected (Jefferson, 2010). If successful treatment with lithium needs to be discontinued for medical reasons or pregnancy (see below), it is highly advisable to taper it over a period of at least 4 weeks, as sudden cessation has been shown to precipitate recurrent mood episodes (Baldessarini *et al.* 1999).

With valproate the major common side effects are sedation and weight gain, as well as hair loss and sometimes tremor. Pancreatitis and thrombocytopenia are rare. Drug interactions that increase levels of lamotrigine and of warfarin require careful attention. Controversy surrounds a possible association with polycystic ovary disease (Rasgon *et al.* 2005) leading some guidelines to recommend avoidance if possible in young women.

Carbamazepine's principal liability is drug interactions from induction of cytochrome P450 liver enzymes. It reduces levels of lamotrigine, many antidepressants, antipsychotics, and benzodiazepines, as well as estrogen in oral contraceptives that may lead to unexpected pregnancy, and many other medications used in health care. For this reason, plus a smaller evidence base, it is not a first-line medication.

Safe use of medication in pregnant women with bipolar disorder is covered in greater detail in Chapter 15. The traditional mood stabilizers, lithium, valproate, and carbamazepine, are teratogenic, particularly in the first trimester, although the risk of cardiovascular malformation with lithium is thought by some to have been overestimated (Yonkers *et al.* 2004). In general FGAs, SGAs, and, if necessary ECT, are preferred for mania in pregnancy.

Practical recommendations

Review of published guidelines

In the past 10 years a number of organizations have assembled evidence-based treatment guidelines (American Psychiatric Association, 2002, Yatham *et al.* 2005, Goodwin 2009, Grunze *et al.* 2009, Yatham *et al.* 2009) and consensus-based guidelines (Keck *et al.* 2004, National Institute for Clinical Excellence, 2005, Suppes *et al.* 2005). Adjusted for inclusion of new data, they are fairly similar in their algorithms.

For acute phase, guidelines follow a structure of sequential trials moving from monotherapy to successive combinations, usually reserving initial combined medication for severe mania. First-line choices are SGAs, lithium, and valproate, with a slight tilt toward SGAs for monotherapy. All guidelines agree that antidepressants should be stopped in bipolar I mania. The ideal of evidence-based medicine is limited by the design of most clinical trials, which are conducted to bring new drugs to market rather than to answer real-world questions about selection and sequence (Fountoulakis *et al.* 2005). Hence, guidelines differ slightly in opinion-based nuances such as top choices amongst SGAs, how quickly to use combined therapy, duration of each step, and when to consider clozapine, FGAs, or ECT (e.g., whether they are "second" or "third" line).

For continuation and maintenance, all guidelines recommend staying with what worked acutely, with simplification of combined therapy to reduce side effects, unless by history the combination is needed to prevent further recurrences. This circles back to the desirability of anticipating long-term treatment when choosing acute agents. There is consensus that medication should be continued indefinitely following two manic episodes, or one episode if severe, or if there is a clear bipolar family history (Frances *et al.* 1996). Guidelines differ in recommending only lithium and valproate as first-line choices (American Psychiatric Association, 2002, Hirschfeld, 2005) or including the SGAs (Yatham *et al.* 2009).

Initial assessment for mania and hypomania

1. Determine appropriate level of care – hospital or outpatient – based on severity of illness, level of insight and co-operation, and social supports.
2. Assess current psychiatric medications: taking or not taking mood stabilizers, antidepressants, or other psychiatric medications.
3. Obtain psychiatric history, including past medication responses, adherence problems, and family history of psychiatric disorders and treatment responses.
4. Screen for other medical or physical factors that could precipitate an episode:
   a. All other prescribed medications
   b. Substances of abuse (consider toxicology screen)
   c. Medical conditions, e.g., neurological, endocrine, using tests appropriate to the patient's medical history and physical examination.

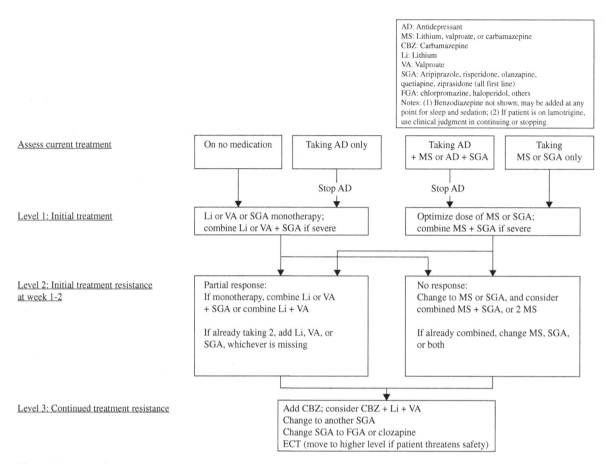

AD: Antidepressant
MS: Lithium, valproate, or carbamazepine
CBZ: Carbamazepine
Li: Lithium
VA: Valproate
SGA: Aripiprazole, risperidone, olanzapine,
quetiapine, ziprasidone (all first line)
FGA: chlorpromazine, haloperidol, others
Notes: (1) Benzodiazepine not shown; may be added at any
point for sleep and sedation; (2) If patient is on lamotrigine,
use clinical judgment in continuing or stopping.

Assess current treatment

| On no medication | Taking AD only | Taking AD + MS or AD + SGA | Taking MS or SGA only |

Stop AD — Stop AD

Level 1: Initial treatment

Li or VA or SGA monotherapy; combine Li or VA + SGA if severe

Optimize dose of MS or SGA; combine MS + SGA if severe

Level 2: Initial treatment resistance at week 1-2

Partial response:
If monotherapy, combine Li or VA + SGA or combine Li + VA

If already taking 2, add Li, VA, or SGA, whichever is missing

No response:
Change to MS or SGA, and consider combined MS + SGA, or 2 MS

If already combined, change MS, SGA, or both

Level 3: Continued treatment resistance

Add CBZ; consider CBZ + Li + VA
Change to another SGA
Change SGA to FGA or clozapine
ECT (move to higher level if patient threatens safety)

Figure 8.1

5. Assess medical conditions that could influence treatment:

   a. Hydration and nutritional status related to general health as well as manic overactivity
   b. Heart, kidney, endocrine, and liver function
   c. Obesity, metabolic syndrome, or diabetes
   d. Medication interactions.

6. Practical recommendations for medical laboratory evaluation: use initial tests appropriate to the patient's age, medical history, and physical examination, but in general obtain an EKG in older patients or anyone with cardiac risks, and in all patients, blood tests for BUN, creatinine, electrolytes, calcium, thyroid functions, fasting glucose and lipids, hepatic enzymes. Consider brain imaging during a first episode, and urine toxicology when substance abuse is suspected. In emergency rooms and hospitals these are all readily available. Outpatients may need to begin treatment before results can be obtained. If patients have no overt medical risks and have baseline labs within the recent past, it may be safe and in the patient's interest to begin medication first and obtain new laboratory tests (and initial blood levels of medication) as soon thereafter as practical.

Acute phase [see Figure 8.1]

Initial treatment: Level 1

Patients may present with a well-known bipolar treatment history, or for the first time with no prior treatment of mania. They may already be taking mood stabilizers alone, antidepressants alone, the combination, or no medication at all.

If currently taking medication: Dose of current mood stabilizer or antipsychotic should be increased if not optimal; if already maximized, a different antimanic medicine should be added or substituted.

In bipolar I disorder antidepressants should be stopped as quickly as possible. In bipolar II disorder judgment can be exercised as to whether to continue, reduce, or stop the antidepressant based on severity of current hypomania and past depressions.

If currently on no medication: In patients who stopped medication due to intolerability or lack of efficacy, begin a different antimanic drug. If a previous medication was known to be both effective and tolerable, it should be resumed.

In first-time mania, initial options are an SGA, lithium or valproate, or a combination of an SGA plus lithium or valproate. Valproate should be given as a loading dose of 20 to 30 mg/kg for more rapid effect (Hirschfeld *et al.* 1999). Lithium is adjusted more gradually.

Monotherapy is usually advised for mild to moderate mania, and combination therapy in severe mania, as would be the case in a hospital setting. Combinations are also a logical way to reduce initial treatment failure, analogous to initiating two antibiotics for infections in the intensive care unit to cover unknown pathogens. Combination therapy also makes sense when the clinician expects to continue a nonantipsychotic for maintenance, but wishes to use an antipsychotic early on for rapid tranquilization.

For monotherapy, some guidelines prefer an SGA due to more rapid onset of action. The choice amongst SGAs is highly individualized. Based on recent comparative efficacy data (Cipriani *et al.* 2011), olanzapine or risperidone may be preferred amongst the SGAs for initial therapy. One guideline recommends aripiprazole, risperidone, and ziprasidone, but not olanzapine or quetiapine, amongst first choices, due to metabolic concerns (Grunze *et al.* 2009). Intramuscular aripiprazole, olanzapine, or quetiapine can be given for severe agitation in emergencies (Allen *et al.* 2005). A reasonable stance is to use more robust, sedating SGAs such as olanzapine, risperidone, and quetiapine in more severe mania, while reserving aripiprazole and ziprasidone for milder mania or hypomania where rapid sedation is less important and for patients where metabolic side effects are of special concern.

In all situations, adjunctive benzodiazepines may be prescribed for sleep and sedation, though tolerance may develop quickly and abuse is a concern with some patients.

Lack of initial response: Level 2

There is no clear evidence for how quickly to step up dosing, or how long to wait for an initial monotherapy or combined treatment to take hold, although RCTs demonstrate drug/placebo separation at about 1 week. Expert consensus suggests making a change within a week if there is little or no response, or 2 weeks if there is a partial response that has plateaued (Keck *et al.* 2004). The options are either to switch completely from ineffective or poorly tolerated medication that has been adequately dosed, or adding a second medication to boost a partial response. If Level 1 monotherapy with an SGA, lithium, or valproate is not working, then the next step in Level 2 should be to try a different monotherapy with another SGA or mood stabilizer, or combine an SGA, lithium, or valproate if warranted by severity. If combination therapy was used in Level 1, one of the medicines should be changed if there is no response, or a third medicine may be added if there has been a partial response. It is generally wise to avoid using more than one SGA at a time, aside from transitional periods.

Continued lack of response: Level 3

For insufficient response to the second monotherapy or combination, choices include changing to a third monotherapy or trying an as-yet untried combination, including an SGA plus two or even three of lithium, valproate, or carbamazepine, based on a combination that has not already been used. Further medication choices include oxcarbazepine, FGAs, clozapine, or a newer SGA such as asenapine. As in Level 2, it is not generally advised to combine two antipsychotics within or across SGAs and FGAs, but when medications are cross-tapered, such combinations naturally evolve and can be maintained for a time if a patient is finally stabilizing. ECT may also be considered in Level 3. It is the author's experience that ECT is extraordinarily effective for mania when hospitalized patients remain in a severely agitated or aggressive state that has not responded to high doses of combined medications (Robinson *et al.* 2011). ECT offers a safe, humane path compared to the medical risks of prolonged, extreme doses of antipsychotics and benzodiazepines, as well as the danger of violent injury to self and others over weeks of unchecked manic behavior.

Continuation phase

Following stabilization, the key decisions are whether to add new medication or subtract current medication. The answers depend on two goals: eradicating residual symptoms, and establishing the safest, most tolerable long-term regimen.

Residual or newly emergent symptoms predict a threefold higher risk of relapse compared with full remission (Judd *et al*. 2008). While there is concern after mania about cycling into depression, relapse is more often in the same direction as the most recent episode (Goodwin *et al*. 2004). It may be appropriate to add or change antimanic medication if the remission is fragile. Concern about depressive cycling, if this seems likely based on past history, may warrant judiciously adding back antidepressant medication or lamotrigine.

It is essential as well to establish a regimen that is safe and tolerable for longer-term use. Traditionally, patients who achieve full resolution of mania on combined medications are weaned down from at least one, for example, tapering an antipsychotic while optimizing the dose of lithium, or tapering an antipsychotic while optimizing an anticonvulsant mood stabilizer. Past history and medical concerns about particular side effects guide the choice of the best and simplest regimen. If an antipsychotic is to be tapered off, it should be done gradually, over months (Keck *et al*. 2004). In contrast, if a patient received monotherapy with an SGA acutely, but needs long-term maintenance, consideration may be given to introducing a nonantipsychotic to avoid long-term neurological or metabolic side effects. Lithium, valproate, or carbamazepine may be added, and the SGA then gradually tapered.

Even taking side effects into account, there may be hesitation to change from a medication that was effective for the acute episode. However, given the potential for decades of future treatment here, the clinician must balance the risks and benefits to determine, for each individual, the best program. For example, severe psychosis during the acute episode might favor continuing with an SGA, while obesity might steer the choice away from olanzapine or quetiapine, even if effective in the acute phase.

Maintenance phase

Mood stabilization

As mentioned earlier, long-term medication is strongly recommended after two manic episodes, or one if severe, or in the presence of a strong family history. Lithium, valproate, olanzapine, quetiapine (alone or combined with lithium or valproate), risperidone, and adjunctive ziprasidone are all first-line treatments that protect against mania and to a lesser extent against depression. Aripiprazole is effective against mania only, and lamotrigine against depression only.

The long-term neurological toxicity of SGAs is not completely known, and the short-term metabolic problems can be quite serious. With careful monitoring, lithium and valproate may represent safer, more tolerable choices when contemplating decades of use.

Carbamazepine and oxcarbazepine may be considered when other treatments have failed or been poorly tolerated, e.g., due to weight gain. Depot injectable antipsychotics are valuable for nonadherence. Clozapine or maintenance ECT, while arduous, can be utilized when standard approaches have failed.

Lamotrigine does not prevent mania, and is thus inappropriate as monotherapy for bipolar I maintenance. It can be combined with a first-line antimanic medication to prevent depression in bipolar I patients. Depending on history, it may added after a manic episode when there is a history of cycling into depression, or held while waiting to see if a depression occurs. In contrast, in bipolar II disorder lamotrigine may be a reasonable choice for monotherapy in carefully selected patients who have not had frequent or seriously consequential hypomania, though in most patients it should probably be combined with a standard mood stabilizer to prevent recurrence of cycles.

Antidepressants

Standard antidepressants should never be used as monotherapy in bipolar I or II maintenance. However, they are often employed for patients with histories of recurrent depression that are not prevented by mood stabilizers. There appears to be a sub-set of "depression-prone" bipolar I patients who do well for long periods after index episodes of depression on combined antidepressants and mood stabilizers. This has been shown in an RCT with lithium and imipramine (Shapiro *et al*. 1989), as well as a naturalistic study of outcomes during combined treatment with a variety of mood stabilizers and modern antidepressants (Altshuler *et al.* 2001). However, it is not clear how to block a switch to depression after mania. Adding or resuming an antidepressant during euthymia after mania or hypomania to prevent future depressions may be considered if warranted by history, and there is adequate antimanic medication on board.

Rapid cycling

Rapid cycling between mania or hypomania and depression poses another difficult maintenance problem. Though its hallmark is often severe depressions lasting far longer than manic or hypomanic upswings, rapid cycling is thought sometimes to paradoxically worsen with prolonged use of antidepressants and to remit more readily when antidepressants are withheld. In fact, there is some evidence that rapid cycling is actually a time-limited phenomenon, resolving within 2 years for 80% who stay on continuous mood stabilizers, with uncertainty as to the need for antidepressants after resolution (Coryell *et al.* 2003). To break the pattern and achieve stability it may be necessary to experiment systematically over many months or years with various combinations of lithium, the three anticonvulsants, SGAs, and adjunctive treatments, such as thyroid hormone (Kilzieh and Akiskal, 1999) or maintenance ECT, often withholding antidepressants or using them cautiously and with close monitoring. Lifestyle and circadian rhythm adjustments coupled with strong psychosocial support are important to pursue at the same time.

References

Allen, M.H., Currier, G.W., Carpenter, D., Ross, R.W., and Docherty, J.P. (2005). The expert consensus guideline series. Treatment of behavioral emergencies 2005. *Journal of Psychiatric Practice*, 11 Suppl 1, 5–108; quiz 110–112.

Altshuler, L., Kiriakos, L., Calcagno, J. *et al.* (2001). The impact of antidepressant discontinuation versus antidepressant continuation on 1-year risk for relapse of bipolar depression: A retrospective chart review. *Journal of Clinical Psychiatry*, 62, 612–616.

American Psychiatric Association (2002). Practice guideline for the treatment of patients with bipolar disorder (revision). *American Journal of Psychiatry*, 159, 1–50.

Aronson, T.A., Shukla, S., and Hirschowitz, J. (1989). Clonazepam treatment of five lithium-refractory patients with bipolar disorder. *American Journal of Psychiatry*, 146, 77–80.

Asenjo Lobos, C., Komossa, K., Rummel-Kluge, C. *et al.* (2010). Clozapine versus other atypical antipsychotics for schizophrenia. *Cochrane Database of Systematic Reviews*, CD006633.

Baldessarini, R.J., Tondo, L., and Viguera, A.C. (1999). Discontinuing lithium maintenance treatment in bipolar disorders: Risks and implications. *Bipolar Disorders*, 1, 17–24.

Barbini, B., Scherillo, P., Benedetti, F. *et al.* (1997). Response to clozapine in acute mania is more rapid than that of chlorpromazine. *International Clinical Psychopharmacology*, 12, 109–112.

Bauer, M.S. and Mitchner, L. (2004). What is a "mood stabilizer"? An evidence-based response. *American Journal of Psychiatry*, 161, 3–18.

Berwaerts, J., Xu, H., Nuamah, I., Lim, P., and Hough, D. (2012). Evaluation of the efficacy and safety of paliperidone extended-release in the treatment of acute mania: A randomized, double-blind, dose-response study. *Journal of Affective Disorders*, 136, e51–e60.

Bowden, C.L. (2011). The role of ziprasidone in adjunctive use with lithium or valproate in maintenance treatment of bipolar disorder. *Neuropsychiatric Disease and Treatment*, 7, 87–92.

Bowden, C.L., Calabrese, J.R., McElroy, S.L. *et al.* (2000). A randomized, placebo-controlled 12-month trial of divalproex and lithium in treatment of outpatients with bipolar I disorder. Divalproex Maintenance Study Group. *Archives of General Psychiatry*, 57, 481–489.

Bowden, C.L., Vieta, E., Ice, K.S. *et al.* (2010). Ziprasidone plus a mood stabilizer in subjects with bipolar I disorder: A 6-month, randomized, placebo-controlled, double-blind trial. *Journal of Clinical Psychiatry*, 71, 130–137.

Calabrese, J.R., Shelton, M.D., Rapport, D.J. *et al.* (2005). A 20-month, double-blind, maintenance trial of lithium versus divalproex in rapid-cycling bipolar disorder. *American Journal of Psychiatry*, 162, 2152–2161.

Canuso, C.M., Schooler, N., Carothers, J. *et al.* (2010). Paliperidone extended-release in schizoaffective disorder: A randomized, controlled study comparing a flexible dose with placebo in patients treated with and without antidepressants and/or mood stabilizers. *Journal of Clinical Psychopharmacology*, 30, 487–495.

Ceron-Litvoc, D., Soares, B.G., Geddes, J., Litvoc, J., and De Lima, M.S. (2009). Comparison of carbamazepine and lithium in treatment of bipolar disorder: A systematic review of randomized controlled trials. *Human Psychopharmacology*, 24, 19–28.

Cipriani, A., Barbui, C., Salanti, G. *et al.* (2011). Comparative efficacy and acceptability of antimanic drugs in acute mania: A multiple-treatments meta-analysis. *Lancet*, 378, 1306–1315.

Colombo, C., Benedetti, F., Barbini, B., Campori, E., and Smeraldi, E. (1999). Rate of switch from depression into mania after therapeutic sleep deprivation in bipolar depression. *Psychiatry Research*, 86, 267–270.

Correll, C.U. and Schenk, E.M. (2008). Tardive dyskinesia and new antipsychotics. *Current Opinion in Psychiatry*, 21, 151–156.

Coryell, W., Solomon, D., Turvey, C. *et al.* (2003). The long-term course of rapid-cycling bipolar disorder. *Archives of General Psychiatry*, 60, 914–920.

Curtin, F. and Schulz, P. (2004). Clonazepam and lorazepam in acute mania: A Bayesian meta-analysis. *Journal of Affective Disorders*, 78, 201–208.

Fink, M. (2006). ECT in therapy-resistant mania: does it have a place? *Bipolar Disorders*, 8, 307–309.

Fountoulakis, K.N., Vieta, E., Sanchez-Moreno, J. *et al.* (2005). Treatment guidelines for bipolar disorder: A critical review. *Journal of Affective Disorders*, 86, 1–10.

Frances, A., Docherty, J.P., and Kahn, D.A. (1996). Treatment of bipolar disorder. The Expert Consensus Panel for Bipolar Disorder. *Journal of Clinical Psychiatry*, 57 Suppl 12A, 3–88.

Frye, M.A., Ketter, T.A., Leverich, G.S. *et al.* (2000). The increasing use of polypharmacotherapy for refractory mood disorders: 22 years of study. *Journal of Clinical Psychiatry*, 61, 9–15.

Goodnick, P.J. (2000). The use of nimodipine in the treatment of mood disorders. *Bipolar Disorders*, 2, 165–173.

Goodwin, F.K., Jamison, K.R., and Ghaemi, S.N. (2007). *Manic-Depressive Illness: Bipolar Disorders and Recurrent Depression*. New York, NY: Oxford University Press.

Goodwin, G.M. (2009). Evidence-based guidelines for treating bipolar disorder: Revised second edition–recommendations from the British Association for Psychopharmacology. *Journal of Psychopharmacology*, 23, 346–388.

Goodwin, G.M., Bowden, C.L., Calabrese, J.R. *et al.* (2004). A pooled analysis of 2 placebo-controlled 18-month trials of lamotrigine and lithium maintenance in bipolar I disorder. *Journal of Clinical Psychiatry*, 65, 432–441.

Green, A.I., Tohen, M., Patel, J.K. *et al.* (2000). Clozapine in the treatment of refractory psychotic mania. *American Journal of Psychiatry*, 157, 982–986.

Grunze, H., Vieta, E., Goodwin, G.M. *et al.* (2009). The World Federation of Societies of Biological Psychiatry (WFSBP) guidelines for the biological treatment of bipolar disorders: Update 2009 on the treatment of acute mania. *World Journal of Biological Psychiatry*, 10, 85–116.

Grunze, H., Vieta, E., Goodwin, G.M. *et al.* (2010). The World Federation of Societies of Biological Psychiatry (WFSBP) Guidelines for the Biological Treatment of Bipolar Disorders: Update 2010 on the treatment of acute bipolar depression. *World Journal of Biological Psychiatry*, 11, 81–109.

Hirschfeld, R.M., Allen, M.H., McEvoy, J.P., Keck, P.E., Jr, and Russell, J.M. (1999). Safety and tolerability of oral loading divalproex sodium in acutely manic bipolar patients. *Journal of Clinical Psychiatry*, 60, 815–818.

Hirschfeld, R.M.A. (2005). *Guideline Watch: Practice Guideline for the Treatment of Patients with Bipolar Disorder, Second Edition*. Arlington, VA: American Psychiatric Association.

Jefferson, J.W. (2010). A clinician's guide to monitoring kidney function in lithium-treated patients. *Journal of Clinical Psychiatry*, 71, 1153–1157.

Judd, L.L., Schettler, P.J., Akiskal, H.S. *et al.* (2008). Residual symptom recovery from major affective episodes in bipolar disorders and rapid episode relapse/recurrence. *Archives of General Psychiatry*, 65, 386–394.

Keck, P.E., Jr, McElroy, S.L., Strakowski, S.M., and Soutullo, C.A. (2000). Antipsychotics in the treatment of mood disorders and risk of tardive dyskinesia. *Journal of Clinical Psychiatry*, 61 Suppl 4, 33–38.

Keck, P.E., Perlis, R.H., Otto, M.W. *et al.* (2004). The Expert Consensus Guideline Series: Treatment of Bipolar Disorder. *Postgraduate Medical Journal*, Supplement.

Ketter, T.A. and Calabrese, J.R. (2002). Stabilization of mood from below versus above baseline in bipolar disorder: A new nomenclature. *Journal of Clinical Psychiatry*, 63, 146–151.

Kilzieh, N. and Akiskal, H.S. (1999). Rapid-cycling bipolar disorder: An overview of research and clinical experience. *Psychiatric Clinics of North America*, 22, 585–607.

MacFadden, W., Alphs, L., Haskins, J.T. *et al.* (2009). A randomized, double-blind, placebo-controlled study of maintenance treatment with adjunctive risperidone long-acting therapy in patients with bipolar I disorder who relapse frequently. *Bipolar Disorders*, 11, 827–839.

MacRitchie, K.A., Geddes, J.R., Scott, J., Haslam, D.R., and Goodwin, G.M. (2001). Valproic acid, valproate and divalproex in the maintenance treatment of bipolar disorder. *Cochrane Database of Systematic Reviews*, CD003196.

Mallinger, A.G., Thase, M.E., Haskett, R. *et al.* (2008). Verapamil augmentation of lithium treatment improves outcome in mania unresponsive to lithium alone: Preliminary findings and a discussion of therapeutic mechanisms. *Bipolar Disorders*, 10, 856–866.

Mantere, O., Suominen, K., Valtonen, H.M. *et al.* (2008). Differences in outcome of DSM-IV bipolar I and II disorders. *Bipolar Disorders*, 10, 413–425.

McIntyre, R.S. (2011). Asenapine: A review of acute and extension phase data in bipolar disorder. *CNS Neuroscience and Therapeutics*, 17, 645–648.

Meyer, J.M., Davis, V.G., Goff, D.C. *et al.* (2008). Change in metabolic syndrome parameters with antipsychotic treatment in the CATIE Schizophrenia Trial: Prospective data from phase 1. *Schizophrenia Research*, 101, 273–286.

Mukherjee, S., Sackeim, H.A., and Schnur, D.B. (1994). Electroconvulsive therapy of acute manic episodes: A review of 50 years' experience. *American Journal of Psychiatry*, 151, 169–176.

Muller, P. and Heipertz, R. (1977). Treatment of manic psychosis with clozapine [authors' translation]. *Fortschritte der Neurologie, Psychiatrie, und ihrer Grenzgebiete*, 45, 420–424.

National Institute for Clinical Excellence (2005). *Bipolar Disorder: NICE Clinical Guideline 38.* http://www.nice.org.uk/CG38 (accessed 11/1/2011).

Phelps, J. (2008). Dark therapy for bipolar disorder using amber lenses for blue light blockade. *Medical Hypotheses*, 70, 224–229.

Prien, R.F., Caffey, E.M., Jr, and Klett, C.J. (1974). Factors associated with treatment success in lithium carbonate prophylaxis. Report of the Veterans Administration and National Institute of Mental Health collaborative study group. *Archives of General Psychiatry*, 31, 189–192.

Rasgon, N.L., Reynolds, M.F., Elman, S. *et al.* (2005). Longitudinal evaluation of reproductive function in women treated for bipolar disorder. *Journal of Affective Disorder*, 89, 217–225.

Robinson, L.A., Penzner, J.B., Arkow, S., Kahn, D.A., and Berman, J.A. (2011). Electroconvulsive therapy for the treatment of refractory mania. *Journal of Psychiatric Practice*, 17, 61–66.

Sachs, G.S., Dupuy, J.M., and Wittmann, C.W. (2011). The pharmacologic treatment of bipolar disorder. *Journal of Clinical Psychiatry*, 72, 704–715.

Scherk, H., Pajonk, F.G., and Leucht, S. (2007). Second-generation antipsychotic agents in the treatment of acute mania: A systematic review and meta-analysis of randomized controlled trials. *Archives of General Psychiatry*, 64, 442–455.

Shapiro, D.R., Quitkin, F.M., and Fleiss, J.L. (1989). Response to maintenance therapy in bipolar illness. Effect of index episode. *Archives of General Psychiatry*, 46, 401–405.

Sikdar, S., Kulhara, P., Avasthi, A., and Singh, H. (1994). Combined chlorpromazine and electroconvulsive therapy in mania. *British Journal of Psychiatry*, 164, 806–810.

Small, J.G., Klapper, M.H., Kellams, J.J. *et al.* (1988). Electroconvulsive treatment compared with lithium in the management of manic states. *Archives of General Psychiatry*, 45, 727–732.

Smith, L.A., Cornelius, V., Warnock, A., Tacchi, M.J., and Taylor, D. (2007a). Acute bipolar mania: A systematic review and meta-analysis of co-therapy vs. monotherapy. *Acta Psychiatrica Scandinavica*, 115, 12–20.

Smith, L.A., Cornelius, V., Warnock, A., Tacchi, M.J., and Taylor, D. (2007b). Pharmacological interventions for acute bipolar mania: A systematic review of randomized placebo-controlled trials. *Bipolar Disorders*, 9, 551–560.

Strech, D., Soltmann, B., Weikert, B., Bauer, M., and Pfennig, A. (2011). Quality of reporting of randomized controlled trials of pharmacologic treatment of bipolar disorders: A systematic review. *Journal of Clinical Psychiatry*, 72, 1214–1221.

Suppes, T., Vieta, E., Liu, S., Brecher, M., and Paulsson, B. (2009). Maintenance treatment for patients with bipolar I disorder: Results from a North American study of quetiapine in combination with lithium or divalproex (trial 127). *American Journal of Psychiatry*, 166, 476–488.

Suppes, T., Dennehy, E.B., Hirschfeld, R.M. *et al.* (2005). The Texas implementation of medication algorithms: Update to the algorithms for treatment of bipolar I disorder. *Journal of Clinical Psychiatry*, 66, 870–886.

Tohen, M., Goldberg, J.F., Gonzalez-Pinto Arrillaga, A.M. *et al.* (2003). A 12-week, double-blind comparison of olanzapine vs haloperidol in the treatment of acute mania. *Archives of General Psychiatry*, 60, 1218–1226.

Tohen, M., Bowden, C.L., Calabrese, J.R. *et al.* (2006). Influence of sub-syndromal symptoms after remission from manic or mixed episodes. *British Journal of Psychiatry*, 189, 515–519.

Tohen, M., Bowden, C.L., Smulevich, A.B. *et al.* (2008). Olanzapine plus carbamazepine v. carbamazepine alone in treating manic episodes. *British Journal of Psychiatry*, 192, 135–143.

Vaidya, N.A., Mahableshwarkar, A.R., and Shahid, R. (2003). Continuation and maintenance ECT in treatment-resistant bipolar disorder. *Journal of ECT*, 19, 10–16.

Vasudev, A., MacRitchie, K., Watson, S., Geddes, J.R., and Young, A.H. (2008). Oxcarbazepine in the maintenance treatment of bipolar disorder. *Cochrane Database of Systematic Reviews*, CD005171.

Vieta, E., T'Joen, C., McQuade, R.D. *et al.* (2008). Efficacy of adjunctive aripiprazole to either valproate or lithium in bipolar mania patients partially nonresponsive to valproate/lithium monotherapy: A placebo-controlled study. *American Journal of Psychiatry*, 165, 1316–1325.

Weisler, R.H., Nolen, W.A., Neijber, A., Hellqvist, A., and Paulsson, B. (2011). Continuation of quetiapine versus switching to placebo or lithium for maintenance treatment of bipolar I disorder (trial 144: a randomized controlled study). *Journal of Clinical Psychiatry*, 72, 1452–1464.

Woods, S.W., Morgenstern, H., Saksa, J.R. *et al.* (2010). Incidence of tardive dyskinesia with atypical versus conventional antipsychotic medications: a prospective cohort study. *Journal of Clinical Psychiatry*, 71, 463–474.

Yatham, L.N., Grossman, F., Augustyns, I., Vieta, E., and Ravindran, A. (2003). Mood stabilisers plus risperidone or placebo in the treatment of acute mania. International, double-blind, randomised controlled trial. *British Journal of Psychiatry*, 182, 141–147.

Yatham, L.N., Kennedy, S.H., O'Donovan, C. *et al.* (2005). Canadian Network for Mood and Anxiety Treatments (CANMAT) guidelines for the management of patients with bipolar disorder: Consensus and controversies. *Bipolar Disorders*, 7 Suppl 3, 5–69.

Yatham, L.N., Kennedy, S.H., Schaffer, A. *et al.* (2009). Canadian Network for Mood and Anxiety Treatments (CANMAT) and International Society for Bipolar Disorders (ISBD) collaborative update of CANMAT guidelines for the management of patients with bipolar disorder: update 2009. *Bipolar Disorders*, 11, 225–255.

Yazici, O., Kora, K., Polat, A., and Saylan, M. (2004). Controlled lithium discontinuation in bipolar patients with good response to long-term lithium prophylaxis. *Journal of Affective Disorders*, 80, 269–271.

Yildiz, A., Guleryuz, S., Ankerst, D.P., Ongur, D., and Renshaw, P.F. (2008). Protein kinase C inhibition in the treatment of mania: A double-blind, placebo-controlled trial of tamoxifen. *Archives of General Psychiatry*, 65, 255–263.

Yonkers, K.A., Wisner, K.L., Stowe, Z. *et al.* (2004). Management of bipolar disorder during pregnancy and the postpartum period. *American Journal of Psychiatry*, 161, 608–620.

Young, R.C., Biggs, J.T., Ziegler, V.E., and Meyer, D.A. (1978). A rating scale for mania: Reliability, validity and sensitivity. *British Journal of Psychiatry*, 133, 429–435.

Zarate, C.A., Jr., Tohen, M., and Baraibar, G. (1997). Combined valproate or carbamazepine and electroconvulsive therapy. *Annals of Clinical Psychiatry*, 9, 19–25.

Zarate, C.A., Jr., Tohen, M., Banov, M.D., Weiss, M.K., and Cole, J.O. (1995). Is clozapine a mood stabilizer? *Journal of Clinical Psychiatry*, 56, 108–112.

Zarate, C.A., Jr., Singh, J.B., Carlson, P.J. *et al.* (2007). Efficacy of a protein kinase C inhibitor (tamoxifen) in the treatment of acute mania: A pilot study. *Bipolar Disorders*, 9, 561–570.

Treatment of mood disorders in late life

Steven P. Roose and Davangere P. Devanand

Introduction

Society is aging. By the year 2030, over 70 million people in the United States will be over the age of 65 years, and the group over the age of 85 years will be the most rapidly growing segment of the population. The aging of society is a global phenomenon; the rate of increase in the proportion of the population over 65 in the United States and Europe will be equaled, if not exceeded, in Africa, Asia, and South America. Thus, the prevalence of late-life depression and the need for effective therapeutics for this vulnerable population represent critical challenges for psychiatry.

The influence of age on illness presentation and the problem of diagnosis

Patients with late-life depression, generally defined as over age 65, and patients over 85 are often referred to as the old-old, are different in important dimensions from younger adult depressed patients. These differences may result from age-associated physiological changes, the impact of a lifetime of episodic or chronic depressive illness (the ravages of a depressed life), and/or the impact of co-morbid medical conditions (Sheline, 1999, Roose and Krishnan, 2004). For example, the manifestation of functional impairment is different depending on age: adolescents present with poor performance in school or antisocial behavior, young adults with failures at work or troubled relationships, and older patients with hypochondrias and increased utilization of medical resources (Unutzer, 2002).

The physiological changes that are part of aging may significantly influence the vulnerability to,

phenomenology of, and the course of depressive illness. Dysfunction in the prefrontal areas is associated with instability of temperament, intensification of the experience of distress, and loss of coping mechanisms. Any one of these factors may result in increased social isolation and/or loss of independence, which are states that can precipitate, intensify, or prolong a depressive episode. Changes in brain structure and function may, in part, explain the increased frequency of the melancholic and delusional sub-type of depressive episodes in late life or the degree of cognitive impairment.

Of significant clinical concern is that age-associated changes in presenting symptoms undoubtedly contribute to underdiagnosis and inadequate treatment of depression in late-life patients. Older patients are more likely to present with cognitive and somatic symptoms, e.g., apathy, sleep disturbance, appetite loss, pain, and memory complaints. They may never complain of, or indeed may deny, a "depressed mood." This presentation of late life depression, specific to late life, has been designated as "depression without sadness" (Gallo, 1999).

Another feature of depression in late life is the appearance of sub-types that are different in etiology, pathophysiology, and prognosis, and which may be specific to older adults. An example is depression that is associated with cerebrovascular disease.

Stroke occurs most commonly in late life and can be followed by a depressive syndrome in patients with no prior history of mood disorder. The pathophysiology is distinct and patients with post-stroke depression have a different response pattern to antidepressant medications than patients with late-life depressive syndromes not associated with a vascular event (Robinson, 1982). In addition to the well-documented syndrome of post-stroke depression,

---

Clinical Handbook for the Management of Mood Disorders, ed. J. John Mann, Patrick J. McGrath, and Steven P. Roose.
Published by Cambridge University Press. © Cambridge University Press 2013.

another ischemic-related sub-type of depression in late life is "vascular depression."

This syndrome was first proposed by Hickie *et al.* (1995) who wrote that "cerebral vascular insufficiency in elderly people leads to major changes in their subcortical and basal ganglia structure. The resultant late-onset depressive disorders are characterized by deficits in functions that are dependent on intact cortical striatal connections (e.g., psychomotor speed), as well as subcortical hyperintense lesions and reduced basal ganglia volumes." The stimulus for this hypothesis was the higher rates of hyperintensities on MRI in patients with late-onset depression (first episode after the age of 60) compared to patients of comparable age, but whose first episode of depression occurred as a young adult. (Hickie *et al.* 1995, Krishnan *et al.* 1997). Another characteristic feature of this syndrome is deficits on neuropsychological testing, including, but not limited to, deficits in executive function that are postulated to result from ischemic-related damage to frontostriatal tracts (Alexopoulos, 2002a). In contrast to post-stroke depression, "vascular" depression results from small-vessel disease and there are typically no accompanying motor deficits. The vascular depression syndrome is associated with poorer response to antidepressants and potential progression to vascular dementia (Krishnan, 1993).

As a result of age-associated differences in phenomenology and sub-types unique to late life, it is to be expected that there is a particular set of patient and study design variables that affect treatment response in older patients. These include, sub-type (e.g., melancholic or delusional), medical burden, social support, hyperintensities on MRI indicating vascular disease, and neurocognitive deficits, including both mild cognitive impairment and executive dysfunction.

Treatment

The mainstay of treatment for late-life depression is antidepressant medication, although recently there have been some psychotherapies that have been developed specifically for the older patient, e.g., problem-solving therapy, that have proved effective (Areán, 2010). Furthermore, electroconvulsive therapy (see Chapter 24) is critically important in this population because of its unique effectiveness and relative safety.

There are a number of issues that must be considered when prescribing an antidepressant to a patient in late life, specifically age-associated pharmacokinetic and pharmacodynamic changes. Pharmacokinetic changes may be due to changes in absorption, distribution, metabolism, or elimination of a drug that result in higher and more variable drug concentrations. Pharmacodynamic differences may result from the fact that homeostatic mechanisms, such as postural control, water balance, orthostatic circulatory responses, and thermoregulation, are frequently less robust in the older person. Consequently, older patients are more sensitive to adverse effects of psychotropics at lower concentrations (Pollock, 1999). Selective serotonin reuptake inhibitors (SSRIs), may increase the risk of falls and hip fracture (Liu *et al.* 1998) and the syndrome of inappropriate antidiuretic hormone secretion has been reported as an age-associated adverse effect of all SSRIs and of venlafaxine (Kirby and Ames, 2001).

There are three widely held clinical beliefs about the pharmacological treatment of late-life depression that have dominated clinical decisions. First, it is believed that older patients do not respond at the same rate or as robustly as younger patients. However, there are no prospective studies that address this question and an analysis comparing rates of response in late-life vs. younger adults with depression did not indicate a difference in response rates (Sackeim, 2005). It may be that some sub-types of depression prevalent in the elderly, e.g., vascular depression or depression with mild cognitive impairment, may be less responsive to monotherapy, and this may account for this clinical impression, but that remains to be proven.

Second, it is believed that older patients are more sensitive to the side effects of medication and a lower starting dose and slower dose escalation of antidepressant medication will improve tolerability, i.e., the "start low–go slow" dosing strategy. There is, however, little evidence indicating that this strategy increases tolerability of either the TCAs or the SSRIs in the elderly, and this approach can obviously delay response and/or result in inadequate dosing (Roose, 1990). Nonetheless it is customary, and not unreasonable, to begin patients over 70 years on a lower starting dose, as long as dose increase to an established effective dose is not unreasonably delayed.

Third, it is believed that older patients take longer to respond to antidepressant medication, and therefore a 12-week trial is mandatory (Young, 1992). Do all patients really require a 12-week trial before being declared nonresponders? The evidence suggests that the answer is no. Supporting the argument for longer treatment trials in older depressed patients are the results of two 12-week, randomized controlled trials of SSRIs (Bondareff, 2000, Newhouse, 2000), indicating a higher response rate at week 12 compared to week 8. The conclusion was that patients are still getting better at week 8 and so at least 12 weeks is warranted. This conclusion, however, does not address whether a 12-week trial is mandatory in all patients. Patients who did not meet response criteria by week 8 but do so by week 12 may represent two different groups: (1) patients who were close to response criteria by week 8 and crossed the threshold by week 12 and (2) patients who had little or no significant symptom reduction by week 8 but then improved dramatically over the next four weeks to meet response criteria at week 12, so-called "late responders." If the higher response rate at week 12 resulted primarily from patients in group two, it would imply that all patients deserve a 12-week trial, even those who have no significant improvement by week 8. However, if the new responders at week 12 have already shown significant improvement by week 8, it means that we can identify by week 8, or earlier, who will benefit from a longer trial and therefore extend the treatment duration only in those patients. Thus trial duration is defined by time to response (how long it must be) and the identification of nonresponders (how short it can be).

An innovative analysis of data from a number of 12-week antidepressant trials in late-life depression helped define the time boundaries of antidepressant treatment in the clinical setting and also addressed some of the beliefs enumerated previously about remission, defined as a final HRSD score less than or equal to 10 (the criteria commonly used in late-life antidepressant trials). The median time to onset of sustained remission was only 31 days, not significantly different from mean time to sustained remission in younger patients. This finding does not support the belief that older patients (over age 60) with depression take longer to respond than younger patients (Sackeim, 2005).

With respect to trial duration, 36% of late-life patients who achieved sustained remission required 8 or more weeks to do so, but the vast majority these patients had significant improvement by the end of week 8. This pattern of time to remission in late-life patients is very similar to the pattern of time to remission found in the STAR-D study including the percentage of patients who reached sustained remission between weeks 8 and 12 of treatment. There is strong

predictive power that allows for the early identification on nonresponders; by week 6, if a patient did not achieve a 30% reduction from baseline HRSD then they had only a 22% chance of being in remission at the end of the study (Sackeim, 2005). Thus a 12-week (or longer) trial of medication is not necessary for all late-life depressed patients. The clinician can make an evidence-based decision at 6 weeks whether to change medication or continue the current treatment based on the probability that given the patient's improvement to date they will or will not meet remission criteria by week 12.

Pharmacological treatments for late-life depression

Tricyclic antidepressants

Although TCAs are used much less frequently in younger patients, they still have a very important role in the treatment of late-life depression. Most of the placebo-controlled trials involving TCAs were done before the use of plasma-level measurements to ensure optimal TCA treatment. Subsequent RCTs compared tricyclics with SSRIs, but these studies were predominantly supported by industry and the study design did not compare the sponsor's drug to optimal tricyclic treatment. Of the tricyclics, nortriptyline has emerged as the preferred TCA, based on a "therapeutic window" that permits optimal dosing and the least problems with orthostatic hypotension (Roose et al. 1981). The therapeutic effectiveness in late-life depression is based on two open trials and three randomized comparator trials; there are no rigorous placebo-controlled trials of nortriptyline in late-life depression (Roose et al. 1994, Flint and Rifat, 1996). Three RCTs compared nortriptyline with an SSRI; two studies compared a therapeutic plasma level of nortriptyline to paroxetine, and one study compared flexible-dose nortriptyline with sertraline (Flint and Rifat 1996, Nelson et al. 1999). There was no statistical difference in remission rates between the two medications (57 and 63% for NT, 55 and 61% for paroxetine), but the dropout rate was significantly higher for nortriptyline in both studies.

Though effective in the treatment of late-life depression and still believed by many clinicians to be more effective than SSRIs, the use of TCAs is limited because of tolerability and safety concerns. The anticholinergic effects of TCAs results in dry mouth, constipation, and blurred vision, but more importantly, older patients may develop urinary retention and confusional states. The safety concerns focus on the cardiovascular effects of the TCAs, specifically conduction defects. The TCAs slow cardiac conduction and thus can induce dangerous degrees of heart block in patients with intraventricular conduction (Roose, 1990). TCAs have type 1A antiarrhythmic activity similar to that of quinidine. Use of type 1A antiarrhythmics is associated with increased mortality in patients with ischemic heart disease and it is both reasonable and appropriately cautious to assume that the use of TCAs in depressed patients with ischemic heart disease is associated with an increased rate of mortality as well. Furthermore, the tricyclics are potentially lethal on overdose, and as little as three times the daily therapeutic dose can result in death from heart block or arrhythmias (Barbey and Roose, 1998).

SSRIs

The SSRIs are the most prescribed class of antidepressants for late-life depression and no differences have been demonstrated in efficacy or side effects between different SSRIs.

Fluoxetine

Four studies of fluoxetine in late-life depression have been done: (1) a placebo-controlled RCT study of 671 patients (Tollefson *et al.* 2002) reported a 23% remission rate for fluoxetine and 13% for placebo. The strict remission criterion of final HRSD < 7 (generally a final HRSD < 10 is the remission criteria use in studies of late-life depression), low dose of 20 mg, and short trial duration of 6 weeks, may have kept the remission rates for both cells lower than expected. (2) A three-cell study comparing venlafaxine, placebo, and fluoxetine found no superiority of either drug over placebo. As usual, when two active treatments are included, the study was underpowered to find a difference between the two active treatments, but it was sufficiently powered to compare either active drug to placebo. (3) An RCT comparing 12 weeks' treatment with fluoxetine, 20–40 mg, to sertraline, 50–100 mg (Newhouse *et al.* 2000) found no difference in remission rates (46 to 45%) or dropout rates (33 to 32%). (4) In an open trial, 308 patients meeting criteria for major depressive disorder were treated with 20 mg of fluoxetine for 8 weeks (Mesters *et al.* 1992) and found the remission rate was 35%, and the dropout rate was 29%, which is comparable to rates found in younger patients.

Sertraline

In addition to the two comparator RCTs of fluoxetine vs. sertraline previously discussed and nortriptyline vs. sertraline discussed under nortriptyline, a large, N = 716, placebo-controlled trial of sertraline in late-life depression reported a remission rate of 29% for sertraline compared with 23% for placebo (p < 0.05) (Schneider, 2003).

Paroxetine

In addition to the two RCTs comparing NT to paroxetine, a third RCT compared mirtazapine with paroxetine (Schatzberg *et al.* 2002) in 255 patients treated for 8 weeks; remission rates, 38% for mirtazapine and 28% for paroxetine, were not statistically different, but as usual the study was underpowered to compare the two active treatments.

Citalopram

A placebo-controlled study of citalopram is unique because to date it has treated the oldest, mean age 80 years, depressed population (Roose, 2004). The response rate was 41% for the citalopram group and 39% for placebo. In a single-blind comparison study comparing citalopram to a therapeutic plasma level of nortriptyline in 58 patients, the remission rates were 69% for citalopram and 93% for nortriptyline. The remission rates for both medications were strikingly high in comparison to those in other trials; whether this results from differences in patient population or study design is not obvious. It is important to note that the FDA has issued a warning about QTC prolongation in patients treated with more than 40 mg/d of citalopram and has recommend that the dose not exceed 20 mg/d in a late-life population.

Escitalopram

There are two placebo-controlled RCTs that have focused on escitalopram and neither showed a significant difference in effectiveness of drug compared to placebo. In the first study, 517 patients were randomized to escitalopram, fluoxetine, or placebo and in the second study, 264 patients were randomized to escitalopram or placebo (Kasper *et al.* 2005).

In a well-executed meta-analysis of ten SSRI–placebo RCTs that included 2377 patients on medication and 1788 on placebo, response and dropout due to side effects were significantly greater in the medication group; the mean response rates were 44% on medication and 34.7% on placebo and response was greater in a trial of 10–12 weeks compared to 6–8 weeks (Nelson, 2011).

The SSRIs have the same side-effect profile in older patients as in younger patients, though; as discussed previously, older patients may be more vulnerable to some adverse events. However, the SSRIs do offer an improved safety profile compared to the TCAs, specifically with respect to cardiovascular effects. The SSRIs are relatively benign on overdose (Barbey and Roose, 1998) and in contrast to TCAs, do not have an effect on blood pressure, heart rate, or cardiac conduction. Most importantly, there are now many studies that have shown that SSRIs are relatively safe in patients post-myocardial infarction, and their use may be associated with increased survival. (Barbey and Roose, 1998, Berkman et al. 2003). This may be due in part to the "antiplatelet" effect of the SSRIs; the SSRIs exert this effect above and beyond aspirin, but SSRI use is also associated with a small increased risk of GI bleed.

Venlafaxine

One study reported meaningful information about venlafaxine in a geriatric population (Schatzberg and Cantillon, 2000). In an a RCT comparing venlafaxine, fluoxetine, and placebo in an 8-week trial the remission rates, 42% for venlafaxine, 29% for fluoxetine, and 38% for placebo, were not statistically significantly different. The dropout rates for patients treated with venlafaxine (27%) and fluoxetine (19%) were significantly greater compared with placebo (9%).

Duloxetine

Two RCTs for duloxetine found that it was significantly more effective than placebo. In the first trial, 90 patients were randomized; the remission rate was 44% on duloxetine and 16% on placebo. In the second trial, 311 patients were randomized; the remission rate was 27% on duloxetine and 15% on placebo.

Mirtazapine

In addition to the comparator study with paroxetine cited earlier, there was an open study of mirtazapine for depressed patients residing in a skilled nursing facility. The medication was effective and well tolerated, and in this population the side effects of sedation and weight gain were not seen as disadvantageous (Roose, 2003).

Bupropion

The only data available on bupropion in late-life depression are from an RCT comparing bupropion to paroxetine, where there was a response rate of 71% for bupropion and 77% for paroxetine (Weihs et al. 2000).

Summary

The number of studies that demonstrate a significant difference when comparing any antidepressant medication to placebo is disconcerting. The ratio of studies that show a drug–placebo difference compared to those that do not may not be different in young vs. late-life depressed patients, but the number of clinical trials done in the late-life population is so much less and thus negative trials may make a greater impression. When selecting an antidepressant for a late-life patient with depression, it is reasonable to begin with either an SSRI or an SNRI. Citaolpram used to be perhaps the most popular first-choice antidepressant of geriatric psychiatrists, but this is now undoubtedly impacted by the FDA warning about QTC prolongation. Since escitalopram is now generic, it may be the clinician's drug of choice unless the QTC warning is extended to this drug as well. Given comparable efficacy, it is reasonable that the potential for drug–drug interactions and concern over potential hypertensive effects, when many of the patients are being treated for hypertension, should guide medication selection.

The need to select a medication primarily on safety grounds raises the issue of what is the recommended pretreatment work-up before any antidepressant medication is begun in a late-life patient. Most late-life patients do see a primary care doctor on a regular basis and so it is imperative that a psychiatrist consult this physician to get a complete understanding of the patient's health and to avoid duplicating blood tests. Before beginning antidepressant treatment the psychiatrist should review a complete set of laboratory tests that include CBC, chemistries, electrolytes, thyroid profile, B12 and folate levels, cardiogram, and weight and blood pressure measurements. In patients with significant vascular risk factors, e.g., hypertension, diabetes, smoking, strong family history, it is reasonable to get an MRI, especially if there is any suggestion of memory difficulties.

Augmentation

Given the number of patients with late-life depression who do not respond to a trial of an antidepressant there is considerable opportunity to study augmentation strategies. To date, only information from open studies are available. In one study patients who were nonresponders to a trial of an SSRI were augmented with nortriptyline, buproprion, or lithium. About 50% of patients responded to augmentation, but the numbers were too small to compare the augmentation treatments.

With respect to augmentation with atypical antipsychotics, there have been two relatively small open trials (Rutherford *et al.* 2007, Sheffrin *et al.* 2009). The response rate is about 50% without significant side effects. However, the number of patients studied is limited, and with respect to augmentation strategies, as with all treatments for late-life depression, much more study is needed.

It is established that there is a small risk of increased mortality when the atypicals are given to patients with dementia and behavioral problems. However, to date there are no data on the adverse event profile when atypicals are used in the treatment of late-life depression.

Psychotherapy

In a meta-analysis comparing the efficacy of psychotherapy for the treatment of depression in younger vs. older adults there was a comparable moderate effect size for the effectiveness of treatment in both age groups. However, this meta-analysis included a wide range of treatments identified as psychotherapy, many unpublished studies, and by the authors own admission many studies of poor quality. In a second meta-analysis the same authors considered only psychotherapy studies of depressed patients over the age of 50 years, but again the confidence in the results of this study is delimited by poor study selection, inclusion of a range of mood disorders, and no definition of psychotherapy. Although frequently cited, these reports provide no useful information for the clinician and serve as cautions about the limitations of the meta-analysis technique.

What role does psychotherapy have in the treatment of late-life depression as a stand-alone treatment or in combination with medication? In an attempt to establish consensus guidelines for the treatment of late-life depression, 50 experts were asked about their recommended treatment approach and psychotherapy, primarily CBT and IPT, alone for mild depression, or in combination with medication for more severe illness, which was widely endorsed. However, the evidence supporting the recommendations of the experts would seem to call for more limited conclusions. As might be expected there is not an abundance of well-controlled studies, but there are some older studies concluding that ITP in combination with antidepressants is a more effective treatment than medication alone in the prevention of relapse, and recently some excellent studies of problem-solving therapy.

As previously discussed, patients with executive dysfunction (ED), which is strongly associated with vascular depression, have a lower response rate to antidepressant treatment than patients without ED. In an RCT, 221 patients with MDD and ED, mean age 73, were randomized to treatment with either problem-solving therapy or supportive psychotherapy for 12 weeks. The remission rate was significantly higher in the PST group, 38%, compared to the supportive therapy group, 22%. Patients were not on antidepressant medication and there was no comparator medication group.

Psychotherapy is probably an underutilized treatment for late-life MDD. Studies that compare open medication treatment to psychotherapy alone or in combination would provide evidenced-based guidance to the clinician, but such studies are unlikely to be done. Given the current state of knowledge, clinicians who routinely do specific psychotherapies with older patients might select a psychotherapy treatment as a first option in a mild-moderately depressed older patient. Medication should be favored over psychotherapy in the more severe cases and should be added if a psychotherapy is not fully effective

Dysthymic disorder in late life

Dysthymic disorder is defined in the DSM classification system as a specific syndrome of depression of mild or moderate severity that lasts at least 2 years. Dysthymia may begin early in life and extend into late life, and episodes of major depression may occur during the course of dysthymic disorder. In these patients, the term "chronic depression" has been used to indicate the co-morbid or sequential occurrence of major depression and dysthymic disorder (Kocsis *et al.* 1998). However, in the elderly, nearly all patients with dysthymic disorder have late onset by DSM criteria (age of onset > 21 years) and the majority of patients have an age of onset above the age of 50 years (Devanand *et al.* 1994). In young adults, most patients with dysthymia have concurrent or intervening episodes of major depression, so that the term chronic depressive disorder is likely to replace the term dysthymic disorder in the DSM-5 classification scheme (Chapter 2). However, this classification will apply only to a small minority of elderly patients with dysthymic disorder, because the majority of older patients have relatively "pure" dysthymic disorder with a late age of onset and without concurrent or prior major depression (Devanand *et al.* 1994, 2004a). They also do not have increased family history of depressive illness (Devanand *et al.* 2004a). There is considerable evidence that patients with late-onset major depression (onset after 50 to 60 years of age; definitions of late-onset vary in older patients) have less family history of affective disorder and more evidence of cerebrovascular disease and cerebral atrophy than elderly patients with early-onset depressive illness (Alexopoulos *et al.* 1997, Sneed *et al.* 2006). These features also appear to be present in elderly patients with dysthymic disorder (Devanand *et al.* 1994, Kumar *et al.* 1998, Devanand *et al.* 2003) who often have a "pure" dysthymia uncomplicated by a history of major depression (Devanand *et al.* 1994).

In the National Comorbidity Survey, co-morbid depressive and anxiety disorders in the elderly appeared to be as common as in young adults (King-Kallimanis *et al.* 2009). However, there may be a difference between early- and late-onset dysthymic patients: co-morbid Axis I disorders, particularly anxiety disorders, are common in early-onset but not in late-onset patients with dysthymic disorder (Devanand *et al.* 1994, 2003). There is an equal gender distribution in late-onset dysthymic disorder, unlike the predominance of females in most types of affective disorder (Devanand *et al.* 2004a). Personality disorders in elderly dysthymic patients are less common than in young adults with dysthymic disorder, and are more commonly the obsessive compulsive and avoidant sub-types. Borderline, histrionic, narcissistic, and antisocial personality disorders are rare in the elderly (Devanand *et al.* 1994, 2003).

Co-morbid general medical conditions, cognitive disorders, and frequent adverse life events, e.g., bereavement, can complicate the diagnosis of dysthymic disorder. Dysthymia before myocardial infarction has been shown to predict poor cardiac outcome at 2.5 years of follow-up (Rafanelli *et al.* 2010). Associated features in dysthymia may include the presence of major chronic stressors, increased physical impairment, and symptoms of anxiety (Kirby *et al.* 1999). Of note, most patients with dysthymia are seen in primary care settings rather than by psychiatrists (Bellino *et al.* 2000). Mild to moderate symptoms of depression in these patients are often unrecognized in primary care. Even when such depression is recognized in older patients, it is too often erroneously ascribed to being alone, elderly, frail, impaired in terms of hearing, vision, gait, balance, and having medical problems. As a result, the depression typically remains untreated.

DSM-IV describes the symptoms of dysthymic disorder as being similar to those in major depression with the distinction being the presence of fewer symptoms of lesser severity. However, the DSM-IV field trials revealed a high prevalence of cognitive and social symptoms in patients with dysthymic disorder, and neurovegetative symptoms were less frequent. This led to the alternate symptom criteria for dysthymic disorder that were listed in the DSM-IV appendix. These symptoms include low self-esteem, hopelessness, social withdrawal and lack of interest, fatigue, low productivity, poor concentration, and indecisiveness. These symptoms are also more common than classical neurovegetative symptoms in elderly patients with dysthymic disorder (Devanand *et al.* 2003). The assessment of dysthymic disorder in the elderly can benefit from the use of the Cornell Dysthymia Rating Scale that emphasizes cognitive, and social and motivational difficulties (Mason *et al.* 1993).

The optimal treatment of dysthymic disorder in the elderly remains uncertain. Fluoxetine showed marginal superiority over placebo in a large-scale study, but overall response rates were low (Devanand *et al.* 2005). There is initial evidence from an open treatment trial that venlafaxine may have some efficacy (Devanand *et al.* 2004b). In two pilot trials, there were suggestions of efficacy in the sub-set of elderly male patients with dysthymic disorder who had low testosterone levels (Seidman *et al.* 2009, Shores *et al.* 2009). There is equivocal evidence on whether psychotherapy or SSRIs should be the first-line treatment in older patients with dysthymic disorder (Williams *et al.* 2000). Problem-solving therapy may be useful in late-life depression, but there appears to be considerable variability in treatment response when therapy is not administered by experts (Williams *et al.* 2000,

Areán *et al.* 2008). A pragmatic consideration is that most patients with dysthymia are seen in primary care, and if the depression is recognized, physicians are more likely to use an antidepressant medication than psychotherapy. Long-term disability is a key feature of chronic depression that exceeds the disability from most medical illnesses (Moussavi *et al.* 2007), but there is little evidence from treatment studies about the impact of specific treatments on long-term functioning and disability in older depressed patients.

Other sub-syndromal depressive disorders

Sub-syndromal depression is defined as the presence of depressive symptoms that do not qualify for a mood disorder syndrome like major depression or dysthymic disorder. Sub-syndromal depressive disorder is a heterogenous group of milder forms of depression with symptom patterns qualitatively distinct from more severe forms such as major depression. Sub-syndromal depression is often used to describe patients with occasional depressed mood in the absence of other depressive symptoms, and the term "minor depression" has also been used (Tamburrino *et al.* 2009). Sub-syndromal depressive states can be associated with adverse medical outcomes (Lin *et al.* 2003). Minor depression in elderly people is associated with functional disability, and about 25% of patients develop major depression within 2 years. These sub-syndromal depressive disorders commonly occur in patients with co-morbid medical illness, cognitive impairment, and other Axis I and II psychiatric disorders. There have been few treatment studies in the elderly, partly because the inherent heterogeneity of this set of syndromes makes it difficult to identify consistent treatment effects. Another argument is that these patients' symptoms are too mild to require treatment, but the higher than expected likelihood of progression to major depression and the possible detrimental impact of even low levels of depression on medical outcomes (Lin *et al.* 2003) suggest that treatment may often be warranted. Most older patients with sub-syndromal depression present to primary care physicians who typically do not recognize low to moderate levels of depression, and these patients with sub-syndromal depression typically do not receive treatment.

Depression with cognitive impairment

In the elderly, the most common neuropsychiatric disorders are depression and cognitive impairment. Their co-occurrence may exceed chance. Apathetic, withdrawn behavior is common to both depression and dementia. Paucity of speech with long latency is characteristic of major depression, particularly the melancholic sub-type. There are many symptoms common to both depression and mild cognitive impairment (MCI) or early dementia: apathy, anhedonia, insomnia, agitation, irritability, memory loss, and difficulty concentrating. This overlap in symptoms often makes it difficult to make an accurate diagnosis and can confound prognosis and treatment.

In patients with depression and cognitive decline, several cognitive symptoms are common: difficulties in memory or thinking or concentration, forgetting recent events, forgetting where things are located, problems in finding the right word to say, getting lost in familiar places, not remembering appointments and to take medications, and difficulty in managing finances like balancing the checkbook or paying for items in a store. These symptoms, especially problems with financial management, and remembering appointments or remembering to take medications, may be the first indicators of dementia (Brown *et al.* 2011). The symptom of forgetting names of books, movies, and people is common during the normal aging process and by itself does not indicate dementia. Common cognitive screens include the Mini Mental State Exam (MMSE) and the Montreal Cognitive Assessment (MOCA). In these and related test instruments, orientation and short-term recall are key measures of cognitive abilities, and these features should be given priority in addition to evaluating the total score. Clock-drawing is another brief screening test, but some training is required for accurate scoring. For patients who show clear deficits on one of these instruments, further work-up is indicated and typically begins with neuropsychological testing.

On neuropsychological testing, deficits in memory, especially short-term verbal episodic memory, and executive function deficits are indicators of early dementia. Focal neurological signs are indicative of brain pathology, but by themselves may not be sufficient to make a definitive diagnosis.

A variety of neurobiological markers have been shown to predict future conversion to Alzheimer's disease in patients with mild cognitive impairment. These include odor identification deficits, hippocampal and entorhinal cortex atrophy on MRI (Devanand *et al.* 2008), decreased metabolism in the temporal and parietal regions with ^{18}FDG PET (Silverman *et al.* 2001), and increased uptake with amyloid imaging agents using PET (Klunk *et al.* 2004, Mintun *et al.* 2006). An increase in tau protein and decrease in amyloid beta components in cerebrospinal fluid are strongly associated with a diagnosis of Alzheimer's disease (Visser *et al.* 2009). None of these measures individually can be used to definitely make the diagnosis, but when combined with clinical assessment, these measures improve diagnostic accuracy and the prediction of likely conversion to dementia during follow-up. Although these measures have not yet been tested systematically in older depressed patients with cognitive impairment, it is likely that these measures will be abnormal in the sub-group of patients with Alzheimer's brain pathology.

Several epidemiological and clinical studies show that depression in patients with cognitive impairment leads to a high conversion rate to dementia (Alexopoulos *et al.* 1993, Devanand *et al.* 1996, Bassuk *et al.* 1998, Wilson *et al.* 2002), with limited dissenting data (Chen *et al.* 1999). Most converters to dementia are diagnosed with Alzheimer's disease. There is some evidence that this relationship holds even after adjusting for vascular risk factors and stroke (Luchsinger *et al.* 2009), but other studies suggest that cerebrovascular disease does contribute to conversion to dementia in cognitively impaired patients (Honig *et al.* 2005). At autopsy, a majority of depressed subjects who have moderate to severe cognitive impairment have pathological diagnoses of Alzheimer's disease, vascular dementia, or Lewy body dementia (Sweet *et al.* 2004).

While some patients with depression and cognitive impairment have Alzheimer's disease brain pathology, other patients show evidence of cerebrovascular disease. "Vascular depression" (VaD) refers to major depression in older patients who have high rates of leukoencephalopathy on MRI and executive function deficits (Alexopoulos *et al.* 1997). Cluster analysis of the proposed criteria to diagnose vascular depression suggests that MRI evidence of leukoencephalopathy is particularly important in making the diagnosis, and that age of onset may be a less important variable (Sneed *et al.* 2006). Part of the difficulty is that age of onset is difficult to ascertain accurately in many patients.

Treatment of depression with cognitive impairment

In patients with depression and cognitive impairment, there is a need to understand pathophysiology, determine early prognostic indicators, and develop optimal treatment strategies. Since depression in patients with cognitive deficits increases the risk of conversion to dementia, treatment strategies in these patients have longer-term implications beyond acute antidepressant treatment response. However, in this group of patients there is a lack of data on treatment response of mood symptoms to antidepressant treatment and of cognitive deficits to cognitive enhancer treatment, and the long-term prognosis remains unclear.

In a pilot study of patients with major depression or dysthymia, most of whom also met criteria for mild cognitive impairment, open treatment with sertraline showed improvement in depression with little improvement in cognitive deficits (Devanand *et al.* 2003). In another pilot study in a similar patient sample, adding donepezil, a cholinesterase inhibitor, to antidepressant treatment led to improvement in cognitive test performance compared to placebo plus antidepressant treatment (Pelton *et al.* 2008). There are no large-scale studies directly addressing treatment of depression with co-morbid cognitive impairment. In a reanalysis of the study that compared donepezil, vitamin E, and placebo in 769 amnestic MCI patients, only the depressed sub-group, identified by high Beck Depression Inventory scores, showed an advantage for donepezil over placebo (Lu *et al.* 2009). In contrast, in nondepressed subjects, survival curves did not differ among treatment groups after the first year, and at 2 years the conversion rates were nearly identical in the treatment groups (Lu *et al.* 2009). The results suggest that donepezil moderates the increased risk of AD (may delay conversion) conferred by even mild depressive symptoms in patients with MCI. In contrast, in elderly depressed patients without MCI, donepezil does not show an advantage over placebo in improving cognition (Reynolds *et al.* 2011).

Another sub-group of patients with depression and cognitive impairment is characterized by executive function deficits, which indicate difficulty in performing tasks that require actions to complete multiple components in sequence or require changing one's strategy when the rules of the task are changed. The presence of these types of deficits, especially in isolation, is associated with cerebrovascular disease (hyperintensities, lacunes, infarcts) on an MRI scan of the brain. However, executive function deficits in the presence of objectively identified memory impairment are more likely to be due to Alzheimer's disease. There is some evidence that antidepressant treatment is not very effective in these patients (Alexopoulos *et al.* 2000b) and initial evidence that problem-solving therapy may be helpful to a small degree (Areán *et al.* 2008). In these studies, patients who met criteria for amnestic MCI were excluded, thereby decreasing the likelihood of including patients with incipient Alzheimer's disease. The variable results in treatment studies of older depressed patients with cognitive impairment highlight two issues that need to be addressed in future research: (1) to improve clinical applicability, inclusion/exclusion criteria in research studies need to include all patients with depression plus cognitive impairment without exclusion of amnestic MCI or other specific categories of cognitive impairment so that more clinically applicable data is generated on the efficacy of antidepressant treatment, and (2) the therapeutic effects of antidepressants, cognitive enhancers, and therapies such as problem-solving therapy, singly and in combination, need to be clarified in these patients. A pilot study suggested that stimulants may be effective in older adults with major depression (Lavretsky *et al.* 2006), but large-scale systematic trials are lacking, and patients with depression and cognitive impairment have not been studied.

In the absence of definitive data on the optimal treatment strategy, current clinical practice in depressed patients with cognitive impairment is to first treat with antidepressants and then evaluate if cognition improves along with antidepressant response. Of note, "pseudodementia" which indicates that the patient presents with cognitive impairment, but in fact has an underlying depression, is very rare. The literature on the treatment of depression in patients with an established diagnosis of dementia, primarily Alzheimer's disease, suggests a marginal positive effect for antidepressant medication in some studies, while other studies show no advantage of medication over placebo, and methodological inadequacies in many trials may account for these variable findings (Nelson and Devanand, 2011). A recent discontinuation trial of antidepressants in patients with dementia showed significantly increased relapse on placebo compared to continuation antidepressant, indirectly suggesting that antidepressants were effective in treating depression (Bergh *et al.* 2012).

Clinical case

A 72-year-old black male comes to his primary care doctor complaining of less energy and trouble sleeping. Initially he was treated with a hypnotic, but after 3 weeks he returned, now adding loss of appetite to his complaints. He has a history of hypertension that is controlled by medication, and recent physical exam and laboratory tests were normal.

The patient was referred to a geriatric psychiatrist and, during the consultation, symptoms of depressed mood, ruminations about past life events, feelings of hopelessness, and concerns about memory led to a diagnosis of major depressive disorder. The patient had no history of depression and MMSE exam score was 29/30.

How should this patient be treated? Currently, in the absence of data to the contrary, the general approach to treatment of late-life depression should parallel the approach established for younger adults by the STAR-D study, i.e., careful, systematic, sequential trials of antidepressant treatments alone or in combination. There are two important exceptions: (1) the use of problem-solving therapy for patients with executive dysfunction, and (2) the use of nortriptyline for patients with no medical contraindication should be considered after the first failed trial. ECT is also often used sooner than might be for younger patients because of medication nonresponse.

Clinical case of depression with cognitive impairment

A 74-year-old woman was brought by her daughter for the assessment. The daughter was concerned about depression and memory loss. The patient accepted that she may have some of these symptoms, but minimized them and did not find them to be disturbing or problematic. SCID evaluation confirmed a diagnosis of dysthymic disorder. On cognitive testing, she scored 27 out of 30 on the Folstein MMSE with recall of one out of three objects at 5 minutes. Upon further inquiry, the patient revealed that she occasionally had trouble in her work in sales at a department store, and that her younger colleagues sometimes needed to help her out. Her depression improved on sertraline, 100 mg/d, but she continued to have cognitive deficits on testing. She was unable to continue her job after another

2 years, by which time she had received a clinical diagnosis of Alzheimer's disease with further progression in her cognitive deficits. She showed initial response to donepezil, but disease progression continued over the next 7 years and at that stage she was admitted to a nursing home.

This case illustrates some points that are common in patients with depression and cognitive impairment:

1. Family members often identify the problem, not the patient, and they bring the patient for evaluation.
2. Objective cognitive testing is important to establish the nature of cognitive impairment, and performance on recall after 5 minutes rather than the total MMSE score is important in these patients.
3. Both depression and cognition need to be assessed thoroughly without any assumptions about one set of symptoms being causative for the other set of symptoms.
4. Functional impairment is typically not reported spontaneously by the patient, and further specific inquiries, as well as independent history obtained from a knowledgeable informant may be needed.
5. If successful treatment of depression does not lead to remission of cognitive deficits, the patient may have an incipient dementia that can be treated with cholinesterase inhibitors (or memantine in more advanced cases).

References

Alexopoulos, G.S., Meyers, B.S., Young, R.C., Mattis, S., and Kakuma, T. (1993). The course of geriatric depression with "reversible dementia": A controlled study. *American Journal of Psychiatry*, 150, 1693–1699.

Alexopoulos, G.S., Kiosses, D.N., Choi, S.J., Murphy, C.F., and Lim, K.O. (2002a). Frontal white matter microstructure and treatment response of late-life depression: A preliminary study. *American Journal of Psychiatry*, 159, 1929–1932.

Alexopoulos, G.S., Kiosses, D.N., Klimstra, S., Kalayam, B., and Bruce, M.L. (2002b). Clinical presentation of the "depression-executive dysfunction syndrome" of late life. *American Journal of Geriatric Psychiatry*, 10, 98–106.

Alexopoulos, G.S., Meyers, B.S., Young, R.C. et al. (1997). Clinically defined vascular depression. *American Journal of Psychiatry*, 154, 562–565.

Alexopoulos, G.S., Meyers, B.S., Young, R.C. et al. (2000). Executive dysfunction and long-term outcomes of geriatric depression. *Archives of General Psychiatry*, 57, 285–290.

Areán, P., Raue, P., Mackin, R.S., and Alexopoulos, G. (2010). Problem-solving therapy and supportive therapy in older adults with major depression and executive dysfunction. *American Journal of Psychiatry*, 167, 1391–1398.

Areán, P., Hegel, M., Vannoy, S., Fan, M.Y., and Unutzer, J. (2008). Effectiveness of problem-solving therapy for older, primary care patients with depression: Results from the IMPACT project. *Gerontologist*, 48, 311–323.

Barbey, J.T. and Roose, S.P. (1998). SSRI safety in overdose. *Journal of Clinical Psychiatry*, 59 Suppl 15, 42–48.

Bassuk, S.S., Berkman, L.F., and Wypij, D. (1998). Depressive symptomatology and incident cognitive decline in an elderly community sample. *Archives of General Psychiatry*, 55, 1073–1081.

Bellino, S., Bogetto, F., Veschetto, P., et al. (2000). Recognition and treatment of dysthymia in elderly patients. *Drugs Aging*, 16, 107–121.

Bergh, S., Selbæk, G., and Engedal, K. (2012). Discontinuation of antidepressants in people with dementia and neuropsychiatric symptoms (DESEP study): Double blind, randomised, parallel group, placebo controlled trial. *British Medical Journal*, 344, e1566.

Berkman, L.F., Blumenthal, J., Burg, M., et al. (2003). Effects of treating depression and low perceived social support on clinical events after myocardial infarction: The Enhancing Recovery in Coronary Heart Disease Patients (ENRICHD) Randomized Trial. *Journal of the American Medical Association*, 289, 3106–3116.

Bondareff, W., Alpert, M., Friedhoff, A.J. et al. (2000). Comparison of sertraline and nortriptyline in the treatment of major depressive disorder in late-life. *American Journal of Psychiatry*, 157, 729–736.

Brown, P.J., Devanand, D.P., Liu, X., and Caccappolo, E. (2011). Functional impairment in elderly patients with mild cognitive impairment and mild Alzheimer disease. *Archives of General Psychiatry*, 68, 617–626.

Chen, P., Ganguli, M., Mulsant, B.H., and DeKosky, S.T. (1999). The temporal relationship between depressive symptoms and dementia: A community-based prospective study. *Archives of General Psychiatry*, 56, 261–266.

Devanand, D.P., Nobler, M.S., Singer, T. et al. (1994). Is dysthymia a different disorder in the elderly? *American Journal of Psychiatry*, 151, 1592–1599.

Devanand, D.P., Sano, M., Tang, M.X. et al. (1996). Depressed mood and the incidence of Alzheimer's disease in the elderly living in the community. *Archives of General Psychiatry*, 53, 175–182.

Devanand, D.P., Kim, M.K., Nobler, M.S. (1997). Fluoxetine discontinuation in elderly dysthymic patients. *American Journal of Geriatric Psychiatry*, 5, 83–87.

Devanand, D.P., Pelton, G.H., Marston, K. *et al.* (2003). Sertraline treatment of elderly patients with depression and cognitive impairment. *International Journal of Geriatric Psychiatry*, 18, 123–130.

Devanand, D.P., Adorno, E., Cheng, J., *et al.* (2004a). Late onset dysthymic disorder and major depression differ from early onset dysthymic disorder and major depression in elderly outpatients. *Journal of Affective Disorders*, 78, 259–267.

Devanand, D.P., Juszczak, N., Nobler, M.S., *et al.* (2004b). An open treatment trial of venlafaxine for elderly patients with dysthymic disorder. *Journal of Geriatric Psychiatry and Neurology*, 17, 219–224.

Devanand, D.P., Nobler, M.S., Cheng, J., *et al.* (2005). Randomized, double-blind, placebo-controlled trial of fluoxetine treatment for elderly patients with dysthymic disorder. *American Journal of Geriatric Psychiatry*, 13, 59–68.

Devanand, D.P., Liu, X., Tabert, M.H. *et al.* (2008). Combining early markers strongly predicts conversion from mild cognitive impairment to Alzheimer's disease. *Biological Psychiatry*, 64, 871–879.

Flint, A.J. and Rifat, S.L. (1996). The effect of sequential antidepressant treatment on geriatric depression. *Journal of Affective Disorders*, 36, 95–105.

Gallo, J.J. and Rabins, P.V. (1999). Depression without sadness: Alternative presentations of depression in late life. *American Family Physician*, 60, 820–826.

Hickie, I., Scott, E., Mitchell, P. *et al.* (1995). Subcortical hyperintensities on magnetic resonance imaging: Clinical correlates and prognostic significance in patients with severe depression. *Biological Psychiatry*, 37, 151–160.

Honig, L.S., Kukull, W., and Mayeux, R. (2005). Atherosclerosis and AD: Analysis of data from the US National Alzheimer's Coordinating Center. *Neurology*, 64, 494–500.

Kasper, S., de Swart, H., and Andersen, H.F. (2005). Escitalopram in the treatment of depressed elderly patients. *American of Geriatric Psychiatry* 13, 884–891.

King-Kallimanis, B., Gum, A.M., and Kohn, R. (2009). Comorbidity of depressive and anxiety disorders for older Americans in the national comorbidity survey-replication. *American Journal of Geriatric Psychiatry*, 17, 782–792.

Kirby, M., Bruce, L., Coakley, D., and Lawlor, B.A. (1999). Dysthymia among community-dwelling elderly. *International Journal of Geriatric Psychiatry*, 14, 440–445.

Klunk, W.E., Engler, H., Nordberg, A. *et al.* (2004). Imaging brain amyloid in Alzheimer's disease with Pittsburgh Compound-B. *Annals of Neurology*, 55, 306–319.

Kocsis, J.H. (1998). Geriatric dysthymia. *Journal of Clinical Psychiatry*, 59, 13–15.

Krishnan, K.R. and McDonald, W.M. (1995). Arteriosclerotic depression. *Medical Hypotheses*, 44, 111–115.

Krishnan, K.R., Hays, J.C., and Blazer, D.G. (1997). MRI-defined vascular depression. *American Journal of Psychiatry*, 154, 497–501.

Krishnan, K.R., McDonald, W.M., Doraiswamy, P.M. *et al.* (1993). Neuroanatomical substrates of depression in the elderly. *European Archives of Psychiatry and Clinical Neuroscience*, 243, 41–46.

Kumar, A., Jin, Z., Bilker, W., Udupa, J., and Gottlieb, G. (1998). Late-onset minor and major depression: Early evidence for common neuroanatomical substrates detected by using MRI. *Proceedings of the National Academy of Sciences, 23*, 95, 7654–7658.

Lavretsky, H., Park, S., Siddarth, P., Kumar, A., and Reynolds, C.F., III. (2006). Methylphenidate-enhanced antidepressant response to citalopram in the elderly: A double-blind, placebo-controlled pilot trial. *American Journal of Geriatric Psychiatry*, 14, 181–185.

Lin, E.H., Katon, W., Von Korff, M. *et al.* (2003). Effect of improving depression care on pain and functional outcomes among older adults with arthritis: A randomized controlled trial. *Journal of the American Medical Association*, 290, 2428–2429.

Liu, B., Anderson, G., Mittmann, N. *et al.* (1998). Use of selective serotonin-reuptake inhibitors or tricyclic antidepressants and risk of hip fractures in elderly people. *Lancet*, 351, 1303–1307.

Lu, P.H., Edland, S.D., Teng, E. *et al.* (2009). Donepezil delays progression to AD in MCI subjects with depressive symptoms. *Neurology*, 72, 2115–2121.

Luchsinger, J.A., Honig, L.S., Tang, M.X., and Devanand, D.P. (2009). Depressive symptoms, vascular risk factors, and Alzheimer's disease. *International Journal of Geriatric Psychiatry*, 9, 922–928.

Mason, B.J., Kocsis, J.H., Leon, A.C. *et al.* (1993). Measurement of severity and treatment response in dysthymia may have been limited by the structure and format of existing rating instruments. *Psychiatric Annals*, 23, 625–631.

Mesters, P., Ansseau, M., Brasseur, R., *et al.* (1992). An open multicentre study to evaluate the efficacy and tolerance of fluoxetine 20 mg in depressed ambulatory patients. *Acta Psychiatrica Belgica*, 92, 232–245.

Mintun, M.A., Larossa, G.N., Sheline, Y.I. *et al.* (2006). [11C]PIB in a nondemented population: Potential antecedent marker of Alzheimer disease. *Neurology*, 67, 446–452.

Moussavi, S., Chatterji, S., Verdes, E. *et al.* (2007). Depression, chronic diseases, and decrements in health: Results from the World Health Surveys. *Lancet Neurology*, 370, 851–858.

Nelson, J.C. and Devanand, D.P. (2011). A systematic review and meta-analysis of placebo-controlled antidepressant studies in patients with depression and dementia. *Journal of the American Geriatric Society*, 59, 577–585.

Nelson, J.C., Kennedy, J.S., Pollock, B.G. *et al.* (1999). Treatment of major depression with nortriptyline and paroxetine in patients with ischemic heart disease. *American Journal of Psychiatry*, 156, 1024–1028.

Newhouse, P.A., Krishnan, K.R., Doraiswami, P.M. *et al.* (2000). A double blind comparison of sertraline and fluoxetine in depressed elderly outpatients. *Journal of Clinical Psychiatry*, 61, 559–568.

Pelton, G.H., Harper, O.L., Tabert, M.H., *et al.* (2008). Randomized double-blind placebo-controlled donepezil augmentation in antidepressant-treated elderly patients with depression and cognitive impairment: A pilot study. *International Journal of Geriatric Psychiatry*, 23, 670–676.

Pollock, B.G. (1999). Adverse reactions of antidepressants in elderly patients. *Journal of Clinical Psychiatry*, 60 Suppl, 4–8.

Rafanelli, C., Milaneschi, Y., Roncuzzi, R., and Pancaldi, L.G. (2010). Dysthymia before myocardial infarction as a cardiac risk factor at 2.5-year follow-up. *Psychosomatics*, 51, 8–13.

Reynolds, C.F., III, Butters, M.A., Lopez, O. *et al.* (2011). Maintenance treatment of depression in old age: A randomized, double-blind, placebo-controlled evaluation of the efficacy and safety of donepezil combined with antidepressant pharmacotherapy. *Archives of General Psychiatry*, 68, 51–60.

Robinson, R.G. and Price, T.R. (1982). Post-stroke depressive disorders: A follow-up study of 103 outpatients. *Stroke*, 13, 635–641.

Roose, S.P. (1990). Methodological issues in the diagnosis, treatment and study of refractory depression. In Roose, S.P. and Glassman, A.H., eds., *Treatment Strategies for Refractory Depression*. Washington, DC: American Psychiatric Press, 3–9.

Roose, S.P. and Glassman, A.H. (1990). Cardiovascular effects of tricyclic antidepressants in depressed patients with and without heart disease. In Amsterdam, J.D., ed., *Antidepressant Therapy*. New York: Marcel Dekker, Inc., 151.

Roose, S.P. and Glassman, A.H. (1994). Antidepressant choice in the patient with cardiac disease: Lessons from the Cardiac Arrhythmia Suppression Trial (CAST) studies. *Journal of Clinical Psychiatry*, 55, 83–87.

Roose, S.P. and Krishnan, R. (2004). Depression comorbid with other illness. In Charney, D.S. and Nestler, E.J., eds., *Neurobiology of Mental Illness, Second Edition*. Oxford: Oxford University Press.

Roose, S.P., Glassman, A.H., Attia, E., and Woodring, S. (1994). Comparative efficacy of the selective serotonin reuptake inhibitors and the tricyclics in the treatment of melancholia. *American Journal of Psychiatry*, 151, 1735–1739.

Roose, S.P., Nelson, J.C., Salzman, C., Hollander, S.B., and Rodrigues, H. (2003). Mirtazapine in the Nursing Home Study Group. Open-label study of mirtazapine orally disintegrating tablets in depressed patients in the nursing home. *Current Medical Research Opinions*, 19, 737–746.

Roose, S.P., Glassman, A.H., Siris, S.G. *et al.* (1981). Comparison of imipramine and nortriptyline induced orthostatic hypotension: A meaningful difference. *Journal of Clinical Psychopharmacology*, 1, 316–319.

Roose, S.P., Glassman, A.H., Attia, E. *et al.* (1998). Cardiovascular effects of fluoxetine in depressed patients with heart disease. *American Journal of Psychiatry*, 155, 660–665.

Roose, S.P., Sackeim, H.A., Krishnan, K.R., *et al.* (2004). Old-Old Depression Study Group. Antidepressant pharmacotherapy in the treatment of depression in the very old: A randomized, placebo-controlled trial. *American Journal of Psychiatry*, 161, 2050–2059.

Rutherford, B., Roose, S., Sneed, J., *et al.* (2007). An open trial of aripiprazole augmentation for SSRI nonremitters. *International Journal of Geriatric Psychiatry*, 22, 986–991.

Sackeim, H.A., Roose, S.P., and Lavori, P.W. (2005). Determining the duration of antidepressant treatment: Application of signal detection methodology and the need for duration adaptive designs (DAD). *Biological Psychiatry*, 59, 483–492.

Schatzberg, A. and Cantillon, M. (2000). *Antidepressant Early Response and Remission with Venlafaxine or Flouxetine in Depressed Geriatric Outpatients*. Presented at the European College of Neuropsychopharmacology Meeting, Nice, France.

Schatzberg, A.F., Kremer, C., Rodrigues, H.E. *et al.* (2002). Double-blind randomized comparison of mirtazapine and paroxetine in elderly depressed patients. *American Journal of Geriatric Psychiatry*, 10, 541–550.

Schneider, L.S., Nelson, J.C., Clary, C.M. *et al.* (2003). Sertraline Elderly Depression Study Group: An 8-week multicenter, parallel-group, double-blind, placebo-controlled study of sertraline in elderly outpatients with major depression. *American Journal of Psychiatry*, 160, 1277–1285.

Seidman, S.N., Araujo, A.B., Roose, S.P., *et al.* (2002). Low testosterone levels in elderly men with dysthymic disorder. *American Journal of Psychiatry*, 159, 456–459.

Seidman, S.N., Orr, G., Raviv, G., *et al.* (2009). Effects of testosterone replacement in middle-aged men with dysthymia: A randomized, placebo-controlled clinical trial. *Journal of Clinical Psychopharmacology*, 29, 216–221.

Sheffrin, M., Driscoll, H.C., Lenze, E.J. *et al.* (2009). Getting to remission: Use of aripiprazole for incomplete response in late-life depression. *Journal of Clinical Psychiatry*, 70, 208–213.

Sheline, Y.I., Sanghavi, M., Mintun, M.A., and Gado, M.H. (1999). Depression duration but not age predicts hippocampal volume loss in medically healthy women with recurrent major depression. *Journal of Neuroscience*, 19, 5034–5043.

Shores, M.M., Kivlahan, D.R., Sadak, T.I., Li, E.J., and Matsumoto, A.M. (2009). A randomized, double-blind, placebo-controlled study of testosterone treatment in hypogonadal older men with subthreshold depression (dysthymia or minor depression). *Journal of Clinical Psychiatry*, 70, 1009–1016.

Silverman, D.H., Small, G.W., Chang, C.Y., *et al.* (2001). Positron emission tomography in evaluation of dementia: Regional brain metabolism and long-term outcome. *Journal of the American Medical Association*, 286, 2120–2127.

Sneed, J.R., Roose, S.P., and Sackeim, H.A. (2006). Vascular depression: A distinct diagnostic subtype? *Biological Psychiatry*, 60, 1295–1298.

Sweet, R.A., Hamilton, R.L., Butters, M.A. *et al.* (2004). Neuropathologic correlates of late-onset major depression. *Neuropsychopharmacology*, 29, 2242–2250.

Tabert, M., Liu, X., Doty, R.I. *et al.* (2005). A 10-item smell identification scale related to risk for Alzheimer's disease. *Annals of Neurology*, 58, 155–160.

Tamburrino, M.B., Lynch, D.J., Nagel, R.W., and Smith, M.K. (2009). Primary Care Evaluation of Mental Disorders (PRIME-MD) screening for minor depressive disorder in primary care. Prim care companion. *Journal of Clinical Psychiatry*, 11, 339–343.

Toffefson, G.D., Bosomworth, J.C., Heligeenstein, J.H. *et al.* (2002). A double-blind, placebo-controlled clinical trial of fluoxetine in geriatric patients with major depression. *International Psychogeriatrics*, 7, 89–104.

Unutzer, J., Katon, W., Callahan, C.M. *et al.* (2002). Collaborative care management of late-life depression in the primary care setting: A randomized controlled trial. *Journal of the American Medical Association*, 288, 2836–2845.

Visser, P.J., Verhey, F., Knol, D.L. *et al.* (2009). Prevalence and prognostic value of CSF markers of Alzheimer's disease pathology in patients with subjective cognitive impairment or mild cognitive impairment in the DESCRIPA study: a prospective cohort study. *Lancet Neurology*, 8, 619–627.

Weihs, K.L., Settle, E.C., Jr., Batey, S.R. *et al.* (2002). Bupropion sustained release versus paroxetine for the treatment of depression in the elderly. *Journal of Clinical Psychiatry*, 61, 196–202.

Williams, J.W., Jr., Barrett, J., Oxman, T. *et al.* (2000). Treatment of dysthymia and minor depression in primary care: A randomized controlled trial in older adults. *Journal of the American Medical Association*, 284, 1519–1526.

Wilson, R.S., Barnes, L.L., Mendes de Leon, C.F. *et al.* (2002). Depressive symptoms, cognitive decline, and risk of AD in older persons. *Neurology*, 59, 364–370.

Young, R.C. and Meyers, B.S. (1992). Psychopharmacology. In Sadavoy, J., Lazarus, L.W., and Jarvik, L.F., eds., *Comprehensive Review of Geriatric Psychiatry*. Washington, DC: American Psychiatric Press, 435–467.

Chapter

10

Chronic depression

James H. Kocsis and Benjamin D. Brody

Introduction

Once conceptualized as a uniformly episodic illness, major depressive disorder has now long been recognized to have a chronic course in up to 20% of those who become depressed, affecting 3% of the adult US population (Weissman *et al.* 1988, Kessler *et al.* 1994). Defined by convention and in the DSM IV-TR as the presence of depressive symptoms for 2 years, these states represent a disproportionately high amount of the overall disease burden caused by major depressive disorder, as they begin earlier in life, are associated with a higher degree of occupational and psychosocial maladjustment and more frequent suicide attempts than episodic forms of the illness (Keller *et al.* 2000). In subjects in the STAR-D trial, the largest ever clinical trial for treatments of major depression, the subjects with chronic forms of depression were also significantly older, more likely to be unemployed, to have more co-morbid medical conditions, to have less educational achievement, and be more likely to a be a racial minority (Gilmer *et al.* 2005). Despite the significant morbidity associated with the diagnosis, it is also a condition that remains notably undertreated: only 33% of 801 subjects who participated in a treatment study for chronic depression had ever had a prior adequate antidepressant trial (Kocsis *et al.* 2008). As such, chronic depression should not be confused with treatment-resistant depression, which has been defined as depression that is refractory to adequate prior treatment (Thase and Rush, 1997).

In this chapter, we will review how concepts of chronic depression have evolved in modern psychiatry, describe the evaluation of patients who present with depressive symptoms that are 2 years or longer in duration, review the evidence base for the management of these conditions, and present an illustrative case.

Historical perspectives: the evolution of diagnosis

In *Manic-Depressive Insanity and Paranoia*, Emil Kraeplin offered one of the early descriptions of what he characterized as the depressive temperament, a "fundamental state" that he also described as "constitutional moodiness."

The depressive temperament is characterized by a permanent gloomy emotional stress in all the experiences of life…[T]he patients, as a rule, have to struggle with all sorts of internal obstructions…They take everything seriously, and in every occurrence feel small disagreeables much more strongly than the elevating and satisfying aspects of untroubled and cheerful enjoyment…Frequently, therefore, a capricious, irritable, unfriendly, repellant behavior is developed. (Kraeplin 1976)

Kraeplin noted that such a condition generally had an early onset and persisted throughout life.

Early versions of the DSM labeled these patients as "cyclothymic personality" or "depressive neurosis" and they were classified as suffering from a neurosis or personality disorder. Reviewing these earlier perspectives nearly 25 years ago, one of us concluded that chronic depressive states "have been viewed variously as inherent temperaments, acquired character tendencies, attenuated variants of classic manic depressive disorder, or complications of other mental disorders, physical illnesses, or environmental stressors" (Kocsis and Frances, 1987).

By 1980, the concept of chronic depression began to evolve. Akiskal and colleagues made an attempt to sub-classify chronic forms of depression in a retrospective chart review of 50 outpatients with greater than 5 years of depressive symptoms (Akiskal *et al.* 1980). In a sub-set for whom sleep EEG data were available, they compared REM latency data between those subjects that had responded to antidepressant medication and those whose symptoms were refractory to medication. They found that medication responders, a group they called "sub-affective dysthymia," had a mean REM latency time of 57.6 min, which was similar to a group of unipolar depressed control subjects, who had a mean REM latency of 59 min. Medication nonresponders, whom they termed "character spectrum depression," on the other hand, had a mean REM latency of 98.8 min, which was similar to a mean time of 101 min in healthy control subjects. This study was influential in spurring research into the treatment of chronic depression.

Chronic forms of depression were shown to be responsive to a variety of antidepressant medications, first in open-label and subsequently in a placebo-controlled trial (Kocsis *et al.* 1988a). *Dysthymia* was introduced in DSM-III, to describe a mild chronic form of depression and, in a notably reclassification, the disorder was moved from a personality disorder on Axis II to affective disorder on Axis I. It was proposed that chronic forms of depression may resemble personality disorders, because such patients may exhibit pessimistic cognitive styles, occupational impairments and social maladjustments, characteristics that resemble personality traits. However, such impairments can all be viewed as downstream sequellae of a chronic affective illness and are responsive to treatment with antidepressants (Kocsis *et al.* 1988b). Fluoxetine and other SSRI antidepressants were approved for use in major depression in the United States during this decade. Their widespread popularity for the treatment of milder forms of depression lead some observers to reconceptualize the boundaries of "static" character traits or temperaments, most notably Peter Kramer, in his book *Listening to Prozac* (Kramer 1993). Efforts to sub-categorize chronic depressive states continued over the next decade. Keller and others first described the phenomenon of "double depression," or acute major depressive episodes that are superimposed on a pre-existing dysthymic state. The DSM-IV field trial for major depression, minor depression, and depressive personality found that among 432 subjects with major depression, 22% had a recurrent course, with antecedent dysthymia and without full recovery (Keller *et al.* 1995). Recognition of such a frequency of recurrent episodes with incomplete recovery led to up to five separate sub-types ultimately described in the chronic depression literature: (1) chronic major depression (meeting full criteria for 2 years), (2) dysthymia (meeting minor depressive criteria for 2 years), (3) double depression (dysthymia punctuated by major depressive episodes), (4) chronic major depression with periods of partial recovery, and (5) recurrent major depression with periods of incomplete recovery.

More recently, McCullough and colleagues have suggested that such sub-types are not reliably distinct (McCullough *et al.* 2003). On the basis of their work and others, the Depressive Disorders Work Group for DSM-5 considered merging dysthymia and chronic depression, but ultimately maintained separate diagnostic entities. "We believe it important to distinguish from dysthymic disorder the relatively high illness severity implicit in the DSM-IV definition of chronic MDD, a definition that requires the continuous presence of the full major depressive syndrome over a two-year period," they noted (DSM-5, 2012).

The diagnostic evaluation

The initial priority in the evaluation of a patient with chronic depressive symptoms includes establishing safety, with specific attention to risk factors for suicide. Prior suicide attempts, active substance abuse, the presence of suicidal ideation (particularly ideation that includes a specific plan), as well as demographic risk factors, such as being elderly, single, living alone, and male, should all be taken into consideration as the clinician makes the initial decision about initiating treatment on an inpatient or outpatient basis. In addition to evaluating safety, the clinician's initial task is to rule out the possibility that the symptoms are secondary to a medical illness or other psychiatric condition such as bipolar disorder, complicated grief, substance abuse, or a personality disorder. Patient preference and history of early-life adversity should also be assessed as they may impact responsiveness to pharmacotherapy vs. psychotherapy (Nemeroff *et al.* 2003, Kocsis *et al.* 2009).

The exclusion of a depressive disorder secondary to a general medical condition

A comprehensive review of the myriad general medical conditions that can present insidiously with depressive symptoms is beyond the scope of this chapter. However, medical conditions should be considered when evaluating anyone who presents with these symptoms. Basic laboratory tests, including thyroid studies, should be strongly considered. Hematologic conditions, such as anemia, electrolyte disturbances, such as hyponatremia, certain types of tumors, like pancreatic or lung cancer, and autoimmune disturbances should be considered and may present across the life cycle and in diverse backgrounds. The differential diagnosis for other possible general medical conditions is very broad, and laboratory testing and imaging studies should be tailored to the level of clinical suspicion and demographics of the patient in question. These judgments are complicated by the tendency of some depressed patients towards somatic symptoms and alexithymia.

Special populations warrant particular attention. Geriatric patients should be screened for cognitive symptoms to rule out mild cognitive impairment or frank dementia. Older men presenting with chronic depressive symptoms, especially low mood in combination with low sex drive and fatigue, should be screened for low testosterone. Similarly, perimenopausal women with mood symptoms that are accompanied by classic menopausal complaints should be evaluated for the possibility of hormone replacement therapy to address both mood and somatic symptoms. Many primary neurological conditions, such as epilepsy, Parkinson's disease, multiple sclerosis, intracranial mass lesions, or infections can be accompanied by long-term disturbances in mood, but can be largely ruled out by a careful review of systems, neurologic examination, and brain imaging.

Side effects of medications are another important potential etiology for depressed mood. Commonly prescribed medications that can lead to iatrogenic mood disturbance include antihypertensives, oral contraceptives, steroids, analgesics, antimicrobials, and some dermatologic preparations such as retinoic acid. Psychotropic medications such as benzodiazepines and other CNS agents are also possible causes of iatrogenic depressed mood. A temporal correlation between the onset of the mood symptoms and the initiation of a medication may warrant a trial off the medication as an initial approach. Clearly this must be done in co-operation with the physician prescribing the other medication. While many drugs of abuse can also cause mood symptoms, alcohol abuse, prescription narcotic, and benzodiazepine abuse are seen frequently in depressed patients and should be routinely screened for during the interview, and with serum or urine toxicology when suspicion is high. Please see Table 10.1 for a more comprehensive differential diagnosis for mood disorder secondary to general medical condition.

The exclusion of a bipolar spectrum disorder

Patients with bipolar spectrum disorders spend the majority of their symptomatic time depressed, much of it in sub-threshold states (Judd *et al.* 2002). They may not actively report a history of mania or hypomania, which they may not subjectively experience as psychopathology. As such, careful history-taking in all patients with depressive symptoms is critical, with specific attention to periods of notable changes in energy, sleep requirement, talkativeness, risk-taking behaviors around sexual behavior and financial expenditures, irritability, and goal-directed activity such as starting businesses or new hobbies. One patient who presented with a chief complaint of chronic depressive symptoms, when a full history was taken, revealed that his illness was punctuated by periods of increased energy and intense interest in food canning: in fact, he had a garage filled with thousands of jars of pickled vegetables.

Prior periods of episodic change in baseline personality characteristics, rapid thought processes, or increased talkativeness are all clues that a patient complaining of sustained depressive symptoms may be manifesting a bipolar spectrum disorder. If there is any question about a possible history of manic or hypomanic symptoms, prior treatment records and collateral information from family, friends, or colleagues of the patient who can provide longitudinal perspective become all the more paramount. The diagnosis of a bipolar spectrum disorder has important treatment implications. Antidepressants are more likely to induce mania or rapid cycling in this group, and lithium augmentation may be more effective.

Chronic depression in the setting of a co-morbid personality disorder

As noted above, early versions of the DSM characterized chronic forms of major depression as a personality disorder. With the introduction of the dysthymia diagnosis in DSM-III, some attention shifted to the prevalence of co-morbidity between chronic depression and other personality disorders. Russell *et al.* (2003) examined the prevalence of an Axis II

Table 10.1 Reprinted from Williams, E. and Shepherd, S. Medical clearance of psychiatric patients. *Emergency Medicine Clinics of North America*, 18, 193, with permission from Elsevier

Medical/Toxic Effects	CNS	Infections	Metabolic/Endocrine	Cardiopulmonary	Miscellaneous
Alcohol and drug abuse	Subdural hematoma	Pneumonia	Thyroid disease	Arrhythmias	SLE
Drugs of abuse	Tumor	Urinary tract infection	Adrenal disease	Myocardial infarction	Vasculitis
Cocaine	Intracranial aneurysm		Renal disease	Congestive heart failure	Temporal artheritis
Marijuana	Hypertensive encephalopathy	Sepsis	Pituitary dysfunction	COPD/asthma	Anemia
PCP		Malaria		Pulmonary embolism	
LSD	Primary CNS infection	Legionnaire's	Diabetic ketoacidosis		
Heroin	Normal pressure	Syphilis	Hypoglycemia		
Amphetamines	Hydrocephalus	Typhoid fever	Hepatic encephalopathy		
Jimson weed	Seizure disorders postictal nonconvulsive status	Diphtheria			
GHB		Rocky Mountain spotted fever	Wilson's disease		
Benzodiazepines			Imbalances of Na, K, Ca		
Prescription medications (common offenders)		Acute rheumatic fever	Vitamin deficiencies		
Digitalis					
Tricyclics					
Steroids					
Anticonvulsants					
Cimetidine					
Propanolol					

diagnosis as defined by the SCID-II, the Structured Clinical Interview for Personality Disorders, DSM-III-R, in 633 patients with chronic forms of depression. They found that 46% of that population had at least one co-occurring personality disorder. Patients with antisocial personality disorder and severe forms of borderline personality disorder were excluded from the sample; therefore the true prevalence would have been higher if such subjects had been offered enrollment. Cluster C personality disorders were the most commonly represented in the sample, with 25% meeting criteria for avoidant personality disorder and 18% meeting criteria for obsessive compulsive personality disorder. Notably, when these subjects were treated with 12 weeks of sertraline or imipramine, those with co-morbid personality disorders achieved response and remission rates that were similar to those subjects who did not have an Axis II co-morbidity (Russell

et al. 2003). Despite long-held concerns that Axis II disorders cannot be reliably diagnosed during cross-sectional observation in depressed patients, a large naturalistic study of over 600 subjects with personality disorder concluded that personality disorders can be accurately diagnosed in patients who are currently depressed (Morey *et al.* 2010). The literature on the effect of personality disorders on response to treatment in depressed patients is limited (Phillips *et al.* 1990 Shea *et al.* 1992). In one study, the presence of the personality disorders did not affect the rate of response to pharmacotherapy for chronic depression. In fact, the rate of response was actually higher in patients with borderline personality disorders than in patients without personality disorder (Hirschfeld *et al.* 1998). It is important to note that those patients with severe borderline personality disorder were excluded from the study.

Complicated grief

Although not recognized in DSM-IV-R, complicated grief is a syndrome of persistent symptoms after the death of a loved one that may appear similar to chronic forms of depression (Lichtenthal *et al.* 2004). Chronic depressive symptoms that evolve from bereavement are thus better conceptualized in this narrower construct, and should be treated with an evidence-based therapy such as complicated grief treatment when possible (Shear *et al.* 2005).

Evidence-based treatments for chronic depression

The acute treatment of chronic depression

Medication monotherapy

In 1988, Kocsis *et al.* reported the results of the first large-scale, randomized, placebo-controlled trial of an antidepressant for chronic forms of depression. A total of 76 subjects were randomized to imipramine or placebo for 6 weeks after a 2-week, single-blind, placebo lead in. The initial placebo-responders were excluded from the randomization. Of the subjects, 84% had been depressed for greater than 5 years, despite 71% having had prior psychotherapy and 33% prior exposure to a tricyclic antidepressant. In this study, 59% of the imipramine arm responded, as defined by a greater than 50% reduction in HAM-D score, while only 13% of the placebo arm responded (Kocsis *et al.* 1988a).

The finding that antidepressants are efficacious in the treatment of chronic depression was consistently replicated over the following decade. In an earlier review of the topic, one of us identified 11 randomized placebo-controlled studies examining the efficacy of monoamine antidepressant medications for the treatment of pure dysthymia and double depression that were published between 1985 and 2000. All of the studies that were powered appropriately showed a significant advantage for the active antidepressant arm over placebo. Importantly, all of the studies that examined social function with the Social Adjustment Scale also showed significantly greater improvement in the subjects in the active drug arms (Kocsis, 2003).

In 2002, Thase *et al.* reported similar results in a Pfizer-sponsored trial of sertraline vs. imipramine for chronic depression. The acute phase of the study randomized 635 subjects in a 2:1 ratio to sertraline or imipramine in order to produce a pool of subjects for subsequent studies of medication switching for non-responders and maintenance therapy for responders. In the intent-to-treat analysis of this group, 52% of the sertraline arm and 51% of the imipramine arm responded to a 12-week medication trial. It is notable that approximately half of the subjects treated in these short-term, acute monotherapy studies failed to remit with treatment or even show significant responses, underscoring the need for additional interventions (Thase *et al.* 2002).

One such additional intervention is simply to switch medications. Thase and colleagues tested this strategy in the Pfizer study when they reported the results of 168 subjects who had failed a double-blinded sertraline or imipramine trial and were subsequently switched to the other medication. During the second prospective medication trial, 60% of the subjects in the sertraline arm responded to the medication and 32% remitted. In the imipramine arm, 44% responded and 23% remitted. A high proportion of the imipramine patients dropped out of the study secondary to intolerable side effects. Significantly, the subjects had been depressed for over 6 years on average. Overall, over half responded to their second medication after failing an initial trial (Thase *et al.* 2002).

Psychotherapy and combined psychotherapy with medication

Early efforts to treat chronic depression with psychotherapy grew out of dominant schools of thought, beginning with psychoanalytic views of chronic depression as conceptualized as a personality disorder. Once formally classified as its own Axis I diagnosis, dysthymia began to be subjected to empirical psychotherapy studies. In 1994, Markowitz reviewed the newly accumulating literature on psychotherapeutic interventions for dysthymia and other forms of chronic depression. He found six small studies of cognitive behavior therapy that enrolled a combined total of 116 patients. Half of the studies included patients with double depression and the remaining studies enrolled only patients with pure dysthymia. Response rates varied from 33 to 100% (Markowitz, 1994).

The most promising of these case series were reported by John McCullough, who developed the first structured psychotherapy specifically aimed to address some of the unique interpersonal challenges of working with chronically depressed patients. He noted that such patients present with "Repeated expressions of misery and helplessness…a submissive and defeated demeanor…Wariness of interpersonal involvement that extends to interactions with the clinician…An entrenched conviction that nothing can be done…[and] rigidly stable behavior patterns that do not appear to be affected by either positive or negative events" (McCullough, 2003). He developed the cognitive behavioral analysis system of psychotherapy, or CBASP, conceptualizing chronically depressed patients in Piagetian terms as arrested in a preoperational developmental stage. The treatment draws on a variety of cognitive and behavioral techniques in addition to use of transference and a therapeutic technique called situational analysis that highlights maladaptive patient behavior in the context of the therapeutic session (McCullough, 2003).

Although the efficacy of this approach was never established in comparisons with appropriate control groups, CBASP was the psychotherapy used in Keller's multi-center study comparing nefazodone, psychotherapy, or combination treatment for chronic depression.

Published in 2000, Keller *et al.* addressed the fundamental question of whether the combination of psychotherapy plus medication is a more robust treatment than either alone for chronic depression. They randomized 681 subjects with chronic nonpsychotic major depression to a three-arm trial of nefazodone, CBASP, or combination treatment for 12 weeks. In the combination treatment group, 73% of the subjects responded, while only 48% responded in both the nefazodone monotherapy and the CBASP monotherapy groups. Several important secondary analyses identified moderator variables, or patient characteristics at the time of presentation for treatment, that help provide guidance for treatment selection (Keller *et al.* 2000).

For example, 429 of the patients enrolled in the study completed surveys at the time of randomization asking if they had a preference for medication, psychotherapy, combination treatment, or no preference at all. The subjects were then randomized without taking these preferences into account. For those subjects who preferred psychotherapy, only 8% achieved remission if they were randomized to medication, whereas 50% achieved remission if they did receive psychotherapy. For those who preferred medication, only 22% remitted if they were randomized to

receive psychotherapy, whereas 46% remitted if they were randomized to medication. Both monotherapies were outperformed by combination treatment in the cohort that preferred combination treatment and in the cohort who expressed no preference at all (Kocsis *et al.* 2009).

Using the same dataset, Nemeroff *et al.* examined the differential effect of whether a subject reported a childhood history of neglect, physical or sexual abuse, parental loss, or other forms of trauma on response rates to medication or psychotherapy. Nearly two-thirds of the subjects reported some type of childhood abuse or trauma. As in the larger sample, combination treatment was more efficacious than either monotherapy in the sub-population of patients who had not reported abuse or trauma. However, the subjects who reported a history of a childhood insult benefited more from psychotherapy in terms of their change in HAM-D scores and remission rates. The addition of medication to psychotherapy did not produce a statistically significant additional benefit (Nemeroff *et al.* 2003).

Other investigators have sought to examine whether other forms of psychotherapy are efficacious in treating chronic depression and whether combination therapy is superior to either intervention alone. Interpersonal therapy (IPT) is one such modality that has been studied with mixed results. IPT is a structured, brief treatment that assigns patients the sick role in a medical model of psychopathology and then focuses on interpersonal difficulties that fall into categories such as complicated bereavement, disagreements with a significant other, significant life transitions or, if none of the above are apparent at the outset of treatment, the patient's more broadly defined interpersonal deficits (Markowtiz and Weissman, 2004). Homework and exercises are not part of the treatment, as in CBT, and the therapist–patient relationship is not a focus of the treatment, as in psychodynamic psychotherapy or CBASP.

In 2005, Markowitz *et al.* compared IPT alone with the combination of IPT and sertraline, sertraline monotherapy, and brief supportive psychotherapy as an active control. A total of 94 subjects were randomized to one of the four treatment arms, which the authors felt left the study underpowered. In the sertraline monotherapy arm 58% responded to treatment, as did 57% of the sertraline plus IPT arm. The response rates for both psychotherapies were significantly lower (Markowtiz *et al.* 2005).

In 2008, a group from Germany randomized inpatients with chronic depression to 5 weeks of pharmacotherapy plus IPT or pharmacotherapy plus case management, which was defined as "psychoeducative, supportive and empathic intervention of 15–20 min in length and was delivered by psychiatric residents." The pharmacotherapy was sertraline, except in the case of subjects who had a documented treatment failure on sertraline, in which case amitryptaline was used as the second-line psychotropic agent. In contrast to the Markowitz IPT study, the German group found that combined pharmacotherapy with IPT yielded a response rate of 71%, whereas pharmacotherapy combined with case management produced a response rate of 38.1%. Remission rates also trended towards a higher efficacy for the IPT combination group but the result was not statistically significant, likely in part due to the small sample size (Schramm et al. 2008).

Noting the high frequency of treatment failure and response without remission in the studies described above, the REVAMP investigators more recently undertook an effort to compare CBASP augmentation with supportive psychotherapy augmentation and continued medication monotherapy in patients with chronic depression who failed to remit during a prospective trial with antidepressant. In this trial, 491 subjects failed to remit to a 12-week trial of an antidepressant medication that was selected on the basis of prior medication exposure. These subjects were then randomized in a 1:2:2 ratio to additional pharmacotherapy alone or to one of the two psychotherapy arms plus continued medication for an additional 12 weeks. Approximately 40% of the subjects in the pharmacotherapy alone group remitted during their second medication trial. Neither form of psychotherapy as an augmentation technique significantly improved this outcome (Kocsis et al. 2009). It is important to highlight that subjects in this large sample had depression that was not only chronic but also *prospectively treatment resistant.*

In a follow-up report from the nefazodone and CBASP study, Schatzberg et al. (2005) examined the nonresponders to both the nefazodone monotherapy arm and the CBASP monotherapy arm after they were switched to the treatment they did not initially receive. This switch study resulted in a second 12-week exposure to an intervention – nefazodone between 100 mg and 600 mg or CBASP up to 16 sessions – after failing the initial treatment. At the end of the second 12-week intervention, 57% of patients who crossed over from CBASP to nefazodone showed a response, which was significantly higher than the 42% response rate in the cohort who switched from nefazodone to CBASP, although the nefazodone had a higher attrition rate. This result underscores the observation that chronic forms of depression are not necessarily treatment resistant and provides an evidence base for this common clinical strategy (Schatzberg et al. 2005).

In 2010, Cuijpers et al. published a meta-analysis of the results of 16 individual studies of psychotherapy for the treatment of chronic major depression and dysthymia. With a total of 2116 subjects, the individual studies that the group drew upon included the aforementioned trials of CBASP and IPT in addition to other, often smaller, trials of CBT and other forms of psychotherapy. The psychotherapy arms in these trials were compared to a variety of controls, ranging from waiting lists to pharmacotherapy and combination treatment. They found that psychotherapy was modestly effective as a monotherapy for chronic depression and that there was an increased effect size with increasing number of sessions. Psychotherapy was less effective, however, than monotherapy with medication or combination medication and psychotherapy. The authors note that their data were significantly impacted by the large fraction of their data pool that was drawn from Keller's nefazodone study, which came to similar conclusions (Cuijpers et al. 2010).

Relapse prevention

For patients who do remit or have a significant response to medication, psychotherapy, or combined treatment, the treating clinician is faced with the question of how to optimally treat the patient to maintain a robust and durable recovery. A number of the larger trials discussed above continued to follow subjects in maintenance phases to provide guidance on longer-term outcomes. A significant body of work suggests that continuing the medication or psychotherapy are both effective relapse-prevention strategies.

In 1996, Kocsis et al. reported the results of the first large placebo-controlled trial to address the efficacy of medication to prevent relapse in chronic depression. In this trial, 129 subjects were treated acutely with up to 200 mg of open-label desipramine for 10 weeks. Of these, 66 subjects experienced remissions or significant symptom improvement, and 53 remained well for an additional 16 weeks. These final 53 subjects were then randomized to continue desipramine or be cross-tapered to placebo for up to 2 years of follow-up. In the placebo arm, 52% of subjects experienced relapses of their depression, whereas only 11% of the subjects in the desipramine arm relapsed (Kocsis *et al.* 1996). A secondary analysis of these data looked at the sub-group of subjects who had pure dysthymia (27 of the total of 53) who entered the 2-year maintenance phase of the trial. Among this population with a more mild form of chronic depression, 46% of the placebo group relapsed over the 2-year maintenance period, while none of the subjects in the desipramine arm relapsed (Miller *et al.* 2001).

In 1998, Keller *et al.* reported results from the maintenance phase of Pfizer's study of sertraline and imipramine for chronic depression. A total of 161 patients who had had a remission or significant response to sertraline were randomized to continue the medication or switch to placebo for 76 weeks of follow-up. In this group, 26% of the sertraline arm suffered a re-emergence of depressive symptoms, whereas 50% of the placebo arm showed a re-emergence of symptoms (Keller *et al.* 1998). This was the first study of an SSRI for maintenance treatment in chronic depression, and the results were a replication of Kocsis' desipramine study results. Several reports examined the long-term outcomes for subjects in Keller's nefazodone and CBASP trial. In total, 165 subjects from the nefazodone monotherapy or combined nefazodone and CBASP arms experienced a response or remission and were subsequently randomized to continue nefazodone or be cross-tapered to placebo for a 1-year follow-up of relapse rates. The investigators noted a significant methodological difficulty: the majority of the subjects (61.9%) in the placebo arm of the study dropped out of the maintenance phase, whereas only 38.2% of the active treatment arm dropped out over the course of the 1-year study. To address this confound, the investigators used a " 'competing risk' analytic strategy" that emphasized the later part of the year-long maintenance period. In this model 30.3% of the nefazodone-treated patients, compared to 47.5% of the placebo controls, experienced a significant relapse of depressive symptoms (Gelenberg *et al.* 2003). In the same trial, 82 subjects responded to CBASP monotherapy or responded after being crossed over to CBASP monotherapy after failing a trial of nefazodone. These subjects were then randomized to a monthly CBASP session or only monthly assessment, for 1 year of maintenance. Over the course of the year of maintenance treatment, the CBASP group continued to

show a mean improvement on HAM-D scores while the assessment-only arm showed a gradual increase in their depressive symptoms, as measured by the HAM-D. Depending on the measures used to define recurrence, the CBASP arm subjects suffered recurrence rates between 2.6 and 10.7%, while the assessment-only arm relapsed at rates between 20.9 and 32.0% (Klein *et al.* 2004).

Taken in aggregate, these maintenance studies are unequivocal: patients who recover from chronic depression are at lower risk of relapse if they continue treatment beyond their acute recovery.

Clinical vignette

Ms. K was a 37-year-old Hispanic woman who presented to the outpatient psychiatry department of New York Presbyterian Hospital/Weill Cornell Medical Center in 2008 with complaints of depressed mood, low energy, and interpersonal problems that interfered with her work in human resources for a large corporation. We have changed some details of her case to protect her identity. She reported that although she had been depressed for much of her adult life, her symptoms had worsened over the previous 3 months without an antecedent stressor. She now found it hard to complete basic tasks at work and had tearful outbursts over minor disappointments. Over the 2 weeks prior to presentation she had experienced intrusive suicidal thoughts about jumping off the Manhattan Bridge, which she crossed daily on the subway for her commute to work. The thoughts frightened her and prompted her to schedule the initial evaluation. She had a medical history of hypothyroidism and was maintained on 75 μg of synthroid; recent thyroid studies were within normal limits. She had no other medical problems and took no other medications. She rarely drank alcohol and used no other substances.

The patient reported three prior major depressive episodes. The first episode occurred when she was an undergraduate in college and included a suicide attempt by an overdose of over-the-counter sleep medication. This suicide attempt led to her only lifetime psychiatric hospitalization. She reported being treated with fluoxetine and having a rapid improvement of her symptoms. She quickly discontinued the medication after discharge. She "never really felt like a normal person" in that she was socially withdrawn during college, dated infrequently, and was involved in few other significant social activities. She developed a sense that she "didn't fit" and "couldn't understand why everyone else seemed to be having so much fun." These thoughts solidified after her graduation and in her 20s into a sense of herself as a person with a "fundamental flaw." She had no history of mania, hypomania, or psychosis.

Ms. K grew up in a suburb of Los Angeles, the second daughter of a working class family, and her parents divorced when she was in grade school. She was sexually abused between the ages of 9 and 11 by a distant relative. She was a talented student and won a scholarship to a prestigious Californian university, which her family did not support her accepting, because they felt it would be "too far away from home." She accepted the scholarship anyhow and subsequently had her first depressive episode during her freshman year. After college she moved to New York to take the first of a series of jobs in corporate marketing, communications, and public relations. On several occasions her career trajectory had not progressed at the expected pace, and she had been told in performance reviews that she appeared "quiet," "too passive," "not enough of a self-starter," and that she "seemed unengaged."

Ms. K had had two prior significant relationships with men, but had not dated in approximately 3 years at the time of the initial evaluation. She stated that the men she had dated previously had ended the relationships "because I wasn't the right one for them," which in both cases had come as a surprise to her and led to a worsening of her baseline dysphoria. These perceived failures had made her apprehensive about dating. She had few friends and engaged in few leisure activities other than reading and participating in a food co-operative close to her home in Brooklyn. She was in touch with her family and closest with her older sister, a property manager in Los Angeles. She reported that the last time she really felt "normal" was in high school.

On the basis of this presentation, Ms. K was diagnosed with chronic depression. She had no preference in terms of the choice of medication, psychotherapy, or both, and felt that she was able to maintain her safety as an outpatient. The resident physician treating her began her on fluoxetine in conjunction with weekly supportive psychotherapy for a proposed course of 16 weeks. The fluoxetine was titrated up to 40 mg/d, and the psychotherapy focused on her interpersonal difficulties at work and avoidant social posture outside of work. Her mood and energy improved notably with a complete resolution of her suicidal thoughts by the end of the first month of treatment. Ms. K was able to complete a work assignment that seemed overwhelming at the onset of treatment. Despite these initial successes, she continued to hold a persistent belief that she was "defective," and had ruminative worries about what her colleagues and other members of her food co-operative thought of her. The therapist made supportive interventions around the management of her relationship with her boss, a more assertive younger woman whom the patient found intimidating, and towards the end of the psychotherapy these interactions became less strained. The patient also met a man through her food co-operative and had several dates at the end of the treatment. At follow-up 3 months later, they were in a relationship and the patient had few residual symptoms.

This case is illustrative of some of the challenges of working with chronic depression patients, in that her symptoms had led to notable work and social impairment in addition to her cognitive and emotional symptoms. She had a history of childhood sexual abuse, her symptoms began early in her life, and she had had only a limited exposure to antidepressant medication at the time of the initial evaluation. These accumulated difficulties led to the recommendation for medication in addition to psychotherapy, which is supported by the evidence reviewed above.

Clinical pearls of diagnostic wisdom

As indicated by the scholarship reviewed in this chapter, there is a considerable evidence base that clinicians can draw upon when making treatment recommendations for patients with chronic forms of depression. Pharmacotherapy alone or combined medication and psychotherapy are clearly well supported in the literature as initial approaches. Patient preference for psychotherapy or a history of early-life adversity or abuse should lead clinicians to consider psychotherapy, either alone or in combination with medication, as an initial approach. While there is no evidence that a specific antidepressant or class of medication is most efficacious, SSRIs have become the mainstay first-line treatment due to their low side-effect burden. Medication algorithms such as those from the STAR*D trial or the Texas Medication Algorithm Project can aid in medication selection. As many patients with chronic depression have not had adequate pharmacotherapy in the past, reports of prior medication failures should be corroborated from treatment records or with the aid of the Antidepressant Treatment History Form (Sackheim, 2001), to help ensure that prior trials have

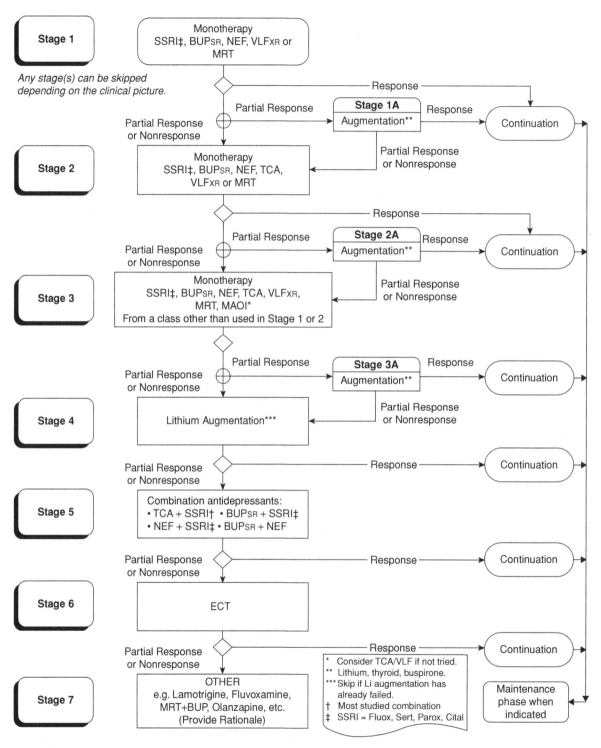

Figure 10.1 Texas Medication Algorhithm Project – Non-Psychotic Major Depression. (Reproduced with permission from Algorithms for optimizing the treatment of depression: making the right decision at the right time. Adli, M., Rush, A.J., Möller, H.J., and Bauer, M. (2003). *Pharmacopsychiatry*, 36 Suppl 3, S222–S229.)

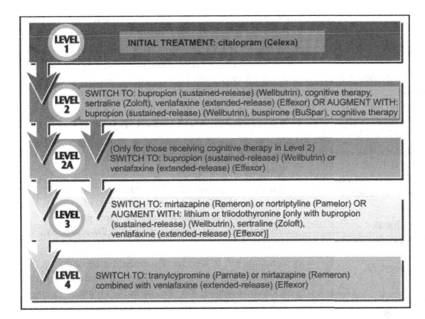

Figure 10.2 STAR-D. (Reprinted from Vieweg, W.V., Levy, J.R., Fredrickson, S.K. *et al.* (2008). Psychotropic drug considerations in depressed patients with metabolic disturbances. *American Journal of Medicine*, 121, 647–655, with permission from Elsevier.)

been of an adequate dose for an adequate duration. When depressed patients do not show a preference for a particular form of treatment or have a history of early-life adversity, a reasonable approach would be to either recommend combined medication and psychotherapy or to attempt what Akiskal has described as "pharmacologic dissection:" exposing the chronically depressed patient to adequate pharmacotherapy to "dissect out" those patients who remit from those who remain depressed and maladjusted, who could then go on combined treatment. Given the pessimistic cognitive and interpersonal styles that have long been noted in patients with chronic depression, we have found that is useful to tell such patients at the outset of treatment that although there is good reason to be optimistic about their prognosis, there is also a reasonable chance that they will not remit during the initial weeks of treatment or with the first treatment trial *and that this is not a reason to discontinue treatment.* Such measured optimism on the part of the treating clinician can facilitate establishing a good therapeutic alliance that is central to any form of treatment.

References

Akiskal, H.S., Rosenthal, T.L., Haykal, R.F. *et al.* (1980). Characterological depressions. Clinical and sleep EEG findings separating 'subaffective dysthymias' from 'character spectrum disorders'. *Archives of General Psychiatry*, 37, 777–783.

Cuijpers, P., van Straten, A., Schuurmans, J. *et al.* (2010). Psychotherapy for chronic major depression and dysthymia: A meta-analysis. *Clinical Psychology Reviews*, 30, 51–62.

DSM-5 (2012). *Chronic Depressive Disorder (Dysthymia). Proposed Revision.* http://www.dsm5.org/ProposedRevision/Pages/proposedrevision.aspx?rid=46# (assessed).

Gelenberg, A.J., Trivedi, M.H., Rush, A.J. *et al.* (2003). Randomized, placebo-controlled trial of nefazodone maintenance treatment in preventing recurrence in chronic depression. *Biological Psychiatry*, 54, 806–817.

Gilmer, W.S., Trivedi, M.H., Rush, A.J. *et al.* (2005). Factors associated with chronic depressive episodes: a preliminary report from the STAR-D project. *Acta Psychiatrica Scandinavica*, 112, 425–433.

Hirschfeld, R.M., Russell, J.M., Delgado, P.L. *et al.* (1998). Predictors of response to acute treatment of chronic and double depression with sertraline or imipramine. *Journal of Clinical Psychiatry*, 59, 669–775.

Judd, L.L., Akiskal, H.S., Schettler, P.J., *et al.* (2002). The long-term natural history of the weekly symptomatic status of bipolar I disorder. *Archives of General Psychiatry*, 59, 530–537.

Kramer, P.D. (1993). *Listening to Prozac.* New York, NY: Viking.

Keller, M.B., Klein, D.N., Hirschfeld, R.M. *et al.* (1995). Results of the DSM-IV mood disorders field trial. *American Journal of Psychiatry*, 152, 843–849.

Keller, M.B., Kocsis, J.H., Thase, M.E. *et al.* (1998). Maintenance phase efficacy of sertraline for chronic depression: A randomized controlled trial. *Journal of the American Medical Association*, 280, 1665–1672.

Keller, M.B., McCullough, J.P., Klein, D.N. *et al.* (2000). A comparison of nefazodone, the cognitive behavioral-analysis system of psychotherapy, and their combination for the treatment of chronic depression. *New England Journal of Medicine*, 342, 1462–1470.

Kessler, R.C., McGonagle, K.A., Zhao, S. *et al.* (1994). Lifetime and 12-month prevalence of DSM-III-R psychiatric disorders in the United States. Results from the National Comorbidity Survey. *Archives of General Psychiatry*, 51, 8–19.

Klein, D.N., Santiago, N.J., Vivian, D. *et al.* (2004). Cognitive-behavioral analysis system of psychotherapy as a maintenance treatment for chronic depression. *Journal of Consulting and Clinical Psychology*, 72, 681–688.

Kocsis, J.H. (2003). Pharmacotherapy for chronic depression. *Journal of Clinical Psychology*, 59, 885–892.

Kocsis, J.H. and Frances, A.J. (1987). A critical discussion of DSM-III dysthymic disorder. *American Journal of Psychiatry*, 144, 1534–1542.

Kocsis, J.H., Frances, A.J., Voss, C. *et al.* (1988a). Imipramine treatment for chronic depression. *Archives of General Psychiatry*, 45, 253–257.

Kocsis, J.H., Frances, A.J., Voss, C. *et al.* (1988b). Imipramine and social-vocational adjustment in chronic depression. *American Journal of Psychiatry*, 145, 997–999.

Kocsis, J.H., Friedman, R.A., Markowitz, J.C. *et al.* (1996). Maintenance therapy for chronic depression: A controlled clinical trial of desipramine: *Archives of General Psychiatry*, 53, 769–774.

Kocsis, J.H., Gelenberg, A.J., Rothbaum, B. *et al.* (2008). Chronic forms of major depression are still undertreated in the 21st century: Systematic assessment of 801 patients presenting for treatment. *Journal of Affective Disorders*, 110, 55–61.

Kocsis, J.H., Gelenberg, A.J., Rothbaum, B.O. *et al.* (2009a). Cognitive behavioral analysis system of psychotherapy and brief supportive psychotherapy for augmentation of antidepressant nonresponse in chronic depression: The REVAMP Trial. *Archives of General Psychiatry*, 66, 1178–1188.

Kocsis, J.H., Leon, A.C., Markowitz, J.C. *et al.* (2009b). Patient preference as a moderator of outcome for chronic forms of major depressive disorder treated with nefazodone, cognitive behavioral analysis system of psychotherapy, or their combination. *Journal of Clinical Psychiatry*, 70, 354–361.

Kraeplin, E. (1976). *Manic-Depressive Insanity and Paranoia*. New York, NY: Arnow Press (reprint).

Lichtenthal, W.G., Cruess, D.G., and Prigerson, H.G. (2004). A case for establishing complicated grief as a distinct mental disorder in DSM-V. *Clinical Psychology Reviews*, 24, 637–662.

Markowitz, J.C. (1994). Psychotherapy of dysthymia. *American Journal of Psychiatry*, 151, 1114–1121.

Markowitz, J.C. and Weissman, M.M. (2004). Interpersonal psychotherapy: Principles and applications. *World Psychiatry*, 3, 136–139.

Markowitz, J.C., Kocsis, J.H., Bleiberg, K.L., Christos, P.J., and Sacks, M. (2005). A comparative trial of psychotherapy and pharmacotherapy for "pure" dysthymic patients. *Journal of Affective Disorders*, 89, 167–175.

McCullough, J.P., Jr. (2003a). Treatment for chronic depression using Cognitive Behavioral Analysis System of Psychotherapy (CBASP). *Journal of Clinical Psychology*, 59, 833–846.

McCullough, J.P., Jr. (2003b). *Treatment for Chronic Depression: The Cognative Behavioral Analysis System of Psychotherapy (CBASP)*. New York, NY: The Guilford Press.

McCullough, J.P., Jr., Klein, D.N., Borian, F.E. *et al.* (2003). Group comparisons of DSM-IV subtypes of chronic depression: Validity of the distinctions, part 2. *Journal of Abnormal Psychology*, 112, 614–622.

Miller, N.L., Kocsis, J.H., Leon, A.C. *et al.* (2001). Maintenance desipramine for dysthymia: A placebo-controlled study. *Journal of Affective Disorders*, 64, 231–237.

Morey, L.C., Shea. M.T., Markowitz, J.C. *et al.* (2010). State effects of major depression on the assessment of personality and personality disorder. *American Journal of Psychiatry*, 167, 528–535.

Nemeroff, C.B., Heim, C.M., Thase, M.E. *et al.* (2003). Differential responses to psychotherapy versus pharmacotherapy in patients with chronic forms of major depression and childhood trauma. *Proceedings of the National Academy of Sciences USA*, 100, 14293–14296.

Phillips, K.A., Gunderson, J.G., Hirschfeld, R.M., and Smith, L.E. (1990). A review of the depressive personality. *American Journal of Psychiatry*, 147, 830–837.

Russell, J.M., Kornstein, S.G., Shea, M.T. *et al.* (2003). Chronic depression and comorbid personality disorders: response to sertraline versus imipramine. *Journal of Clinical Psychiatry*, 64, 554–561.

Sackeim, H.A. (2001). The definition and meaning of treatment-resistant depression. *Journal of Clinical Psychiatry*, 62 Suppl 16, 10–17.

Schatzberg, A.F., Rush, A.J., Arnow, B.A. *et al.* (2005). Chronic depression: Medication (nefazodone) or psychotherapy (CBASP) is effective when the other is not. *Archives of General Psychiatry*, 62, 513–520.

Schramm, E., Schneider, D., Zobel, I. *et al.* (2008). Efficacy of interpersonal psychotherapy plus pharmacotherapy in chronically depressed inpatients. *Journal of Affective Disorders*, 109, 65–73.

Shea, M.T., Widiger, T.A., and Klein, M.H. (1992). Comorbidity of personality disorders and depression: Implications for treatment. *Journal of Consulting and Clinical Psychology*, 60, 857–868.

Shear, K., Frank, E., Houck, P.R., and Reynolds, C.F., III (2005). Treatment of complicated grief: A randomized controlled trial. *Journal of the American Medical Association*, 293, 2601–2608.

Thase, M.E. and Rush, A.J. (1997). When at first you don't succeed: sequential strategies for antidepressant nonresponders. *Journal of Clinical Psychiatry*, 58 Suppl 13, 23–29

Thase, M.E., Rush, A.J., Howland, R.H. *et al.* (2002). Double-blind switch study of imipramine or sertraline treatment of antidepressant-resistant chronic depression. *Archives of General Psychiatry*, 59, 233–239.

Weissman, M.M., Leaf, P.J., Tischler, G.L. *et al.* (1988). Affective disorders in five United States communities. *Psychological Medicine*, 18, 141–153.

11

Pediatric depression

David A. Brent

Introduction

This chapter reviews the developmental epidemiology, and determinants of course and outcome of child and adolescent depression. Guidelines for the assessment, the acute and continuation treatment of depression, and the clinical management of partial response and treatment resistance are articulated. This chapter concludes with recommendations for further research.

Phenomenology and developmental epidemiology

The spectrum of clinically significant unipolar depressive disorders in children and adolescents includes major depression, dysthymic disorder, and depression not otherwise specified. Sub-syndromal depression and dysthymic disorder are impairing and strongly predict the development of major depression in clinical and community samples (Kovacs et al. 1994, Gonzalez-Tejera et al. 2005, Georgiades et al. 2006). Although clinical trials have mainly empanelled those with major depression, both cognitive behavior therapy and interpersonal therapy have been shown to reduce symptomatology and prevent the development of major depression in children and adolescents with sub-syndromal symptoms of depression (Weisz et al. 1997, Horowitz et al. 2007, Garber et al. 2009). The point prevalence of major depression in children is 1–2% and in adolescents 3–8% (Lewinsohn et al. 1998). By the end of adolescence, one in five youths will have experienced at least one major depressive episode (Lewinsohn et al. 1998).

Depression has been reported even in preschool youngsters, usually associated with a very strong family history (Stalets and Luby, 2006). In clinical samples, preadolescent depression is more likely to present with psychotic symptoms, somatic complaints, and separation anxiety, whereas in adolescent depression, hypersomnia, weight gain, and suicidal behavior are more common (Ryan et al. 1987). Preadolescent-onset depression, compared to depression with onset in adolescence, is more likely to be characterized by parental criminality and family discord (Harrington et al. 1997). Follow-up studies into adulthood show that those with a preadolescent onset of their depression have a threefold increased risk for suicide attempt and a fourfold increased risk for substance abuse compared to healthy controls, but no increased risk for recurrent depression, except if there is increased family loading for mood disorder (Weissman et al. 1999a). Adolescent-onset depressives, when followed into adulthood, showed a twofold increased risk for recurrence of depression, a fivefold increased risk for suicide attempt, and a very high (7.7%) risk for completed suicide, but no increased risk for substance abuse compared to healthy controls (Weissman et al. 1999b). Depression in parents conveys a two- to sixfold increased risk for depression in offspring, and early-onset, familial depression may be co-transmitted with anxiety disorder (Weissman et al. 2005).

Among preadolescent youths, the risk for depression is equal across genders, whereas after puberty, females with depression outnumber males 2–3:1 (Angold and Costello, 2006). While the mechanism to explain the increased risk of depression in postpubertal females is not known, girls' increased vulnerability to depression may be due to their higher risk for anxiety, greater sensitivity to stressful, interpersonal life events, increased likelihood of engaging in rumination, and possible mediation by increases in

Clinical Handbook for the Management of Mood Disorders, ed. J. John Mann, Patrick J. McGrath, and Steven P. Roose. Published by Cambridge University Press. © Cambridge University Press 2013.

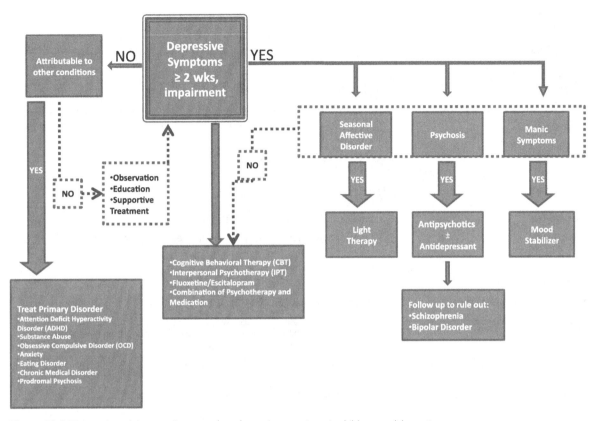

Figure 11.1 Diagnostic and therapeutic approach to depressive symptoms in children or adolescents

testosterone and estradiol (Angold and Costello, 2006, Nolen-Hoeksema, 2011). Puberty may contribute to increased rates of depression through changes in sleep patterns, more rapid maturation of circuitry associated with drives and reward relative to those for inhibitory control, or through increased capacity to formulate complex, long-term goals, which, if not achieved, may lead to depression (Davey *et al.* 2008, Dahl, 2011, Forbes and Dahl, 2012).

Course

Untreated, depressive episodes last between 4 and 8 months (Birmaher *et al.* 2002). A more prolonged course is predicted by greater clinical severity, co-morbid dysthymic, disruptive, and/or substance-use disorders, suicidal ideation, hopelessness, family discord, history of abuse or peer victimization, bereavement, and concurrent parental depression; risk of recurrence is up to 40% within 5 years (Birmaher *et al.* 2002). Early-onset depression conveys significantly increased risk, compared to later-onset depression (around 20%) for the development of

bipolar spectrum disorder. Specific risk factors among those with depressive disorders for bipolar disorder are family history of mania, psychotic depression, a history of sub-clinical hypomania, the development of pharmacologically induced mania, and earlier age of onset of mood disorder (Strober and Carlson, 1982, Geller *et al.* 1994, 2004, Martin *et al.* 2004). Symptoms of mania may overlap with those of attention deficit hyperactivity disorder (ADHD), particularly irritability, distractibility, hyperactivity, and rapid speech. In contrast, symptoms of elation, grandiosity, racing thoughts and flight of ideas, inappropriate sexuality, and decreased need for sleep most strongly differentiate youths with bipolar disorder from those with ADHD (Geller *et al.* 2002).

Approach to the depressed patient

Assessment (see Figure 11.1)

First, the patients should be assessed for conditions that either masquerade as depression, or may

Table 11.1 Differential diagnosis of pediatric depression

Disorder	Differential
Attention Deficit Hyperactivity Disorder	Demoralization due to peer, school, family problems, improves with treatment
Asperger's Syndrome	Demoralization due to peer rejection
Anxiety Disorder	Dysphoria only in anxiogenic situations
Obsessive Compulsive Disorder (OCD)	Upset by obsessive thoughts, impairment due to rituals, or inability to complete them
Eating Disorder	Secondary to nutritional issues, reverses with weight restoration; may also be sad because being forced to gain weight
Conduct Disorder	Precipitated by legal/disciplinary difficulties, but also peer and family conflict, erosion in developmental competencies
Substance use	Can mimic affective symptoms, so need to assess temporal order, mood may change with abstinence
Pre-psychosis	Abnormal development prior to onset, family history, course
Medical illness	Fatigue, concentration, anhedonia secondary to illness or treatment

Table 11.2 Treatment-resistant depression

Barriers to treatment efficacy	Recommendations
Sub-therapeutic dose and/or duration	Psychotherapy: >9 sessions; therapist with expertise Medication: 8 weeks SSRI; 4 weeks $\geq$ 40 mg. Establish blood level is in therapeutic range. Switch to second selective serotonin reuptake inhibitor.
Nonadherence	Psychotherapy: Verify session attendance; outside practice of skills Medication: Pill count to establish adherence; blood level of drug and metabolites
Co-morbidity	Alcohol/substance: Motivational interviewing for abstinence
Sleep difficulties	Review sleep hygiene, melatonin
Sub-syndromal manic symptoms	Mood stabilizer
Anxiety, pain syndrome	Selective norepinephrine reuptake inhibitor, exercise
Anhedonia-concentration-motivation	Bupropion, exercise, behavior activation
Lability, irritability	Mood stabilizer, exercise, mindfulness

Psychosocial stressors:
   Family discord
   Parental depression
   Peer victimization
   Gay-lesbian-bisexual-transgender
	
	Family therapy
	Referral for treatment
	Social support, school consultation
	Therapy, increase support, family and school intervention

adversely affect functioning, course, and treatment response (Brent *et al.* 1998, Birmaher *et al.* 2002, Curry *et al.* 2006, Asarnow *et al.* 2009) (see Table 11.1). Second, patients should be assessed for bipolar, seasonal, or psychotic depression, each of which requires a therapeutic approach distinct from the treatment of unipolar depression. Third, family and contextual factors that can adversely affect outcome should be assessed (see Table 11.2). Finally, the clinician must determine the required intensity and restrictiveness of treatment, based on level of function, and threat to self or others (Birmaher *et al.* 2007).

Collaborating with parents and schools

Parents have a right to know the goals and progress of treatment. While personal details discussed with the clinician need not be shared, both patients and parents should understand that confidentiality will be overridden if there is a threat to the patient's or another person's safety. School problems are often part of the presenting complaint, and can influence treatment response, so the clinician should help parents advocate for the patient's needs with respect to academic demand, social issues, or peer victimization (Shamseddeen *et al.* 2011).

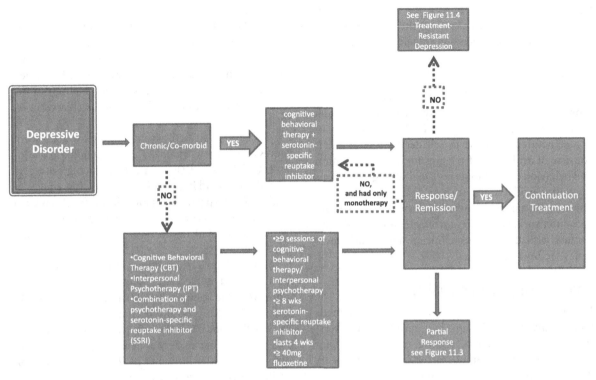

Figure 11.2 Acute treatment of unipolar depression

Acute treatment (see Figure 11.2)

Depression severity

A patient who has mild depressive symptoms, e.g., minor depression or an adjustment disorder of duration less than 1 month, and who is not psychotic or suicidal, can be treated with supportive psychotherapy and education. A significant portion (30–50%) of depressed youths will respond quickly to support. In a meta-analysis of clinical antidepressant trials for pediatric depression, the placebo response rate showed a strong inverse correlation with clinical severity, ranging from around 60% for those who were rated as "moderately ill" to 35% for those who were "markedly ill" (Bridge *et al.* 2009). Also, in a clinical psychotherapy trial of adolescent depression, 31/107 (29%) showed a 50% or greater clinical improvement in depressive symptoms within two treatment sessions (Renaud *et al.* 1998). For those with "mild" depression that does not respond to supportive psychotherapy, or those with moderate depressive symptomatology, psychotherapy, medication, or the combination of

medication and psychotherapy is indicated (Birmaher *et al.* 2007).

Education

The patient and parent should learn about the manifestations, cause, care, and expectable course of depressive disorders, so that they can more effectively collaborate in care. Patients and families who understand that depression is a treatable illness are more hopeful. Knowledgeable and hopeful patients are more likely to adhere to treatment and to have better outcomes (Brent *et al.* 1998, Fristad *et al.* 2009). Presenting depression as an illness helps parents and the patient to understand that depression is "no one's fault" (Koplewicz, 1997). Patients with long-standing depression should be prepared for a more lengthy course of treatment because the greater the duration of depression, the longer the time to recovery (Curry *et al.* 2006, Bridge *et al.* 2007, Maalouf *et al.* 2012). Specifically, in the Treatment of SSRI-Resistant Depression in Adolescents (TORDIA), a latent classification analysis of the course of depressive symptom trajectories revealed those with the longest times to response and remission entered the study with the longest duration of depression (Maalouf et al. 2012).

Safety plan

A high proportion of clinically referred youth with mood disorders have clinically significant suicidal ideation or behavior (Bridge et al. 2006). A safety plan is a structured response to self-destructive urges. It consists of avoidance of triggers for suicidal ideation and behavior, use of simple personal strategies for coping with suicidal urges, such as distraction; reaching out to peers, parents, or other adults within the youth's social network; and if these strategies are insufficient, contact with the patient's clinician and/or an emergency facility (Stanley et al. 2009).

Choose a treatment modality

For moderate depression, the combination of medication and psychotherapy will result in the most functional improvement, relative to monotherapies (March et al. 2004a, Brent et al. 2008, Dubicka et al. 2010). In the Treatment of Adolescent Depression Study (TADS), at 12 weeks, the combination of CBT and fluoxetine resulted in a response rate of 71%, fluoxetine alone, 61%, CBT, 43%, and placebo, 35%; combination treatment was not significantly different than fluoxetine, but both of these conditions were superior to CBT alone and to placebo, while CBT was not different than placebo (March et al. 2004a). In TADS, combination treatment resulted in the most rapid and complete improvement (March et al. 2004a). In the TORDIA study, combination of CBT and medication resulted in a significantly better response rate at 12 weeks than medication monotherapy (54% vs. 41%; Brent et al. 2008). However, in the Adolescent Drug and Psychotherapy Treatment (ADAPT) study, which enrolled youth who were more severely depressed than either TADS or TORDIA, the addition of CBT to fluoxetine did not boost response rate vs. fluoxetine alone. Also, CBT did not add to medication monotherapy in the more severely ill participants in TADS and TORDIA (Curry et al. 2006, Goodyer et al. 2007, Maalouf et al. 2012).

Cognitive behavior therapy (CBT), a brief, focused psychotherapy that targets the recognition and correction of distorted information processing resulting in negative mood, has been shown to be more efficacious than either a wait-list control, family therapy, relaxation therapy, or nondirective supportive therapy (Wood et al. 1996, Brent et al. 1997, Weisz et al. 2006) Some other components of CBT include problem-solving, behavioral activation, social skills training, and emotion regulation. In TADS, while CBT lagged behind fluoxetine at 12 weeks, it did catch up to the other intervention groups by 18 weeks (March et al. 2004a).

A second indicated psychotherapy for adolescent depression is interpersonal therapy adapted for adolescents (IPT-A). IPT-A targets reducing interpersonal discord, and improving the rewarding aspects of important interpersonal relationships. IPT-A has been shown to be superior to clinical management, and to treatment as usual in a school-based clinic (Mufson et al. 1999, 2004).

Two studies have compared IPT and CBT for depressed adolescents; the first study found a more favorable response to IPT, and the second study favored CBT (Rossello and Bernal, 1999, Rossello et al. 2008). CBT appears to perform particularly well in the patient with either anxiety or behavioral comorbidities (Brent et al. 1998, Rohde et al. 2006, Asarnow et al. 2009), but is less effective in the face of parent–child conflict, a history of abuse, or current parental depression (Brent et al. 1998, Lewinsohn et al. 1998, Rohde et al. 2006, Asarnow et al. 2009, Feeny et al. 2009, Lewis et al. 2010). IPT shows a stronger response relative to comparison treatments for patients with co-morbid anxiety, high levels of parent–child conflict, social role impairment, and those with high sociotropy (i.e., placing a high importance on social relationships and pleasing others). (Horowitz et al. 2007, Young et al. 2009, Gunlicks-Stoessel et al. 2010). Effective treatment with either IPT or CBT requires a therapist with the relevant training and expertise, a patient who can focus on a treatment agenda, attend treatment regularly and practice the skills learned between sessions. A minimum effective dose of CBT is around nine sessions (Kennard et al. 2009). If expertise in both CBT and IPT is available, IPT may be preferable for patients with high levels of parent–child discord, whereas CBT may be preferable for patients with behavior disorder co-morbidities.

Combination treatment

Combination of CBT and antidepressant medication appears to be superior to medication alone for those with co-morbid anxiety and/or behavioral disorders, but does not add to medication alone for those with severe depression, high levels of family conflict, parental depression, or a history of abuse, and in meta-analyses does not appear to protect against suicidal events (Brent *et al.* 1998 Asarnow *et al.* 2009. Feeny *et al.* 2009, Dubicka *et al.* 2010). Combination treatment also is superior to medication alone as a continuation treatment in preventing depressive relapse (Kennard *et al.* 2008). Therefore, the combination of CBT and antidepressant medication is most strongly indicated in those with moderate depression and for those with co-morbid anxiety and/or behavioral disorders.

Multi-family psychoeducation (often added to medication management) and family-based attachment therapy, while not as extensively studied as CBT or IPT, show promise in randomized clinical trials (Diamond *et al.* 2002, Fristad *et al.* 2009, Diamond *et al.* 2010). In preadolescent community youths with mild to moderate depression, primary and secondary control enhancement therapy (PASCET), a variant of CBT (Weisz *et al.* 1997), was superior to no treatment. Two other promising psychotherapies for preadolescent depression that actively involve parents in treatment are contextual emotion regulation therapy (CERT) and family-based interpersonal therapy (FBIPT). CERT teaches parents how to coach their depressed child in the use of more effective and adaptive emotion regulation therapies (Kovacs *et al.* 2006). FBIPT focuses directly on the parent–child interaction using the principles of IPT (Dietz *et al.* 2008).

Medication

Two selective serotonin reuptake inhibitors, fluoxetine and escitalopram are approved for use in adolescent depression by the Federal Drug Administration (FDA); fluoxetine is also approved for use in preadolescent patients. Fluoxetine outperformed placebo in one single-site and two multi-site studies (Emslie *et al.* 1997, 2002, 2009), and most recently, in TADS (March *et al.* 2004a, Kennard *et al.* 2006). Escitalopram has been shown in two randomized clinical trials to be superior to placebo in terms of the reduction of depressive symptoms in adolescents, but not in children (Wagner *et al.* 2006, Emslie *et al.* 2009). Other SSRIs have shown efficacy in the treatment of adolescent depression, with the exception of paroxetine, which is no longer recommended for adolescent depression because meta-analyses of all extant clinical trials, including those that had been unpublished, failed to show evidence of efficacy over placebo (Bridge *et al.* 2007). In the TORDIA study, which is the only head-to-head comparison of newer antidepressants, venlafaxine resulted in a similar response rate compared to SSRIs, and within the SSRI group, fluoxetine and citalopram had similar response rates (Brent *et al.* 2008).

Initial medication titration

Begin with a dosage of 10 mg of fluoxetine or its equivalent for the first week, to see if the patient can tolerate the SSRI. Then, increase the daily dosage to 20 mg and observe for another 3 weeks. If the patient is still depressed and not experiencing significant side effects, then the dosage should be increased to the equivalent of 40 mg of fluoxetine and the patient observed for 4 weeks, based on clinical trial and pharmacokinetic data supporting the efficacy of a dose increase in nonresponders (Heiligenstein *et al.* 2006, Sakolsky *et al.* 2011). Ideally, appointments should be weekly for the first 4 weeks, since early in treatment is the most critical time for the occurrence of suicidal and other adverse events (Brent *et al.* 2009). For the next 8 weeks, patients can be seen biweekly, and less frequently thereafter.

Preadolescent depression

Fluoxetine is the only antidepressant that has an indication for preadolescent depression; the number needed to treat (NNT) for fluoxetine is 5, similar to adolescents. For other antidepressants, the NNT is 14, twice the NNT for adolescents (Bridge *et al.* 2007). This disparity could be due to developmental differences in pharmacokinetics and pharmacodynamics, but that explanation is not consistent with similar response rates between preadolescents and adolescents treated for anxiety or for obsessive compulsive disorder (Bridge *et al.* 2007). Alternatively, the superior showing of fluoxetine in preadolescent youth could be due to the higher quality of studies of fluoxetine and the greater severity of depressed youth in these studies, resulting in a lower placebo response rate compared to other treatment studies in this age group (Bridge *et al.* 2007, 2009). One small, randomized clinical trial showed that omega-3 fatty acids were more efficacious than placebo for the treatment of preadolescent depression (Nemets *et al.* 2006).

Suicidal events

The Federal Drug Administration (FDA) issued a Black-Box Warning for all antidepressants for individuals under the age of 25, since the increased risk for suicidal events in drug vs. placebo is only found in this age group (Stone et al. 2009). The most complete meta-analysis of suicidal events and antidepressants in pediatric depression found a rate of suicide events of 2.9% on antidepressant and 1.7% on placebo, a difference that was *not* statistically significant even though this meta-analysis included 3405 youth in total (Bridge et al. 2007). The difference in the rates of suicide attempts and/or preparatory actions towards an attempt between drug and placebo was also not significantly different between antidepressant and placebo (1.7% vs. 0.6%) (Bridge et al. 2007). For all antidepressants, the number needed to treat (NNT) for pediatric depression was 10, whereas the number needed to harm (e.g., for suicidal events) (NNH) was 112, meaning that 11 times more youth will benefit from an antidepressant than will experience a suicidal event (Bridge et al. 2007).

In meta-analyses of placebo-controlled antidepressant studies that assessed studies in both depressed youth and adults, Gibbons et al. (2012) reported that while both youths and adults reported similar improvement in depressive symptoms, that depressed youths, unlike adults, did not show a close relationship between improvement in depression and improvement in suicidal ideation. Therefore, antidepressant medications may help depression in youth without ameliorating risk for suicidal behavior. However, findings from TADS and TORDIA suggest that suicidal events *are* related to poor response to treatment and continued high depressive symptomatology (Brent et al. 2009, Vitiello et al. 2009). Suicide events in depressed youths tend to occur within the first 3–5 weeks in treatment, and are predicted by high baseline suicidal ideation, drug and alcohol use, family conflict, poor response to treatment, and a history of nonsuicidal self-injury (Brent et al. 2009, Vitiello et al. 2009, Asarnow et al. 2011, Wilkinson et al. 2011). In the TORDIA study, sub-syndromal manic symptoms were associated with treatment resistance and a higher risk for suicidal events (Maalouf et al. 2012).

Because depressed youth have a high risk for increases in suicidal ideation and actual suicidal behavior, the clinician should develop a safety plan in collaboration with the patient and family (see above),

and reduce the risk for suicidal events by working to achieve a reduction in depressive symptoms as quickly as possible, ameliorate family conflict, and encourage the patient to abstain from alcohol and substances (Brent et al. 2009).

Management of adverse effects

The FDA has recently issued a safety warning about citalopram, recommending that it not be used in doses higher than 40 mg due to its tendency to result in a prolonged QTc interval (Sala et al. 2005). Patients who are treated with citalopram should have a baseline ECG, and serial ECGs prior to and following dose increases, and be monitored for concomitant medications that could have an additive effect on cardiac conduction.

The risk of medication-induced mania is inversely proportional to the age of the patient, probably because the earlier the onset of major depression, the greater the risk for eventual bipolar disorder (Martin et al. 2004). If mania ensues, antidepressant medication should be stopped immediately or tapered quickly. Other side effects include headache, nausea, agitation, anxiety, and akathisia; often patients with these side effects need to be switched to an alternative SSRI or another class of medication. Headaches are half as common in adolescents treated with bupropion, compared to those treated with SSRIs, whereas SNRI use is associated with triple the risk for headache compared to SSRIs (Anderson et al. 2012). Because SSRIs and SNRIs can increase clotting time, bleeding problems may occur with trauma or surgery or when these medications are combined with other agents that prolong bleeding time (Weinrieb et al. 2005). Therefore, other physicians involved with the patient's care need to be informed of antidepressant treatment. Although not specifically studied in adolescents, the risk for osteoporotic fracture is about double in drugs with a high affinity for the serotonin transporter (Verdel et al. 2010). Weight gain of around 1–2.5 kg in 12 months has been reported in SSRIs and SNRIs, with only bupropion associated with weight loss (Nihalani et al. 2011). In adults, sexual side effects tend to be more common in SSRIs and SNRIs than in those treated with bupropion (Anderson et al. 2012). Little is known about the incidence of sexual side effects in adolescents treated with SSRIs, in part because adolescents are reluctant to disclose sexual activity and clinicians are reluctant to ask (Scharko, 2004). The clinician should, in private, review these side effects with the adolescent, so that the patient can make an informed choice about the use of medication.

Other antidepressants

Tricyclic antidepressants (TCAs) have been found *not* to be efficacious for child or adolescent depression, with the possible exception of clomipramine, which, in one small trial given intravenously (IV), was superior to IV saline for treatment-resistant depression in adolescents (Sallee *et al.* 1997, Hazell *et al.* 2002). TCAs should be avoided in child and adolescents not only because of their lack of efficacy but because they are much more likely to result in a fatality when used in an overdose compared to SSRIs (Kapur *et al.* 1992, White *et al.* 2008). Post-hoc analyses in other studies of the treatment of depression, found that venlafaxine has efficacious in adolescents, but not in preadolescents, although venlafaxine has showed similar efficacy for anxiety disorders in both groups (Emslie *et al.* 2007). One trial supported the use of nefazodone, but due to increased risk of hepatotoxicity, only the generic form is available. Mirtazapine, in one clinical trial, did not appear efficacious. Its hypnotic side effects make it a useful second-line option for the treatment of insomnia, although it is more likely than other agents to cause weight gain (Bridge *et al.* 2007).

Common problems in the acute management of depression

Decline in diagnosis of depression and prescriptions for SSRIs after the FDA Black Box Warning

After the Black Box Warning, young people with depression are now less likely to receive treatment for any type of depression, and less likely to have antidepressants prescribed, compared to the period prior to the warning (Libby *et al.* 2009). Primary care physicians are also much more reluctant to prescribe these agents, and one possible unintended repercussion of this change has been a reversal in the decade-long decline in adolescent suicide seen in the United States, Canada, and Western Europe (Gibbons *et al.* 2007, Katz *et al.* 2008). Clinicians should present parents and patients with the facts, including the nonsignificant increased risk for suicidal events in

adolescents treated with antidepressants and the favorable benefit–risk ratio, that 11 adolescents will show an improvement in their depression for everyone who experiences a suicidal event. Strategies for family education and for supporting evidence-based treatment in primary care should be studied.

Sleep difficulties

Subjective complaints of difficulty falling asleep, staying asleep, hypersomnia, and "poor quality sleep" are common in depressed patients (Forbes *et al.* 2008). SSRIs may lead to vivid dreams, and if disturbing to the patient, may require a switch to another medication. Poor sleep can predispose to depression, predict relapse, and interfere with treatment response (Gregory *et al.* 2009, Emslie *et al.* 2012).

In patients with sleep concerns, the clinician should screen for narcolepsy (sudden onset of daytime sleep), sleep apnea (history of snoring, observed episodes of apnea), and restless legs syndrome (discomfort and urge to move legs once in bed). If the patient has difficulty falling asleep, review sleep hygiene, and check that the patient is not overstimulated (e.g., on cell phone, computer) prior to going to bed, is not taking in caffeine close to bedtime, and is not napping in the afternoon. Some patients with comorbid anxiety may have ruminative thoughts at bedtime that interfere with sleep. For these patients, a specific relaxation and distraction plan can bring relief. If the sleep difficulty began with the onset of depression, treating the depression alone may improve sleep. A brief, school-based intervention to improve sleep in primary school students resulted in improved functioning and reduction in depressive symptoms (Quach *et al.* 2011). For persistent sleep problems not responsive to psychosocial interventions, melatonin about an hour before bedtime has been shown to be efficacious in patients with ADHD and is commonly used in adolescent depression (Bendz and Scates, 2010). SSRIs should usually be taken in the morning because they can sometimes cause sleep disruption. However, if a patient reports fatigue that follows the pharmacokinetic trajectory of an SSRI, then either divide the dosage between morning and evening, or switch the dosage entirely to the evening.

Case example

An obese 15-year-old girl with chronic depression is referred because of nonresponse to fluoxetine, 20 mg.

Due to sleep difficulties, she is also maintained on tra-zodone, 50 mg. The patient reports that, while the fluox-etine did not help, she actually feels worse since the tra-zodone was added. What are the possible explanations for her nonresponse to fluoxetine, and what should be done next?

The patient may be nonresponsive to fluoxetine simply because 40–50% of people do not respond to any one antidepressant. Since the patient's like-lihood of response is enhanced with higher blood concentration of fluoxetine and norfluoxetine, and concentration is inversely proportional to weight, it is possible that this patient may have been treated at what might be an inadequate dose of an antidepres-sant (Sakolsky *et al.* 2011). Also, her antidepressant treatment may have contributed to her obesity (Smits *et al.* 2010). *She may also have become more dysphoric because of a drug interaction between trazodone and fluoxetine.* Trazodone is the most commonly used sleep agent in pediatric mood disorder (Owens *et al.* 2010). Surprisingly, in TORDIA, its use was associated with a much poorer response rate (15%) compared to those treated with other sleep aids (e.g., diphenhydramine (60%), or those who received no medication for sleep (51%) (Shamseddeen *et al.* 2012). None (0/13) of those youths who received both trazodone and either fluoxetine or paroxetine responded, perhaps because these antidepressants are potent inhibitors of CYP 2D6, resulting in an accumulation of methylchloropiperazine (mCPP), a breakdown product of trazodone that has anxiogenic and dysphorogenic properties (Shamseddeen *et al.* 2012).

Therefore, the trazodone should be discontinued to see if its interaction with fluoxetine might be con-tributing to the patient's nonresponse. Other clinical suggestions include:

1. Get more clinical information about sleep (e.g., history of snoring, sleep apnea).
2. Draw blood level of fluoxetine/norfluoxetine and depending on level, either increase or switch to a different antidepressant.
3. She also has never had CBT, and so psychotherapy should be added to her treatment.
4. Examine the patient's weight trajectory before and since she has been on this antidepressant to determine if the patient's antidepressant treatment may have contributed to her obesity.

Co-morbid ADHD

A 12-year-old boy presents with a long-standing history of ADHD and dysphoric mood, poor concentration, poor sleep, low self-esteem, and sense of worthlessness.

ADHD and depression often co-occur. However, some symptoms (like poor sleep and concentra-tion) are found in both conditions, and sometimes dysphoria and low self-esteem are a consequence of the ADHD, rather than attributable to *bona fide* depression. Clinical guidelines recommend treating the most impairing condition first (Bond *et al.* 2012). If the two conditions are equally impairing, start with a stimulant because it will result in a more rapid response of ADHD than an antidepressant will for depressive symptoms, some of the depressive symp-toms may be secondary to the ADHD, and stimulants have mild antidepressant properties in any case (Biederman *et al.* 2004). However, patients treated with stimulants, particularly those given mixtures of dextroamphetamine and amphetamine may become dysphoric as a side effect in around 5% of those treated. Bupropion, while not an established treat-ment for pediatric depression, has some efficacy against ADHD as well as depression, although it should not be used in patients with co-morbid eating disorders (Daviss *et al.* 2006). Atomoxetine, while effective for ADHD, was not better than placebo for treatment of co-morbid depression (Atomoxetine ADHD and Comorbid MDD Study Group *et al.* 2007). In addition, stimulants and SSRIs can be safely combined, although the combination may result in higher antidepressant concentrations (Findling, 1996).

Co-morbid anxiety or OCD

Patients with co-morbid anxiety or OCD can usually be treated with the same antidepressant as that used for the depression, although higher dosages may be needed to treat anxiety or OCD (Bandelow, 2008). In addition, specific therapeutic interventions involving graduated exposure are an important component of treatment (March *et al.* 2004b, Walkup *et al.* 2008). Anxiety is frequently co-morbid with unipolar depression, but the presence of panic disorder is more specifically associated with an increased risk for bipolar disorder (Diler *et al.* 2004).

Seasonal affective disorder (SAD)

Ideally, patients with SAD should be treated with light therapy, although many youths will not sit in front of a light box daily for the recommended time of at least 30 minutes. Light therapy may also be helpful for patients with late luteal phase dysphoria (Pail *et al.* 2011).

Bipolar diathesis

Patients with a clear history of mania should be treated with a mood stabilizer prior to attempting to use an antidepressant. In patients with a history of hypomania or with a family history of bipolar disorder, initially treat with psychotherapy and/or with light, both of which are less likely to induce mania than antidepressants. Some reports in adults suggest that of the commonly used antidepressants, selective norepinephrine reuptake inhibitors (SRNIs) are the most likely to induce manic conversion, and that bupropion is the least likely to do so (Leverich *et al.* 2006). Two open trials in adolescents suggest that lamotrigine is helpful in the treatment of bipolar depression (Chang *et al.* 2006, Biederman *et al.* 2010) and one randomized clinical trial of aripiprazole showed efficacy relative to placebo in bipolar youth, some of whom had mixed states of depression and mania.

Case example

A 16-year-old boy presents with treatment-resistant depression and a strong family history of bipolar disorder. He is treated with citalopram and responds well, but then becomes irritable, disinhibited, sexually preoccupied, and engages in inappropriate humor.

This patient has symptoms of hypomania. His citalopram should be tapered quickly (to avoid withdrawal symptoms) and he should be observed. If manic symptoms persist, he should be treated with either a second-generation antipsychotic (SGA), as SGAs have been shown to be better than placebo, lithium, and divalproex for the treatment of pediatric mania (Findling *et al.* 2009, Geller *et al.* 2012). If the patient's bipolar symptoms recede and depression recurs, open trials suggest that lamotrigine may be helpful. For the treatment of bipolar depression, another accepted, although untested alternative, is to first treat with an antipsychotic, and if the depression does not lift, add either bupropion or an SSRI.

Psychotic depression

Youths with psychotic depression are at increased risk to develop bipolar disorder, and, if a combination of antipsychotics and antidepressants are not successful, such patients are good candidates for electroconvulsive therapy (ECT; see below). However, the treatment of psychotic depression in youth has not been well studied.

Depression co-morbid with alcohol or substance-use disorder

In TORDIA, nonresponders showed patterns of alcohol or substance use below the DSM-IV diagnostic threshold, but compared to responders, their use either began high, or increased substantially during the course of treatment, whereas responders' use either stayed low, or showed a decline during treatment (Goldstein *et al.* 2009). Clinical trials for youths with both depression and either alcohol- or substance-abuse disorders have found some positive effects of CBT focused on substance abuse for both conditions, but a less clear impact of fluoxetine, compared to placebo (Riggs *et al.* 2007, Cornelius *et al.* 2009, Cornelius *et al.* 2010).

Partial response (see Figure 11.3)

Partial response occurs when a patient shows improvement in symptomatology and functioning, but still has significant residual symptomatology after 8–12 weeks of treatment, with the most common residual symptoms being anhedonia, irritability, sleep difficulties, and fatigue (Vitiello *et al.* 2010). The patient and family should be reassessed to rule out inadequate dosage, nonadherence, psychosocial stressors, or co-morbid conditions (see Table 11.2). If the patient is not at the maximum dosage for a drug, one can consider increasing the current medication. If an increase is not feasible, or has already been attempted, then the patient and family should be given a choice of starting a new medication ("switching"), or adding one ("augmentation"). The choice between switching and augmentation should be based on the degree of improvement achieved with the "base" medication, the likelihood that a new agent will yield a better result, and the relative likelihood of drug interactions and adverse events. In adults, augmentation with lithium, neuroleptics, thyroxine, and bupropion have all been shown to be

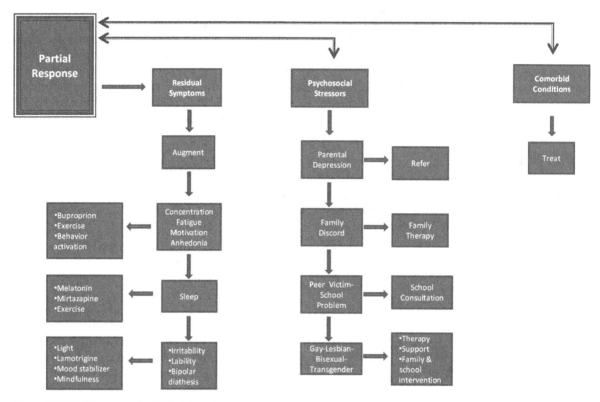

Figure 11.3 Partial response to child/adolescent depression

efficacious for treatment-resistant depression (Nelson and Papakostas, 2009).

If a patient shows residual fatigue, low motivation, anhedonia, and/or poor concentration, in the absence of other medical explanations, augmentation with bupropion, which has noradrenergic and dopaminergic properties is recommended. For depressed patients with residual irritability, emotional lability, or a bipolar diathesis, consider the use of lithium, atypical antipsychotics, or lamotrigine (Inoue *et al.* 2011).

Aerobic exercise and/or yoga are recommended for all youths with partial response or treatment-resistant depression, in light of their beneficial effects on depression (Larun *et al.* 2006, Saeed *et al.* 2010).

Continuation treatment

While around 60% of patients will respond to treatment in 12 weeks (e.g., show a 50% decrease in depressive symptoms), it takes an additional 3 months of treatment for many patients to achieve remission (March *et al.* 2007, Vitiello *et al.* 2010). Once a patient

has been symptom-free for 2 months, an additional 6–12 months of continuation treatment at the same dosage of medication is necessary to prevent symptom recurrence, as has been demonstrated in placebo-controlled trials with fluoxetine (Emslie *et al.* 2008). The addition of a wellness-orientated CBT to fluoxetine continuation resulted in even better protection against recurrence than fluoxetine continuation alone (Kennard *et al.* 2008). For those treated with CBT, monthly boosters may prolong time to recurrence (Kroll *et al.* 1996). Patients with more severe, chronic, or recurrent depression may require a longer period of prophylaxis, based on studies in adults (Kupfer *et al.* 1992). When tapering successful continuation treatment, the developmental needs of the youth should be considered. For example, it is preferable to taper a patient from an antidepressant during the summer, rather than during the school year. For those patients who are going off to college, we recommend continuation on the same medication for the first year of college because the risk of depression during that first year is substantial.

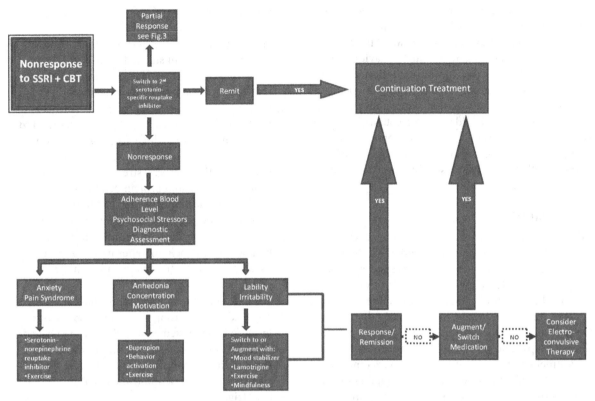

Figure 11.4 Treatment-resistant depression

Prevention

Group CBT using an adaptation of Lewinsohn's "Coping with Depression" model, and more recently, group IPT, have been shown to prevent onset or recurrences of depression in adolescents at risk for depression that is either due to a previous episode, parental depression, and/or sub-syndromal depression (Horowitz *et al.* 2007, Garber *et al.* 2009).

Treatment-resistant depression

For the patient who has not showed a significant decrease in depressive symptoms, revisit and address any likely barriers to treatment efficacy (see Table 11.2).

Third-step switch (see Figure 11.4)

If the patient's depression has not responded to two adequate trials with SSRIs, then the patient could be switched to an SNRI, bupropion or lamotrigine. Based on a mixture of clinical experience and empirical evidence in adults, we tend to use an SNRI for patients with pain syndromes, bupropion for those with difficulty with fatigue, anhedonia, and attentional difficulties, and lamotrigine for those with emotional lability, sub-syndromal manic symptoms, or a bipolar diathesis. Monoamine oxidase inhibitors (MAOI) have not been rigorously assessed in adolescent depression, but are useful in those adults with "atypical" or bipolar depression (Mallinger *et al.* 2009).

Electroconvulsive therapy (ECT)

A recent review citing the overall efficacy of ECT in children and adolescents finds response rates of 80% in catatonia and 63% in depression (Wachtel *et al.* 2011). ECT is probably underutilized for adolescent depression, given that over one-fourth of child and adolescent psychiatrists indicated that they thought ECT was not safe for adolescent patients. Negative portrayals of ECT in the media and restrictive laws for its use in some states may also have served as impediments, despite evidence supporting safety, absence of long-term cognitive effects, and efficacy (Wachtel *et al.* 2011). Although the profile of responders is similar in adults and in adolescents, adults were most often referred for ECT due to lack of response to pharmacotherapy, whereas adolescents were most often referred due to catatonia or suicidal behavior (Bloch *et al.* 2008). In patients who have continued severe depression and have not responded to 3–4 adequate trials of antidepressants and/or augmentations, ECT should be strongly considered. The extant data suggest that ECT has a much better outcome in adolescents with bipolar or psychotic depression compared to those with co-morbid personality disorder (Walter and Rey, 2003).

Conclusions

Adolescent depression is a treatable illness with two indicated psychotherapies, IPT and CBT, and two FDA-approved antidepressants, fluoxetine and escitalopram. As noted above, there is also evidence to support the efficacy of citalopram, sertraline, and venlafaxine for the treatment of adolescent depression. Goals of treatment should be remission, and prevention of relapse and recurrence. Assessment is the key to treatment, both for identifying salient treatment targets, but also identifying other forms of depression and contributing co-morbid disorders that require a different or complementary therapeutic approach. The advantages and disadvantages of each treatment step should be discussed with the patient so that treatment decisions can be decided collaboratively.

Future directions

1. Because of a lack of published clinical trials, there are no established psychotherapies for youths with preadolescent depression. Some promising interventions that may be useful for this population are attachment-based family therapy, contextual emotion regulation therapy (CERT), and family-based IPT (Kovacs *et al.* 2006, Dietz *et al.* 2008).

2. Depressed youths with a history of abuse are common in clinical populations. In TORDIA, an abuse history predicted poorer response to combination treatment than to medication monotherapy, despite a low rate of PTSD and/or acute symptoms of trauma (Asarnow *et al.* 2009). It is important to try to understand why CBT is not efficacious in these youths, and to evaluate alternative interventions that may be robust to a history of trauma, such as behavioral activation, special adaptations of CBT or IPT, or attachment-based family therapy.

3. Slow response to antidepressants is associated with a higher risk of suicidal events. Are there pharmacological or psychosocial interventions that can accelerate treatment response?

4. Conversely, are there ways to identify early in treatment which patients are going to respond to antidepressants and which are likely to have a suicidal event? Studies that examine changes in neurocognitive markers, stress responsivity, gene expression, and protein products may shed light on the mechanisms that lead to these outcomes and suggest alternative approaches.

5. Similarly, can we identify neurocognitive or other biomarkers that help to better match patient to psychotherapeutic treatment and monitor progress?

6. Sub-syndromal manic symptoms have been reported to be a strong predictor of nonresponse in severely depressed youths. Studies are needed to clarify the clinical significance of these sub-syndromal symptoms, and whether they signal the need for a mood stabilizer or lamotrigine.

7. Although sleep difficulties are common precursors, correlates, and residual symptoms of depression, there are few empirical studies of either psychotherapies or medication for the management of sleep difficulties in depression, nor on the impact of treatment of sleep difficulties on depression outcome (Emslie *et al.* 2012).

8. Pain syndromes, especially chronic headache are very common in clinical populations of depressed youth, yet no study has looked at the co-treatment of depression and pain in this age group.

9. There are a number of interventions that have not been carefully evaluated in youths and may expand our therapeutic armamentarium, either alone, or in combination with other treatments: lamotrigine, bupropion, omega-3 fatty acids, S-adenosyl methionine (SAM-E), and transcranial magnetic stimulation.

10. Given that chronicity is a risk factor for poor response to acute treatments, population-based studies should be conducted that evaluate the efficacy of early identification and prevention in school and primary care settings in reducing the burden of chronic depression.

11. Personality disorders and alcohol- and substance-abuse disorders may be consequences of early-onset depression (Lewinsohn *et al.* 1997, 1998, Curry *et al.* 2012). Is early identification and treatment sufficient to prevent these possible consequences, or are more specific psychosocial treatments targeted to self-regulation and interpersonal effectiveness necessary?

References

Anderson, H.D., Pace, W.D., Libby, A.M., West, D.R., and Valuck, R.J. (2012). Rates of 5 common antidepressant side effects among new adult and adolescent cases of depression: A retrospective US claims study. *Clinical Therapeutics*, 34, 113–123.

Angold, A. and Costello, E.J. (2006). Puberty and depression. *Child and Adolescent Psychiatric Clinics of North America*, 15, 919–937.

Asarnow, J.R., Emslie, G., Clarke, G. *et al.* (2009). Treatment of selective serotonin reuptake inhibitor-resistant depression in adolescents: Predictors and moderators of treatment response. *Journal of the American Academy of Child and Adolescent Psychiatry*, 48, 330–339.

Asarnow, J.R., Porta, G., Emslie, G. *et al.* (2011). Suicide attempts and nonsuicidal self-injury in the Treatment of Resistant-Depression in Adolescents (TORDIA) study: Findings from the TORDIA trial. *Journal of the American Academy of Child and Adolescent Psychiatry*, 50, 772–781.

Atomoxetine ADHD and Comorbid MDD Study Group, Bangs, M.E., Emslie, G.J. *et al.* (2007). Efficacy and safety of atomoxetine in adolescents with attention-deficit/hyperactivity disorder and major depression. *Journal of Child and Adolescent Psychopharmacology*, 17, 407–420.

Bandelow, B. (2008). The medical treatment of obsessive-compulsive disorder and anxiety. *CNS Spectrums*, 13, 37–46.

Bendz, L.M. and Scates, A.C. (2010). Melatonin treatment for insomnia in pediatric patients with attention-deficit/hyperactivity disorder. *Annals of Pharmacotherapy*, 44, 185–191.

Biederman, J., Spencer, T., and Wilens, T. (2004). Evidence-based pharmacotherapy for attention-deficit hyperactivity disorder. *The International Journal of Neuropsychopharmacology / Official Scientific Journal of the Collegium Internationale Neuropsychopharmacologicum (CINP)*, 7, 77–97.

Biederman, J., Joshi, G., Mick, E. *et al.* (2010). A prospective open-label trial of lamotrigine monotherapy in children and adolescents with bipolar disorder. *CNS Neuroscience and Therapeutics*, 16, 91–102.

Birmaher, B., Arbelaez, C., and Brent, D. (2002). Course and outcome of child and adolescent major depressive disorder. *Child and Adolescent Psychiatric Clinics of North America*, 11, 619–637.

Birmaher, B., Brent, D., AACAP Work Group on Quality Issues *et al.* (2007). Practice parameters for the assessment and treatment of children and adolescents with depressive disorders. *Journal of the American Academy of Child and Adolescent Psychiatry*, 46, 1503–1526.

Bloch, Y., Sobol, D., Levkovitz, Y., Kron, S., and Ratzoni, G. (2008). Reasons for referral for electroconvulsive therapy: A comparison between adolescents and adults. *Australasian Psychiatry*, 16, 191–194.

Bond, D.J., Hadjipavlou, G., Lam, R.W. *et al.* (2012). The Canadian Network for Mood and Anxiety Treatments (CANMAT) task force recommendations for the management of patients with mood disorders and comorbid attention-deficit/hyperactivity disorder. *Annals of Clinical Psychiatry*, 24, 23–37.

Brent, D., Emslie, G., Clarke, G. *et al.* (2008). Switching to another SSRI or to venlafaxine with or without cognitive behavioral therapy for adolescents with SSRI-resistant depression: The TORDIA randomized controlled trial. *Journal of the American Medical Association*, 299, 901–913.

Brent, D., Emslie, G., Clarke, G. *et al.* (2009). Predictors of spontaneous and systematically assessed suicidal adverse events in the treatment of SSRI-resistant depression in adolescents (TORDIA) study. *American Journal of Psychiatry*, 166, 418–426.

Brent, D.A., Holder, D., Kolko, D. *et al.* (1997). A clinical psychotherapy trial for adolescent depression comparing cognitive, family, and supportive treatments. *Archives of General Psychiatry*, 54, 877–885.

Brent, D.A., Kolko, D., Birmaher, B. *et al.* (1998). Predictors of treatment efficacy in a clinical trial of three psychosocial treatments for adolescent depression. *Journal of the American Academy of Child and Adolescent Psychiatry*, 37, 906–914.

Bridge, J., Iyengar, S., Salary, C.B. *et al.* (2007). Clinical response and risk for reported suicidal ideation and suicide attempts in pediatric antidepressant treatment: A meta-analysis of randomized controlled trials. *Journal of the American Medical Association*, 297, 1683–1696.

Bridge, J.A., Goldstein, T.R., and Brent, D.A. (2006). Adolescent suicide and suicidal behavior. *Journal of Child Psychology and Psychiatry*, 47, 372–394.

Bridge, J.A., Birmaher, B., Iyengar, S., Barbe, R.P., and Brent, D.A. (2009). Placebo response in randomized controlled trials of antidepressants for pediatric major depressive disorder. *American Journal of Psychiatry*, 166, 42–49.

Chang, K., Saxena, K., and Howe, M. (2006). An open-label study of lamotrigine adjunct or monotherapy for the treatment of adolescents with bipolar depression. *Journal of the American Academy of Child and Adolescent Psychiatry*, 45, 298–304.

Cornelius, J.R., Bukstein, O.G., Wood, D.S. *et al.* (2009). Double-blind placebo-controlled trial of fluoxetine in adolescents with comorbid major depression and an alcohol use disorder. *Addictive Behaviors*, 34, 905–909.

Cornelius, J.R., Bukstein, O.G., Douaihy, A.B. *et al.* (2010). Double-blind fluoxetine trial in comorbid MDD-CUD youth and young adults. *Drug and Alcohol Dependence*, 112, 39–45.

Curry, J., Rohde, P., Simons, S. *et al.* (2006). Predictors and moderators of acute outcome in the Treatment for Adolescents with Depression Study (TADS). *Journal of the American Academy of Child and Adolescent Psychiatry*, 45, 1427–1439.

Curry, J., Silva, S., Rohde, P. *et al.* (2012). Onset of alcohol or substance use disorders following treatment for adolescent depression. Journal of Consulting and Clinical Psychology, 80, 299–312.

Dahl, R. (2011). Understanding the risky business of adolescence. *Neuron*, 69, 837–839.

Davey, C.G., Yucel, M., and Allen, N.B. (2008). The emergence of depression in adolescence: Development of the prefrontal cortex and the representation of reward. *Neuroscience and Biobehavioral Reviews*, 32, 1–19.

Daviss, W.B., Perel, J.M., Brent, D.A. *et al.* (2006). Acute antidepressant response and plasma levels of bupropion and metabolites in a pediatric-aged sample: an exploratory study. *Therapeutic Drug Monitoring*, 28, 190–198.

Diamond, G.S., Reis, B.F., Diamond, G.M., Siqueland, L., and Isaacs, L. (2002). Attachment-based family therapy for depressed adolescents: A treatment development study. *Journal of the American Academy of Child and Adolescent Psychiatry*, 41, 1190–1196.

Diamond, G.S., Wintersteen, M.B., Brown, G.K. *et al.* (2010). Attachment-based family therapy for adolescents with suicidal ideation: A randomized controlled trial. *Journal of the American Academy of Child and Adolescent Psychiatry*, 49, 122–131.

Dietz, L.J., Mufson, L., Irvine, H., and Brent, D.A. (2008). Family-based interpersonal psychotherapy for depressed preadolescents: An open-treatment trial. *Early Intervention in Psychiatry*, 2, 154–161.

Diler, R.S., Birmaher, B., Brent, D.A. *et al.* (2004). Phenomenology of panic disorder in youth. *Depression and Anxiety*, 20, 39–43.

Dubicka, B., Elvins, R., Roberts, C. *et al.* (2010). Combined treatment with cognitive-behavioural therapy in adolescent depression: Meta-analysis. *British Journal of Psychiatry*, 197, 433–440.

Emslie, G., Rush, J.A., Weinberg, W.A. *et al.* (1997). A double-blind, randomized placebo-controlled trial of fluoxetine in depressed children and adolescents with depression. *Archives of General Psychiatry*, 54, 1031–1037.

Emslie, G., Heiligenstein, J.H., Wagner, K.D. *et al.* (2002). Fluoxetine for acute treatment of depression in children and adolescents: A placebo-controlled, randomized clinical trial. *Journal of the American Academy of Child and Adolescent Psychiatry*, 41, 1205–1215.

Emslie, G.J., Ventura, D., Korotzer, A., and Tourkodimitris, S. (2009). Escitalopram in the treatment of adolescent depression: A randomized placebo-controlled multisite trial. *Journal of the American Academy of Child and Adolescent Psychiatry*, 48, 721–729.

Emslie, G.J., Findling, R.L., Yeung, P.P., Kunz, N.R., and Li, Y. (2007). Venlafaxine ER for the treatment of pediatric subjects with depression: Results of two placebo-controlled trials. *Journal of the American Academy of Child and Adolescent Psychiatry*, 46, 479–488.

Emslie, G.J., Kennard, B.D., Mayes, T.L. *et al.* (2008). Fluoxetine versus placebo in preventing relapse of major depression in children and adolescents. *American Journal of Psychiatry*, 165, 459–467.

Emslie, G.J., Kennard, B.D., Mayes, T.L. *et al.* (2012). Insomnia moderates outcome of serotonin-selective reuptake inhibitor treatment in depressed youth. *Journal of Child and Adolescent Psychopharmacology*, 22, 21–28.

Feeny, N.C., Silva, S.G., Reinecke, M.A. *et al.* (2009). An exploratory analysis of the impact of family functioning on treatment for depression in adolescents. *Journal of Clinical Child and Adolescent Psychology*, 38, 814–825.

Findling, R.L. (1996). Open-label treatment of comorbid depression and attentional disorders with co-administration of serotonin reuptake inhibitors and psychostimulants in children, adolescents, and adults: A case series. *Journal of Child and Adolescent Psychopharmacology*, 6, 165–175.

Findling, R.L., Nyilas, M., and Forbes, R.A. *et al.* (2009). Acute treatment of pediatric bipolar I disorder, manic or mixed episode, with aripiprazole: A randomized, double-blind, placebo-controlled study. *Journal of Clinical Psychiatry*, 70, 1441–1451.

Forbes, E.E. and Dahl, R.E. (2012). Research review: Altered reward function in adolescent depression: What, when and how? *Journal of Child Psychology and Psychiatry, and Allied Disciplines*, 53, 3–15.

Forbes, E.E., Bertocci, M.A., Gregory, A.M. *et al.* (2008). Objective sleep in pediatric anxiety disorders and major depressive disorder. *Journal of the American Academy of Child and Adolescent Psychiatry*, 47, 148–155.

Fristad, M.A., Verducci, J., Walters, K., and Young, M. (2009). Impact of multifamily psychoeducational psychotherapy in treating children aged 8 to 12 years with mood disorders. *Archives of General Psychiatry*, 66, 1013–1021.

Garber, J., Clarke, G., Weersing, R. *et al.* (2009). Prevention of depression in at-risk adolescents: A randomized controlled trial. *Journal of the American Medical Association*, 301, 2215–2224.

Geller, B., Fox, L.W., and Clark, K.A. (1994). Rate and predictors of prepubertal bipolarity during follow-up of 6- to 12-year-old depressed children. *Journal of the American Academy of Child and Adolescent Psychiatry*, 33, 461–468.

Geller, B., Tillman, R., Craney, J.L., and Bolhofner, K. (2004). Four-year prospective outcome and natural history of mania in children with a prepubertal and early adolescent bipolar disorder phenotype. *Archives of General Psychiatry*, 61, 459–467.

Geller, B., Zimerman, B., Williams, M. *et al.* (2002). DSM-IV mania symptoms in a prepubertal and early adolescent bipolar disorder phenotype compared to attention-deficit hyperactive and normal controls. *Journal of Child Psychology and Psychiatry and Allied Disciplines*, 12, 11–25.

Geller, B., Luby, J.L., Joshi, P. *et al.* (2012). A randomized controlled trial of risperidone, lithium, or divalproex sodium for initial treatment of bipolar I disorder, manic or mixed phase, in children and adolescents. *Archives of General Psychiatry*, 69, 515–528.

Georgiades, K., Lewinsohn, P.M., Monroe, S.M., and Seeley, J.R. (2006). Major depressive disorder in adolescence: The role of subthreshold symptoms. *Journal of the American Academy of Child and Adolescent Psychiatry*, 45, 936–944.

Gibbons, R.D., Brown, C.H., Hur, K., Davis, J.M., and Mann, J.J. (2012). Suicidal thoughts and behavior with antidepressant treatment: Reanalysis of the randomized placebo-controlled studies of fluoxetine and venlafaxine. *Archives of General Psychiatry*, 69, 580–587.

Gibbons, R.D., Brown, C.H., Hur, K. *et al.* (2007). Early evidence on the effects of regulators' suicidality warnings on SSRI prescriptions and suicide in children and adolescents. *American Journal of Psychiatry*, 164, 1356–1363.

Goldstein, B.I., Shamseddeen, W., Spirito, A. *et al.* (2009). Substance use and the treatment of resistant depression in adolescents. *Journal of the American Academy of Child and Adolescent Psychiatry*, 48, 1182–1192.

Gonzalez-Tejera, G., Canino, G., Ramirez, R. *et al.* (2005). Examining minor and major depression in adolescents.

Journal of Child Psychology and Psychiatry and Allied Disciplines, 46, 888–899.

Goodyer, I., Dubicka, B., Wilkinson, P. *et al.* (2007). Selective serotonin reuptake inhibitors (SSRIs) and routine specialist care with and without cognitive behaviour therapy in adolescents with major depression: Randomised controlled trial. *British Medical Journal*, 335, 106–107.

Gregory, A.M., Caspi, A., Moffitt, T.E., and Poulton, R. (2009). Sleep problems in childhood predict neuropsychological functioning in adolescence. *Pediatrics*, 123, 1171–1176.

Gunlicks-Stoessel, M., Mufson, L., Jekal, A., and Turner, J.B. (2010). The impact of perceived interpersonal functioning on treatment for adolescent depression: IPT-A versus treatment as usual in school-based health clinics. *Journal of Consulting and Clinical Psychology*, 78, 260–267.

Harrington, R., Rutter, M., Weissman, M. *et al.* (1997). Psychiatric disorders in the relatives of depressed probands. I. Comparison of prepubertal, adolescent and early adult onset cases. *Journal of Affective Disorders*, 42, 9–22.

Hazell, P., O'Connell, D., Heathcote, D., and Henry, D.A. (2002). Tricyclic drugs for depression in children and adolescents. *Cochrane Database of Systematic Reviews*, 2, CD002317.

Heiligenstein, J., Hoog, S.L., Wagner, K.D. *et al.* (2006). Fluoxetine 40–60 mg versus fluoxetine 20 mg in the treatment of children and adolescents with a less-than-complete response to nine-week treatment with fluoxetine 10–20 mg: A pilot study. *Journal of Child and Adolescent Psychopharmacology*, 16, 207–217.

Horowitz, J.L., Garber, J., Ciesla, J.A., Young, J.F., and Mufson, L. (2007). Prevention of depressive symptoms in adolescents: A randomized trial of cognitive-behavioral and interpersonal prevention programs. *Journal of Consulting and Clinical Psychology*, 75, 693–706.

Inoue, T., Abekawa, T., Nakagawa, S. *et al.* (2011). Long-term naturalistic follow-up of lithium augmentation: Relevance to bipolarity. *Journal of Affective Disorders*, 129, 64–67.

Kapur, S., Mieczkowski, T., and Mann, J. (1992). Antidepressant medications and the relative risk of suicide attempt and suicide. *Journal of the American Medical Association*, 268, 3441–3445.

Katz, L.Y., Kozyrskyj, A.L., Prior, H.J. *et al.* (2008). Effect of regulatory warnings on antidepressant prescription rates, use of health services and outcomes among children, adolescents and young adults. *Canadian Medical Association Journal*, 178, 1005–1011.

Kennard, B., Silva, S., Vitiello, B. *et al.* (2006). Remission and residual symptoms after short-term treatment in the

Treatment of Adolescents with Depression Study (TADS). *Journal of the American Academy of Child and Adolescent Psychiatry*, 45, 1404–1411.

Kennard, B.D., Emslie, G.J., Mayes, T.L. *et al.* (2008). Cognitive-behavioral therapy to prevent relapse in pediatric response to pharmacotherapy for major depressive disorder. *Journal of the American Academy of Child and Adolescent Psychiatry*, 47, 1395–1404.

Kennard, B.D., Clarke, G.N., Weersing, V.R. *et al.* (2009). Effective components of TORDIA cognitive behavioral therapy for adolescent depression. *Journal of Consulting and Clinical Psychology*, 77, 1033–1041.

Koplewicz, H.S. (1997). *It's Nobody's Fault: New Hope and Help for Difficult Children and Their Parents*. New York, NY: Three Rivers Press.

Kovacs, M., Akiskal, H.S., Gatsonis, C., and Parrone, P.L. (1994). Childhood-onset dysthymic disorder: Clinical features and prospective naturalistic outcome. *Archives of General Psychiatry*, 51, 365–374.

Kovacs, M., Sherrill, J., George, C.J. *et al.* (2006). Contextual emotion-regulation therapy for childhood depression: Description and pilot testing of a new intervention. *Journal of the American Academy of Child and Adolescent Psychiatry*, 45, 892–903.

Kroll, L., Harrington, R., Jayson, D., and Fraser, J. (1996). Pilot study of continuation cognitive-behavioral therapy for major depression in adolescent psychiatric patients. *Journal of the American Academy of Child and Adolescent Psychiatry*, 35, 1156–1161.

Kupfer, D.J., Frank, E., Perel, J.M. *et al.* (1992). Five-year outcome for maintenance therapies in recurrent depression. *Archives of General Psychiatry*, 49, 769–773.

Larun, L., Nordheim, L.V., Ekeland, E., Hagen, K.B., and Heian, F. (2006). Exercise in prevention and treatment of anxiety and depression among children and young people. *Cochrane Database of Systematic Reviews*, 3, CD004691.

Leverich, G.S., Altshuler, L.L., Frye, M.A. *et al.* (2006). Risk of switch in mood polarity to hypomania or mania in patients with bipolar depression during acute and continuation trials of venlafaxine, sertraline, and bupropion as adjuncts to mood stabilizers. *American Journal of Psychiatry*, 163, 232–239.

Lewinsohn, P.M., Rohde, P., and Seeley, J.R. (1998a). Treatment of adolescent depression: Frequency of services and impact on functioning in young adulthood. *Depression and Anxiety*, 7, 47–52.

Lewinsohn P.M., Rohde, P., and Seeley, J.R. (1998b). Major depressive disorder in older adolescents: Prevalence, risk factors, and clinical implications. *Clinical Psychology Review*, 18, 765–794.

Lewinsohn, P.M., Rohde, P., Seeley, J.R., and Klein, D.N. (1997). Axis II psychopathology as a function of Axis I disorders in childhood and adolescence. *Journal of the American Academy of Child and Adolescent Psychiatry*, 36, 1752–1759.

Lewis, C.C., Simons, A.D., Nguyen, L.J. *et al.* (2010). Impact of childhood trauma on treatment outcome in the Treatment for Adolescents with Depression Study (TADS). *Journal of the American Academy of Child and Adolescent Psychiatry*, 49, 132–140.

Libby, A.M., Orton, H.D., and Valuck, R.J. (2009). Persisting decline in depression treatment after FDA warnings. *Archives of General Psychiatry*, 66, 633–639.

Maalouf, F.T., Porta, G., Vitiello, B. *et al.* (2012). Do sub-syndromal manic symptoms influence outcome in treatment resistant depression in adolescents? A latent class analysis from the TORDIA study. *Journal of Affective Disorders*, 138, 86–95.

Mallinger, A.G., Frank, E., Thase, M.E. *et al.* (2009). Revisiting the effectiveness of standard antidepressants in bipolar disorder: Are monoamine oxidase inhibitors superior? *Psychopharmacology Bulletin*, 42, 64–74.

March, J., Silva, S., Petrycki, S. *et al.* (2004a). Fluoxetine, cognitive-behavioral therapy, and their combination for adolescents with depression: Treatment for Adolescent Depression Study (TADS) randomized controlled trial. *Journal of the American Medical Association*, 292, 807–820.

March, J.S., Foa, E., Gammon, P. *et al.* (2004b). Cognitive-behavior therapy, sertraline and their combination for children and adolescents with obsessive-compulsive disorder: The Pediatric OCD Treatment Study (POTS) randomized controlled trial. *Journal of the American Medical Association*, 292, 1969–1976.

March, J.S., Silva, S., Petrycki, S. *et al.* (2007). The Treatment for Adolescents with Depression Study (TADS): Long-term effectiveness and safety outcomes. *Archives of General Psychiatry*, 64, 1132–1144.

Martin, A., Young, C., Leckman, J.F. *et al.* (2004). Age effects on antidepressant-induced manic conversion. *Archives of Pediatrics and Adolescent Medicine*, 158, 773–780.

Mufson, L., Weissman, M.M., Moreau, D., and Garfinkel, R. (1999). Efficacy of interpersonal psychotherapy for depressed adolescents. *Archives of General Psychiatry*, 56, 573–579.

Mufson, L., Dorta, K.P., Wickramaratne, P. *et al.* (2004). A randomized effectiveness trial of interpersonal psychotherapy for depressed adolescents. *Archives of General Psychiatry*, 61, 577–584.

Nelson, J.C. and Papakostas, G.I. (2009). Atypical antipsychotic augmentation in major depressive disorder: A meta-analysis of placebo-controlled randomized trials. *American Journal of Psychiatry*, 166, 980–991.

Nemets, H., Nemets, B., Apter, A., Bracha, Z., and Belmaker, R.H. (2006). Omega-3 treatment of childhood depression: A controlled, double-blind pilot study. *American Journal of Psychiatry*, 163, 1098–1100.

Nihalani, N., Schwartz, T.L., Siddiqui, U.A., and Megna, J.L. (2011). Weight gain, obesity, and psychotropic prescribing. *Journal of Obesity*, Article ID 893629, doi: 10.1155/2011/893629 (Accessed March 2, 2012).

Nolen-Hoeksema, S. (2011). Emotion regulation and psychopathology: The role of gender. *Annual Review of Clinical Psychology*, 8, 161–187.

Owens, J.A., Rosen, C.L., Mindell, J.A., and Kirchner, H.L. (2010). Use of pharmacotherapy for insomnia in child psychiatry practice: A national survey. *Sleep Medicine*, 11, 692–700.

Pail, G., Huf, W., Pjrek, E. *et al.* (2011). Bright-light therapy in the treatment of mood disorders. *Neuropsychobiology*, 64, 152–162.

Quach, J., Hiscock, H., Ukoumunne, O.C., and Wake, M. (2011). A brief sleep intervention improves outcomes in the school entry year: A randomized controlled trial. *Pediatrics*, 128, 692–701.

Renaud, J., Brent, D.A., Baugher, M. *et al.* (1998). Rapid response to psychosocial treatment for adolescent depression: A two-year follow-up. *Journal of the American Academy of Child and Adolescent Psychiatry*, 37, 1184–1190.

Riggs, P.D., Mikulich-Gilbertson, S.K., Davies, R.D. *et al.* (2007). A randomized controlled trial of fluoxetine and cognitive behavioral therapy in adolescents with major depression, behavior problems, and substance use disorders. *Archives of Pediatric and Adolescent Medicine*, 161, 1026–1034.

Rohde, P., Seeley, J.R., Clarke, G.N., Kaufman, N.K., and Stice, E. (2006). Predicting time to recovery among depressed adolescents treated in two psychosocial group interventions. *Journal of Consulting and Clinical Psychology*, 74, 80–88.

Rossello, J. and Bernal, G. (1999). The efficacy of cognitive-behavioral and interpersonal treatments for depression in Puerto Rican adolescents. *Journal of Consulting and Clinical Psychology*, 67, 734–745.

Rossello, J., Bernal, G., and Rivera-Medina, C. (2008). Individual and group CBT and IPT for Puerto Rican adolescents with depressive symptoms. *Cultural Diversity and Ethnic Minority Psychology*, 14, 234–245.

Ryan, N.D., Puig-Antich, J., Ambrosini, P. *et al.* (1987). The clinical picture of major depression in children and adolescents. *Archives of General Psychiatry*, 44, 854–861.

Saeed, S.A., Antonacci, D.J., and Bloch, R.M. (2010). Exercise, yoga, and meditation for depressive and anxiety disorders. *American Family Physician*, 81, 981–986.

Sakolsky, D.J., Perel, J.M., Emslie, G.J. *et al.* (2011). Antidepressant exposure as a predictor of clinical outcomes in the Treatment of Resistant Depression in Adolescents (TORDIA) study. *Journal of Clinical Psychopharmacology*, 31, 92–97.

Sala, M., Vicentini, A., Brambilla, P. *et al.* (2005). QT interval prolongation related to psychoactive drug treatment: A comparison of monotherapy versus polytherapy. *Annals of General Psychiatry*, 4, 1.

Sallee, F.R., Vrindavanam, N.S., Deas-Nesmith, D., Carson, S.W., and Sethuraman, G. (1997). Pulse intravenous clomipramine for depressed adolescents: Double-blind, controlled trial. *American Journal of Psychiatry*, 154, 668–673.

Scharko, A.M. (2004). Selective serotonin reuptake inhibitor-induced sexual dysfunction in adolescents: A review. *Journal of the American Academy of Child and Adolescent Psychiatry*, 43, 1071–1079.

Shamseddeen, W., Clarke, G., Wagner, K.D. *et al.* (2011). Treatment-resistant depressed youth show a higher response rate if treatment ends during summer school break. *Journal of the American Academy of Child and Adolescent Psychiatry*, 50, 1140–1148.

Shamseddeen, W., Clarke, G., Keller, M.B. *et al.* (2012). Adjunctive sleep medications and depression outcome in the Treatment of SSRI Resistant Depression in Adolescents (TORDIA) study. *Journal of Child and Adolescent Psychopharmacology*, 22, 29–36.

Smits, J.A., Rosenfield, D., Mather, A.A. *et al.* (2010). Psychotropic medication use mediates the relationship between mood and anxiety disorders and obesity: Findings from a nationally representative sample. *Journal of Psychiatric Research*, 44, 1010–1016.

Stalets, M.M. and Luby, J.L. (2006). Preschool depression. *Child and Adolescent Psychiatric Clinics of North America*, 15, 899–917.

Stanley, B., Brown, G., Brent, D. *et al.* (2009). Cognitive Behavior Therapy for Suicide Prevention (CBT-SP): Treatment model, feasibility and acceptability. *Journal of the American Academy of Child and Adolescent Psychiatry*, 48, 1005–1013.

Stone, M., Laughren, T., Jones, M.L. *et al.* (2009). Risk of suicidality in clinical trials of antidepressants in adults: Analysis of proprietary data submitted to US Food and Drug Administration. *British Medical Journal*, 11, 339–342.

Strober, M. and Carlson, G. (1982). Bipolar illness in adolescents with major depression: Clinical, genetic, and psychopharmacologic predictors in a three- to four-year prospective follow-up investigation. *Archives of General Psychiatry*, 39, 549–555.

Verdel, B.M., Souverein, P.C., Egberts, T.C. *et al.* (2010). Use of antidepressant drugs and risk of osteoporotic and non-osteoporotic fractures. *Bone*, 47, 604–609.

Vitiello, B., Silva, S.G., Rohde P. *et al.* (2009). Suicidal events in the Treatment of Adolescents with Depression Study (TADS). *Journal of Clinical Psychiatry*, 70, 741–747.

Vitiello, B., Emslie, G., Clarke, G. *et al.* (2011). Long-term outcome of adolescent depression initially resistant to selective serotonin reuptake inhibitor treatment: A follow-up study of the TORDIA sample. *Journal of Clinical Psychiatry*, 72, 388–396.

Wachtel, L.E., Dhossche, D.M., and Kellner, C.H. (2011). When is electroconvulsive therapy appropriate for children and adolescents? *Medical Hypotheses*, 76, 395–399.

Wagner, K.D., Jonas, J., Findling, R.L., Ventura, D., and Saikali, K. (2006). A double-blind randomized, placebo-controlled trial of escitalopram in the treatment of pediatric depression. *Journal of the American Academy of Child and Adolescent Psychiatry*, 45, 280–288.

Walkup, J.T., Albano, A.M., Piacentini, J. *et al.* (2008). Cognitive behavioral therapy, sertraline, or a combination in childhood anxiety. *New England Journal of Medicine*, 359, 2753–2766.

Walter, G. and Rey, J.M. (2003). Has the practice and outcome of ECT in adolescents changed? Findings from a whole-population study. *Journal of ECT*, 19, 84–87.

Weinrieb, R.M., Auriacombe, M., Lynch, K.G., and Lewis, J.D. (2005). Selective serotonin re-uptake inhibitors and the risk of bleeding. *Expert Opinion on Drug Safety*, 4, 337–344.

Weissman, M., Wolk, S., Goldstein, R. *et al.* (1999a). Depressed adolescents grown up. *Journal of the American Medical Association*, 281, 1707–1713.

Weissman, M.M., Wolk, S., Wickramaratne, P. *et al.* (1999b). Children with prepubertal onset major depressive disorder and anxiety grown up. *Archives of General Psychiatry*, 56, 794–801.

Weissman, M.M., Wickramaratne, P., Nomura, Y. *et al.* (2005). Families at high and low risk for depression: A 3-generation study. *Archives of General Psychiatry*, 62, 29–36.

Weisz, J.R., McCarty, C.A., and Valeri, S.M. (2006). Effects of psychotherapy for depression in children and adolescents: A meta-analysis. *Psychological Bulletin*, 132, 132–149.

Weisz, J.R., Thurber, C.A., Sweeney, L., Proffitt, V.D., and LeGagnoux, G.L. (1997). Brief treatment of mild-to-moderate child depression using primary and secondary control enhancement training. *Journal of Consulting and Clinical Psychology*, 65, 703–707.

White, N., Litovitz, T., and Clancy, C. (2008). Suicidal antidepressant overdoses: A comparative analysis by antidepressant type. *Journal of Medical Toxicology*, 4, 238–250.

Wilkinson, P., Kelvin, R., Roberts, C., Dubicka, B., and Goodyer, I. (2011). Clinical and psychosocial predictors of suicide attempts and nonsuicidal self-injury in the Adolescent Depression Antidepressants and Psychotherapy Trial (ADAPT). *American Journal of Psychiatry*, 168, 495–501.

Wood, A., Harrington, R., and Moore, A. (1996). Controlled trial of a brief cognitive-behavioural intervention in adolescent patients with depressive disorders. *Journal of Child Psychology and Psychiatry*, 37, 737–746.

Young, J.F., Gallop, R., and Mufson, L. (2009). Mother-child conflict and its moderating effects on depression outcomes in a preventive intervention for adolescent depression. *Journal of Clinical Child and Adolescent Psychology*, 38, 696–704.

Chapter

12

Therapeutics of pediatric bipolar disorder

Robert A. Kowatch, Melissa P. DelBello, and Barbara L. Gracious

Bipolar disorders are increasingly being recognized and diagnosed in children and adolescents. There has also been an increase in the number of large, well-controlled medication trials in this group of patients. In this chapter we review the diagnostic features of these patients, co-morbidity, and review the evidence for various medications, including complementary treatments, and offer a treatment algorithm.

Introduction

Pediatric bipolar disorders (BPD) are prevalent psychiatric disorders that seriously disrupt the lives of children, adolescents, and their families (Lewinsohn *et al.* 1995, Geller and Luby, 1997, Fristad and Goldberg-Arnold, 2002). Numerous studies have shown that children and adolescents with BPD have significantly higher rates of morbidity and mortality, including psychosocial morbidity with impaired family and peer relationships (Geller *et al.* 2000a); impaired academic performance with increased rates of school failure and school dropouts (Weinberg and Brumback, 1976); increased levels of substance-use disorders, increased rates of suicide attempts and completion, legal difficulties, and multiple hospitalizations (Akiskal *et al.* 1985, Geller and Luby, 1997). It is important that these disorders be diagnosed accurately and reliably so that appropriate treatments are provided and these patients receive the psychological and educational services they need.

The *population* prevalence of bipolar disorder in adolescents appears to be similar to the adult rate of approximately 1.5% (Lewinsohn *et al.* 1995, Merikangas *et al.* 2010). But, in *clinical* settings the prevalence of BPD or "base rate" is much higher, approximately 15% (Wozniak *et al.* 1995). Youngstrom and

Duax (2005) recently reported that the rate of bipolar disorder in children and adolescents varied from 0–0.6% in epidemiological samples to 17–30% in clinical samples.

Diagnosis

The diagnosis of a child or adolescent with BPD is often difficult because of the pediatric differences in symptom expression, frequent co-morbid disorders, and the lack of biologic tests to confirm this disorder. It is important to realize that the DSM-IV criteria for mania/hypomania were developed for adults and none of these criteria take into account developmental differences between bipolar adults and bipolar children or adolescents. Clinicians who evaluate such children often attempt to use the DSM-IV course modifier "rapid cycling," but find that this description does not fit children very well, as they often do not have clearly delineated episodes of mania, but appear to be chronically "cycling" (Wozniak and Biederman 1997, Geller *et al.* 2000b, Findling *et al.* 2001, Geller *et al.* 2001).

Dr. Barbara Geller, MD at Washington University was one of the leaders in the diagnosis and phenomenology of pediatric BPD and developed and validated a structured interview, the Washington University K-SADS (WASH-U K-SADS). Geller *et al.* reported the results of a 4-year longitudinal study of a sample of 93 consecutively ascertained outpatients with BPD. During the course of this study the WASH-U KSADS was blindly administered by research nurses to the subjects' mothers and to children/adolescents about themselves. In this study, Geller and colleagues elected to require current DSM-IV mania or hypomania with elated mood

Clinical Handbook for the Management of Mood Disorders, ed. J. John Mann, Patrick J. McGrath, and Steven P. Roose.
Published by Cambridge University Press. © Cambridge University Press 2013.

and/or grandiosity as their inclusion criterion for BPD (Geller *et al.* 2004). Geller and colleagues defined a manic episode as the entire length of the illness and cycling as mood changes within an episode. They reported that the BPD subjects in this study were aged 10.9 ± 2.6 years, had a current episode length of 3.6 ± 2.5 years, with an age of onset at 7.3 ± 3.5 years. No effects were found for gender, puberty, or co-morbid ADHD on rates of mania criteria, mixed mania, psychosis, rapid cycling, suicidality, or co-morbid oppositional defiant disorder (ODD). This first longitudinal study of children with mania verifies that children with bipolar I disorder present differently than adults, with episodes that are longer, mixed in nature, and chronic in course.

When evaluating a child or adolescent for a possible bipolar disorder there are two questions that become important – does the patient have a bipolar disorder and if so, how severe is it? The former is important for predication of course and the latter for planning and monitoring treatment. When determining the presence or absence of manic symptoms, clinicians can use a variation of the FIND (frequency, intensity, number, and duration) strategy to make this determination. The original FIND guidelines were developed by Mary Fristad (Quinn and Fristad, 2004) at Ohio State University and modified here to include:

- *Frequency* – of symptoms – how many days in a week is the patient symptomatic?
- *Intensity* – are the patient's symptoms severe enough to cause severe dysfunction in one domain or moderate disturbance in two or more domains?
- *Number* – of DSM-IV manic symptoms.
- *Duration* – how long is the patient symptomatic for, on an average day, when manic or hypomanic?

There are also a number of medications and medical disorders that may exacerbate or mimic bipolar symptoms and it is important to assess these potential confounds before initiating treatment. Potential medical disorders and medications that should be evaluated before making the diagnosis of a bipolar disorder in children and adolescents are listed in Table 12.1.

Co-morbid disorders

Co-morbid disorders are the rule rather than the exception among children and adolescents with bipolar disorder. These co-morbid disorders often

Table 12.1 Medical conditions that may mimic mania in children and adolescents

Hyperthyroidism

Closed or open head injury

Temporal lobe epilepsy

Multiple sclerosis

Systemic lupus erythematosus (SLE)

Fetal alcohol spectrum disorder/alcohol-related neurodevelopmental disorder

Wilson's disease

Table 12.2 Estimated rates of frequent co-morbid disorders

Disorder	Prepubertal	Adolescent
ADHD	70–90%	30–60%
Anxiety disorders	20–30%	30–40%
Conduct disorders	30–40%	30–60%
Oppositional defiant disorder	60–90%	20–30%
Substance abuse	10%	40–50%
Learning disabilities	30–40%	30–40%

complicate the presentation and treatment response. The most common co-morbid diagnosis among children and adolescents with BPD is attention deficit hyperactivity disorder (ADHD). Several studies have determined that ADHD is more common in prepubertal-onset bipolar disorder than in adolescent-onset bipolar disorder (West *et al.* 1995, Faraone *et al.* 1997). The rate of co-morbid ADHD in prepubertal children is around 60–90%, whereas in adolescents the rate is 30–40%. Children with ADHD do not demonstrate the elated mood, grandiosity, hypersexuality, decreased need for sleep, racing thoughts, and other manic symptoms that are present in children with mania and co-morbid ADHD (Geller *et al.* 1998b). Another disorder that is frequently co-morbid in children with bipolar disorder is conduct disorder. Kovacs and Pollock found a 69% rate of conduct disorder among 26 bipolar children and adolescents (Kovacs and Pollock, 1995) independent of their mood disorder. Moreover, adolescents with bipolar disorder are 4–5 times more likely to develop a substance-use disorder than those without bipolar disorder (Wilens *et al.* 2004). Children and adolescents with pervasive developmental disorders may be at increased risk for developing mania (Wozniak *et al.* 1997). Common co-morbid disorders found in patients with pediatric bipolar disorders are listed in Table 12.2.

Treatment of mania/hypomania

Mood stabilizers

Lithium

Lithium is the oldest mood stabilizer and has significant data supporting its use for BD in adults (Cade 1949, Geddes *et al.* 2004). A recent review of adult placebo-controlled studies revealed an effect size of 0.40 (95% confidence interval (CI): 0.28, 0.53) and an overall NNT of 6 (95% CI: 4, 13) for lithium in the treatment of acute mania in adults (Storosum *et al.* 2007). Lithium is the only mood stabilizer approved by the United States Food and Drug Administration (FDA) for use in the treatment of mania in adolescents (ages 12–18 years).

In the first prospective, placebo-controlled trial of lithium in children and adolescents with bipolar disorders and co-morbid substance abuse, subjects treated with lithium for 6 weeks showed a significant improvement in global assessment of functioning (46% response rate in the lithium treated group vs. 8% response rate in the placebo group; Geller *et al.* 1998a).

In an open, prospective study of 100 adolescents 12–18 years of age, with an acute manic episode treated with lithium, 63 met response criteria and 26 achieved remission of manic symptoms at a 4-week assessment (Kafantaris *et al.* 2003). Prominent depressive features, age at first mood episode, severity of mania, and co-morbidity with ADHD did not distinguish responders from nonresponders to lithium. Kafantaris *et al.* (2004) subsequently reported the results of a placebo-controlled, discontinuation study of lithium in adolescents with mania (N = 40, mean age 15). During the first part of this study, subjects received open treatment with lithium at therapeutic serum levels (mean 0.99 mEq/L) for at least 4 weeks. Responders to lithium were then randomly assigned to continue or discontinue lithium during a 2-week double-blind, placebo-controlled phase. Of these subjects, 58% experienced a clinically significant symptom exacerbation during the 2-week double-blind phase. However, the slightly lower exacerbation rate in the group maintained on lithium (53%) vs. the group switched to placebo (62%) did not reach statistical significance. This study did not appear to support a large effect for lithium continuation treatment of adolescents with acute mania, but with only a two-week discontinuation period, it is hard to draw definitive conclusions about efficacy. It is very possible that if the discontinuation period had been longer, a clear separation between the lithium and placebo groups would have been observed.

Kowatch, Findling, Scheffer, and Stanford (Kowatch *et al.* 2007) presented the results of a large, NIMH-funded controlled trial of lithium vs. divalproex vs. placebo in subjects ages 7–17 years with BD I, the "Pediatric Bipolar Collaborative Trial" (PBC). In this trial, 153 outpatients between the ages of 7–17 (mean 10.6 years) were randomized in a double-blind to treatment with lithium, divalproex, or placebo. The total trial length was 24 weeks. During the first 8 weeks, subjects were treated with lithium, divalproex, or placebo in a double-blind fashion; no other psychotropic medications were allowed other than short-term "rescue" agents. At the end of 8 weeks, divalproex demonstrated efficacy on both a priori outcome measures, whereas lithium did not. The response rates based on a Clinical Global Impression (CGI) improvement score of "1 or 2" (much or very much improved) were: divalproex 54%, lithium 42%, and placebo 29%. There was a definite trend towards efficacy for lithium, but it did not clearly separate from placebo on the primary outcome measures.

Based on the studies reviewed it appears that lithium is a mood stabilizer with a moderate effect size in children and adolescents, similar to the effect size found in adult lithium studies. However, lithium may cause renal, hematological, thyroid, and other endocrine changes that must be monitored. Common side effects of lithium, potentially problematic for children and adolescents, include nausea, polyuria, polydipsia, tremor, acne, and weight gain.

Valproate

Valproic acid (VPA) is a chemical compound that has found clinical use as an anticonvulsant and mood stabilizer. Related drugs include the sodium salts of valproic acid, sodium valproate, and divalproex sodium (Depakote), which consists of a compound of sodium valproate and valproic acid. For many years valproate has been used to treat adults with mania. A review of the five controlled studies of valproate for the acute treatment of mania in adults showed an average response rate of 54% demonstrating efficacy for valproate vs. placebo (McElroy and Keck, 2000). In many of these studies, positive results were obtained even though patients were selected from a population previously refractory to lithium treatment and were characterized by rapid cycling, mixed affective states, and irritability.

A discontinuation trial of lithium and divalproex was conducted to determine whether divalproex was superior to lithium in the maintenance monotherapy of BD youth who had been previously stabilized on the combination of lithium and divalproex (Findling *et al.* 2005). Children with bipolar I or II disorder (N = 139) with a mean age of 10.8 ± 3.5 years were treated with lithium and divalproex for a mean duration of 10.7 weeks initially. Patients meeting remission criteria for 4 consecutive weeks were then randomized in a double-blind fashion to treatment with lithium (n = 30) or divalproex (n = 30) for up to 76 weeks. At the end of the study period, the lithium and divalproex treatment groups did not differ in survival time until emerging symptoms of relapse or until discontinuation for any reason. The authors concluded that lithium was not superior to divalproex as maintenance treatment in youths who had stabilized on combination lithium and divalproex pharmacotherapy. This trial also demonstrated that monotherapy was not sufficient for maintenance treatment of the children and adolescents with BD in this trial.

Wagner and colleagues (2009) recently reported the results of an industry-funded, randomized, placebo-controlled, double-blind, multi-center study to evaluate the safety and efficacy of Depakote ER in the treatment of bipolar I disorder, manic or mixed episode, in children and adolescents. During this trial, 150 children aged 10–17 with a current clinical diagnosis of bipolar I disorder were enrolled at 20 study sites. Subjects were outpatients with a manic or mixed episode with a Young Mania Rating Scale (YMRS) score of greater than or equal to 20 at screening and baseline. Subjects were randomized in a 1:1 ratio to receive active study medication (250 mg and/or 500 mg tablets of Depakote ER) or matching placebo tablets. The duration of this study was 6 weeks, including a screening period lasting 3–14 days, a 4-week treatment period, and an optional 1-week taper period.

There were no statistically significant differences between the valproate and placebo arms on any of the efficacy variables. This trial may have been negative because of differences in the absorption and distribution of the extended-release formulation of valproate that was used. Moreover, the active treatment period of 4 weeks may not have been long enough to detect a drug–placebo difference. The mean daily dose of divalproex ER was 24.3 mg/kg (1286 mg) with a mean dose of 27.1 mg/kg on day 28 of the study. Mean (SD) serum

valproate concentrations (μg/mL) was 79.9 (43.7) at the last visit.

In contrast to the results of the Wagner and colleagues trial (2009), the PBC trial, previously discussed, found that valproate was superior to lithium over 8 weeks. The PBC trial used the immediate-release formulation of valproate; the acute treatment period was 8 weeks; and the mean serum levels of valproate were 100 ng/L, as opposed to the Wagner *et al.* study where the mean level was 79.9 ng/L.

Common side effects of valproate in children and adolescents include nausea, increased appetite, weight gain, sedation, thrombocytopenia (low blood platelets), transient hair loss, tremor, and vomiting. Rarely, pancreatitis (Sinclair *et al.* 2004, Werlin and Fish, 2006) and liver failure (Konig *et al.* 1994, Treem, 1994, Ee *et al.* 2003) can occur in children treated with valproate. Fetal exposure to valproate is associated with an increased rate of neural tube defects (Ketter *et al.* 2006). Valproate-induced hyperammonemia (abnormally high levels of blood ammonia) has been observed in children and adolescents treated with valproate, as it has in adults (Raskind and El-Chaar, 2000, Carr and Shrewsbury, 2007). It can present as lethargy, disorientation, and reversible cognitive deficits, which may progress to marked sedation, coma, and even death. It is a transient and asymptomatic phenomenon, but can become chronic if undetected and the valproate is not stopped.

There are increasing concerns about the association between valproate and polycystic ovarian syndrome (PCOS). PCOS is an endocrine disorder characterized by ovulatory dysfunction and hyperandrogenism, affecting between 3% and 5% of women who are not taking psychotropic medications (Rasgon, 2004). Common symptoms of PCOS include irregular or absent menstruation, lack of ovulation, weight gain, hirsutism, and/or acne. The initial reports of the association between PCOS and divalproex exposure were in women with epilepsy. The association was particularly strong if their exposure was during adolescence (Isojarvi *et al.* 1993). In a recent report on adults with BD there was a sevenfold increased risk of new-onset oligoamenorrhea with hyperandrogenism in women treated with valproate (Joffe *et al.* 2006). The current recommendations are that females treated with valproate should have a baseline assessment of menstrual cycle patterns and be continually monitored for menstrual irregularities, weight gain, hirsutism, and/or acne during treatment (Buchsbaum *et al.* 1997). If symptoms of PCOS develop, referral to a pediatric endocrinologist should be considered.

Carbamazepine

Carbamazepine is an anticonvulsant agent structurally similar to imipramine that was first introduced in the USA in 1968 for the treatment of seizures. Two controlled studies of a long-acting preparation of carbamazepine in adults with BD demonstrated efficacy for carbamazepine as monotherapy for mania (Weisler *et al.* 2006). There have been no controlled studies of carbamazepine for the treatment of children and adolescents with BD; the majority of reports in the literature concern its use in children and adolescents with ADHD or conduct disorder (Puente, 1975, Evans *et al.* 1987, Kafantaris *et al.* 1992, Cueva *et al.* 1996). Pleak *et al.* reported the worsening of behavior in 6 of 20 child and adolescent patients treated with carbamazepine for ADHD and conduct disorder (Pleak *et al.* 1988). There is no good evidence to support the use of carbamazepine as a first-line agent for children and adolescents with bipolar disorder and this drug's numerous P450 drug interactions make its clinical use difficult.

Carbamazepine should not be used in patients with a history of previous bone marrow depression, hypersensitivity to the drug, or known sensitivity to any of the tricyclic compounds. Common side effects of carbamazepine in children and adolescents include sedation, ataxia, dizziness, blurred vision, nausea, and vomiting. Uncommon side effects of carbamazepine include aplastic anemia and hyponatremia. Serious and sometimes fatal dermatological reactions, notably Stevens–Johnson syndrome and toxic epidermal necrolysis have been reported in about 1 to 6 per 10 000 new users in countries with mainly Caucasian populations (Keating and Blahunka, 1995, Devi *et al.* 2005). Carbamazepine can cause fetal harm and is therefore contraindicated during pregnancy (Ciraulo *et al.* 1995). The FDA recommends, but does not require, genetic testing of patients from at-risk populations prior to initiating treatment with carbamazepine. Studies have shown that, in patients of Chinese ancestry, there is a strong association between presence of one or two copies of the HLA-B*1502 allele and the risk of developing SJS/TEN (Stevens–Johnson syndrome/toxic epidermal necrolysis; Locharernkul *et al.* 2011). The HLA-B*1502 allele has been reported to be present in greater than 15% of the population in Hong Kong, Thailand, Malaysia,

and parts of the Philippines, with lower prevalence in other parts of Asia. Not all Asian patients carrying HLA-B*1502 develop SJS/TEN, and, infrequently, HLA-B*1502-negative patients of any ethnicity do experience these reactions. This same caution applies to children and adolescents of Chinese ancestry treated with carbamazepine.

Novel antiepileptic agents

There have been several new antiepileptic drugs (AEDs) that have been developed for the treatment of epilepsy that may be useful for the treatment of BD, although the data are presently limited regarding the efficacy and tolerability of these agents for pediatric BD. Additionally, there have been several negative trials of these agents in manic or mixed adults (Bowden and Karren, 2006).

Lamotrigine

Lamotrigine (Lamictal) has a novel mechanism of action by blocking voltage-sensitive sodium channels, and secondarily inhibiting the release of excitatory neurotransmitters, particularly glutamate and aspartate (Ketter *et al.* 2003). Lamotrigine also inhibits serotonin reuptake, suggesting it might possess antidepressant properties. In 2003 the FDA approved lamotrigine for the long-term maintenance treatment of bipolar type I disorder in adults.

Several prospective studies in adults with BD suggest that lamotrigine may be beneficial for the treatment of mood symptoms in BD (Calabrese *et al.* 1999, Bowden *et al.* 2003). Chang *et al.* (2006) conducted an 8-week, open-label trial of lamotrigine alone or as adjunctive therapy for the treatment of 20 adolescents aged 12–17 years (mean age 15.8 years) with BD (I, II, and NOS), who were experiencing a depressive or mixed episode. The mean final dose was 131.6 mg/d. Of these subjects, 84% were rated as much or very much improved on the CGI. Larger, placebo-controlled studies of lamotrigine in bipolar children and adolescents are needed.

The most common side effects of lamotrigine are dizziness, tremor, somnolence, nausea, asthenia, and headache. Benign rashes develop in 12% of adult patients, typically within the first 8 weeks of lamotrigine therapy (Calabrese *et al.* 2002). Rarely, severe cutaneous reactions such as Stevens–Johnson syndrome and toxic epidermal necrolysis have been described. The risk of developing a serious rash is approximately three times greater in children and adolescents less than 16 years old compared with adults. Adolescent patients on oral contraceptives may require increased lamotrigine doses since estrogen induces the metabolism of lamotrigine. If the contraceptives are discontinued or the patient is postpartum, the dose of lamotrigine has to be decreased (Reimers *et al.* 2005).

Alternative mood stabilizers

Gabapentin (Neurontin) is structurally similar to GABA, increases GABA release from glia, and may modulate sodium channels. Double-blind controlled studies of gabapentin as adjunctive therapy to lithium or valproate, and as monotherapy, suggest it is no more effective than placebo for the treatment of mania in adults (Pande *et al.* 2000). However, gabapentin may be useful in combination with other mood-stabilizing agents for the treatment of anxiety disorders in individuals with BD (Keck *et al.* 2006).

Topiramate (Topamax) is a sulfamate-substituted monosaccharide, with several potential mechanisms of action, including blockade of voltage-gated sodium channels, antagonism of the kainate/AMPA sub-type of glutamate receptor, enhancement of GABA activity, and carbonic anhydrase inhibition. There has been one double-blind, placebo-controlled study of topiramate for children and adolescents with manic or mixed episodes associated with bipolar disorder (ages 6–17 years, N = 56) that was inconclusive because it was discontinued early when adult mania trials with topiramate failed to show efficacy (DelBello *et al.* 2005).

Wagner and colleagues (2006) have reported the results of a multi-center, industry-funded, controlled study of oxcarbazepine (Trileptal) in 116 bipolar youth (mean age 11.1 years). The difference in the primary outcome variable, change in YMRS mean scores, between the treatment and placebo groups was not statistically or clinically significant. Therefore, there is little evidence to support the use of oxcarbazepine for the treatment of children and adolescents with BD.

Atypical antipsychotics

The atypical antipsychotics are widely used in child, adolescent, and adult psychiatry. A recent meta-analysis of controlled atypical antipsychotic trials in adults with BD concluded that all of the five newer atypical antipsychotics (aripiprazole, olanzapine, quetiapine, risperidone, and ziprasidone) were superior to placebo for the treatment of mania in adults with BD (Perlis *et al.* 2006). All of the atypical

antipsychotics (except clozapine, which is generic) have received FDA approval for the treatment of acute mania associated with bipolar disorder in adults. Olanzapine, aripiprazole, and quetiapine have also received FDA approval as maintenance treatment for adults with bipolar disorder. Industry-sponsored trials are currently underway with asenapine and lurasidone for patients with mania, aged 10–17 years.

There are five, large, well-designed, placebo-controlled trials that have studied the efficacy of atypical antipsychotics in children and adolescents with BD and the results of these trials are summarized in Table 12.3.

Risperidone and olanzapine are indicated by the FDA for the short-term treatment of acute manic or mixed episodes associated with BD I in children and adolescents aged 10–17 years. Quetiapine is indicated for the treatment of bipolar mania in ages 10–17 years and aripiprazole is indicated for the acute and maintenance treatment of manic and mixed episodes associated with BD I with or without psychotic features in pediatric patients, 10–17 years of age.

Risperidone's efficacy for short-term treatment of mania in children and adolescents was demonstrated in a 3-week, randomized, double-blind, placebo-controlled, multi-center study of 169 patients aged 10–17 who were experiencing a manic or mixed episode of bipolar I disorder (Haas *et al.* 2009). Subjects in this trial were assigned to either low-dose risperidone, 0.5–2.5 mg/d, or high-dose risperidone, 3.0–6.0 mg/d. In both active medication groups, treatment with risperidone significantly decreased the total YMRS score. No evidence of increased efficacy was observed at doses >2.5 mg/d. Subjects in the high-dose group had significantly more extrapyramidal side effects than those in the low-dose group, 25% vs. 5%, indicating the lower dose is preferable.

A large, industry-sponsored, double-blind placebo controlled study of olanzapine (Tohen *et al.* 2007) included 159 children and adolescents (aged 10–17 years) with BD who were randomized to placebo or olanzapine (1:2 ratio) for 3 weeks. There was a statistically significant greater reduction in manic symptoms in the olanzapine group as compared to the placebo group. However, 42% of the children and adolescents gained ≥ 7% of their baseline body weight. Other side effects of olanzapine included lipid profile abnormalities and elevated prolactin levels. Given that the need for medication can be long-term, these medication effects on weight and lipids are a major concern.

Table 12.3 Summary of atypical controlled trials in pediatric bipolar disorder

Study/ sponsor	Reference	N	Sites	Age range (years)	DX	Design	Duration (days)	Dose (mg/d)	Response rate (YMRS)	Mean weight gain (kg)
Olanz./ Lilly	(Tohen et al. 2007)	161	26	10–17	BPD I Manic, mixed	DBPCRT 2:1	21	10.4 ± 4.5	49%	3.66 ± 2.18
Risper./ Janssan	(Haas et al. 2009)	169	M	10–17	BPD I Manic, mixed	DBPCRT 1:1:1	21	0.5–2.5 3–6	59% 63%	1.9 1.4
Aripip/ BMS	(Findling et al. 2009)	296	M	10–17	BPD I Manic, mixed	DBPCRT 1:1:1	28	10 30	45% 64%	0.9 0.54
Que/ Astra-Zeneca	(DelBello et al. 2007)	284	M	10–17	BPD I Manic	DBPCRT 1:1:1	21	400 600	64% 58%	1.7
Zipras/ Pfizer	(DelBello et al. 2007)	238	M	10–17	BPD I Manic, mixed	DBPCRT 2:1	28	80–160	−13.83 (Zipras) −8.61 (PBO)	–

There is a controlled trial of quetiapine in which 277 subjects with a BD I manic episode were assigned to quetiapine 400 mg/d, 600 mg/d, or placebo in a double-blind for 3 weeks (DelBello et al. 2007). Both doses of quetiapine demonstrated efficacy as compared to placebo. The most common adverse effects noted with quetiapine were somnolence, sedation, dizziness, and weight gain (1.7 kg).

There was also a large industry-supported, multisite trial of aripiprazole in which 296 subjects with BD I mixed or manic episodes were randomized to aripiprazole or placebo for 4 weeks (Wagner et al. 2007). During this trial, subjects were randomized to either 10 mg/d or 30 mg/d of aripiprazole, or placebo in a 1:1:1 ratio. Both doses of aripiprazole demonstrated clinical and statistical superiority to placebo with 45% in the low-dose group vs. 64% in the high-dose group demonstrating a ≥ 50% drop in their baseline YMRS scores. The most common adverse events reported during this trial were somnolence (23%), extrapyramidal disorder (18%), and fatigue (11%).

Lastly, ziprasidone was studied in a large multisite trial during which 238 pediatric subjects with BD I, manic or mixed, were randomized in a 2:1 ratio in a double-blinded fashion to treatment with flexible-dose ziprasidone (80–160 mg/d) or placebo (DelBello et al. 2008). In the intent-to-treat analysis, ziprasidone demonstrated an effect that was clinically and statistically significant in children and adolescents

with BD I. No significant changes in mean body mass index scores, or lipids, liver enzymes, or glucose levels were reported. Ziprasidone appears to be the only atypical antipsychotic that causes little or no weight gain in bipolar children and adolescents, but it also the only atypical antipsychotic that did not receive an FDA indication for the treatment of mania in children or adolescents. This was because of methodological problems during their pediatric registration trials.

Geller et al. recently published the results of the "Treatment of Early Age Mania" (TEAM) trial in which 290 children aged 6–15 years diagnosed with bipolar I disorder (having mixed or manic symptoms) were randomized in a double-blind to treatment with lithium, divalproex sodium, or risperidone for 8 weeks (Geller et al. 2012). They reported that after 8 weeks, 68% of the children taking risperidone showed improvement in manic symptoms, compared to 35% of those taking lithium and 24% of those taking divalproex sodium. Overall, 24% discontinued the trial, but more children taking lithium, 32%, discontinued the trial compared to those taking risperidone (15% discontinued) or divalproex sodium (26% discontinued). Bipolar subjects treated with risperidone gained more weight than those on the other medications, an average of more than 7 lb compared to 3 lb for those taking lithium and 3.7 lb for those taking divalproex sodium. The investigators concluded that risperidone was significantly more effective than lithium or divalproex sodium for initial treatment of pediatric mania. In addition, the subjects were less likely to discontinue the drug compared to those taking lithium or divalproex sodium, indicating a higher tolerance for it.

Combination treatment strategies

Kafantaris and colleagues (2001) evaluated acutely manic adolescents with psychotic features following treatment with lithium to assess whether adjunctive antipsychotics are necessary to stabilize psychotic mania. Antipsychotics were gradually tapered and discontinued after 4 weeks of therapeutic lithium levels in patients whose psychotic symptoms resolved. These patients were maintained with lithium monotherapy for up to 4 weeks. Significant improvement was seen in 64% of the sample with psychotic features after 4 weeks of combination treatment. However, 43% did not maintain their mood response after discontinuation of the antipsychotic medication, suggesting that greater than 4 weeks of antipsychotic treatment is required for some adolescents with psychotic mania. Variables associated with successful discontinuation of antipsychotic medication were first episode status, shorter duration of psychosis, and the presence of thought disorder at baseline (Kafantaris et al. 2001).

One study found that the combination of mood stabilizers and atypical antipsychotics was more effective than mood stabilizer alone for adolescent mania (DelBello et al. 2002). A 6-month open trial compared the efficacy of two combination therapies for manic or mixed episodes of pediatric BD (Pavuluri et al. 2004). This study examined divalproex and risperidone vs. lithium and risperidone in 37 subjects aged 5–18 years with a mixed or manic episode. Effect sizes based on change in YMRS scores from baseline to endpoint were 4.36 for the divalproex and risperidone combination group and 2.82 for the lithium and risperidone combination group. Response rates based on a $\geq 50\%$ decrease from baseline in YMRS score were 80% for the divalproex and risperidone group and 82.4% for the lithium and risperidone group; both combination treatments were well tolerated. Results of this open trial suggest that either treatment strategy may be used for adolescents with mania, although the findings must be confirmed in randomized designs, and side effects increase when patients are treated with combination therapy.

In the first comparison study of a mood stabilizer to an atypical antipsychotic for the treatment of mania in adolescents, DelBello and colleagues randomized 50 adolescents (ages 12–18 years) with bipolar I disorder, manic or mixed episode, to quetiapine (400–600 mg/d) or divalproex (serum level 80–120 µg/mL) for 28 days in a double-blind study and found that patients receiving quetiapine had faster resolution of their manic symptoms and higher rates of remission than those treated with divalproex. Additionally, both medications were well tolerated (DelBello et al. 2006).

In a double-blind, placebo-controlled study of an atypical antipsychotic for the treatment of bipolar adolescents, quetiapine in combination with divalproex resulted in a greater reduction of manic symptoms than divalproex monotherapy, suggesting that the combination of a mood stabilizer and an atypical antipsychotic is more effective than a mood stabilizer alone for the treatment of adolescent mania. In this study, quetiapine was titrated to a dose of 450 mg/d in 7 days and was well tolerated (Delbello et al. 2002).

Medication algorithm for treatment of mania

There are four main factors to consider when choosing a medication for mania in a child or adolescent: efficacy, safety, tolerability, and cost. The ideal medication will have demonstrated efficacy as compared to placebo, demonstrate no adverse medical effects, be tolerable by most patients, which increases adherence, and be relatively affordable – patients will only take medicine that they can afford. The second-generation antipsychotics, though efficacious, may also cause significant side effects that must be recognized and managed effectively. These side effects include extrapyramidal effects, tardive dyskinesia, obesity, hyperlipidemia, increased prolactin levels, and cardiac QTc changes. There is emerging evidence that children and adolescents may be more susceptible to these side effects than adults (Correll, 2005). A review of these adverse effects is beyond the scope of this chapter but Correll and colleagues have published several recent reviews on this topic (Correll, 2008a, b).

Based upon the adult and pediatric evidence reviewed above, safety, tolerability, and clinical experience, we offer the following treatment algorithm for treating mania/hypomania.

For a child or adolescent with a mixed or manic episode, Stage 1A of this algorithm recommends monotherapy with quetiapine, aripiprazole, or

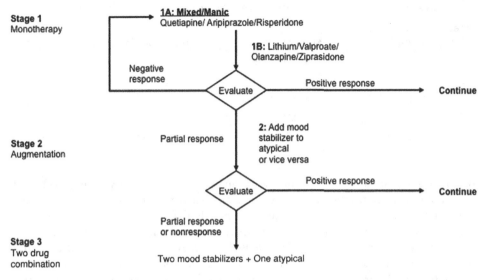

Figure 12.1 Treatment algorithm for mania/hypomania in children and adolescents

risperidone. The particular medication chosen at this stage will depend upon the patient's past experiences with these medications, their metabolic profile, and FDA indication. Quetiapine has the advantage of low risk of EPS and TD, aripiprazole also has a relatively low weight-gain risk. Risperidone, though very potent at low doses, will increase prolactin levels and the long-term significance of this is unknown, as discussed above. Lithium and valproate are considered as second-line choices, "1B," because of their lower potency compared to atypicals, and olanzapine, though very potent, causes significant weight gain and was also considered as a Stage 1B agent. Ziprasidone has not received an FDA indication for the treatment of mania in this age group and is also considered second line.

If a patient is not able to tolerate the first atypical agent chosen because of lack of response or intolerable side effects, then the option is to cycle back up through an alternative agent from 1A or 1B. Stage 2 of this algorithm is for patients who show a partial response, "mild to moderately improved," to monotherapy, but who are not "much or very much improved." Stage 3 of this algorithm recommends combination treatment with two mood stabilizers, e.g., lithium and valproate, and an atypical antipsychotic. Alternatively, two atypicals together or, two atypicals with a mood stabilizer are possible treatment combinations with the understanding that there is no evidence at this time about the efficacy of these combinations in bipolar children and adolescents. Two atypicals may increase the metabolic syndrome risk. Table 12.4 summarizes dosing and monitoring information for the use of atypical antipsychotics in children and adolescents with manic or hypomanic symptoms.

Bipolar depression

Adolescents with BD whose index episode is major depression are more likely to experience a poorer outcome compared with those with an index episode of mania or mixed mania (Strober *et al.* 1995). Despite the severe morbidity and mortality associated with bipolar depression, there are limited data regarding the treatment of depression in children and adolescents with BD.

Treatment of bipolar depression can be complicated because of the often necessary use of combinations of medications, including antidepressants, that may induce mania, hypomania, or rapid cycling (Compton and Nemeroff, 2000). A retrospective study assessing treatment of depressed children and adolescents with BD suggests that selective serotonin reuptake inhibitors (SSRIs) may be effective for acute bipolar depression, but these agents may be associated with mood destabilization and exacerbation of manic symptoms (Biederman *et al.* 2000). Specifically, in this study, depressive symptoms were 6.7 times more likely to improve when subjects received an SSRI. However, SSRIs were associated with a threefold greater

Table 12.4 Summary of the use of atypical antipsychotics in children and adolescents with manic or hypomanic symptoms

Atypical antipsychotic	Start at (mg/d)	Target dose (mg/d)	Monitor	Watch out for
Aripiprazole	2.5–5	5–20	Weight/height/BMI	EPS
Olanzapine	5	5–20	Weight/height/BMI	Weight (Choles/FAs)
Quetiapine	50–100	300–600	Weight/height/BMI	Weight
Risperidone	0.25–0.50	1–3	Weight/height/BMI	EPS/TD/weight
Ziprasidone	20–40	80–160	Weight/height/BMI, ECG	Take with food; assess cardiac risk factors

probability of relapse of manic symptomatology. In patients with active manic symptoms, the concomitant use of SSRIs with mood stabilizer treatment did not significantly inhibit the improvement of manic symptoms associated with mood stabilizer treatment. Thus, further studies of antidepressants in combination with mood stabilizers or atypical antipsychotics are needed. Antidepressant medications should be used with caution in children and adolescents with BD because of the potential risk for increased mood instability and for the emergence of suicidal ideation. On the other hand, depression is a major cause of morbidity and suicide risk, and so effective treatment of the depression is critical to giving the patient the quality of life in social and educational domains that are so important at this stage of life. Our clinical experience is that it is optimal to treat first with a mood stabilizer like lithium and if there is no antidepressant response after 6–8 weeks, to add a low dose of an SSRI.

As previously described, there have been two recent prospective open-label studies assessing lithium and lamotrigine for bipolar depression in adolescents (Chang et al. 2006, Patel et al. 2006). Methodological differences between the studies make it difficult to compare the results. Specifically, Chang et al. included adolescents with depression or mixed episodes, and bipolar disorder, type I or II, and lamotrigine was used as monotherapy or adjunctive to other medication (Chang et al. 2006). In contrast, Patel et al. included only adolescents with bipolar disorder, type I, and depressed, and lithium was used as monotherapy (Patel et al. 2006). Nonetheless, these studies suggest that both medications may be useful for depression associated with bipolar disorder in adolescents.

Recent placebo-controlled studies suggest that atypical antipsychotics, specifically, quetiapine and olanzapine, are useful for the treatment of depression in bipolar adults (Calabrese et al. 2005). In contrast, a double-blind, placebo-controlled study revealed that quetiapine may be no more effective than placebo for depression associated with bipolar disorder in adolescents, although the response rate to placebo in this study was large and the sample was small (N = 32) (DelBello et al. 2009). Additional controlled trials of various medications effective for adult bipolar depression, e.g., the olanzapine–fluoxetine combination medication (Symbyax), are needed in children and adolescents with bipolar disorder.

Maintenance treatment

In addition to the treatment of acute affective episodes, lithium may also be useful for the prevention of recurrent affective episodes in children and adolescents with BD. One early maintenance treatment study for pediatric bipolar disorder (Strober et al. 1990) prospectively evaluated 37 adolescents whose mood had been stabilized with lithium while hospitalized. After 18 months of follow-up, 35% of these patients discontinued lithium, and 92% of those who discontinued subsequently relapsed, as compared to 38% of those who were lithium-compliant, supporting the potential utility of lithium for maintenance treatment for adolescent BD.

Findling and colleagues (2006) published the results of an open trial of lithium combined with divalproex. The participants (N = 38, mean age of 10.5 years) had initially responded to lithium combined with divalproex, but had relapsed during monotherapy with either medication. All were treated with lithium and divalproex as outpatients for 8 weeks and 89% of subjects responded to restabilization with this combination. Based on these findings, the authors concluded that youths who had initially responded to a combination of lithium with divalproex may be effectively restabilized on this combination if they relapse during maintenance monotherapy with either medication.

Treatment of co-morbid disorders

Children and adolescents with bipolar disorder commonly present with co-occurring psychiatric disorders (Pavuluri *et al.* 2005), the most common of which is ADHD. Treatment of children with BD and co-occurring ADHD requires stabilization with a traditional mood stabilizer or an atypical antipsychotic as a necessary prerequisite to initiating stimulant medications (Biederman *et al.* 1999). However, controlled studies are lacking to support this common clinical practice. A randomized controlled trial of 40 bipolar children and adolescents with ADHD demonstrated that low-dose mixed-salts amphetamines are effective and well tolerated for the treatment of co-morbid ADHD symptoms following mood stabilization with divalproex (Scheffer *et al.* 2005). None of these patients experienced any mood destabilization while treated with stimulants and our clinical experience has been that if you stabilize a bipolar patient's mood first with a mood stabilizer or atypical antipsychotic, then it is safe to add a stimulant for ADHD. Sustained-release psychostimulants may be more effective at reducing rebound symptoms in bipolar children and adolescents compared with immediate-release formulations of stimulant mediations.

Disruptive behavior disorders also commonly co-occur in children and adolescents with BD. One study suggested that divalproex may be effective to treat aggressive symptoms associated with bipolar disorder in adolescents (DelBello *et al.* 2004) Additionally, in a post-hoc analysis of a controlled prospective study, quetiapine was found to reduce aggression in bipolar adolescents with co-occurring disruptive behavior disorders (Barzman *et al.* 2006), suggesting that in the sub-set of youths with BD and co-occurring disruptive behavior disorders, atypical antipsychotics may be warranted.

Up to 40% of bipolar adolescents have co-occurring substance-use disorders (Wilens *et al.* 2004). Despite this high co-occurrence there has been only one small treatment study of bipolar adolescents with substance-use disorders (Geller *et al.* 1998a), which suggested lithium may be more effective than placebo. Results from recent studies suggest that topiramate may be useful for the treatment of disorders related to poor impulse control in adults, including alcohol dependence (Johnson *et al.* 2003), binge eating (McElroy *et al.* 2004), and bulimia nervosa (Hoopes

et al. 2003). Alternatively, children and adolescents who are earlier in their illness course may respond differently than older patients, who typically have a history of multiple treatment failures. Specifically, the relationship between acute affective episodes and cellular stress has been well documented (Manji and Zarate, 2002). Stress-induced cortisol elevation results in excessive neuronal glutamate release that typically occurs following a major stressor (e.g., onset of an illness). Therefore, bipolar youth who are closer to illness onset may be more likely than adults, who are further along in illness course, to respond to medications that block acute glutamanergic release. Indeed, topiramate inhibits the excitatory effects of glutamanergic receptors. These findings highlight the importance of evaluating new treatment options for BD in age-specific controlled trials.

Other treatment alternatives

It is important for clinicians to be familiar with complementary and alternative medicine (CAM) and integrative therapies for bipolar disorder, as parents may well be using them for their affected children, with or without informing the clinician. Reasons patients and families may be interested in CAM and integrative therapy use include incomplete response to conventional treatments, concern about conventional treatment side effects and perceived safety of CAM, as well as greater accessibility, particularly for those with limited access to mental health, insurance, or distrust of traditional medicine. Families may thus turn to over-the-counter products with potentially lower cost than conventional treatments, as well as holistic practitioners. A good psychiatric history will include a formal inquiry of alternative approaches, including both oral agents and other techniques such as acupuncture.

A literature review by Sarris *et al.* (2011) on the use of complementary and alternative treatments (CAM) for bipolar disorder found evidence for nutritional supplements adjunctive to conventional first-line pharmacotherapy for bipolar depression, as well as for branched chain amino acids and magnesium for mania. Overall severity of illness may be influenced by diet quality, including micronutrients (vitamins and minerals) and quality protein sources providing adequate amino acid intake. More details on CAMs may be found in Chapter 18.

Clinical pearls

1. ADHD with ODD is common, bipolar disorder is not.
2. The most common cause of "mood swings" in children and adolescents is an anxiety disorder that has been overlooked.
3. The atypical antipsychotics are powerful first-line treatments for mania but they come with a high cost – weight gain and all of its consequences.
4. The traditional mood stabilizers, lithium and valproate, have been relegated to second-line treatments for bipolar disorder due to their smaller effect sizes and need for more frequent blood draws.
5. There are no great treatments for bipolar depression in children and adolescents.
6. It is important to diagnose and treat the frequent co-morbid disorders of pediatric bipolar disorder.

Future directions

The diagnosis and treatment of children and adolescents can be difficult due to developmental differences in symptom presentation, frequent co-morbidities, and phases of the illness. When considering the initial plan after assessing a child or adolescent with symptoms resembling mania, one of the most important decisions to be made is whether treatment with medication commonly utilized for pediatric BPD is indicated. There are now sufficient evidence-based studies that demonstrate the effectiveness of atypical antipsychotics for the treatment of manic or mixed episodes in bipolar children and adolescents that these agents have become first-line agents for this disorder. Another emerging area of interest is the use of two atypical antipsychotics together or an atypical antipsychotic with a typical antipsychotic. One area for further research is how to best combine atypical antipsychotics with the traditional mood stabilizers, lithium and divalproex, and how long patients should be treated for with any agent.

But, the potential adverse effects of these agents must be recognized, monitored, and managed. Also, there is, for some CAM and integrative techniques, scientific rationale to suspect that they may be shown in future prospective controlled research to be definitively helpful; such studies will likely need to include appropriate screening to determine whether certain patients display genetic allelic variants or dietary aberrancies that may increase or decrease their likelihood of response to both conventional and non-conventional treatments. Such research is critical to the future of integrative care in mental health and may add significantly to the ability to assist patients with expeditious and safe improvement in their bipolar illness.

References

Akiskal, H.S., Downs, J., Jordan, P. *et al.* (1985). Affective disorders in referred children and younger siblings of manic-depressives. Mode of onset and prospective course. *Archives of General Psychiatry*, 42, 996–1003.

Barzman, D.H., DelBello, M.P., Adler, C.M., Stanford, K.E., and Strakowski, S.M. (2006). The efficacy and tolerability of quetiapine versus divalproex for the treatment of impulsivity and reactive aggression in adolescents with co-occurring bipolar disorder and disruptive behavior disorder(s). *Journal of Child and Adolescent Psychopharmacology*, 16, 665–670.

Biederman, J., Mick, E., Spencer, T.J., Wilens, T.E., and Faraone, S.V. (2000). Therapeutic dilemmas in the pharmacotherapy of bipolar depression in the young. *Joural of Child and Adolescent Psychopharmacology*, 10, 185–192.

Biederman, J., Mick, E., Prince, J. *et al.* (1999). Systematic chart review of the pharmacologic treatment of comorbid attention deficit hyperactivity disorder in youth with bipolar disorder. *Journal of Child and Adolescent Psychopharmacology*, 9, 247–256.

Bowden, C.L. and Karren, N.U. (2006). Anticonvulsants in bipolar disorder. *Australian and New Zealand Journal of Psychiatry*, 40, 386–393.

Bowden, C.L., Calabrese, J.R., Sachs, G. *et al.* (2003). A placebo-controlled 18-month trial of lamotrigine and lithium maintenance treatment in recently manic or hypomanic patients with bipolar I disorder. *Archives of General Psychiatry*, 60, 392–400.

Buchsbaum, M.S., Wu, J., Siegel, B.V. *et al.* (1997). Effect of sertraline on regional metabolic rate in patients with affective disorder. *Biological Psychiatry*, 41, 15–22.

Cade, J.F. (1949). Lithium salts in the treatment of psychotic excitement. *Medical Journal of Australia*, 36, 349–352.

Calabrese, J., Bowden, C., Sachs, G. *et al.* (1999). A double-blind placebo-controlled study of lamotrigine monotherapy in outpatients with bipolar I depression. *Journal of Clinical Psychiatry*, 60, 79–88.

Calabrese, J.R., Elhaj, O., Gajwani, P., and Gao, K. (2005). Clinical highlights in bipolar depression: Focus on atypical antipsychotics. *Journal of Clinial Psychiatry*, 66 Suppl 5, 26–33.

Calabrese, J.R., Sullivan, J.R., Bowden, C.L. *et al.* (2002). Rash in multicenter trials of lamotrigine in mood disorders: Clinical relevance and management. *Journal of Clinical Psychiatry*, 63, 1012–1019.

Carr, R.B. and Shrewsbury, K. (2007). Hyperammonemia due to valproic acid in the psychiatric setting. *American Journal of Psychiatry*, 164, 1020–1027.

Chang, K., Saxena, K., and Howe, M. (2006). An open-label study of lamotrigine adjunct or monotherapy for the treatment of adolescents with bipolar depression. *Journal of the American Academy of Child and Adolescent Psychiatry*, 45, 298–304.

Ciraulo, D.A., Shader, R.J., Greenblatt, D.J., and Creelman, W.L. (eds.) (1995). *Drug Interactions in Psychiatry*. Baltimore, MD: Williams and Wilkins.

Compton, M.T. and Nemeroff, C.B. (2000). The treatment of bipolar depression. *Journal of Clinical Psychiatry*, 61 Suppl 9, 57–67.

Correll, C.U. (2005). Metabolic side effects of second-generation antipsychotics in children and adolescents: A different story? *Journal of Clinical Psychiatry*, 66, 1331–1332.

Correll, C.U. (2008a). Antipsychotic use in children and adolescents: Minimizing adverse effects to maximize outcomes. *Journal of the American Academy of Child and Adolescent Psychiatry*, 47, 9–20.

Correll, C.U. (2008b). Assessing and maximizing the safety and tolerability of antipsychotics used in the treatment of children and adolescents. *Journal of Clinical Psychiatry*, 69, 26–36.

Cueva, J.E., Overall, J.E., Small, A.M. *et al.* (1996). Carbamazepine in aggressive children with conduct disorder: a double-blind and placebo-controlled study. *Journal of the American Academy of Child and Adolescent Psychiatry*, 35, 480–490.

DelBello, M., Findling, R.L., Earley, W., Acevedo, L., and Stankowski, J. (2007). *Efficacy of quetiapine in children and adolescents with bipolar mania: A 3-week, double-blind, randomized, placebo-controlled trial.* 54th Annual Meeting of the American Academy of Child and Adolescent Psychiatry, Boston, MA.

DelBello, M., Findling, R.L., Wang, P., Gundapaneni, B., and Versavel, M. (2008). *Safety and Efficacy of Ziprasidone in Pediatric Bipolar Disorder*. Washington, DC: American Psychiatric Assocation.

DelBello, M.P., Adler, C., and Strakowski, S.M. (2004). Divalproex for the treatment of aggression associated with adolescent mania. *Journal of Child and Adolescent Psychopharmacology*, 14, 325–328.

DelBello, M.P., Schwiers, M.L., Rosenberg, H.L., and Strakowski, S.M. (2002). A double-blind, randomized, placebo-controlled study of quetiapine as adjunctive treatment for adolescent mania. *Journal of the American Academy of Child and Adolescent Psychiatry*, 41, 1216–1223.

DelBello, M.P., Findling, R.L., Kushner, S. *et al.* (2005). A pilot controlled trial of topiramate for mania in children and adolescents with bipolar disorder. *Journal of the American Academy of Child and Adolescent Psychiatry*, 44, 539–547.

DelBello, M.P., Kowatch, R.A., Adler, C.M. *et al.* (2006). A double-blind randomized pilot study comparing quetiapine and divalproex for adolescent mania. *Journal of the American Academy of Child and Adolescent Psychiatry*, 45, 305–313.

DelBello, M.P., Chang, K., Welge, J.A. *et al.* (2009). A double-blind, placebo-controlled pilot study of quetiapine for depressed adolescents with bipolar disorder. *Bipolar Disorders*, 11, 483–493.

Devi, K., George, S., Criton, S., Suja, V., and Sridevi, P.K. (2005). Carbamazepine–the commonest cause of toxic epidermal necrolysis and Stevens–Johnson syndrome: A study of 7 years. *Indian Journal of Dermatology, Venereology and Leprology*, 71, 325–328.

Ee, L.C., Shepherd, R.W., Cleghorn, G.J. *et al.* (2003). Acute liver failure in children: A regional experience. *Journal of Paediatrics and Child Health*, 39, 107–110.

Evans, R.W., Clay, T.H., and Gualtieri, C.T. (1987). Carbamazepine in pediatric psychiatry. *Journal of the American Academy of Child and Adolescent Psychiatry*, 26, 2–8.

Faraone, S.V., Biederman, J., Wozniak, J. *et al.* (1997). Is comorbidity with ADHD a marker for juvenile-onset mania? *Journal of the American Academy of Child and Adolescent Psychiatry*, 36, 1046–1055.

Findling, R.L., Gracious, B.L., McNamara, N.K. *et al.* (2001). Rapid, continuous cycling and psychiatric co-morbidity in pediatric bipolar I disorder. *Bipolar Disorders*, 3, 202–210.

Findling, R.L., McNamara, N.K., Youngstrom, E.A. *et al.* (2005). Double-blind 18-month trial of lithium versus divalproex maintenance treatment in pediatric bipolar disorder. *Journal of the American Academy of Child and Adolescent Psychiatry*, 44, 409–417.

Findling, R.L., McNamara, N.K., Stansbrey, R. *et al.* (2006). Combination lithium and divalproex sodium in pediatric bipolar symptom re-stabilization. *Journal of the American Academy of Child and Adolescent Psychiatry*, 45, 142–148.

Findling, R.L., Nyilas, M., Forbes, R.A. *et al.* (2009). Acute treatment of pediatric bipolar I disorder, manic or mixed episode, with aripiprazole: A randomized, double-blind, placebo-controlled study. *Journal of Clinical Psychiatry*, 70, 1441–1451.

Fristad, M.A. and Goldberg-Arnold, J.S. (2002). Working with families of children with early-onset bipolar disorder. In Geller, B. and DelBello, M., eds., *Child and Early Adolescent Bipolar Disorder: Theory, Assessment and Treatment.* New York, NY: Guilford Publications, Inc.

Geddes, J.R., Burgess, S., Hawton, K., Jamison, K., and Goodwin, G.M. (2004). Long-term lithium therapy for bipolar disorder: systematic review and meta-analysis of randomized controlled trials. *American Journal of Psychiatry*, 161, 217–222.

Geller, B. and Luby, J. (1997). Child and adolescent bipolar disorder: a review of the past 10 years. *Journal of the American Academy of Child and Adolescent Psychiatry*, 36, 1168–1176.

Geller, B., Tillman, R., Craney, J.L., and Bolhofner, K. (2004). Four-year prospective outcome and natural history of mania in children with a prepubertal and early adolescent bipolar disorder phenotype. *Archives of General Psychiatry*, 61, 459–467.

Geller, B., Cooper, T.B., Sun, K. *et al.* (1998a). Double-blind and placebo-controlled study of lithium for adolescent bipolar disorders with secondary substance dependency. *Journal of the American Academy of Child and Adolescent Psychiatry*, 37, 171–178.

Geller, B., Williams, M., Zimerman, B. *et al.* (1998b). Prepubertal and early adolescent bipolarity differentiate from ADHD by manic symptoms, grandiose delusions, ultra-rapid or ultradian cycling. *Journal of Affective Disorders*, 51, 81–91.

Geller, B., Bolhofner, K., Craney, J. *et al.* (2000a). Psychosocial functioning in a prepubertal and early adolescent bipolar disorder phenotype. *Journal of the American Academy of Child and Adolescent Psychiatry*, 39, 1543–1548.

Geller, B., Zimerman, B., Williams, M. *et al.* (2000b). Diagnostic characteristics of 93 cases of a prepubertal and early adolescent bipolar disorder phenotype by gender, puberty and comorbid attention deficit hyperactivity disorder. *Journal of Child and Adolescent Psychopharmacology*, 10, 157–164.

Geller, B., Zimerman, B., Williams, M. *et al.* (2001). Reliability of the Washington University in St. Louis Kiddie Schedule for Affective Disorders and Schizophrenia (WASH-U-KSADS) mania and rapid cycling sections. *Journal of the American Academy of Child and Adolescent Psychiatry*, 40, 450–455.

Geller, B., Luby, J.L., Joshi, P. *et al.* (2012). A randomized controlled trial of risperidone, lithium, or divalproex sodium for initial treatment of bipolar I disorder, manic or mixed phase, in children and adolescents. *Archives of General Psychiatry*, 69, 515–528.

Haas, M., DelBello, M.P., Pandina, G. *et al.* (2009). Risperidone for the treatment of acute mania in children

and adolescents with bipolar disorder: A randomized, double-blind, placebo-controlled study. *Bipolar Disorders*, 11, 687–700.

Hoopes, S.P., Reimherr, F.W., Hedges, D.W. *et al.* (2003). Treatment of bulimia nervosa with topiramate in a randomized, double-blind, placebo-controlled trial, part 1: Improvement in binge and purge measures. *Journal of Clinical Psychiatry*, 64, 1335–1341.

Isojarvi, J.I., Laatikainen, T.J., Pakarinen, A.J., Juntunen, K.T., and Myllyla, V.V. (1993). Polycystic ovaries and hyperandrogenism in women taking valproate for epilepsy. *New England Journal of Medicine*, 329, 1383–1388.

Joffe, H., Cohen, L.S., Suppes, T. *et al.* (2006). Valproate is associated with new-onset oligoamenorrhea with hyperandrogenism in women with bipolar disorder. *Biological Psychiatry*, 59, 1078–1086.

Johnson, B.A., Ait-Daoud, N., Bowden, C.L. *et al.* (2003). Oral topiramate for treatment of alcohol dependence: A randomised controlled trial. *Lancet*, 361, 1677–1685.

Kafantaris, V., Coletti, D.J., Dicker, R., Padula, G., and Kane, J.M. (2001). Adjunctive antipsychotic treatment of adolescents with bipolar psychosis. *Journal of the American Academy of Child and Adolescent Psychiatry*, 40, 1448–1456.

Kafantaris, V., Coletti, D.J., Dicker, R., Padula, G., and Kane, J.M. (2003). Lithium treatment of acute mania in adolescents: A large open trial. *Journal of the American Academy of Child and Adolescent Psychiatry*, 42, 1038–1045.

Kafantaris, V., Campbell, M., Padron-Gayol, M.V. *et al.* (1992). Carbamazepine in hospitalized aggressive conduct disorder children: An open pilot study. *Psychopharmacological Bulletin*, 28, 193–199.

Kafantaris, V., Coletti, D.J., Dicker, R. *et al.* (2004). Lithium treatment of acute mania in adolescents: A placebo-controlled discontinuation study. *Journal of the American Academy of Child and Adolescent Psychiatry*, 43, 984–993.

Keating, A. and Blahunka, P. (1995). Carbamazepine-induced Stevens–Johnson syndrome in a child. *Annals of Pharmacotherapy*, 29, 538–539.

Keck, P.E., Jr., Strawn, J.R., and McElroy, S.L. (2006). Pharmacologic treatment considerations in co-occurring bipolar and anxiety disorders. *Journal of Clinical Psychiatry*, 67 Suppl 1, 8–15.

Ketter, T.A., Nasrallah, H.A., and Fagiolini, A. (2006). Mood stabilizers and atypical antipsychotics: Bimodal treatments for bipolar disorder. *Psychopharmacological Bulletin*, 39, 120–146.

Ketter, T.A., Wang, P.W., Becker, O.V., Nowakowska, C., and Yang, Y.S. (2003). The diverse roles of anticonvulsants in bipolar disorders. *Annals of Clinical Psychiatry*, 15, 95–108.

Konig, S.A., Siemes, H., Blaker, F. *et al.* (1994). Severe hepatotoxicity during valproate therapy: An update and report of eight new fatalities. *Epilepsia*, 35, 1005–1015.

Kovacs, M. and Pollock, M. (1995). Bipolar disorder and comorbid conduct disorder in childhood and adolescence. *Journal of the American Academy of Child and Adolescent Psychiatry*, 34, 715–723.

Kowatch, R., Findling, R., Scheffer, R., and Stanford, K. (2007). *Placebo controlled trial of divalproex versus lithium for bipolar disorder.* 54th Annual Meeting of the American Academy of Child and Adolescent Psychiatry, October 26, 2007, Boston, MA.

Lewinsohn, P.M., Klein, D.N., and Seeley, J.R. (1995). Bipolar disorders in a community sample of older adolescents: prevalence, phenomenology, comorbidity, and course. *Journal of the American Academy of Child and Adolescent Psychiatry*, 34, 454–463.

Locharernkul, C., Shotelersuk, V., and Hirankarn, N. (2011). Pharmacogenetic screening of carbamazepine-induced severe cutaneous allergic reactions. *Journal of Clinical Neuroscience*, 18, 1289–1294.

Manji, H.K. and Zarate, C.A. (2002). Molecular and cellular mechanisms underlying mood stabilization in bipolar disorder: Implications for the development of improved therapeutics. *Molecular Psychiatry*, 7 Suppl 1, S1–S7.

McElroy, S. and Keck, P.J. (2000). Pharmacologic agents for the treatment of acute bipolar mania. *Biological Psychiatry*, 48, 539–557.

McElroy, S.L., Shapira, N.A., Arnold, L.M. *et al.* (2004). Topiramate in the long-term treatment of binge-eating disorder associated with obesity. *Journal of Clinical Psychiatry*, 65, 1463–1469.

Merikangas, K.R., He, J.P., Burstein, M. *et al.* (2010). Lifetime prevalence of mental disorders in U.S. adolescents: results from the National Comorbidity Survey Replication–Adolescent Supplement (NCS-A). *Journal of the American Academy of Child and Adolescent Psychiatry*, 49, 980–989.

Pande, A.C., Crockatt, J.G., Janney, C.A., Werth, J.L., and Tsaroucha, G. (2000). Gabapentin in bipolar disorder: A placebo-controlled trial of adjunctive therapy. *Bipolar Disorders*, 2, 249–255.

Patel, N.C., DelBello, M.P., Bryan, H.S. *et al.* (2006). Open-label lithium for the treatment of adolescents with bipolar depression. *Journal of the American Academy of Child and Adolescent Psychiatry*, 45, 289–297.

Pavuluri, M.N., Birmaher, B., and Naylor, M.W. (2005). Pediatric bipolar disorder: A review of the past 10 years. *Journal of the American Academy of Child and Adolescent Psychiatry*, 44, 846–871.

Pavuluri, M.N., Henry, D.B., Carbray, J.A. *et al.* (2004). Open-label prospective trial of risperidone in combination with lithium or divalproex sodium in pediatric mania. *Journal of Affective Disorders*, 82 Suppl 1, S103–S111.

Perlis, R.H., Welge, J.A., Vornik, L.A., Hirschfeld, R.M., and Keck, P.E. (2006). Atypical antipsychotics in the treatment of mania: A meta-analysis of randomized, placebo-controlled trials. *Journal of Clinical Psychiatry*, 67, 509–516.

Pleak, R.R., Birmaher, B., Gavrilescu, A., Abichandani, C., and Williams, D.T. (1988). Mania and neuropsychiatric excitation following carbamazepine. *Journal of the American Academy of Child and Adolescent Psychiatry*, 27, 500–503.

Puente, R.M. (1975). The use of carbamazepine in the treatment of behavioural disorders in children. In Birkmayer, W. (ed.) *Epileptic Seizures – Behaviour – Pain.* Baltimore, MD: University Park Press.

Quinn, C.A. and Fristad, M.A. (2004). Defining and identifying early onset bipolar spectrum disorder. *Current Psychiatry Reports*, 6, 101–107.

Rasgon, N. (2004). The relationship between polycystic ovary syndrome and antiepileptic drugs: A review of the evidence. *Journal of Clinical Psychopharmacology*, 24, 322–334.

Raskind, J.Y. and El-Chaar, G.M. (2000). The role of carnitine supplementation during valproic acid therapy. *Annals of Pharmacotherapy*, 34, 630–638.

Reimers, A., Helde, G., and Brodtkorb, E. (2005). Ethinyl estradiol, not progestogens, reduces lamotrigine serum concentrations. *Epilepsia*, 46, 1414–1417.

Sarris, J., Lake, J., and Hoenders, R. (2011). Bipolar disorder and complementary medicine: Current evidence, safety issues, and clinical considerations. *Journal of Alternative and Complementary Medicine*, 17, 881–890.

Scheffer, R., Kowatch, R., Carmody, T., and Rush, A. (2005). A randomized placebo-controlled trial of adderall for symptoms of comorbid ADHD in pediatric bipolar disorder following mood stabilization with divalproex sodium. *American Journal of Psychiatry*, 162, 58–64.

Sinclair, D.B., Berg, M., and Breault, R. (2004). Valproic acid-induced pancreatitis in childhood epilepsy: Case series and review. *Journal of Child Neurology*, 19, 498–502.

Storosum, J.G., Wohlfarth, T., Schene, A. *et al.* (2007). Magnitude of effect of lithium in short-term efficacy studies of moderate to severe manic episode. *Bipolar Disorders*, 9, 793–798.

Strober, M., Morrell, W., Lampert, C., and Burroughs, J. (1990). Relapse following discontinuation of lithium maintenance therapy in adolescents with bipolar I illness: A naturalistic study. *American Journal of Psychiatry*, 147, 457–461.

Strober, M., Schmidt-Lackner, S., Freeman, R. *et al.* (1995). Recovery and relapse in adolescents with bipolar affective illness: A five-year naturalistic, prospective follow-up. *Journal of the American Academy of Child and Adolescent Psychiatry*, 34, 724–731.

Tohen, M., Kryzhanovskaya, L., Carlson, G. *et al.* (2007). Olanzapine versus placebo in the treatment of adolescents with bipolar mania. *American Journal of Psychiatry*, 164, 1547–1556.

Treem, W.R. (1994). Inherited and acquired syndromes of hyperammonemia and encephalopathy in children. *Seminars in Liver Disease*, 14, 236–258.

Wagner, K., Nyilas, M., Forbes, R. *et al.* (2007). *Acute Efficacy of Aripiprazole for the Treatment of Bipolar I Disorder, Mixed or Manic, in Pediatric Patients*. Boca Raton, FL: American College of Neuropharmacology.

Wagner, K.D., Kowatch, R.A., Emslie, G.J. *et al.* (2006). A double-blind, randomized, placebo-controlled trial of oxcarbazepine in the treatment of bipolar disorder in children and adolescents. *American Journal of Psychiatry*, 163, 1179–1186.

Wagner, K.D., Redden, L., Kowatch, R.A. *et al.* (2009). A double-blind, randomized, placebo-controlled trial of divalproex extended-release in the treatment of bipolar disorder in children and adolescents. *Journal of the American Academy of Child and Adolescent Psychiatry*, 48, 519–532.

Weinberg, W.A. and Brumback, R.A. (1976). Mania in childhood: Case studies and literature review. *American Journal of Diseases of Children*, 130, 380–385.

Weisler, R.H., Cutler, A.J., Ballenger, J.C., Post, R.M., and Ketter, T.A. (2006). The use of antiepileptic drugs in bipolar disorders: a review based on evidence from controlled trials. *CNS Spectrums*, 11, 788–799.

Werlin, S.L. and Fish, D.L. (2006). The spectrum of valproic acid-associated pancreatitis. *Pediatrics*, 118, 1660–1663.

West, S.A., McElroy, S.L., Strakowski, S.M., Keck, P.E., Jr. and McConville, B.J. (1995). Attention deficit hyperactivity disorder in adolescent mania. *American Journal of Psychiatry*, 152, 271–273.

Wilens, T.E., Biederman, J., Kwon, A. *et al.* (2004). Risk of substance use disorders in adolescents with bipolar disorder. *Journal of the American Academy of Child and Adolescent Psychiatry*, 43, 1380–1386.

Wozniak, J. and Biederman, J. (1997). Childhood mania: Insights into diagnostic and treatment issues. *Journal of the Association for Academic Minority Physicians*, 8, 78–84.

Wozniak, J., Biederman, J., Kiely, K. *et al.* (1995). Mania-like symptoms suggestive of childhood-onset bipolar disorder in clinically referred children. *Journal of the American Academy of Child and Adolescent Psychiatry*, 34, 867–876.

Wozniak, J., Biederman, J., Faraone, S.V. *et al.* (1997). Mania in children with pervasive developmental disorder revisited. *Journal of the American Academy of Child and Adolescent Psychiatry*, 36, 1552–1559; discussion 1559–1560.

Youngstrom, E. A. and Duax, J. (2005). Evidence-based assessment of pediatric bipolar disorder, part I: Base rate and family history. *Journal of the American Academy of Child and Adolescent Psychiatry*, 44, 712–717.

Depression in the context of physical illness

Emily Gastelum, Philip R. Muskin, and Peter A. Shapiro

Defining the scope

Connections between abnormal mood states and abnormalities of bodily function have interested clinicians for centuries. There is a bidirectional association between depression and medical illness. Depression is associated with a higher risk of developing diabetes (Eaton *et al.* 1996), coronary heart disease (Wulsin and Singal, 2003), hypertension (Patten *et al.* 2009), and stroke (Pan *et al.* 2011). Depression predicts lower quality of life and increased morbidity and mortality in patients with diabetes (de Groot *et al.* 2001, Black *et al.* 2003), cardiac disease (Spertus *et al.* 2000, Faris *et al.* 2002, van Melle *et al.* 2004), and neurological disorders (House *et al.* 2001, Global Parkinson's Disease Survey Steering Committee, 2002, Hesdorffer *et al.* 2006).

Major depressive disorder (MDD) is common in patients with medical illness, though precise depression prevalence rates vary widely across studies and depend upon the population sampled, rating scales used, and the inclusion of a wider or narrower spectrum of depressive disorders (Li and Rodin, 2011). For example, point prevalence rates for diagnoses of MDD in heart disease patients have been estimated to be in the range of 17–27% (Rudisch and Nemeroff, 2003), for stroke 14–23% (Robinson, 2003), and for Parkinson's disease from 4–75% (McDonald *et al.* 2003). Prevalence rates of major depression in various medical illnesses are listed in Table 13.1. The prevalence of minor depression and dysthymic disorder is even higher. These *point* prevalence rates are remarkable in comparison to the 16.6% *lifetime* prevalence rate and 6.7% *12-month* prevalence rate of major depression in the general population in the United States (Kessler *et al.* 2005a, b).

The high prevalence of depression in medically ill patients may be accounted for at least in part by both

Table 13.1 Prevalence of major depressive disorder in selected medical conditions

Medical Illness	Prevalence (%)
Cancer	0–38
Diabetes	9–26
Heart disease	17–27
HIV/AIDS	14–19
Stroke	14–23
Epilepsy	20–55
Parkinson's disease	4–75

Data from Li and Rodin (2011) and Robinson (2003)

psychological reactions to illness and direct biological effects of illness or treatment on brain function.

Thinking about depression in the medically ill with the biopsychosocial model

The complexity of patients presenting with co-morbid psychiatric and medical symptoms demands thorough assessment and thoughtful integration of relevant clinical data. The biopsychosocial model offers a useful approach to this population.

Biological factors

A genetic-constitutional propensity for depressive disorders is suggested by a positive family history of mood disorder. Early age of onset of a depressive syndrome may also be an indicator of biological vulnerability to primary mood disorders. Early childhood traumas such as physical or sexual abuse, parental neglect, and abandonment have long-lasting effects on hypothalamic pituitary adrenal axis function,

Table 13.2 Medical conditions associated with depression secondary to a general medical condition

Disease	Examples
Cerebrovascular disease	
Degenerative neurological disease	Alzheimer's disease, Parkinson's disease, Huntington's disease
Hypothalamic pituitary adrenal Axis disorders	Addison's disease, Cushing's syndrome
Parathyroid disease	
Testosterone deficiency	
Hyper- and hypothyroid states	
Viral infections	HIV/AIDS, mononucleosis

resulting in tonic elevation of corticotrophin releasing hormone and heightened rates of depressive illness.

Medical causes of depression

In addition to evaluating biological risk factors for primary depressive disorders, clinicians evaluating and treating a medically ill patient for depression must consider whether depression is secondary to medical illness. Treating an underlying medical illness may result in resolution of depression, so the psychiatrist must explore whether underdiagnosis or undertreatment of medical disorders could account for a patient's mood syndrome. Depression secondary to medical illness is an appropriate diagnosis when the physiological effects of the illness on the brain directly result in depressive symptoms. Several medical disorders are associated with depressive symptoms in this way (Table 13.2). Occult hypothyroidism, though unusual, exemplifies disorders in which recognition and treatment of the underlying condition may alleviate depression symptoms. Therefore, contact with a patient's medical provider is essential and may shed light upon how well understood and managed the patient's medical illness has been, and identify barriers to care.

Drugs and substances

Depression is listed in textbooks and manufacturers' prescribing information materials as a possible adverse effect of a very large number of medications, but epidemiological evidence of a substantial risk for major depressive disorder associated with medications is lacking for most of these agents. Worsening of depressed mood and associated symptoms has been convincingly linked to a few specific medications, including corticosteroids, interferon-alpha, gonadotropin-releasing hormone agonists and progestin-releasing implanted contraceptives, and reserpine (Patten and Barbui, 2004). Data on the impact of beta-blockers on depression is unconvincing (Steffensmeier *et al.* 2006). Intoxication and withdrawal from alcohol and illicit substances can also cause or exacerbate transient dysphoric states, and chronic depressed mood and associated symptoms of depressive disorder occur frequently in alcohol-dependent patients during the early weeks and months of attempted sobriety after alcohol detoxification.

Psychosocial factors

In addition to organic causes of depression in the medically ill, other relevant factors to consider and explore with patients include: the meaning of the illness to the patient, the patient's causal attributions about illness, distorted cognitions or maladaptive behavioral responses to illness, coping mechanisms, and strengths or weaknesses which may be imbedded in patients' premorbid personality traits and style. These factors may affect how individuals manage their medical and psychiatric illnesses and can be important targets for treatment in the depressed medically ill. Other psychosocial stressors may be present independent of, but coinciding with, the patient's medical illness. Clinicians must be cautious not to assume that physical disease is the main or most important stressor facing a depressed, medically ill patient. Patients sometimes experience stressors or events that are external to their illness (e.g., marital problems, financial issues) as more distressing.

Example

An elderly, divorced woman admitted to the hospital with an infected foot ulcer and diabetic ketoacidosis endorsed several weeks of depressive symptoms and poor self-care. Her symptoms arose after her only daughter married and moved away from home. This patient may not identify diabetes as her most distressing problem. Treatment for her depression would require addressing social and interpersonal factors that are intertwined with her mood and ability to manage her medical illness. A careful personal and family psychiatric history will guide clinicians in understanding and addressing social and psychological stressors and vulnerability.

Diagnosing depression in the context of co-morbid medical illness

Despite the significant rates of depression among medically ill patients, depression is underdiagnosed and undertreated in these co-morbid populations (Fallowfield *et al.* 2001, Katon *et al.* 2004a). Assessing depression in the context of medical illness is challenging because somatic symptoms that are part of the diagnostic criteria for depression may overlap with symptoms commonly seen in medical illnesses (i.e., disturbances in sleep, appetite, concentration, energy, and psychomotor functioning). The DSM-IV does not provide specific advice to practitioners on how to differentiate MDD from mood disturbance secondary to a general medical condition or substance, beyond stating that to make a diagnosis of MDD, symptoms and signs must not be due to a general medical condition or substance (including medications) (McDonald *et al.* 2003). The problem is further complicated by the high prevalence of sub-syndromal depression, which surpasses that of MDD in medically ill patients (Tandberg *et al.* 1996, Fisher *et al.* 2008).

In practice, most consultation–liaison psychiatrists would, and we recommend it, take an inclusive approach to diagnosis, such that if a depressive symptom might also be ascribed to the patient's medical illness, it is nevertheless counted toward a depression diagnosis. We would hesitate to make a diagnosis of depression in the absence of sad or depressed mood, or pervasive loss of interest. We also recommend assessing the severity of sad or depressed mood, anhedonia, and difficulty participating in role responsibilities, including treatment of the co-morbid medical illness, as adjunctive factors to weigh in making the diagnosis of depression. When we are not sure whether to ascribe symptoms to depression or to another "medical" problem, we may aim to treat both the medical problem and the depression symptoms simultaneously.

Validated rating scales for assessing depression symptoms in patients with acute or chronic medical illnesses include the Center for Epidemiologic Studies Depression Scale, the Hospital Anxiety and Depression Scale, the Beck Depression Inventory-II and the Patient Health Questionnaire depression module. In primary care, the PHQ-2 and the PHQ-9, which mirror DSM-IV criteria for major depression, have been widely validated (Kroenke *et al.* 2001).

General principles of treatment

To treat or not to treat

Whether or not to treat depression in medically ill patients is an important question for both consultation–liaison and general psychiatrists. Severity of depression, patient preferences, risks associated with antidepressant therapy, and overall goals of care will all inform the decision-making process about whether and how to treat depression in a medically ill patient (including the risks of not treating depression). The course of depression is such that mood episodes may resolve without treatment and, in particular, depressive symptoms of mild severity and briefer duration are more likely to ameliorate without treatment. Sadness and depressive syndromes arising in the context of receiving bad medical news are more likely to remit, particularly in a patient with strong social supports, than a severe major depressive episode with onset preceding that of the patient's medical problem. Clinical history and structured rating scales to assess symptom severity may help providers in making determinations about urgency of active treatment instead of watchful waiting. Patient perception of psychopathology is another important factor to consider. Patients who meet criteria for dysthymia or even major depression may not perceive a need for psychiatric treatment, and data suggest that these patients make an appropriate estimation of their need for care (van Beljouw *et al.* 2010). At times, a patient's denial of mood problems is at odds with a medical provider's impression that depression is interfering with the patient's medical care. A common example of this would be the consultation called for "depression" in a debilitated post-surgical patient who is not participating actively in physical therapy and not eating enough to maintain calorie and protein intake needs for recovery. Here, the psychiatrist plays an important role in working with both parties to negotiate whether there is a problem that merits treatment.

Patient preferences affect treatment acceptability, ongoing treatment alliance, and treatment retention, and may improve depression treatment outcomes (Davidson *et al.* 2010, Gelhorn *et al.* 2011). In the medically ill, psychiatrists must weigh with patients the potential benefits of treatment against the potential medical adverse effect hazards. Goals of care are unique for each individual patient, such that specific treatments may be appropriate in some circumstances but not in others. For example, using opiates or stimulants to treat mood disorders might be a reasonable first line in a palliative care setting, but not a recommended first-line option for a long-term depression treatment in a patient who does not have terminal illness.

Psychotherapy, psychopharmacology, or other management (collaborative/ stepped care)

In medically ill patients, for whom psychopharmacologic side effects may be especially problematic, supportive or cognitive behavioral psychotherapeutic interventions may be preferable to drug treatment. Collaborative-care and stepped-care models also have high acceptability and good evidence for efficacy in the treatment of depression, in both primary care outpatient settings and in the treatment of patients with co-morbid depression with heart disease or diabetes (Katon *et al.* 2004b, Rollman *et al.* 2009). These models typically begin with screening, followed by psychoeducation, and may progress, if needed, to include brief supportive counseling or medication prescribed by the primary care provider. Referral for specialty care follows only for those patients who have not responded to first- and second-line interventions. Stepped-care approaches acknowledge that depression is generally first recognized and treated within a primary care setting and may be most efficiently and cost-effectively addressed in this real-world context.

Although some have argued that in patients with mild depressive symptoms antidepressants are no better than placebo (Fournier *et al.* 2010), other analyses have provided compelling evidence that even mild depression syndromes benefit from antidepressant therapy (Gibbons *et al.* 2012, Stewart *et al.* 2012). In patients who meet criteria for major depressive disorder, we do not withhold antidepressant therapy simply because symptoms are below an arbitrary threshold of severity.

General pharmacological issues

Pharmacodynamics and pharmacokinetics

Pharmacodynamics and pharmacokinetics warrant particular consideration in the medically ill. For example, an antidepressant side-effect profile may be used to target and ameliorate symptoms of medical illness in patients with co-morbid depression, and also should

be carefully considered so as not to exacerbate medical problems in this population. Issues relevant to drug absorption, distribution, metabolism, or excretion can be affected by medical illness or concomitant treatments. Drug–drug interactions require careful attention in medically ill depressed patients. An exhaustive review of pharmacodynamic and pharmacokinetic issues relevant to treating depression along with various medical illnesses is beyond the scope of this chapter. However, here we describe a few common and important considerations. Several excellent texts are available, including the *Textbook of Psychosomatic Medicine* (Levenson, 2011), the *Clinical Manual of Drug Interaction Principles for Medical Practice* (Wynn *et al.* 2009), and the *Clinical Handbook of Psychopharmacology in the Medically Ill* (Ferrando *et al.* 2010).

Specific indications and warnings: some clinical pearls

Depressed patients undergoing chemotherapy and suffering from nausea may benefit from mirtazapine rather than a selective serotonin reuptake inhibitor (SSRI) as first-line treatment. Mirtazapine has appetite-stimulating and antiemetic properties, while SSRIs can cause nausea. A patient with a carcinoid tumor may experience worsened symptoms if serotonin load is increased, but tolerate bupropion very well. Conversely, bupropion may elevate blood pressure at higher doses, and may lower the seizure threshold, and should be used cautiously or not at all in an individual with an intracerebral mass. A seizure disorder is considered a contraindication to its use. The addition of SSRIs in patients with bleeding vulnerabilities modestly increases bleeding risk due to a combination of effects on platelets and potential interactions with warfarin and antiplatelet therapies (Labos *et al.* 2011).

Renal failure patients are particularly sensitive to build-up of metabolites normally cleared through the kidneys following hepatic metabolism, and for this reason some authors have recommended using antidepressants at reduced doses in renal failure (Cohen *et al.* 2007). The antibiotic linezolid, commonly used to treat vancomycin- or methicillin-resistant bacterial infections, is an irreversible monoamine oxidase A inhibitor. Patients taking linezolid and serotonergic antidepressants are at increased risk of serotonin syndrome, while co-administration with stimulants elevates the risk of hypertensive crisis. The breast cancer drug tamoxifen is metabolized to its active antiestrogen metabolite, endoxifen, via cytochrome P450 2D6. 2D6 inhibition (e.g., by fluoxetine, paroxetine, duloxetine, and bupropion) decreases time to cancer recurrence in tamoxifen-treated patients, due to decreased availability of the active metabolite of tamoxifen (Goetz *et al.* 2007).

Diabetes

Psychotherapeutic strategies

Three trials have evaluated cognitive behavior therapy (CBT) for treatment of depression in patients with diabetes. The most rigorous of these studies randomized 51 depressed, type 2 diabetic subjects to either CBT and diabetes education or to education alone, and found that those receiving CBT achieved a significantly greater rate of remission from depression at the conclusion of the trial and at 6 months' follow-up than the subjects receiving only diabetic education (Lustman *et al.* 1998). Two more recent and less methodologically rigorous studies found that group CBT improves depression in diabetic patients (Jiménez Chafey and Rosselló, 2006, Georgiades *et al.* 2007). Brief supportive psychotherapy was effective in improving depressive symptoms in patients hospitalized with diabetic foot ulcers (Simson *et al.* 2008). A number of registered trials are in the process of examining CBT for depression with an integrated focus on diabetes education and care (Petrak and Herpertz, 2009).

A recurrent question in the diabetes and depression literature is whether treating depression might lead to improvements in glycemic control. Currently, there is limited data with mixed results. Lustman demonstrated a decrease in HbA1c in patients receiving CBT plus diabetes education 6 months after the intervention. The decline was unrelated to compliance with self-monitoring of blood glucose levels (Lustman *et al.* 1998), raising questions as to the mechanism by which improved mood correlates with better glycemic control. Other trials have not found psychotherapy for depression to result in improvements in HbA1c (Jiménez Chafey and Rosselló, 2006, Georgiades *et al.* 2007). In summary, we believe that, on balance, a trial of cognitive behavior therapy is appropriate to the goal of reducing depression symptoms in patients with diabetes, but we have less confidence that such interventions can robustly improve diabetes care adherence and glycemic control.

Psychopharmacologic strategies

Newer antidepressants are the treatment of choice in patients with co-morbid diabetes and depression, as opposed to tricyclic antidepressants (TCAs), which may exacerbate hyperglycemia (Lustman *et al.* 1997) and weight gain. There are no trials of MAO inhibitors for depression treatment in diabetes. MAO inhibitors cause weight gain in some patients (Rabkin *et al.* 1984). There are few trials to definitively guide treatment. Randomized controlled trials (RCTs) have demonstrated that fluoxetine is effective for moderate to severe depression in the context of co-morbid diabetes in the acute treatment phase (Lustman *et al.* 2000) and that sertraline is superior to placebo in the maintenance phase of antidepressant treatment (Lustman *et al.* 2006). A small RCT (n = 23) found fluoxetine and paroxetine both reduced the severity of depressive symptoms in diabetic patients (Gulseren *et al.* 2005). An open-label trial demonstrated that bupropion is an effective acute and maintenance treatment for depression in diabetic patients (Lustman *et al.* 2007), but this finding has not been clearly demonstrated for those with fewer depressive symptoms or lower scores on depression rating scales (Paile-Hyvarinen *et al.* 2003, 2007). None of these trials has distinguished between patients with a history of mood disorder arising before diabetes and patients whose depression first appeared after onset of diabetes.

Regarding glycemic control, a few studies have shown small improvements in HbA1c within the first year of treatment with SSRIs such as paroxetine (Paile-Hyvarinen *et al.* 2007), fluoxetine (Lustman *et al.* 2000, Gulseren *et al.* 2005), and sertraline (Lustman *et al.* 2006, Echeverry *et al.* 2009). Bupropion shows promise as a medication that may lead to improved glycemic control in diabetic patients who achieve remission of depression (Lustman *et al.* 2007).

In summary, drug treatment for depression in diabetes has not been shown to be different than drug treatment for depression in patients without co-morbid medical illness, except for the heightened need to avoid unwanted side effects of weight gain and worsening of glycemic control. Most SSRIs, venlafaxine, and bupropion would be appropriate choices for drug treatment in this patient population.

Collaborative care

The Pathways Study randomized 329 patients with diabetes and major depression or dysthymia to treatment as usual or a stepped-care approach in which subjects were evaluated by trained nurses with whom they spoke twice monthly. Patients were first offered problem-solving treatment or antidepressant medication. If their depression had not improved in 10–12 weeks, they were offered a change in treatment, augmentation of their treatment, or consultation with a psychiatrist. Persistent symptoms were addressed by referral to specialty psychiatric care. This intervention improved adequacy of antidepressant dosing, and led to a 40% reduction of depressive symptoms at 12 months, as compared to treatment as usual, with a number needed to treat (NNT) of 6.5 (Katon et al. 2004b). Reductions in health care costs were also significant (Simon et al. 2007). The IMPACT study demonstrated similarly robust findings in which a stepped-care approach was more effective at 12 months in decreasing depressive symptoms by ≥40% than treatment as usual in a population of depressed, diabetic patients ≥60 years of age, with NNT 4.3 as well as NNT 6.6 for depression response at 12 months (Williams et al. 2004). A third collaborative-care trial in which the intervention arm included treatment with citalopram or interpersonal therapy for older, depressed diabetic patients led to significantly lower rates of mortality after 5 years than treatment as usual (Bogner et al. 2007). Culturally sensitive, collaborative stepped-care models may also be effective in helping minority groups with co-morbid depression and diabetes to access and stay engaged with quality psychiatric care, resulting in better depression outcomes, but not necessarily differences in diabetic control (Ell et al. 2010).

While stepped-care/collaborative-care models have proven efficacious in treating depression and reducing health care costs, they have not demonstrated robust improvements in glycemic control (Katon et al. 2004b, Williams et al. 2004). These models suggest that psychiatrists can have significant impact in reducing depression in diabetic patients by acting as consultants to primary care providers who see and treat the greatest numbers of depressed patients with co-morbid medical illness.

Cardiovascular disease

Patients with heart disease have elevated risk for new-onset depression, likely due at least in part to the psychosocial stressors inherent in the course of living with illness. Depression is epidemiologically associated with increased risk for both incident coronary artery disease and recurrent cardiac events, and death in patients with established coronary disease (Rugulies, 2002, Barth et al. 2004, van Melle et al. 2004, Wulsin 2004). Patients with major depressive disorder comprise 15–20% of all patients with coronary disease, and have rates of recurrent myocardial infarction, sudden cardiac death, and all-cause mortality two to three times higher than those of patients without depression. This medical morbidity of depression is independent of traditional cardiac risk factors, and of other "medical" prognostic factors following cardiac events, such as severity of heart failure, leading to a search for mediators of the depression–morbidity relationship in coronary disease. Abnormal platelet activation, poor adherence to treatment regimen, and lifestyle modification factors such as exercise, diet, smoking cessation, and antidepressant medications themselves (particularly, tricyclic antidepressants) have been implicated as the most likely potential mediators for heightened coronary disease-related morbidity and mortality. In parallel with the search for mechanisms mediating the depression–coronary heart disease relationship, numerous clinical trials over the past two decades have examined treatment for depression in CAD patients, using both depression and medical morbidity as outcomes.

Psychosocial strategies

Contemporary clinical trials of psychosocial intervention for coronary disease patients date back to the Recurrent Coronary Prevention Project in the 1980s. In this trial, post-MI patients were randomized to usual care or addition of a behavior modification group psychotherapy aimed at reducing aspects of Type A behavior pattern (propensity toward anger, impatience, time urgency, and competitiveness) believed to be associated with coronary disease risk. Although the Recurrent Coronary Prevention Project demonstrated reduced recurrent coronary event rates over 4.5 years follow-up (Friedman et al. 1986), the Type A construct fell into disfavor over subsequent years, and was largely superseded by interest in depression. Of note, however, a recent trial of cognitive behavioral, stress management groups for post-MI patients, also focused on reducing anger, again demonstrated over 40% reduction in both recurrent MI, and fatal and nonfatal cardiac events (Gulliksson et al. 2011). With respect to depression, only a few trials have examined psychotherapeutic approaches to its treatment in patients with cardiovascular disease. The ENRICHD trial randomized 2481 patients with recent acute MI who also suffered from depression and/or low perceived social support to either CBT or care as usual over 6 months. Patients in both treatment arms improved, and the additional effects of the intervention arm on depression and social support were modest, with differences between the two groups attenuating over time, and no significant difference in cardiac outcomes between treatments (Berkman *et al.* 2003). In another study, interpersonal psychotherapy added to clinical management was not superior to clinical management alone for treatment of depressive symptoms in patients with stable coronary artery disease (Lesperance *et al.* 2007). No studies have shown that psychotherapy improves adherence to heart disease treatment or lifestyle modification.

Despite the failure of trials to date to demonstrate significant benefits of psychotherapy for depression in heart disease patients, we believe that psychoeducation, cognitive behavioral psychotherapy, or brief supportive psychotherapy should be offered to depressed heart disease patients, particularly those who express a desire for such treatment, because the evidence base is limited, and because sub-sets of patients, especially those who express a preference for psychotherapy, may experience greater benefit than is reflected in the overall results of trials that do not take patient preferences into account. Evidence for the impact of patient treatment preference on treatment outcome can be seen in the outcome of the COPES trial, in which assignment to psychotherapy or psychopharmacology as first-line treatment for depressive symptoms, according to patient preference, led to substantial improvement in patient satisfaction with depression care, and in both depression and medical outcomes (Davidson *et al.* 2010).

Psychopharmacologic strategies

SSRIs are the first-line pharmacologic treatment for depressed patients with cardiac disease, with efficacy that seems comparable to the benefits seen in depressed individuals without cardiovascular disease. A small RCT found fluoxetine to be effective in reducing mild depression in post-MI patients, with a trend towards superiority (compared to placebo) in patients with higher HAM-D scores (Strik *et al.* 2000). In the SADHART trial, an investigator-initiated safety study sponsored by Pfizer (n = 369), sertraline was efficacious for treating depression in those subjects with a history of recurrent depression, and not significantly better than placebo for patients with new onset of depression after their acute cardiac event (Glassman *et al.* 2002). The CREATE trial demonstrated that citalopram is superior to placebo as a treatment for MDD in patients with stable coronary artery disease (Lesperance *et al.* 2007).

SSRIs are considered to be generally safe in patients with cardiovascular disease. They may decrease heart rate, but rarely by more than a few beats per minute, and they have no effect on blood pressure (Roose *et al.* 1998a, b). For the many heart disease patients who take beta-blockers, caution about the additive effects of SSRIs on heart rate is warranted; there have been a small number of reported cases of combined treatment resulting in symptomatic bradycardia and syncope. In addition to their pharmacodynamic effects on heart rate, SSRIs that inhibit the cytochrome 2D6 system may block metabolism of beta-blockers, further magnifying the negative chronotropic effect. Studies in heart failure patients found no effect of fluoxetine on cardiac conduction, ventricular arrhythmias, or orthostatic blood pressure change. RCTs have demonstrated the cardiovascular safety of both fluoxetine and sertraline in post-MI depression (Strik *et al.* 2000, Glassman *et al.* 2002). Recently, the FDA issued a safety warning about dose-related QTc prolongation for citalopram, and recommended limiting dosing to no more than 40 mg daily. The FDA warned against using citalopram in patients with a history of congenital prolonged QT interval, and highlighted a greater risk of torsade de pointes in patients with congestive heart failure, bradyarrhythmias, or electrolyte abnormalities, and for patients taking other medications which themselves prolong the QTc interval (US Food and Drug Administration, 2011).

Patients with major depressive disorder have above normal levels of platelet activation, as indexed by flow cytometry measures and circulating markers of platelet activity, resulting in a "pro-thrombotic" state that has been proposed as one of the mediators of the risk for CAD events associated with depression. SSRI antidepressants, but not TCAs, have been shown to reduce this increase in platelet activation. Platelets store serotonin, platelet activation is accompanied by release of stored serotonin, and the resulting increase in locally circulating serotonin is a minor agonist for further platelet activation, promoting clot formation. Because SSRIs interfere with platelet serotonin uptake and storage, they may have an antithrombotic effect in general, which may account in part for the increased risk of gastrointestinal bleeding associated with their use. Adding SSRIs to warfarin, aspirin, or antiplatelet therapy may further increase the risk of abnormal bleeding, although overall risk remains low (Kim *et al.* 2009, Sansone and Sansone, 2009, Labos *et al.* 2011). Some investigations now underway are examining the therapeutic potential of SSRIs as antiplatelet agents for coronary disease patients without depression.

Mirtazapine was shown to be modestly effective and safe for acute treatment of patients with depression between 3–12 months post-MI (Honig *et al.* 2007). For venlafaxine, there is a dose-dependent risk of elevated blood pressure, particularly at doses greater than 150 mg/d. This effect is reduced with use of the extended-release formulation of venlafaxine. Venlafaxine has not been specifically studied in cardiovascular disease populations (Shapiro, 2011). Though bupropion can increase blood pressure, one small study found no other adverse effects in patients with cardiovascular disease (Roose *et al.* 1991). We recommend periodic blood pressure monitoring for patients taking bupropion, venlafaxine, and duloxetine; however, if no increase in blood pressure is observed after a month of a therapeutic dose, no further regular monitoring is necessary.

TCAs are efficacious in depressed patients with pre-existing cardiac disease, but have many undesirable cardiovascular effects including orthostatic hypotension, conduction delay with risk of heart block, and, in overdose, ventricular ectopy. TCAs have quinidine-like (type 1A) antiarrhythmic effects (Veith *et al.* 1982), which increase the risk of ventricular fibrillation in post-MI patients, increasing concern about using TCAs in patients with ischemic heart disease (Glassman *et al.* 1993). Among tricyclic agents, nortriptyline has the lowest risk for orthostatic hypotension and undesirable anticholinergic effects. Still, in a comparison of paroxetine and nortriptyline in patients with co-morbid depression and ischemic heart disease, Roose *et al.* (1998b) found that while both treatments were effective, nortriptyline was associated with more undesirable cardiac effects. Despite their unfavorable adverse effect profile, TCAs might be a reasonable treatment option for cardiac patients with severe depression that has not responded to other treatments, or who have had a favorable response to

TCAs in the past; for these patients, risk assessment should include evaluation of pre-existing cardiac conduction problems and arrhythmias, ongoing ischemia, severity of heart failure, and orthostatic hypotension.

Studies investigating whether psychopharmacological treatment of depression improves cardiac outcomes in heart disease patients have had suggestive outcomes. The SADHART trial was designed and powered as a safety study, not to test an effect on cardiac outcomes. Sertraline was associated with a 22% reduction in death and adverse cardiac events over the 6-month follow-up period, which, if confirmed, would be a very meaningful reduction in the event rate, but the total number of events was very small and this effect was not statistically significant. In the ENRICHD trial, patients who had persistent depression at the end of the 6-month intervention period could receive open-label antidepressant therapy; patients who received an SSRI had a rate of recurrent MI and death that was about half the rate seen in patients who received no antidepressant; the effect of other antidepressants was not as strong (Berkman *et al.* 2003, Taylor *et al.* 2005). Since the nonrandomized choice of antidepressants might have been influenced by medical prognostic variables (e.g., preferentially not using antidepressants in patients who had more severe heart disease) these findings must be viewed with caution. Although the ENRICHD and SADHART studies suggest a beneficial effect of SSRIs, we cannot say for sure that antidepressant treatment has been clearly shown to modify cardiovascular adverse events in depressed coronary disease patients. That does not mean that patients with major depressive disorder and cardiovascular disease should not receive appropriate antidepressant treatment, but it does mean we should not promise patients more than the data supports. Moreover, in depressed congestive heart failure patients, in the only trial of its kind to date, sertraline treatment had no effect on recurrent cardiac events and mortality (O'Connor *et al.* 2010).

We recommend SSRIs as first-line pharmacotherapy for patients with co-morbid depression and cardiovascular disease. For patients who do not respond to SSRIs, clinicians might consider SNRIs, or bupropion (measuring key parameters like blood pressure), or mirtazapine. TCAs should be reserved for patients with treatment-refractory depression after careful weighing of benefits and risks with the patient and cardiologist.

Neurological disease

A recent meta-analysis examining the efficacy of antidepressants in treating all forms of depression in neurological disorders found that antidepressants are effective, with a number needed to treat of 7 at 6–8 weeks (Price *et al.* 2011). This lumping of diverse clinical disorders and antidepressant sub-types belies the nature of the limited data in this area. In this meta-analysis, ten studies were included for post-stroke depression, six studies for depressed patients with Parkinson's disease, two for multiple sclerosis, and one each for epilepsy and traumatic brain injury. Subgroup analyses showed that antidepressants (SSRIs and TCAs) are effective in treating post-stroke depression, but more equivocal results were found for depressed patients with co-morbid Parkinson's disease. Antidepressants were well tolerated across studies. Insufficient data was found in these RCTs to examine the impact of antidepressants upon quality of life and cognitive and functional outcomes of patients with neurological disease.

A subsequent trial comparing sertraline (up to 150 mg/d), mirtazapine (up to 45 mg/d), and placebo in depressed patients with possible or probable Alzheimer's dementia found no effect of drug treatment on depression symptoms (Banerjee *et al.* 2011). Pharmacologic treatment for depression in the context of Alzheimer's disease has had very mixed results in the literature, with data seeming to suggest that more severely depressed patients respond to antidepressants better than peers with milder forms of depression (Lee and Lyketsos, 2003, Banerjee *et al.* 2011).

Noteworthy studies have found that post-stroke depression is responsive to nortriptyline (as compared to fluoxetine or placebo), which also has a positive effect upon recovery of activities of daily living (Robinson *et al.* 2000) and perhaps on cognitive functioning (Kimura *et al.* 2000). Citalopram is safe and effective in post-stroke depression (Andersen *et al.* 1994). In patients with a recent stroke, sertraline treatment was effective as prophylaxis against the development of depression in a 2003 study, with a number needed to treat of approximately 7 (Rasmussen *et al.* 2003), but other studies have had a negative outcome, leaving doubts as to whether post-stroke depression can be prevented by prophylactic low-dose SSRI treatment (Almeida *et al.* 2006).

The first RCT evaluating CBT for treatment of depression in Parkinson's disease found a substantial benefit, with NNT of 2.1 (Dobkin *et al.* 2011), but this result has not been replicated.

In summary, we would recommend treating depression co-morbid with neurologic disease. SSRIs should remain first-line treatment, as is generally the rule for other patients with or without medical co-morbidities. There is satisfactory data that antidepressants are effective for post-stroke depression, and even for those disorders in which there is more limited or even negative trials (e.g., Parkinson's disease, epilepsy, TBI). We believe that potential benefits are great enough, and risks relatively small, to at least warrant a trial of antidepressant therapy for patients experiencing a distressing level of sadness or anhedonia, and neurovegetative symptoms. If a medication trial is ineffective, trials of TCAs or even ECT may at times be considered.

Cancer

While some evidence exists to support the use of SSRIs and TCAs for depression in cancer patients, there are few RCTs in the literature addressing this topic. Imipramine was effective in decreasing depressive symptoms in depressed patients with gynecologic malignancies (Evans *et al.* 1988). Other antidepressants which have been found to be effective in reducing depressive symptoms in cancer patients include desipramine (Holland *et al.* 1998), fluoxetine (Fisch *et al.* 2003), and paroxetine (Morrow *et al.* 2003), though there is often a high dropout rate in these patients due to difficulty tolerating antidepressant side effects. Other placebo-controlled trials have not demonstrated antidepressant efficacy when examining despiramine, fluoxetine, paroxetine, or sertraline (Owen and Ferrando, 2010). Mirtazapine has shown promise in decreasing depressive symptoms in both randomized (Cankurtaran *et al.* 2008) and open trials (Kim *et al.* 2008) of depressed cancer patients, with a side-effect profile that can be used to target insomnia and GI distress. When rapid improvement of depressive symptoms is the goal, psychostimulants have been useful in patients with advanced cancer (Olin and Masand, 1996, Homsi *et al.* 2001, Sood *et al.* 2006). Caution is warranted when using antidepressants in patients with thrombocytopenia, hyponatremia, and carcinoid tumors (Massie and Miller, 2011). The suggestion that antidepressants increase the risk of cancer has been refuted (Theoharides and Konstantinidou, 2003). Finally, it is worth considering that depression and fatigue may at times be confused in patients with cancer. Careful delineation of a depression syndrome from disease or treatment-related fatigue, as well as clarification of goals of care (curative vs. palliative) may help to guide clinicians who are considering treatment options such as antidepressants, stimulants, and newer agents such as modafinil or ketamine.

Looking forward

It is striking that although co-morbid depression increases the morbidity of many medical disorders, treating depression has not been demonstrated to have large effects upon medical outcomes. It is not clear why this is the case. Other questions that are worth further exploration include the following. Who are these medically ill patients who develop a mood episode in the context of medical illness? What predisposing factors predict depression in the context of medical illness? Preventative medicine has emerged as a prominent and important area of interest and research. It may be that attempting to improve medical outcomes by addressing depression is too late in the game to meaningfully reverse course. By identifying the medically ill patients at highest risk for a mood episode, we might be able to institute preventative measures, such as more frequent screening, comprehensive review of psychosocial stressors that could be addressed to improve quality of life and health-care behaviors before a depression occurs. This would likely only be cost effective if we could identify the highest risk group of patients with the greatest likelihood of developing depression and intensively intervene to meaningfully address their life stressors and biology. Few if any psychiatric preventative care programs exist, and benefits of risk-stratification for depression, and identification of current depression, by screening of medically ill patient populations, have yet to be realized.

References

Almeida, O.P., Waterreus, A., and Hankey, G.J. (2006). Preventing depression after stroke: Results from a randomized placebo-controlled trial. *The Journal of Clinical Psychiatry*, 67, 1104–1109.

Andersen, G., Vestergaard, K., and Lauritzen, L. (1994). Effective treatment of poststroke depression with the selective serotonin reuptake inhibitor citalopram. *Stroke*, 25, 1099–1104.

Banerjee, S., Hellier, J., Dewey, M. *et al.* (2011). Sertraline or mirtazapine for depression in dementia (HTA-SADD):

a randomised, multicentre, double-blind, placebo-controlled trial. *Lancet*, 378, 403–411.

Barth, J., Schumacher, M., and Herrmann-Lingen, C. (2004). Depression as a risk factor for mortality in patients with coronary heart disease: a meta-analysis. *Psychosomatic Medicine*, 66, 802–813.

Berkman, L.F., Blumenthal, J., Burg, M. *et al.* (2003). Effects of treating depression and low perceived social support on clinical events after myocardial infarction: The Enhancing Recovery in Coronary Heart Disease Patients (ENRICHD) Randomized Trial. *Journal of the American Medical Association*, 289, 3106–3116.

Black, S.A., Markides, K.S., and Ray, L.A. (2003). Depression predicts increased incidence of adverse health outcomes in older Mexican Americans with type 2 diabetes. *Diabetes Care*, 26, 2822–2828.

Bogner, H.R., Morales, K.H., Post, E.P., and Bruce, M.L. (2007). Diabetes, depression, and death: A randomized controlled trial of a depression treatment program for older adults based in primary care (PROSPECT). *Diabetes Care*, 30, 3005–3010.

Cankurtaran, E.S., Ozalp, E., Soygur, H. *et al.* (2008). Mirtazapine improves sleep and lowers anxiety and depression in cancer patients: Superiority over imipramine. *Supportive Care in Cancer*, 16, 1291–1298.

Cohen, S.D., Norris, L., Acquaviva, K., Peterson, R.A., and Kimmel, P.L. (2007). Screening, diagnosis, and treatment of depression in patients with end-stage renal disease. *Clinical Journal of the American Society of Nephrology*, 2, 1332–1342.

Davidson, K.W., Rieckmann, N., Clemow, L. *et al.* (2010). Enhanced depression care for patients with acute coronary syndrome and persistent depressive symptoms: coronary psychosocial evaluation studies randomized controlled trial. *Archives of Internal Medicine*, 170, 600–608.

De Groot, M., Anderson, R., Freedland, K.E., Clouse, R.E., and Lustman, P.J. (2001). Association of depression and diabetes complications: A meta-analysis. *Psychosomatic Medicine*, 63, 619–630.

Dobkin, R.D., Menza, M., Allen, L.A. *et al.* (2011). Cognitive-behavioral therapy for depression in Parkinson's disease: A randomized, controlled trial. *The American Journal of Psychiatry*, 168, 1066–1074.

Eaton, W.W., Armenian, H., Gallo, J., Pratt, L., and Ford, D.E. (1996). Depression and risk for onset of type II diabetes. A prospective population-based study. *Diabetes Care*, 19, 1097–1102.

Echeverry, D., Duran, P., Bonds, C., Lee, M., and Davidson, M.B. (2009). Effect of pharmacological treatment of depression on A1C and quality of life in low-income Hispanics and African Americans with diabetes: A randomized, double-blind, placebo-controlled trial. *Diabetes Care*, 32, 2156–2160.

Ell, K., Katon, W., Xie, B. *et al.* (2010). Collaborative care management of major depression among low-income, predominantly Hispanic subjects with diabetes: A randomized controlled trial. *Diabetes Care*, 33, 706–713.

Evans, D.L., McCartney, C.F., Haggerty, J.J., Jr. *et al.* (1988). Treatment of depression in cancer patients is associated with better life adaptation: A pilot study. *Psychosomatic Medicine*, 50, 73–76.

Fallowfield, L., Ratcliffe, D., Jenkins, V., and Saul, J. (2001). Psychiatric morbidity and its recognition by doctors in patients with cancer. *British Journal of Cancer*, 84, 1011–1015.

Faris, R., Purcell, H., Henein, M.Y., and Coats, A.J. (2002). Clinical depression is common and significantly associated with reduced survival in patients with non-ischaemic heart failure. *European Journal of Heart Failure*, 4, 541–551.

Ferrando, S.J., Levenson, J.L., and Owen, J.A. (eds.) (2010). *Clinical Manual of Psychopharmacology in the Medically Ill*. Washington, DC: American Psychiatric Publishing.

Fisch, M.J., Loehrer, P.J., Kristeller *et al.* (2003). Fluoxetine versus placebo in advanced cancer outpatients: A double-blinded trial of the Hoosier Oncology Group. *Journal of Clinical Oncology*, 21, 1937–1943.

Fisher, L., Skaff, M.M., Mullan, J.T. *et al.* (2008). A longitudinal study of affective and anxiety disorders, depressive affect and diabetes distress in adults with Type 2 diabetes. *Diabetic Medicine*, 25, 1096–1101.

Fournier, J.C., Derubeis, R.J., Hollon, S.D. *et al.* (2010). Antidepressant drug effects and depression severity: A patient-level meta-analysis. *Journal of the American Medical Association*, 303, 47–53.

Friedman, M., Thoresen, C.E., Gill, J.J. *et al.* (1986). Alteration of type A behavior and its effect on cardiac recurrences in post myocardial infarction patients: Summary results of the Recurrent Coronary Prevention Project. *American Heart Journal*, 112, 653–665.

Gelhorn, H.L., Sexton, C.C., and Classi, P.M. (2011). Patient preferences for treatment of major depressive disorder and the impact on health outcomes: A systematic review. *The Primary Care Companion for CNS Disorders*, 13.

Georgiades, A., Zucker, N., Friedman, K.E. *et al.* (2007). Changes in depressive symptoms and glycemic control in diabetes mellitus. *Psychosomatic Medicine*, 69, 235–241.

Gibbons, R.D., Hur, K., Brown, C.H., Davis, J.M., and Mann, J.J. (2012). Benefits from antidepressants: Synthesis of 6-week patient-level outcomes from double-blind placebo-controlled randomized trials of fluoxetine and venlafaxine. *Archives of General Psychiatry*, 69, 572–579.

Glassman, A.H., Roose, S.P., and Bigger, J.T., Jr. (1993). The safety of tricyclic antidepressants in cardiac patients. Risk-benefit reconsidered. *Journal of the American Medical Association*, 269, 2673–2675.

Glassman, A.H., O'Connor, C.M., Califf, R.M. *et al.* (2002). Sertraline treatment of major depression in patients with acute MI or unstable angina. *Journal of the American Medical Association*, 288, 701–709.

Global Parkinson's Disease Survey Steering Committee (2002). Factors impacting on quality of life in Parkinson's disease: Results from an international survey. *Movement Disorders*, 17, 60–67.

Goetz, M.P., Knox, S.K., Suman, V.J. *et al.* (2007). The impact of cytochrome P450 2D6 metabolism in women receiving adjuvant tamoxifen. *Breast Cancer Research and Treatment*, 101, 113–121.

Gulliksson, M., Burell, G., Vessby, B., Lundin, L., Toss, H., and Svardsudd, K. (2011). Randomized controlled trial of cognitive behavioral therapy vs. standard treatment to prevent recurrent cardiovascular events in patients with coronary heart disease: Secondary Prevention in Uppsala Primary Health Care project (SUPRIM). *Archives of Internal Medicine*, 171, 134–140.

Gulseren, L., Gulseren, S., Hekimsoy, Z., and Mete, L. (2005). Comparison of fluoxetine and paroxetine in type II diabetes mellitus patients. *Archives of Medical Research*, 36, 159–165.

Hesdorffer, D.C., Hauser, W.A., Olafsson, E., Ludvigsson, P., and Kjartansson, O. (2006). Depression and suicide attempt as risk factors for incident unprovoked seizures. *Annals of Neurology*, 59, 35–41.

Holland, J.C., Romano, S.J., Heiligenstein, J.H., Tepner, R.G., and Wilson, M.G. (1998). A controlled trial of fluoxetine and desipramine in depressed women with advanced cancer. *Psycho-oncology*, 7, 291–300.

Homsi, J., Nelson, K.A., Sarhill, N. *et al.* (2001). A phase II study of methylphenidate for depression in advanced cancer. *The American Journal of Hospice and Palliative Care*, 18, 403–407.

Honig, A., Kuyper, A.M., Schene, A.H. *et al.* (2007). Treatment of post-myocardial infarction depressive disorder: A randomized, placebo-controlled trial with mirtazapine. *Psychosomatic Medicine*, 69, 606–613.

House, A., Knapp, P., Bamford, J., and Vail, A. (2001). Mortality at 12 and 24 months after stroke may be associated with depressive symptoms at 1 month. *Stroke*, 32, 696–701.

Jiménez Chafey, M.I. and Rosselló, J.M. (2006). Cognitive-behavioral group therapy for depression in adolescents with diabetes: a pilot study. *Revista Interamericana de Psicología*, 40, 219–226.

Katon, W.J., Simon, G., Russo, J. *et al.* (2004a). Quality of depression care in a population-based sample of patients with diabetes and major depression. *Medical Care*, 42, 1222–1229.

Katon, W.J., Von Korff, M., Lin, E.H. *et al.* (2004b). The Pathways Study: A randomized trial of collaborative care in patients with diabetes and depression. *Archives of General Psychiatry*, 61, 1042–1049.

Kessler, R.C., Berglund, P., Demler, O. *et al.* (2005a). Lifetime prevalence and age-of-onset distributions of DSM-IV disorders in the National Comorbidity Survey Replication. *Archives of General Psychiatry*, 62, 593–602.

Kessler, R.C., Chiu, W.T., Demler, O., Merikangas, K.R., and Walters, E.E. (2005b). Prevalence, severity, and comorbidity of 12-month DSM-IV disorders in the National Comorbidity Survey Replication. *Archives of General Psychiatry*, 62, 617–627.

Kim, D.H., Daskalakis, C., Whellan, D.J. *et al.* (2009). Safety of selective serotonin reuptake inhibitor in adults undergoing coronary artery bypass grafting. *The American Journal of Cardiology*, 103, 1391–1395.

Kim, S.W., Shin, I.S., Kim, J.M. *et al.* (2008). Effectiveness of mirtazapine for nausea and insomnia in cancer patients with depression. *Psychiatry and Clinical Neurosciences*, 62, 75–83.

Kimura, M., Robinson, R.G., and Kosier, J.T. (2000). Treatment of cognitive impairment after poststroke depression: A double-blind treatment trial. *Stroke*, 31, 1482–1486.

Kroenke, K., Spitzer, R.L., and Williams, J.B. (2001). The PHQ-9: validity of a brief depression severity measure. *Journal of General Internal Medicine*, 16, 606–613.

Labos, C., Dasgupta, K., Nedjar, H., Turecki, G., and Rahme, E. (2011). Risk of bleeding associated with combined use of selective serotonin reuptake inhibitors and antiplatelet therapy following acute myocardial infarction. *Canadian Medical Association Journal*, 183, 1835–1843.

Lee, H.B. and Lyketsos, C.G. (2003). Depression in Alzheimer's disease: Heterogeneity and related issues. *Biological Psychiatry*, 54, 353–362.

Lesperance, F., Frasure-Smith, N., Koszycki, D. *et al.* (2007). Effects of citalopram and interpersonal psychotherapy on depression in patients with coronary artery disease: The Canadian Cardiac Randomized Evaluation of Antidepressant and Psychotherapy Efficacy (CREATE) trial. *Journal of the American Medical Association*, 297, 367–379.

Levenson, J.L. (ed.) (2011). *Textbook of Psychosomatic Medicine: Psychiatric Care of the Medically Ill*. Arlington, VA: American Psychiatric Publishing.

Li, M. and Rodin, G. (2011). Depression. In Levenson, J.L., ed., *Textbook of Psychosomatic Medicine, Second Edition*. Arlington, VA: American Psychiatric Publishing.

Lustman, P.J., Freedland, K.E., Griffith, L.S., and Clouse, R.E. (2000). Fluoxetine for depression in diabetes: A randomized double-blind placebo-controlled trial. *Diabetes Care*, 23, 618–623.

Lustman, P.J., Griffith, L.S., Freedland, K.E., Kissel, S.S., and Clouse, R.E. (1998). Cognitive behavior therapy for depression in type 2 diabetes mellitus: A randomized, controlled trial. *Annals of Internal Medicine*, 129, 613–621.

Lustman, P.J., Williams, M.M., Sayuk, G.S., Nix, B.D., and Clouse, R.E. (2007). Factors influencing glycemic control in type 2 diabetes during acute- and maintenance-phase treatment of major depressive disorder with bupropion. *Diabetes Care*, 30, 459–466.

Lustman, P.J., Griffith, L.S., Clouse, R.E. *et al.* (1997). Effects of nortriptyline on depression and glycemic control in diabetes: Results of a double-blind, placebo-controlled trial. *Psychosomatic Medicine*, 59, 241–250.

Lustman, P.J., Clouse, R.E., Nix, B.D. *et al.* (2006). Sertraline for prevention of depression recurrence in diabetes mellitus: A randomized, double-blind, placebo-controlled trial. *Archives of General Psychiatry*, 63, 521–529.

Massie, M.J. and Miller, K. (2011). Oncology. In Levenson, J.L., ed., *Textbook of Psychosomatic Medicine: Psychiatric Care of the Medically Ill, Second Edition*. Arlington, VA: American Psychiatric Publishing.

McDonald, W.M., Richard, I.H., and Delong, M.R. (2003). Prevalence, etiology, and treatment of depression in Parkinson's disease. *Biological Psychiatry*, 54, 363–375.

Morrow, G.R., Hickok, J.T., Roscoe, J.A. *et al.* (2003). Differential effects of paroxetine on fatigue and depression: A randomized, double-blind trial from the University of Rochester Cancer Center Community Clinical Oncology Program. *Journal of Clinical Oncology*, 21, 4635–4641.

O'Connor, C.M., Jiang, W., Kuchibhatla, M. *et al.* (2010). Safety and efficacy of sertraline for depression in patients with heart failure: results of the SADHART-CHF (Sertraline Against Depression and Heart Disease in Chronic Heart Failure) trial. *Journal of the American College of Cardiology*, 56, 692–699.

Olin, J. and Masand, P. (1996). Psychostimulants for depression in hospitalized cancer patients. *Psychosomatics*, 37, 57–62.

Owen, J., and Ferrando, S. (2010). Oncology. In Ferrando, S.L., Levenson, J.L., and Owen, J.A., eds., *Clinical Manual of Psychopharmacology in the Medically Ill*. Washington, DC: American Psychiatric Publishing.

Paile-Hyvarinen, M., Wahlbeck, K., and Eriksson, J.G. (2003). Quality of life and metabolic status in mildly depressed women with type 2 diabetes treated with paroxetine: A single-blind randomised placebo controlled trial. *BMC Family Practice*, 4, 7.

Paile-Hyvarinen, M., Wahlbeck, K., and Eriksson, J.G. (2007). Quality of life and metabolic status in mildly depressed patients with type 2 diabetes treated with paroxetine: A double-blind randomised placebo controlled 6-month trial. *BMC Family Practice*, 8, 34.

Pan, A., Sun, Q., Okereke, O.I., Rexrode, K.M., and Hu, F.B. (2011). Depression and risk of stroke morbidity and mortality: A meta-analysis and systematic review. *Journal of the American Medical Association*, 306, 1241–1249.

Patten, S.B. and Barbui, C. (2004). Drug-induced depression: A systematic review to inform clinical practice. *Psychotherapy and Psychosomatics*, 73, 207–215.

Patten, S.B., Williams, J.V., Lavorato, D.H. *et al.* (2009). Major depression as a risk factor for high blood pressure: Epidemiologic evidence from a national longitudinal study. *Psychosomatic Medicine*, 71, 273–279.

Petrak, F. and Herpertz, S. (2009). Treatment of depression in diabetes: An update. *Current Opinion in Psychiatry*, 22, 211–217.

Price, A., Rayner, L., Okon-Rocha, E. *et al.* (2011). Antidepressants for the treatment of depression in neurological disorders: A systematic review and meta-analysis of randomised controlled trials. *Journal of Neurology, Neurosurgery, and Psychiatry*, 82, 914–923.

Rabkin, J., Quitkin, F., Harrison, W., Tricamo, E., and McGrath, P. (1984). Adverse reactions to monoamine oxidase inhibitors. Part I. A comparative study. *Journal of Clinical Psychopharmacology*, 4, 270–278.

Rasmussen, A., Lunde, M., Poulsen, D.L. *et al.* (2003). A double-blind, placebo-controlled study of sertraline in the prevention of depression in stroke patients. *Psychosomatics*, 44, 216–221.

Robinson, R.G. (2003). Poststroke depression: prevalence, diagnosis, treatment, and disease progression. *Biological Psychiatry*, 54, 376–387.

Robinson, R.G., Schultz, S.K., Castillo, C. *et al.* (2000). Nortriptyline versus fluoxetine in the treatment of depression and in short-term recovery after stroke: A placebo-controlled, double-blind study. *The American Journal of Psychiatry*, 157, 351–359.

Rollman, B.L., Belnap, B.H., Lemenager, M.S. *et al.* (2009). Telephone-delivered collaborative care for treating post-CABG depression: A randomized controlled trial. *Journal of the American Medical Association*, 302, 2095–2103.

Roose, S.P., Dalack, G.W., Glassman, A.H. *et al.* (1991). Cardiovascular effects of bupropion in depressed patients with heart disease. *The American Journal of Psychiatry*, 148, 512–516.

Roose, S.P., Glassman, A.H., Attia, E. *et al.* (1998a). Cardiovascular effects of fluoxetine in depressed patients with heart disease. *The American Journal of Psychiatry*, 155, 660–665.

Roose, S.P., Laghrissi-Thode, F., Kennedy, J.S. *et al.* (1998b). Comparison of paroxetine and nortriptyline in depressed patients with ischemic heart disease. *Journal of the American Medical Association*, 279, 287–291.

Rudisch, B. and Nemeroff, C.B. (2003). Epidemiology of comorbid coronary artery disease and depression. *Biological Psychiatry*, 54, 227–240.

Rugulies, R. (2002). Depression as a predictor for coronary heart disease: A review and meta-analysis. *American Journal of Preventive Medicine*, 23, 51–61.

Sansone, R.A. and Sansone, L.A. (2009). Warfarin and antidepressants: Happiness without hemorrhaging. *Psychiatry*, 6, 24–29.

Shapiro, P.A. (2011). Heart disease. In Levenson, J.L., ed., *Textbook of Psychosomatic Medicine: Psychiatric Care of the Medically Ill, Second Edition*. Arlington, VA: American Psychiatric Publishing.

Simon, G.E., Katon, W.J., Lin, E.H. *et al.* (2007). Cost-effectiveness of systematic depression treatment among people with diabetes mellitus. *Archives of General Psychiatry*, 64, 65–72.

Simson, U., Nawarotzky, U., Friese, G. *et al.* (2008). Psychotherapy intervention to reduce depressive symptoms in patients with diabetic foot syndrome. *Diabetic Medicine*, 25, 206–212.

Sood, A., Barton, D.L., and Loprinzi, C.L. (2006). Use of methylphenidate in patients with cancer. *The American Journal of Hospice and Palliative Care*, 23, 35–40.

Spertus, J.A., McDonell, M., Woodman, C.L., and Fihn, S.D. (2000). Association between depression and worse disease-specific functional status in outpatients with coronary artery disease. *American Heart Journal*, 140, 105–110.

Steffensmeier, J.J., Ernst, M.E., Kelly, M., and Hartz, A.J. (2006). Do randomized controlled trials always trump case reports? A second look at propranolol and depression. *Pharmacotherapy*, 26, 162–167.

Stewart, J.A., Deliyannides, D.A., Hellerstein, D.J., McGrath, P.J., and Stewart, J.W. (2012). Can people with nonsevere major depression benefit from antidepressant medication? *The Journal of Clinical Psychiatry*, 73, 518–525.

Strik, J.J., Honig, A., Lousberg, R. *et al.* (2000). Efficacy and safety of fluoxetine in the treatment of patients with major depression after first myocardial infarction: Findings from a double-blind, placebo-controlled trial. *Psychosomatic Medicine*, 62, 783–789.

Tandberg, E., Larsen, J.P., Aarsland, D., and Cummings, J.L. (1996). The occurrence of depression in Parkinson's disease: A community-based study. *Archives of Neurology*, 53, 175–179.

Taylor, C.B., Youngblood, M.E., Catellier, D. *et al.* (2005). Effects of antidepressant medication on morbidity and mortality in depressed patients after myocardial infarction. *Archives of General Psychiatry*, 62, 792–798.

Theoharides, T.C. and Konstantinidou, A. (2003). Antidepressants and risk of cancer: A case of misguided associations and priorities. *Journal of Clinical Psychopharmacology*, 23, 1–4.

US Food and Drug Administration (2011). *FDA Drug Safety Communication: Abnormal Heart Rhythms Associated with High Doses of Celexa (citalopram hydrobromide)* [Online]. Available: http://www.fda.gov/Drugs/DrugSafety/ucm269086.htm (accessed October 26 2011).

Van Beljouw, I.M., Verhaak, P.F., Cuijpers, P., Van Marwijk, H.W., and Penninx, B.W. (2010). The course of untreated anxiety and depression, and determinants of poor one-year outcome: A one-year cohort study. *BMC Psychiatry*, 10, 86.

Van Melle, J.P., De Jonge, P., Spijkerman, T.A. *et al.* (2004). Prognostic association of depression following

myocardial infarction with mortality and cardiovascular events: A meta-analysis. *Psychosomatic Medicine*, 66, 814–822.

Veith, R.C., Raskind, M.A., Caldwell, J.H. *et al.* (1982). Cardiovascular effects of tricyclic antidepressants in depressed patients with chronic heart disease. *The New England Journal of Medicine*, 306, 954–959.

Williams, J.W., Jr., Katon, W., Lin, E.H. *et al.* (2004). The effectiveness of depression care management on diabetes-related outcomes in older patients. *Annals of Internal Medicine*, 140, 1015–1024.

Wulsin, L.R. (2004). Is depression a major risk factor for coronary disease? A systematic review of the epidemiologic evidence. *Harvard Review of Psychiatry*, 12, 79–93.

Wulsin, L.R. and Singal, B.M. (2003). Do depressive symptoms increase the risk for the onset of coronary disease? A systematic quantitative review. *Psychosomatic Medicine*, 65, 201–210.

Wynn, G., Oesterheld, J., Cozza, K., and Armstrong, S. (2009). *Clinical Manual of Drug Interaction Principles for Medical Practice*. Arlington, VA: American Psychiatric Publishing, Inc.

Mood disorders in the context of borderline personality disorder

Eric A. Fertuck, Megan S. Chesin, and Barbara H. Stanley

Overview

Personality disorders, especially borderline personality disorder (BPD), and mood disorders, particularly major depressive disorder and bipolar II disorder, commonly co-occur (Hasin *et al.* 2005, Grant *et al.* 2008). In fact, the high incidence of co-occurrence between BPD and mood disorder have led to concerns about the distinctness of BPD, and ultimately to questions regarding the existence of the disorder (Akiskal, 2004). Recent data from clinical studies suggest that BPD shares some features with mood disorders and there is frequent co-occurrence. At the same time, there are differences in phenomenology, family history, longitudinal and treatment course, and underlying mechanisms between BPD and mood disorder (Zanarini *et al.* 2004, Wilson *et al.* 2007, Benazzi 2008).

In this chapter, we describe the prevalence of mood disorders in the context of BPD. We also discuss how co-occurrence affects the clinical picture, and therefore, prognosis and treatment. In particular, we discuss how co-occurring BPD affects the quality of depression, how the mood reactivity of BPD and bipolar II can be confused, and how chronic dysphoria in BPD can be mistaken for major depression. These distinctions are more than academic. They affect the choice of treatment, the likelihood of treatment response, and the prognosis.

Depressive disorders in the context of BPD

The most common co-occurring psychiatric disorder with BPD is major depressive disorder (MDD). Studies indicate that at least 70% of individuals with BPD experience a depressive episode at some point during their lives (Grunhaus *et al.* 1985, Zimmerman and Mattia, 1999, Zanarini *et al.* 2003, Gunderson *et al.* 2004, Skodol *et al.* 2011). Conversely, BPD is evident in about 25% of individuals diagnosed with MDD (Pfohl *et al.* 1984) or dysthymia (Pepper *et al.* 1995). There has been controversy over whether BPD is a variant of depression (Davis and Akiskal, 1986) or whether it is persistent if depression is successfully treated. The controversy is crystallized in the question: if you successfully treat the major depression does BPD remit? This led to cautions to clinicians and researchers that individuals should never be given the diagnosis of BPD while they were in the midst of a depressive episode. Subsequent research has, however, generally supported the theory that these are two distinct syndromes with different course, familial aggregation, treatment response, and disease markers (Gunderson and Phillips, 1991, New *et al.* 2008), and that BPD could, indeed, be diagnosed in the context of depression. Individuals with BPD and other personality disorders meet criteria after the depressive episode remits at the same rate as those with these personality disorders without major depression (Morey *et al.* 2010). The presence of co-occuring MDD seems to have little influence on the persistence of personality disorder symptoms and traits. This supports the theory that BPD and other personality disorders are not solely an expression of MDD, but represent a distinct syndrome that persists independently of MDD.

When performing diagnostic assessment, it is crucial to make a determination of the presence of co-occurring BPD because there are additional risks to the patient when both conditions are present. Furthermore, knowledge of this co-occurrence helps in developing a realistic picture of the course of illness and likely treatment response. Patients with both MDD and BPD are more likely to engage in suicidal

Clinical Handbook for the Management of Mood Disorders, ed. J. John Mann, Patrick J. McGrath, and Steven P. Roose.
Published by Cambridge University Press. © Cambridge University Press 2013.

behavior, particularly within a depressive episode, relative to those with MDD who do not have BPD (Corbitt *et al.* 1996). A diagnosis of BPD is associated with a longer time to remission from MDD (Skodol *et al.* 2011). Among those whose MDD is in remission, the time to the next major depressive episode is shorter compared to those without (Grilo *et al.* 2010). It is striking that, in a nationally representative sample, co-occurring BPD was present in over half of the cases of persistent major depression over 3 years (Skodol *et al.* 2011).

Contrasting with clinical lore that treating MDD in BPD leads to a resolution of BPD, a longitudinal study found the opposite. Improvements in MDD were predicted by reductions in BPD symptomatology (Gunderson *et al.* 2004). Corresponding with the findings regarding risk and course of illness, co-occurring MDD and BPD appears to respond less robustly to standard treatments for MDD (Soloff, 2000, Joyce *et al.* 2003, Feske *et al.* 2004, Binks *et al.* 2006, New *et al.* 2008, Feurino Iii and Silk, 2011, Silk, 2011). These findings point to the central importance of thoroughly assessing BPD when determining appropriate treatment approaches for MDD.

Clinicians and researchers have also elaborated the ways in which depression in BPD is often qualitatively distinct from depression without BPD. It is important to differentiate depressive affect and mood in BPD from other symptoms that appear to overlap but are, in fact, distinct. The phenomenology of BPD can be particularly confusing in the differential diagnosis between bona fide MDD or bipolar disorder (BD) owing to the following symptom expressions of BPD: (1) affective instability with strong and intense negative affect, (2) self-criticism, (3) chronic dysphoria, or "mental pain," (3) suicidality and nonsuicidal self-injury, experienced both in and out of depressive episodes, and (4) chronic feelings of emptiness that are not only apparent in a depressive episode. Further complicating this differential diagnosis is the fact that while clinicians may rate depression in BPD and non-BPD patients comparably using the clinician-rated scales such as the Hamilton Depression Rating Scale (Hamilton, 1960), patients with co-occurring BPD self-report heightened subjective experience of depression (Beck and Steer, 1993, Stanley and Wilson, 2006). Furthermore, those with BPD report more symptoms in the cognitive domain of depression using a self-report measure (Beck Depression Inventory; Beck and Steer, 1993).

With regard to differentiating depressed mood from affective instability, many clinicians and researchers propose that those with BPD are less able to regulate transient emotions than individuals with episodic mood disorders (Westen *et al.* 1992, Linehan, 1993). Emotional fluctuations in BPD tend to be negative (Stiglmayr *et al.* 2005), very intense, and relatively delayed in returning to baseline levels (see Herpertz, 2003, for review). When assessing mood in BPD patients, it is crucial to determine if negative mood states are relatively transient, and therefore part of affective instability, or whether depressed or elevated mood episodes are sustained, a presentation more consistent with a mood disorder.

Mental pain vs. depression in BPD

A pervasive dysphoria, often labeled "mental pain," has recently been conceptualized as a core feature of BPD that is distinct from the symptoms of a major depressive episode (Zanarini *et al.* 1998, Pazzagli and Monti, 2000, Zanarini and Frankenburg, 2007). Mental pain is characterized by an intense, multi-faceted inner pain with both affective and cognitive facets. It can be mistaken for major depression in BPD. In a study comparing mental pain with depression and anxiety in college students, mental pain was moderately associated with self-reported depressive and anxious cognitions (Orbach *et al.* 2003b). There was also evidence that mental pain was a distinct and under-recognized symptom (Orbach *et al.* 2003b). Several studies indicate that those with BPD have heightened mental pain and dysphoric affect and suggest that there is a qualitatively distinct experience of depressive affect in BPD, characterized by diffuse negative affectivity, loneliness, and emptiness (Westen, *et al.* 1992). There is speculation that this construct is related to some of the interpersonal and behavioral symptoms that characterize individuals with BPD (Pazzagli and Monti, 2000, Stanley and Siever, 2010). Some of the current diagnostic criteria in the DSM IV – such as affective instability, chronic feelings of emptiness, intense anger, and recurrent suicidal behavior – suggest the experience of mental pain. However, the criteria seem to focus on its behavioral and emotional consequences without addressing the subjective experience directly (Pazzagli and Monti, 2000). Interpersonal dysfunction and self-destructive behaviors may be maladaptive strategies to regulate emotional suffering in BPD. The affective instability of an individual with BPD can be mistaken for bipolar mood swings (Zanarini and Frankenburgh, 2007). Mental pain in BPD is associated with intense affects, thoughts of destructiveness, fragmentation, and a sense of victimization (Zanarini *et al.* 1998). Individuals with co-occurring BPD and MDD have also been found to be more ruminative, more hopeless, and to have lower self-esteem than patients with MDD only, and to have a greater cognitive vulnerability to depression (Abela *et al.* 2003). Depressed adolescents with BPD are particularly prone to self-condemnation and negative self-view when compared with those who have only depression without BPD (Rogers *et al.* 1995).

Rejection sensitivity, atypical depression, and BPD

Atypical depression is characterized by mood reactivity in the context of a depressive episode and at least one of the following symptoms: increased sleep, increased appetite, leaden paralysis, and rejection sensitivity (Quitkin *et al.* 1993). According to Nierenberg *et al.* (1998), it is the most common form of depression in outpatients, but is much less studied than melancholic depression. Owing to the common elements of mood reactivity and rejection sensitivity in both atypical depression and BPD, some have speculated that BPD is a form of atypical depression. Although BPD may share some symptoms with atypical depression, the depressive features are likely to persist after the depressive episode subsides in BPD, but not in atypical depression (Morey *et al.* 2010, Bassett, 2012). Thus, BPD is characterized by a unique quality of depressive affect that is pervasive and multi-faceted.

Suicidal and self-injurious behaviors in MDD with co-occurring BPD

Suicide attempters with co-occurring BPD and MDD have more lifetime suicide attempts, make their first attempt at a younger age, report more interpersonal triggers to attempts, and have higher levels of lifetime aggressive behaviors, hostility, and impulsivity than depressed attempters without BPD (Brodsky *et al.* 2006, Fertuck *et al.* 2007). In BPD without MDD, depressive moods and affects are reactive to interpersonal and other environmental stressors and are usually of briefer duration. By contrast, in BPD with MDD, the severity of depression and suicidal feelings build up more gradually and can persist for weeks or

months. Suicide attempts in MDD with BPD are thus more premeditated and occur after extended periods of consistently depressed mood (Soloff *et al.* 2000a). A subjective perception that the only choice is to end one's life often precedes a suicide attempt in MDD (Oldham, 2006). The prognostic importance of depression severity on suicide is less clear in BPD than in MDD (Kernberg, 2001). In one prospective study, severity of depression did not predict future suicidal behaviors in BPD. Instead, emotional dysregulation was the strongest predictor of future suicidality (Yen *et al.* 2004). Despite this finding, severity of depression in BPD is predictive of increased risk for a greater number of suicide attempts (Kelly *et al.* 2000) and higher medical lethality of suicide attempt (Runeson and Beskow, 1991, Soloff *et al.* 2000a). Further, even moderate depression and hopelessness can increase suicide attempt risk in BPD. Consequently, assessment of the severity of depressive symptoms is crucial when assessing suicidal risk in BPD.

In keeping with the interpersonal sensitivity characteristic of BPD, precipitants of highly lethal suicide attempts among those with BPD and MDD, as opposed to those with MDD only, are more likely to be interpersonal in nature (Brodsky *et al.* 2006). At the same time, lethality of suicide attempts in BPD is comparable to that of MDD, highlighting the fact that the nature of the precipitant is not associated with the lethality of the suicidal behavior. It is essential, then, for clinicians to assess environmental precipitants to suicide when evaluating suicidality in BPD.

Clinical vignette

Ms. M is a 24-year-old Caucasian female who graduated college with honors, but was unable to support herself. She found herself securing good positions but losing them or quitting very quickly after being hired. She got into arguments with co-workers or supervisors and had trouble getting to work on time because of insomnia, which led to oversleeping in the morning. She became increasingly depressed and disappointed in herself for her lack of success. Following another job loss, she went home, swallowed a "handful" of acetaminophen with the thought that, "It was just too hard to go on." She called her father and told him what she'd done, and he took her to the local emergency department. On examination, she was crying and somewhat agitated, reported increasing depression over the past 3 months, serious sleep disturbance, and increased irritability. She told the ED staff that, although she never told anyone before, she had taken several low lethality overdoses in the past with suicide intent when she became very upset with herself. This time she took more pills. On further examination, she revealed that she had been viewed as a difficult child because she was so highly strung, she had difficulty maintaining friendships, and had frequent bouts of depression. More detailed assessment led to the diagnosis of major depression and borderline personality disorder.

Bipolar disorder and BPD: spectrum or distinct disorders?

As mentioned earlier, there are high rates of co-occurrence between BPD and BD and overlap in the clinical characteristics of BPD and BD (e.g., affective lability and impulsivity). This has led some to suggest that BPD is on a spectrum with BD I and II (e.g., Akiskal, 2004, Smith *et al.* 2004). In clinical studies, rates of co-occurring BD among BPD patients are observed to be as high as 20–30% (Gunderson *et al.* 2006, Paris *et al.* 2007, for a review). Rates are even higher when hypomanic behaviors are more thoroughly assessed and "soft" hypomanic symptoms, such as cyclothymic temperament, are considered. In a small study of BPD patients, Deltito *et al.* (2001) found evidence of bipolar spectrum illness among 45% of sample members. Due to the high rate of co-occurrence, studies have sought to determine whether BD and BPD are on the same spectrum of disorders.

In partial support of the spectrum hypothesis, Gunderson *et al.* (2006) found significantly more BPD patients than patients with other personality disorders developed BD over the course of a 4-year period. This finding was consistent with results from an earlier study by Akiskal *et al.* (1985), though the 15% BD-onset rate observed by Akiskal *et al.* was twice the rate observed by Gunderson *et al.* (2006). Furthermore, Akiskal *et al.* (1985) found rates of BD among first-degree family members of BPD probands were similar to rates among family members of bipolar probands and greater than rates among family members of probands with other personality disorders or MDD. The aggregation of BPD and BD in families suggests a possible common etiological factor to the disorders, though definitive conclusions await additional

twin and genetic studies (MacKinnon and Pies, 2006, Goodman *et al.* 2010). Riso *et al.* (2000), in a methodologically rigorous family study comparing rates of BD among family members of BPD, mood-disordered, and normal probands, found first-degree relatives of BPD patients were no more likely to have BD than relatives of normal probands. Loranger *et al.* (1982) similarly found relatives of BPD probands were at relatively low risk for BD compared to relatives of bipolar probands. Loranger *et al.* (1982) also found relatives of bipolar probands were at no higher risk for BPD than relatives of schizophrenic patients. Two studies (Loranger *et al.* 1982, Riso *et al.* 2000) attributed differences between their findings and those of previous studies (e.g., Akiskal *et al.* 1985) to differences in the proband sample. High rates of bipolar co-occurrence among BPD probands in the study by Akiskal *et al.* (1985) could have spuriously inflated the prevalence of BD among family members of BPD probands. Paris *et al.* (2007), in reviewing 10 familial studies assessing BD among BPD patients, concluded relatives of BPD patients are not at increased risk for BD as the median rate of BD among family members of those with BPD from these studies was not higher than the rate of BD in the general population.

In further efforts to examine the potential BD–BPD spectrum, studies have attempted to distinguish the factors more uniquely associated with BPD, BD, or their co-occurrence. Benazzi (2008), for instance, studied the relationship between BPD symptoms and hypomanic symptoms among treatment-seeking bipolar II outpatients who were currently between mood episodes. He found few associations between BPD traits and bipolar symptoms, only observing a robust and meaningful relationship between self-reported impulsivity, a BPD trait, and clinician-assessed impulsive behavior, which was considered a symptom of hypomania. Wilson *et al.* (2007) more thoroughly investigated impulsivity among BPD and bipolar II patients and found differences in the types of impulsivity reported by BPD and bipolar II patients. Whereas bipolar II patients, regardless of BPD diagnosis, reported greater cognitive impulsivity, BPD patients, regardless of mood-disorder diagnosis, reported greater nonplanning impulsiveness (Wilson *et al.* 2007). Similarly, Henry *et al.* (2001) found BPD and bipolar II patients experience distinct types of affective lability. Both patient groups reported greater affective lability than patients with other personality disorders. BPD patients, however, reported more susceptibility to anger while bipolar II patients reported more feelings of elation and depression (Henry *et al.* 2001). Thus, there are differences in the affective symptoms that are characteristic of both BPD and BD.

Adding further support to conceptualizations of BPD as a psychiatric diagnosis distinct from mood disorder (Magill, 2004, Paris, 2007, New *et al.* 2008, Paris *et al.* 2009, Basset, 2012) is evidence from prospective studies showing BPD neither evolves into nor is specifically associated with BD. Links *et al.* (1995) and Zanarini *et al.* (2004), in two prospective studies which followed BPD patients for 6–7 years, found rates of BD onset were no different among BPD patients than patients with other personality disorders or with no personality disorder.

Outcomes and treatment response in the co-occurring mood disorders and BPD

Bowden and Maier (2003), in reviewing the available literature on outcomes associated with co-occurring BD and personality disorder, found individuals with BD and personality disorder, compared to bipolar patients without personality disorder, were more likely to have made a suicide attempt, been unemployed, and experienced greater mood symptom severity. Treatment response to lithium is also poorer among bipolar patients with personality disorder.

Studies specific to co-occurring BPD and BD replicate these findings. Zimmerman *et al.* (2010) found co-occurring BPD and BD was associated with prolonged unemployment, defined as 2 or more years unemployed in 5. Garno (2005) found patients with co-occurring bipolar and cluster B personality disorder, the majority of whom had BPD, had more lifetime suicide attempts than bipolar patients without cluster B co-occurrence. Further, cluster B diagnosis predicted suicide attempter status among bipolar patients even when childhood abuse, current depression, and substance-use disorder history were controlled, suggesting a robust relationship between risk for suicidal behavior and cluster B personality disorders (i.e., BPD, antisocial, narcissistic, histrionic PD) among bipolar patients. Garno (2005) and Swartz (2005) found bipolar patients with co-occurring BPD were less likely to stabilize than bipolar patients without co-occurring BPD receiving psychotherapy

and psychopharmacotherapy. Furthermore, co-occurring BPD and bipolar patients who stabilized required more mood-stabilizing medications and a longer treatment course than bipolar patients without co-occurring BPD. On the other hand, Gunderson *et al.* (2006), in a prospective study of BPD patients, found co-occurring BD did not predict poorer functioning, treatment response, greater utilization of medication, or inpatient treatment among BPD patients over the course of 4 years. Taken together, these results suggest co-occurring BD and BPD may be a particularly difficult combination to treat effectively.

Guidance for treating patients with co-occurring BPD and BD is limited. Treatments with known efficacy for BPD, e.g., dialectical behavior therapy (Linehan *et al.* 1991, 2006) and selective serotonin reuptake inhibitors (Rinne *et al.* 2002), are not well tested as monotherapies for BD (APA, 2010). Preliminary data suggest DBT is feasible and effective for bipolar adolescents (Goldstein *et al.* 2007). Mood stabilizers, the first-line treatment for BD (APA, 2010), and atypical antipsychotics, a psychopharmacological agent effective for bipolar depression (Calabrese, 2005, APA, 2010), show very limited efficacy for BPD (Frankenburg and Zanarini, 2002, Bowden and Maier, 2003, for reviews). Limitations of the few studies testing atypical antipsychotics and mood stabilizers for BPD are plentiful and include small sample sizes and unblinded outcome assessments. Thus, definitive conclusions regarding their efficacy for co-occurring BD and BPD cannot be drawn (Frankenburg and Zanarini, 2002, Bowden and Maier, 2003, for reviews). Two studies have tested treatments specifically among co-occurring BD and personality disorder patients. Colom *et al.* (2004) found psychoeducation vs. a nonstructured intervention, as an adjunctive to pharmacotherapy, reduced the likelihood and frequency of recurrent mood episodes, reduced inpatient days, and increased the time to relapse among co-occurring bipolar I and personality disorder patients for 2 years post-intervention. Frankenburg and Zanarini (2002) found co-occurring BPD and bipolar II patients receiving divalproex sodium compared to placebo had greater reductions in interpersonal sensitivity, anger/hostility, and aggression, but not depression pre- to post-treatment. In sum, a few promising approaches for treating co-occurring BPD and BD exist. Future studies are needed to confirm preliminary findings (Bowden and Maier, 2003).

Biomarkers of BPD

A number of studies have reported altered brain structure and function in patients with BPD relative to controls. Although these brain imaging findings in BPD may lead to diagnostic biomarkers, many of the altered brain regions and systems associated with BPD overlap with mood disorders and other Axis I disorders (Ressler and Mayberg, 2007). Further, there have been few studies that have directly compared BPD to other mood disorders. Moreover, these findings may be the consequence of the environmental risk factors associated with the development of BPD, such as early maltreatment and attachment disturbances.

In structural imaging studies, individuals with BPD (Driessen *et al.* 2000, Schmahl *et al.* 2003b) have been found to have relative reductions in the volumes of the hippocampus, amygdala, and right anterior cingulate cortex (ACC). Additionally, another study (van Elst *et al.* 2003) found relative reduction of the left orbito-frontal cortex (OFC) in individuals with BPD. Functional findings consistently demonstrate overactive amygdala and other limbic structures and underactive prefrontal activations in BPD patients relative to controls during processing of affective stimuli. This pattern of findings is consistent with impaired inhibitory control over emotional arousal. Specifically, when individuals with BPD are presented with emotional and neutral faces (Donegan *et al.* 2003) and negative emotional pictures (Herpertz *et al.* 2001, Koenigsberg *et al.* 2007), they exhibit greater amygdala activation than controls. In addition, fear stimuli are associated with increased activation of the right amygdala and decreased activation of the bilateral rostral/subgenual ACC in BPD relative to controls (Minzenberg *et al.* 2007). Individuals with BPD also exhibit problems regulating stress and emotion, as evidenced by a dysfunctional network including the ACC and frontal brain regions (Wingenfeld *et al.* 2009).

In a related study, individuals with BPD were instructed to employ distancing strategies to negative social–emotional pictures, instead of simply looking at them (Koenigsberg *et al.* 2009). Compared with controls, these individuals showed less activation change in brain regions associated with cognitive control (dorsal ACC, intraparietal sulcus, superior temporal sulcus, and superior frontal gyrus) and less deactivation in the amygdala when attempting cognitive control (distancing). These findings provide further evidence of impaired inhibitory controls of emotional arousal by frontal regions (e.g., OFC) in BPD.

Several positron emission tomography (PET) and magnetic resonance spectroscopy (MRS) imaging studies of BPD further suggest impairments in inhibitory or cognitive control circuits and structures in BPD. A study using proton MRS to assess neuronal viability via metabolites in individuals with BPD vs. controls found that the BPD group exhibited less metabolite concentration in the dorsolateral prefrontal cortex (DLPFC) compared to controls (van Elst *et al.* 2001). A review of [18 F]-fluorodeoxyglucose (FDG) uptake studies in BPD using PET found support in four of five studies for reduced uptake of FDG in prefrontal regions (particularly the OFC) in individuals with BPD relative to controls (Johnson *et al.* 2003). Two PET fenfluramine (FEN) challenge studies found attenuated FEN response in OFC regions (Siever *et al.* 1999, Soloff *et al.* 2000b). Reduced FEN response is an indicator of blunted serotonin activity and has been associated with impulsivity and depressive emotions, both features of BPD. In one of the few studies that directly compared MDD to MDD with BPD using FEN in PET, individuals with BPD and MDD exhibited more activity in parietotemporal cortical regions prior to and subsequent to FEN compared to MDD without BPD. BPD with MDD individuals also had less baseline serotonergic uptake in the anterior cingulate cortex relative to depressed patients without BPD, and FEN challenge eliminated the difference between BPD and MDD, and MDD without BPD (Oquendo *et al.* 2005). In aggregate, the FDG and FEN studies consistently find that individuals with BPD exhibit impaired frontal cortex (i.e., cognitive control) processing, which may impair the downregulation of negative emotions such as fear, dysphoria, and aggression. Moreover, differential serotonergic functioning may distinguish BPD with MDD from MDD without BPD.

Neuropsychological investigations directly comparing BPD and MDD suggest that performance is comparable in co-occurring MDD and BPD and MDD individuals without personality disorder when both are in a major depressive episode (Fertuck *et al.* 2006b). However, neuropsychological deficits may be related to different underlying mechanisms. When neuropsychological performance was corrected for anxiety, co-occurring BPD–MDD individuals outperformed MDD individuals in key areas that typically reflect the effects of depression. Depression-like deficits in BPD participants may be more closely related to characteristic affective instability than to the effects of depressed mood.

Thus, overall, neuroimaging and neurocognitive findings support a broader dysfunction in the executive controls subserved by these frontal networks in BPD, particularly under conditions of affective arousal (Fertuck et al. 2006a, Silbersweig et al. 2007).

In addition to impairment in the cognitive control of emotion, several brain imaging studies document the neural correlates of interpersonal dysfunction in individuals with BPD. Individuals with BPD were impaired, relative to controls, in their ability to trust their partners in an economic exchange task. This lack of trusting was related to dysregulated activation in the anterior insula in participants with BPD (King-Casas et al. 2008). A PET study of neural response to personalized memories of abandonment and neglect found greater increases in blood flow in bilateral DLPFC and right cuneus in women with BPD compared to controls during distressing memories (Schmahl et al. 2003a). Additionally, there were greater decreases in blood flow in the right ACC area in BPD vs. controls during rejection memories.

A recently proposed model with some supporting data suggests that interpersonal difficulties and self-injurious behaviors in BPD are mediated by dysfunction in neuropeptide activity in the brain and central nervous system (Stanley and Siever, 2010, Stanley et al. 2010). The model identifies neurochemical correlates of the unstable relationships, chronic feeling of emptiness, suspiciousness of others, and intense concern and anxiety over the emotional availability and support of romantic partners, friends, and family. This model does not address differences in co-occurring MDD and BPD.

Conclusion

The presence of BPD in patients with mood disorders complicates the clinical picture, treatment, and prognosis. Co-occurring BPD results in longer time to remission of depression and less efficacy of the standard treatments for depression and bipolar depression. Furthermore, there is some evidence that diminishing symptoms of BPD lead to improved mood rather than the reverse (Gunderson et al. 2004). Therefore, it is important to assess for this co-occurrence at the outset of treatment and to consider initiating treatments that target both the mood disorder and the personality disorder.

References

Abela, J.R., Payne, A.V., and Moussaly, N. (2003). Cognitive vulnerability to depression in individuals with borderline personality disorder. *Journal of Personality Disorders*, 17, 319–329.

Akiskal, H.S. (2004). Demystifying borderline personality: critique of the concept and unorthodox reflections on its natural kinship with the bipolar spectrum. *Acta Psychiatrica Scandinavica*, 110, 401–407.

Akiskal, H.S., Chen, S.E., Davis, G.C. et al. (1985). Borderline: An adjective in search of a noun. *Journal of Clinical Psychiatry*, 46, 7.

APA (2010). *Practice Guidelines for the Treatment of Patients with Bipolar Disorder, Second Edition.* Arlington, VA: American Psychiatric Association.

Bassett, D. (2012). Borderline personality disorder and bipolar affective disorder. Spectra or spectre? A review. *Australian and New Zealand Journal of Psychiatry*, 46, 327–339.

Beck, A.T. and Steer, R.A. (1993). *Beck Depression Inventory Manual.* San Antonio, TX: Psychological Corporation.

Benazzi, F. (2008). A relationship between bipolar II disorder and borderline personality disorder? *Progress in Neuro-Psychopharmacology and Biological Psychiatry*, 32, 1022–1029.

Binks, C.A., Fenton, M., McCarthy, L. et al. (2006). Pharmacological interventions for people with borderline personality disorder. *Cochrane Database of Systematic Reviews*, 25, CD005653.

Bowden, C. and Maier, W. (2003). Bipolar disorder and personality disorder. *European Psychiatry*, 18, 3.

Brodsky, B.S., Groves, B.A., Oquendo, M.A., Mann, J.J., and Stanley, B. (2006). Suicide risk and environmental stressors: Comparing depressed attempters with and without borderline personality disorder. *Suicide and Life Threatening Behavior*, 36, 313–322.

Calabrese, J.R. (2005). Clinical highlights in bipolar depression: Focus on atypical antipsychotics. *Journal of Clinical Psychiatry*, 66, 26.

Colom, F., Vieta, E., Sanchez-Moreno, J. et al. (2004). Psychoeducation in bipolar patients with comorbid personality disorders. *Bipolar Disorders*, 6, 4.

Corbitt, E. M., Malone, K. M., Haas, G.L., and Mann, J.J. (1996). Suicidal behavior in patients with major depression and comorbid personality disorders. *Journal of Affective Disorders*, 39, 61–72.

Davis, G.C. and Akiskal, H.S. (1986). Descriptive, biological, and theoretical aspects of borderline personality disorder. *Hospital and Community Psychiatry*, 37, 685–692.

Deltito, J., Martin, L., Riefkohl, J. *et al.* (2001). Do patients with borderline personality disorder belong to the bipolar spectrum? *Journal of Affective Disorders*, 67, 221–228.

Donegan, N.H., Sanislow, C.A., Blumberg, H.P. *et al.* (2003). Amygdala hyperreactivity in borderline personality disorder: Implications for emotional dysregulation. *Biological Psychiatry*, 54, 1284–1293.

Driessen, M., Herrmann, J., Stahl, K. *et al.* (2000). Magnetic resonance imaging volumes of the hippocampus and the amygdala in women with borderline personality disorder and early traumatization. *Archives of General Psychiatry*, 57, 1115–1122.

Fertuck, E.A., Makhija, N., and Stanley, B. (2007). The nature of suicidality in borderline personality disorder. *Primary Psychiatry*, 14, 40–47.

Fertuck, E.A., Lenzenweger, M.F., Clarkin, J.F., Hoermann, S., and Stanley, B. (2006a). Executive neurocognition, memory systems, and borderline personality disorder. *Clinical Psychology Review*, 26(3), 346–375.

Fertuck, E.A., Marsano-Jozefowicz, S., Stanley, B. *et al.* (2006b). The impact of borderline personality disorder and anxiety on neuropsychological performance in major depression. *Journal of Personality Disorders*, 20, 55–70.

Feske, U., Mulsant, B.H., Pilkonis, P.A. *et al.* (2004). Clinical outcome of ECT in patients with major depression and comorbid borderline personality disorder. *American Journal of Psychiatry*, 161, 2073–2080.

Feurino Iii, L. and Silk, K.R. (2011). State of the art in the pharmacologic treatment of borderline personality disorder. *Current Psychiatry Reports*, 13, 69–75.

Frankenburg, F.R. and Zanarini, M.C. (2002). Divalproex sodium treatment of women with borderline personality disorder and bipolar II disorder: A double-blind placebo-controlled pilot study. *Journal of Clinical Psychiatry*, 63, 442–446.

Garno, J.L. (2005). Bipolar disorder with comorbid cluster B personality disorder features: Impact on suicidality. *Journal of Clinical Psychiatry*, 66, 339.

Goldstein, T.R., Axelson, D.A., Birmaher, B.O.R.I., and Brent, D.A. (2007). Dialectical behavior therapy for adolescents with bipolar disorder: A 1-year open trial. *Journal of the American Academy of Child and Adolescent Psychiatry*, 46, 820–830.

Goodman, M., New, A., Triebwasser, J., Collins, K.A., and Siever, L. (2010). Phenotype, endophenotype, and genotype comparisons between borderline personality disorder and major depressive disorder. *Journal of Personality Disorders*, 24, 38–59.

Grant, B.F., Chou, P.S., Goldstein, R.B. (2008). Prevalence, correlates, disability, and comorbidity of DSM-IV borderline personality disorder: Results from the Wave 2 National Epidemiologic Survey on Alcohol and Related Conditions. *Journal of Clinical Psychiatry*, 69, 533.

Grilo, C.M., Stout, R.L., Markowitz, J.C. (2010). Personality disorders predict relapse after remission from an episode of major depressive disorder: S 6-year prospective study. *Journal of Clinical Psychiatry*, 71, 1629–1635.

Grunhaus, L., King, D., Greden, J.F., and Flegel, P. (1985). Depression and panic in patients with borderline personality disorder. *Biological Psychiatry*, 20, 688–692.

Gunderson, J.G. and Phillips, K.A. (1991). A current view of the interface between borderline personality disorder and depression. *American Journal of Psychiatry*, 148, 967–975.

Gunderson, J.G., Morey, L.C., Stout, R.L. *et al.* (2004). Major depressive disorder and borderline personality disorder revisited: Longitudinal interactions. *Journal of Clinical Psychiatry*, 65, 1049–1056.

Gunderson, J.G., Weinberg, I., Daversa, M.T. *et al.* (2006). Descriptive and longitudinal observations on the relationship of borderline personality disorder and bipolar disorder. *American Journal of Psychiatry*, 163, 1173–1178.

Hamilton, M. (1960). A rating scale for depression. *Journal of Neurology, Neurosurgery and Psychiatry*, 23, 56–62.

Hasin, D.S., Goodwin, R.D., Stinson, F.S., and Grant, B.F. (2005). Epidemiology of major depressive disorder: Results from the National Epidemiologic Survey on Alcoholism and Related Conditions. *Archives of General Psychiatry*, 62, 1097–1106.

Henry, C., Mitropoulou, V., New, A. *et al.* (2001). Affective instability and impulsivity in borderline personality and bipolar II disorders: Similarities and differences. *Journal of Psychiatric Research*, 35, 5.

Herpertz, S.C. (2003). Emotional processing in personality disorder. *Current Psychiatry Reports*, 5, 23–27.

Herpertz, S.C., Dietrich, T.M., Wenning, B. *et al.* (2001). Evidence of abnormal amygdala functioning in borderline personality disorder: A functional MRI study. *Biological Psychiatry*, 50, 292–298.

Johnson, P.A., Hurley, R.A., Benkelfat, C., Herpertz, S.C., and Taber, K.H. (2003). Understanding emotion regulation in borderline personality disorder: Contributions of neuroimaging. *Journal of Neuropsychiatry and Clinical Neuroscience*, 15, 397–402.

Joyce, P.R., Mulder, R.T., Luty, S.E. *et al.* (2003). Borderline personality disorder in major depression: Symptomatology, temperament, character, differential drug response, and 6-month outcome. *Comprehensive Psychiatry*, 44, 35–43.

Kelly, T.M., Soloff, P.H., Lynch, K.G., Haas, G.L., and Mann, J.J. (2000). Recent life events, social adjustment, and suicide attempts in patients with major depression and borderline personality disorder. *Journal of Personality Disorders*, 14, 316–326.

Kernberg, O.F. (2001). The suicidal risk in severe personality disorders: Differential diagnosis and treatment. *Journal of Personality Disorders*, 15, 195–208; discussion 209–215.

King-Casas, B., Sharp, C., Lomax-Bream, L. *et al.* (2008). The rupture and repair of cooperation in borderline personality disorder. *Science*, 321, 806–810.

Koenigsberg, H.W., Fan, J., Ochsner, K.N. *et al.* (2007). *Neural Correlates of Emotion Dysregulation in Borderline Personality Disorder*. Paper presented at the American College of Neuropsychopharmacology.

Koenigsberg, H.W., Fan, J., Ochsner, K.N. *et al.* (2009). Neural correlates of the use of psychological distancing to regulate responses to negative social cues: A study of patients with borderline personality disorder. *Biological Psychiatry*, 66, 854–863.

Linehan, M.M. (1993). *Cognitive-Behavioral Treatment of Borderline Personality Disorder*. New York, NY: Guilford.

Linehan, M.M., Armstrong, H.E., Suarez, A., Allmon, D., and Heard, H.L. (1991). Cognitive-behavioral treatment of chronically parasuicidal borderline patients. *Archives of General Psychiatry*, 48, 1060–1064.

Linehan, M.M., Comtois, K.A., Murray, A.M. *et al.* (2006). Two-year randomized controlled trial and follow-up of dialectical behavior therapy vs therapy by experts for suicidal behaviors and borderline personality disorder. *Archives of General Psychiatry*, 63, 757–766.

Links, P.S., Heslegrave, R.J., Mitton, J.E. *et al.* (1995). Borderline psychopathology and recurrences of clinical disorders. *Journal of Nervous and Mental Disease*, 183, 582–586.

Loranger, A.W., Oldham, J.M., and Tulis, E.H. (1982). Familial transmission of DSM-III borderline personality disorder. *Archives of General Psychiatry*, 39, 795–799.

MacKinnon, D.F. and Pies, R. (2006). Affective instability as rapid cycling: theoretical and clinical implications for borderline personality and bipolar spectrum disorders. *Bipolar Disorders*, 8, 1–14.

Magill, C.A. (2004). The boundary between borderline personality disorder and bipolar disorder: Current concepts and challenges. *Canadian Journal of Psychiatry*, 49, 551.

Minzenberg, M.J., Fan, J., New, A.S., Tang, C.Y., and Siever, L.J. (2007). Fronto-limbic dysfunction in response to facial emotion in borderline personality disorder: An event-related fMRI study. *Psychiatry Research – Neuroimaging*, 155, 231–243.

Morey, L.C., Shea, M.T., Markowitz, J.C. *et al.* (2010). State effects of major depression on the assessment of personality and personality disorder. *American Journal of Psychiatry*, 167, 528–535.

New, A.S., Triebwasser, J., and Charney, D.S. (2008). The case for shifting borderline personality disorder to Axis I. *Biological Psychiatry*, 64, 653–659.

Nierenberg, A.A., Alpert, J.E., Pava, J., Rosenbaum, J.F., and Fava, M. (1998). Course and treatment of atypical depression. *Journal of Clinical Psychiatry*, 59 Suppl 18, 5–9.

Oldham, J.M. (2006). Borderline personality disorder and suicidality. *American Journal of Psychiatry*, 163, 20–25.

Oquendo, M.A., A. Krunic, Parsey, R.V. *et al.* (2005). Positron emission tomography of regional brain metabolic responses to a serotonergic challenge in major depressive disorder with and without borderline personality disorder. *Neuropsychopharmacology*, 30, 1163–1172.

Orbach, I., Mikulincer, M., Gilboa- Schechtman, E., and Sirota, P. (2003a). Mental pain and its relationship to suicidality and life meaning. *Suicide and Life Threatening Behavior*, 33, 231–241.

Orbach, I., Mikulincer, M., Sirota, P., and Gilboa-Schechtman, E. (2003b). Mental pain: A multidimensional operationalization and definition. *Suicide and Life Threatening Behavior*, 33, 219–230.

Paris, J. (2007). The nature of borderline personality disorder: multiple dimensions, multiple symptoms, but one category. *Journal of Personality Disorders*, 21, 457–473.

Paris, J., Gunderson, J., and Weinberg, I. (2007). The interface between borderline personality disorder and bipolar spectrum disorders. *Comprehensive Psychiatry*, 48, 145–154.

Paris, J., Silk, K.R., Gunderson, J., Links, P.S., and Zanarini, M. (2009). The case for retaining borderline personality disorder as a psychiatric diagnosis. *Personality and Mental Health*, 3(2), 96–100.

Pazzagli, A. and Monti, M.R. (2000). Dysphoria and aloneness in borderline personality disorder. *Psychopathology*, 33, 220–226.

Pepper, C.M., Klein, D.N., Anderson, R.L. *et al.* (1995). DSM-III-R axis II comorbidity in dysthymia and major depression. *American Journal of Psychiatry*, 152, 239–247.

Pfohl, B., Stangl, D., and Zimmerman, M. (1984). The implications of DSM-III personality disorders for patients with major depression. *Journal of Affective Disorders*, 7, 309–318.

Quitkin, F.M., Stewart, J.W., McGrath, P.J. *et al.* (1993). Columbia atypical depression: A subgroup of depressives with better response to MAOI than to tricyclic antidepressants or placebo. *The British Journal of Psychiatry*, 163 Suppl 21, 30–34.

Ressler, K.J. and Mayberg, H.S. (2007). Targeting abnormal neural circuits in mood and anxiety disorders: From the laboratory to the clinic. *Nature Neuroscience*, 10, 1116–1124.

Rinne, T., van den Brink, W., Wouters, L., and van Dyck, R. (2002). SSRI treatment of borderline personality disorder: A randomized, placebo-controlled clinical trial for female patients with borderline personality disorder. *American Journal of Psychiatry*, 159, 2048–2054.

Riso, L.P., Klein, D.N., and Anderson, R.L. (2000). A families study of outpatients with borderline personality disorder and no history of mood disorder. *Journal of Personality Disorders*, 14, 208–217.

Rogers, J.H., Widiger, T.A., and Krupp, A. (1995). Aspects of depression associated with borderline personality disorder. *American Journal of Psychiatry*, 152, 268–270.

Runeson, B. and Beskow, J. (1991). Borderline personality disorder in young Swedish suicides. *Journal of Nervous and Mental Disease*, 179, 153–156.

Schmahl, C.G., Elzinga, B.M., Vermetten, E. *et al.* (2003a). Neural correlates of memories of abandonment in women with and without borderline personality disorder. *Biological Psychiatry*, 54, 142–151.

Schmahl, C.G., Vermetten, E., Elzinga, B.M., and Bremner, D.J. (2003b). Magnetic resonance imaging of hippocampal and amygdala volume in women with childhood abuse and borderline personality disorder. *Psychiatry Research*, 122, 193–198.

Siever, L.J., Buchsbaum, M.S., New, A.S. *et al.* (1999). d,l-fenfluramine response in impulsive personality disorder assessed with [18F]fluorodeoxyglucose positron emission tomography. *Neuropsychopharmacology*, 20, 413–423.

Silbersweig, D., Clarkin, J.F., Goldstein, M. *et al.* (2007). Failure of frontolimbic inhibitory function in the context of negative emotion in borderline personality disorder. *American Journal of Psychiatry*, 164, 1832–1841.

Silk, K.R. (2011). The process of managing medications in patients with borderline personality disorder. *Journal of Psychiatric Practice*, 17, 311–319.

Skodol, A.E., Grilo, C.M., Keyes, K.M. *et al.* (2011). Relationship of personality disorders to the course of major depressive disorder in a nationally representative sample. *American Journal of Psychiatry*, 168, 257–264.

Smith, D.J., Muir, W.J., and Blacwood, D.H.R. (2004). Is borderline personality disorder part of the bipolar spectrum? *Harvard Review of Psychiatry*, 12, 133–138.

Soloff, P. (2000). Psychopharmacology of borderline personality disorder. *Psychiatric Clinics of North America*, 23, 169–192.

Soloff, P.H., Lynch K.G., Kelly, T.M., Malone, K.M., and Mann, J.J. (2000a). Characteristics of suicide attempts of patients with major depressive episode and borderline personality disorder: A comparative study. *American Journal of Psychiatry*, 157, 601–608.

Soloff, P.H., Meltzer, C.C., Greer, P.J., Constantine, D., and Kelly, T.M. (2000b). A fenfluramine-activated FDG-PET study of borderline personality disorder. *Biological Psychiatry*, 47, 540–547.

Stanley, B. and Wilson, S.T. (2006). Heightened subjective experience of depression in borderline personality disorder. *Journal of Personality Disorders*, 20, 307–318.

Stanley, B. and Siever, L.J. (2010). The interpersonal dimension of borderline personality disorder: Toward a neuropeptide model. *American Journal of Psychiatry*, 167, 24–39.

Stanley, B., Sher, L., Wilson, S. *et al.* (2010). Non-suicidal self-injurious behavior, endogenous opioids and monoamine neurotransmitters. *Journal of Affective Disorders*, 124, 134–140.

Stiglmayr, C.E., Grathwol, T., Linehan, M.M. *et al.* (2005). Aversive tension in patients with borderline personality disorder: a computer-based controlled field study. *Acta Psychiatrica Scandinavica*, 111, 372–379.

Swartz, H.A. (2005). Acute treatment outcomes in patients with bipolar I disorder and co-occurring borderline personality disorder receiving medication and psychotherapy. *Bipolar Disorders*, 7, 192–197.

van Elst, L.T., Thiel, T., Hesslinger, B. *et al.* (2001). Subtle prefrontal neuropathology in a pilot magnetic resonance spectroscopy study in patients with borderline personality disorder. *Journal of Neuropsychiatry and Clinical Neuroscience*, 13, 511–514.

van Elst, L.T., Hesslinger, B., Thiel, T. *et al.* (2003). Frontolimbic brain abnormalities in patients with borderline personality disorder: A volumetric magnetic resonance imaging study. *Biological Psychiatry*, 54, 163–171.

Westen, D., Moses, M.J., Silk, K.R. *et al.* (1992). Quality of depressive experience in borderline personality disorder and major depression: When depression is not just depression. *Journal of Personality Disorders*, 6, 382–393.

Wilson, S.T., Stanley, B., Oquendo, M.A. *et al.* (2007). Comparing impulsiveness, hostility, and depression in borderline personality disorder and bipolar II disorder. *Journal of Clinical Psychiatry*, 68, 1533.

Wingenfeld, K., Spitzer, C., Rullkvatter, N., and Lowe, B. (2009). Borderline personality disorder: Hypothalamus pituitary adrenal axis and findings from neuroimaging studies. *Psychoneuroendocrinology*, 35, 154–170.

Yen, S., Shea, M.T., Sanislow, C.A. *et al.* (2004). Borderline personality disorder criteria associated with prospectively observed suicidal behavior. *American Journal of Psychiatry*, 161, 1296–1298.

Zanarini, M.C. and Frankenburg, F.R. (2007). The essential nature of borderline psychopathology. *Journal of Personality Disorders*, 21, 518–535.

Zanarini, M.C., Frankenburg, F.R., Hennen, J., and Silk, K.R. (2003). The longitudinal course of borderline psychopathology: 6-year prospective follow-up of the phenomenology of borderline personality disorder. *American Journal of Psychiatry*, 160, 274–283.

Zanarini, M.C., Frankenburg, F.R., DeLuca, C.J. *et al.* (1998). The pain of being borderline: Dysphoric states specific to borderline personality disorder. *Harvard Reviews of Psychiatry*, 6, 201–207.

Zanarini, M.C., Frankenburg, F.R., Hennen, J. *et al.* (2004). Axis I comorbidity in patients with borderline personality disorder: 6-year follow-up and prediction of time to remission. *American Journal of Psychiatry*, 161, 2108–2114.

Zimmerman, M. and Mattia, J.I. (1999). Axis I diagnostic comorbidity and borderline personality disorder. *Comprehensive Psychiatry*, 40, 245–252.

Zimmerman, M., Galione, J.N., Chelminski, I. *et al.* (2010). Sustained unemployment in psychiatric outpatients with bipolar disorder: Frequency and association with demographic variables and comorbid disorders. *Bipolar Disorders*, 12, 720–726.

Chapter 15

Depression in the context of pregnancy

Margaret G. Spinelli and Carolyn Broudy

Introduction

The prevalence of depression during pregnancy is 11.0% in the first trimester and 8.5% in the second and third trimesters (Gaynes *et al.* 2005). The detection and appropriate management of depression among women of reproductive age before or early in pregnancy is critical. Because of the growing need for information on the use of medications for depressed pregnant women, members of the American Psychiatric Association (APA) and the American College of Obstetrics and Gynecology (ACOG) have published guidelines for treating depression during pregnancy (Yonkers *et al.* 2009). Antepartum depression may be treated effectively with psychotherapy, medications, electroconvulsive therapy (ECT), or alternative treatments.

Approximately 4.5% of pregnant women use antidepressants in the period of 3 months before conception until the end of pregnancy (Alwan *et al.* 2011). Concern for adverse outcomes of medication use during pregnancy includes teratogenic effects, adverse effects on the neonate at the time of delivery, developmental effects, and unknown long-term cognitive and behavioral effects on the child. Potential risks of medication must be balanced against the risks for adverse effects of the depression itself on mother and fetus.

This chapter will provide the clinician with current information and evidence on the risks and benefits of different treatment options for perinatal depression. In order to provide the patient with appropriate information to make an informed decision, the clinician must be knowledgeable about the risks of untreated depression as well as the risks of conventional and alternative therapies.

Initial management

Initial evaluation of a depressed pregnant woman should include information on the duration and intensity of current symptoms of major depression, present functioning, social supports, feelings about pregnancy, partner support, and thoughts or plans of suicide or self-harm. In addition to the psychiatric history, the clinician should inquire about past pregnancy-associated depressions, including postpartum depression and history of medication efficacy. It is important to obtain information on the patient's medical history and pregnancy complications, and to document any use of prescribed and over-the-counter medications, environmental exposures, alternative medications or herbal treatments, and the use of alcohol, drugs, or tobacco dating back to conception.

Decisions on treatment must be made on a case-by-case basis. Evaluation and diagnosis are followed by informed consent, whereby the risks and benefits of treatment, and the risks of untreated psychiatric illness, are reviewed. Such a discussion must involve the patient and consideration should be given to including the other parent. Patients with mild symptoms or no symptoms for 6 months may be candidates for medication taper or discontinuation, or alternative treatments for depression such as light therapy or psychotherapy (Yonkers *et al.* 2009). Patients with histories of severe, recurrent major depressive disorders or histories of suicide attempts are candidates for pharmacotherapy. For acute suicidality or psychotic symptoms, medication or even electroconvulsive therapy, as well as hospitalization, should be considered. Before prescribing or implementing a treatment plan, the clinician should document the risk–benefit discussion regarding medication or other

Clinical Handbook for the Management of Mood Disorders, ed. J. John Mann, Patrick J. McGrath, and Steven P. Roose.
Published by Cambridge University Press. © Cambridge University Press 2013.

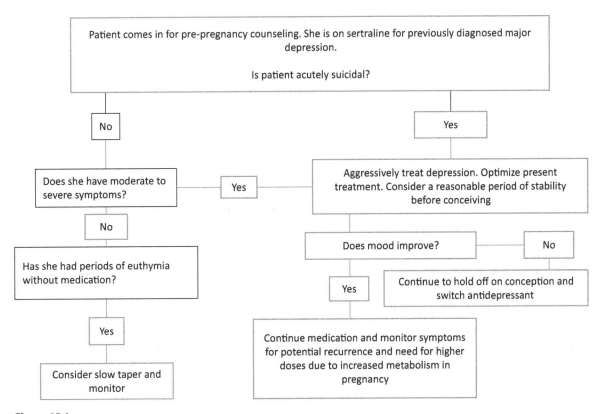

Figure 15.1

therapies and the patient's capacity to understand the informed consent process.

Adverse effects of depression during pregnancy

Untreated antenatal depression poses a number of serious risks to both mother and baby. Evidence suggests untreated depression can directly affect the fetus, or pose secondary risks due to unhealthy maternal behaviors arising from the symptoms of depression. It is also a risk to the mother's health.

In terms of the so-called direct effects, a number of studies have found an association between depression during pregnancy and an increased risk for low-birth-weight infants, preterm delivery, and small-for-gestational-age neonates. A recent meta-analysis of depression during pregnancy and the risk of preterm birth (PTB), low birth weight (LBW), and intrauterine growth restriction (IUGR), found that among prospective studies using a categorical depression measure, pooled effect sizes were 1.39, 1.49, and 1.45, respectively (Grote *et al.* 2010). Untreated depression

during pregnancy also has been associated with an elevated risk of pre-eclampsia (Kurki *et al.* 2000, Shamsi *et al.* 2010), a significant cause of morbidity and mortality.

Higher rates of developmental delay and behavioral problems have also been found in the children of untreated depressed pregnant women. More recent studies show an almost twofold increase in negative developmental outcomes (O'Connor *et al.* 2002, Deave *et al.* 2008).

Not only is depression disruptive to a woman's life and painful to endure, but it can also interfere with her ability to care for herself and the pregnancy. Depressed pregnant women are more likely to receive inadequate prenatal care (Kelly *et al.* 1999), to use tobacco, alcohol, and illicit substances during pregnancy (Horrigan *et al.* 2000), and to not gain sufficient maternal weight (Bennett *et al.* 2004). In severe cases, depression can lead to suicide and death during pregnancy, or attempted suicide which threatens the health of the mother and fetus.

Antenatal depression is also one of the strongest predictors of post-partum depression (Beck, 1996).

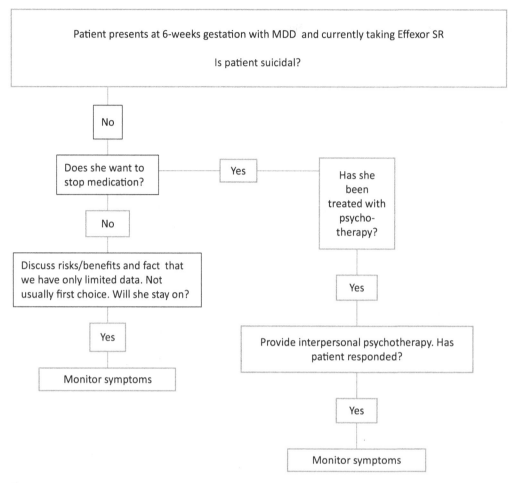

Figure 15.2

The serious adverse consequences of post-partum depression are discussed below.

Medication treatment during pregnancy

Currently, outcomes for >20 000 women exposed to antidepressant medication during pregnancy are available in the literature (Lorenzo *et al.* 2011). Because of ethical concerns, gold-standard prospective, controlled clinical treatment trials do not include pregnant women. Most studies on the use of medications during pregnancy are retrospective and rely on prescription databases, teratology services, birth registries, or population records of congenital defects. Little is known about the actual dosage and gestational timing of exposure, use of other prescribed or over-the-counter drugs, and the medical or psychiatric condition of the mother (Spinelli, 2012). While many studies of the use of medications have contradictory outcomes, emphasis is typically placed on affirmative studies, while negative findings may be disregarded. Given the described inconsistent outcomes and our reliance on peer-reviewed literature, translation of these data into clinical practice remains a challenge for the clinician.

Risk of major congenital malformations associated with antidepressants

Selective serotonin reuptake inhibitors (SSRIs)

The majority of studies have not found an association with major congenital malformations (MCMs) and first-trimester exposure to SSRIs. Data from a teratology information service (Kulin *et al.* 1998) and a population-based study in Finland (Malm *et al.*

2005) indicate no MCMs in first-trimester-exposed infants. A retrospective case control study from the Swedish Medical Birth Registry (Kallen and Otterblad Olousson, 2003) found no cardiac defects in SSRI-exposed infants. In retrospective studies, Davis *et al.* (2007) identified 2201 women who were prescribed an SSRI during pregnancy, and found no increase in MCMs, while Wichman *et al.* (2009) found no increase in congenital heart disease in 808 infants. Similarly, Udechuko *et al.* (2010) reviewed studies on SSRI-exposed infants and found more than 20 additional negative studies in infants exposed to antidepressants.

In contrast, many outcome studies report MCMs in first-trimester-exposed infants. An example of such research describes a Danish population-based cohort study (Pederson *et al.* 2009), in which prescriptions for SSRIs were associated with a twofold (1.99) increase in septal heart defects. Two factors are significant in the interpretation of these findings. First, outcomes must be interpreted in the context of the existing 3% baseline rate of birth defects (CDC, 2008). With reference to risk estimates, most specific defects are rare and absolute risks are small. For example, the baseline prevalence for septal heart defects in unexposed infants is 0.5%. The described elevated risk of 1.99 translates to an absolute risk of 0.9% in infants exposed to SSRIs. A second limitation of this dataset is reliance on prescriptions as evidence of drug exposure. It remains unclear if the medication was actually taken by the mother. Petersen *et al.* (2011) found that pregnancy was a major determinant of cessation of antidepressant medication, and most women do not receive further antidepressant prescriptions beyond 6 weeks of gestation.

Large studies are frequently limited by analyses unadjusted for confounders such as alcoholism or smoking. For example, a recent article suggested that fluoxetine and paroxetine taken during pregnancy increased the risks for cardiac defects and citalopram increased the risk for spina bifida in exposed infants (Malm *et al.* 2011). The authors reported that mothers who took SSRIs during pregnancy also had a 10-fold higher rate of fetal alcohol syndrome. Such a confounder that means alcohol exposure potentially causes the fetal abnormality and not the SSRI, is an important methodological concern for proper interpretation of the findings (Spinelli, 2012).

A fundamental principle in birth defects research is that teratogenic exposures induce specific patterns of malformation and do not increase the incidences of all defects (Chambers, 2009). Yet, selected birth defects often differ from study to study, and findings are seldom replicated. In 2007, the New England Journal of Medicine published two articles in the same issue on the first-trimester use of SSRIs and risk of birth defects. Despite similar sample sets, the authors failed to replicate most findings and commented that multiple tests may have caused significant findings by chance.

Using data from the National Birth Defects Linkage Study, Alwan *et al.* (2007) found that overall SSRI use was associated with a more than twofold increased risk in anencephaly, craniosynostosis, and omphalocele, but found that the absolute risks were small. Data from the Slone Epidemiology Birth Defects Study (Louik *et al.* 2007) failed to replicate Alwan *et al.*'s findings although they found some similar associations with specific SSRIs. If antidepressants are teratogenic, then we would expect to see similar findings for similar drug exposures, and the same specific defects detected in all positive studies.

One finding that was replicated in Alwan *et al.*'s and Louik *et al.*'s data was the increase in right ventricular obstruction outflow defects in infants whose mothers were exposed to paroxetine in the first trimester. Paroxetine has been the most controversial SSRI for use in pregnant women. For example, a recent meta-analysis (Wurst *et al.* 2010) reviewed data on first-trimester paroxetine exposure and found that some studies replicated an increased risk for cardiovascular defects (CVDs), although others found no risk. Conflicting outcomes require clinicians to interpret these findings in the context of the methodological limitations common to birth defects research.

Vignette

Mrs. A was a 24-year-old married woman who presented with her husband for a preconception psychopharmacology consultation. The patient had a history of three major depressive episodes in the last 10 years. She had one psychiatric hospitalization for a suicide attempt and she admits to recent passive suicidal ideation. Mrs. A's depression also placed her at risk for post-partum depression. Although she had a good initial response to sertraline 100 mg/d during the present depression, she has noticed an increase in depressed mood, irritability, loss of appetite, and insomnia in the past week. After discussing with

Mr. and Mrs. A the concern about her worsening symptoms, history of suicide attempt, and risks to a planned pregnancy as well as any potential risks of sertraline during pregnancy, the physician and the patient agreed that she would increase her dose of sertraline to 150 mg/d, stabilize her mood prior to conception, and remain on medication during her pregnancy and throughout delivery into the post-partum period.

Serotonin–norepinephrine reuptake inhibitors (SNRIs) and norepinephrine reuptake inhibitors (NRIs)

Einarson et al. (2001) found no significant increase in MCMs in a total of 171 venlafaxine-exposed infants. Lannestal and Källén (2007) found no increase in MCMs in 732 infants exposed to SNRIs and NRIs. In the largest study to date using the Swedish Medical Birth Registry, Reis and Källén, (2010) found no increased risk for malformations in infants with early SNRI exposure.

Tricyclic Antidepressants (TCAs)

Nortriptyline and desipramine are preferred tricylics for use during pregnancy because they are least likely to cause anticholinergic effects or orthostatic hypotension. In general, studies do not support an association between major malformations in neonates born to mothers who used TCAs during pregnancy (McElhatton et al. 1996). Despite a few early case reports of limb defects (Davis et al. 2007), large studies such as The European Network Teratology Service found no overall increase in the rate of MCMs in TCA-exposed live-born infants (Eberhard-Gran et al. 2005).

Recent findings identified clomipramine as a potential culprit for cardiac defects (Reis and Källén, 2010). A later study from the same registry identified an association between cardiac malformations and TCAs (Reis and Källén, 2010). Of 1662 cases of TCA exposure, 1208 were clomipramine and 379 were amitriptyline, findings that may not be extrapolated to all TCAs. It may be the serotonin transporter inhibition by clomipramine and amitriptyline that explains this association.

Bupropion

The GlaxoSmithKline Bupropion Pregnancy Registry (GlaxoSmithKlein, 2006) suggested a higher than expected frequency of neonatal cardiac malformations, as did Alwan et al. (2010), who observed an increase in left outflow tract heart defect with an absolute risk of 2.1/1000. However, results from a prospective study of pregnancy outcomes among bupropion-exposed children revealed no MCMs above the baseline of 1–3% (Chun-Fai-Chan et al. 2005). Similarly, recent studies found no significant differences in the rate of major malformations between bupropion-exposed groups and control groups (Cole et al. 2007, Einarson et al. 2009). This possible association is important because it would mean that it can potentially be caused by medications that target the noradrenergic system, and not just serotonin-related medications.

Other antidepressants

Non-SSRI and non-TCA antidepressants have been the focus of small studies. These medications include trazodone, mirtazapine, nefazodone, mianserin, and reboxetine. None of these investigations reported higher rates of malformations (Einarson et al. 2001, 2003; Einarson and Einarson, 2005, Djulus et al. 2006; Einarson et al. 2009).

In a study of 21 prenatal exposures to monoamine oxidase inhibitors (MAOIs) in pregnancy, there was a relative risk of 3.4 for congenital malformations (Heinonen et al. 1999). The risk of a hypertensive crisis contributes to recommendations that MAOIs should be avoided in pregnancy.

Spontaneous abortions

Several studies have indicated an increased rate of spontaneous abortion with the use of antidepressants in the first trimester. Broy and Berard (2010) reviewed 15 studies that examined the association between adverse pregnancy outcomes and gestational exposure to antidepressants (TCAs and SSRIs) with data on spontaneous abortions. In unadjusted analyses, fluoxetine (OR 2.0; 95% CI = 1.4–3.0) and bupropion (OR 4.1; 95% CI = 1.5–11.1) were significantly associated with the risk of miscarriage. However in adjusted analyses, paroxetine (OR 1.7; 95% CI = 1.3–2.3) and venlafaxine (2.1; 95% CI = 1.3–3.3) were also confirmed as significantly associated with the risk of spontaneous abortion.

Neonatal outcomes

Persistent pulmonary hypertension of the newborn (PPHN)

While studies report contradictory outcomes on the association between PPHN and prenatal exposure to SSRIs, Occhiogrosso et al. (2012) described the strengths and weaknesses of six studies of SSRI exposure and PPHN. Three studies found no association between PPHN and SSRIs. Of the three studies that did find associations, two of the studies examined the same population database, incorporating additional recent births. Examined together, the six studies identified a total of 50 SSRI-exposed infants with PPHN from approximately 25 000 who had SSRI exposure, less than the estimated rate in the general population. In a more recent study, Kieler et al. (2012) found in a population-based cohort of 11 014 women who were dispensed an SSRI after gestational week 20 that the use of SSRIs in late pregnancy increases the risk of PPHN more than twofold.

Neonatal behavioral syndrome

A neonatal behavioral syndrome (NBS) has been described in neonates exposed to antidepressants *in utero*. Commonly seen symptoms include jitteriness, poor muscle tone, weak or absent cry, respiratory distress, hypoglycemia, low Apgar score, and possible seizures (Moses-Kolko et al. 2005). These symptoms are usually mild, transient, and do not require treatment. Symptoms tend to peak around 48 hours after delivery, and resolve within 3–5 days (Laine et al. 2003, Levinson-Castiel et al. 2006). Some studies suggest NBS can occur in up to 30% of neonates exposed to SSRIs (Chambers et al. 1996, Levinson-Castiel et al. 2006, Oberlander et al. 2006).

Given the data suggesting an association between third-trimester SSRI use and NBS, the FDA stated in 2004 that, "physicians may consider tapering [drug name] in the third trimester (USFDA)." However, many studies supporting this association did not control for important confounders, such as severity of maternal illness and length of exposure to medication. Oberlander and colleagues found that when controlling for several maternal factors, there was no longer a significant difference between early and late exposure (Oberlander et al. 2006, 2008). Interestingly, while the timing of exposure was not associated with NBS, an increased duration of exposure (days) remained significantly associated with respiratory distress.

In an attempt to address the question of whether tapering SSRIs in the third trimester reduces the risk of NBS, Warburton et al. (2010) used population health data, to link maternal health and prenatal SSRI prescriptions to neonatal birth records. When propensity score matching was used to control for potential confounders, there was no significant difference in rates of NBS between neonates exposed in the last 14 days (n = 239) of gestation and those who had not been exposed in the last 14 days (n = 239). Although this study has a number of limitations, it suggests that an acute pharmacological condition such as toxicity or withdrawal may not account for an increased risk of adverse neonatal outcomes, and, as such, tapering SSRIs towards the end of pregnancy may not improve neonatal outcomes.

Prematurity and low birth weight

Antidepressant use during pregnancy has been associated with a reduction in birth weight and preterm delivery; however, not all studies support this association, and maternal depression has also been associated with these outcomes. Several studies have tried to control for maternal depression using propensity score matching, but these studies have a number of methodological limitations. For instance, in a large, retrospective study using population health data, Oberlander et al. (2008) found that with propensity score matching, the incidence of birth weight less than the 10th percentile remained significantly higher among SSRI users, but preterm delivery did not. This study did not control for alcohol and tobacco use during pregnancy, and information obtained from medical records may not accurately reflect the severity of maternal depression, or whether medication was actually taken. In a compelling study, comparing pregnant women with untreated depression to those receiving SSRIs, Wisner and colleagues (2009) found that infants who were continuously exposed to either SSRIs or major depression were more likely to be born preterm than were infants with no exposure.

Long-term developmental effects

Several small studies provide reassuring evidence regarding the safety of antidepressant use on child development. For instance, Nulman et al. (2002) found no effect of neonatal exposure to fluoxetine or tricyclic antidepressants on global IQ, language development, or behavioral development between 15 to 71 months. IQ and language development were, however, significantly and negatively associated with postnatal maternal depression. Similarly, Misri et al. (2006) found that levels of internalizing behaviors did not differ significantly between 22 4-year-old children with prolonged prenatal SSRI exposure, and 14 children born to healthy, nondepressed, nonmedicated mothers. However, as symptoms of maternal anxiety and depression increased, so did reported internalizing behaviors in their children.

Two small studies found significant differences in psychomotor behavior in children prenatally exposed to SSRIs. Casper *et al.* (2003) found that exposed children between the ages of 6 to 40 months, scored lower on the psychomotor indexes (e.g., tremulousness and inappropriate fine motor movement) compared to the unexposed group. A larger, more recent study by Pederson and colleagues (2010) found that at 6 months of age, significantly more children whose mothers took antidepressants were unable to sit without support. However, by 19 months of age there were no differences in milestones measured, except for an association between second- or third-trimester exposure and the inability of the children to occupy themselves for at least 15 minutes. Despite these differences, the ages at which the children in both groups were able to meet their milestones were within the range of normal development.

Based on four cases of attention deficit hyperactivity disorder (ADHD), Figueroa (2010) found that exposure to bupropion was associated with an increased risk of ADHD, but failed to control for parent's mental illness and multiple other factors.

In a recent population-based, case-controlled trial that received widespread media attention (Croen *et al.* 2011), the authors suggested a higher rate of autism spectrum disorders in the children of 15 mothers who were treated with SSRIs in the year before and during pregnancy. In addition to having a small number of case subjects, the study did not control for psychiatric illness in the mother at the time of the study, although the association between psychiatric disorders and autism spectrum disorders is well documented (Daniels *et al.* 2008). Autism spectrum disorder is a heritable disease, but family genetic loading was not reported (Spinelli, 2012).

Taken together, studies on the effects of prenatal exposure to antidepressants on childhood development are generally reassuring. However, the long-term impact of these differences remains unclear. In weighing the possible risks, it is important to keep in mind that antepartum stress, post-partum depression, and concurrent maternal depression all strongly correlate with negative developmental outcomes.

Alternative treatments

The APA/ACOG guidelines recommend psychosocial approaches, such as group or individual therapy, as first-line treatments for mild to moderate antepartum depression (Yonkers *et al.* 2009). Two clinical studies have found interpersonal psychotherapy (IPT), a time-limited therapy focusing on interpersonal relationships, to be effective for the treatment of mild to moderate depression during pregnancy (Spinelli 1997, Spinelli and Endicott, 2003). While other types of psychotherapy such as cognitive behavior therapy (CBT) have yet to be studied in controlled clinical trials in pregnant women, it is reasonable to consider all clinically appropriate psychotherapy options.

There are a number of alternative or adjunctive treatments, but only limited evidence exists to support their use in pregnancy. A small randomized, placebo-controlled trial found that high-dose omega-3 fatty acids (3–4g/d) can reduce depression in women during pregnancy (Su *et al.* 2008). A recent randomized, controlled trial in pregnant women found that acupuncture for depression significantly reduces the severity of symptoms, as compared to sham acupuncture treatment (Manber *et al.* 2010).

Light therapy is another evidence-based treatment option for depression. Recently, a small, randomized, double-blind, placebo-controlled trial found that bright white light treatment for 5 weeks improved depression during pregnancy significantly more than placebo dim red light (Wirz-Justice *et al.* 2011).

Vignette

Ms. B is a 24-year-old mother at 8 weeks' gestation experiencing her first depression. The patient presented as tearful, "exhausted," with hyperphagia and hypersomnia. She had no significant anxiety and no history of bipolar hypomania. After discussing the risks and benefits of all possible treatments, the patient refused medication. In view of her history, first onset of depression, and lack of suicidality she was offered light therapy. Ms. B purchased a 10 000 lux light box and began 30 minutes of light treatment every morning. After 2 weeks there was no improvement in mood, while 1 hour provided minimal improvement. Ultimately 90 minutes was the dose at which her depression remitted after 4 weeks of treatment. When symptoms recurred in the post-partum period, the patient decided to take medication.

Maintenance treatment

Treating depression during pregnancy is an ongoing process. As the pregnancy progresses, new information may shift the risk–benefit analysis so that a change in the treatment plan becomes necessary (Wisner *et al.* 2000). The optimal management is to quickly identify recurrent depressive symptoms through systematic exploration of symptom levels at each gestational month. Medication dose requirements often increase in the second and third trimester due to physiologic changes of pregnancy, such as altered cytochrome activities, plasma volume expansion, decreased plasma protein levels, and hepatic flow, and increased glomerular filtration rate, renal excretion, and volume of distribution (Sit *et al.* 2008). Breastfeeding plans should be discussed during the beginning of the third trimester. This discussion should include an assessment of the patient's preferences, as well as information regarding the risks and benefits of treatment during breastfeeding. After delivery, antidepressants can be continued at the nonpregnant dose of response or two-thirds of the final dose in pregnancy (Sit *et al.* 2008).

Multi-disciplinary care is recommended with involvement of the patient's obstetrician. There are no data to suggest that discontinuing or tapering medications in the weeks before delivery will diminish the potential for neonatal behavioral syndrome (Warburton *et al.* 2010). Should the clinician be inclined to discontinue or taper medications, he/she must be mindful that the pregnant woman is entering the most vulnerable post-partum period in which she is more likely to experience mood symptoms.

Bipolar disorder in pregnancy

Pregnancy does not protect against mood destabilization for bipolar women. Depending on their psychiatric history, some women may slowly taper and discontinue medications. Other women must consider mood stabilizers which may have teratogenetic potential. Bipolar disorder increases the risk for postpartum psychosis, a medical emergency characterized by the sudden onset of confusion, severe mood symptoms, disinhibition, and delusions. Post-partum psychosis occurs at a rate of 0.1–0.2% in the general population, but the risk may be as high as 26% for women with a history of bipolar disorder (Jones and Craddock, 2001).

Mood stabilizers and antipsychotics

Viguera *et al.* (2007) found a twofold greater recurrence risk among women who discontinued maintenance mood-stabilizing treatment proximate to conception, compared to those who continued treatment. For patients who require mood stabilization during pregnancy, there are several medication options, including lithium, anticonvulsants, and antipsychotics. Yonkers *et al.* (2004) reviewed the treatment of pregnant bipolar women. A number of anticonvulsants, most notably sodium valproate and carbamazepine, have been used in the acute treatment of bipolar disorder. Some of these anticonvulsant agents represent more potent teratogenic risks than lithium.

Lithium carbonate

Lithium remains one of the mainstays for acute and maintenance treatment of bipolar disorder. The risk of Ebstein's anomaly among first-trimester-exposed offspring of lithium users is 1:1000 (0.1%) to 2:1000 (0.2%). This cardiac defect involving the tricuspid valve may be identified by a high-resolution ultrasound examination and fetal echocardiography at 16–18 weeks' gestation. Polyhydramnios, prematurity, neonatal hypothyroidism, and nephrogenic diabetes insipidus have also been described in the lithium-exposed pregnancies. The most common toxicity effect in offspring exposed to lithium during labor is the "floppy baby" syndrome, characterized by cyanosis and hypotonicity. As pregnancy progresses, renal lithium excretion increases, generally necessitating an increase in dose. Lithium levels should be taken frequently. Close monitoring of lithium levels in the mother during pregnancy and labor is necessary.

Sodium valproate

Sodium valproate is considered a human teratogen. Use of this compound during the first trimester is associated with neural tube defect (anencephaly and spina bifida) rates of about 5–9%. In addition, intrauterine growth retardation, mental retardation, and severe cognitive impairment are associated with valproate-exposed pregnancies. Adverse outcomes at delivery may include heart rate decelerations, withdrawal symptoms of irritability, jitteriness, feeding difficulties, and abnormal tone. Other complications among neonates include liver toxicity and hypoglycemia. It is recommended that valproate be switched to another mood stabilizer before conception.

Carbamazepine

Carbamazepine is also considered a human teratogen. In one prospective study of 35 women treated with carbamazepine during the first trimester, craniofacial defects (11%), fingernail hypoplasia (26%), and developmental delay (20%) were found in live-born offspring. The rate for neural tube defects in that report and others ranged between 0.5% and 1%. Most experts feel carbamazepine should be used during pregnancy only if other options are lacking. Some researchers have recommended a daily dose of 5 mg of folic acid before and during pregnancy for all women taking antiepileptic drugs in order to decrease the risk of neural tube defects.

Lamotrigine

There have been several registries that have collected information on the use of lamotrigine in the first trimester of pregnancy. Outcomes are conflicting, with some reports of increased MCMs, particularly facial clefts (Reprotox@reprotox.org), while other reports have been negative. Women, who elect to take lamotrigine during the first trimester, should be offered first-trimester screening and a second-trimester level-two ultrasound. There is a significant increase in the clearance rate of lamotrigine during pregnancy, which returns to preconception levels rapidly after delivery, indicating the need for careful dose management throughout pregnancy and in the early post-partum period (Reimers *et al.* 2011).

Atypical antipsychotics

There is limited information on the safety of antipsychotics during pregnancy. A recent review identified only seven studies of antipsychotic exposure during pregnancy; none showed a clear association with any specific malformation (Einarson *et al.* 2009). There was only one prospective trial on the use of atypical antipsychotics with 60 women exposed to olanzapine, 49 to risperidone, 3 to quetiapine, and 6 to clozapine in pregnancy. There were no significant differences in pregnancy outcomes between exposed and comparison groups except for a 10% rate of low birth weight in exposed infants. In general, there is a paucity of data which has primarily been collected by the manufacturers. The number of reported cases and risk of MCMs are too small to make a determination about the safety profile of these drugs.

Recently the FDA updated warnings on antipsychotic drug labels to include the potential risk for extrapyramidal and withdrawal symptoms in newborns exposed during the third trimester of pregnancy. This warning was based on 69 cases of neonatal withdrawal, most with exposure to older typical antipsychotics and a number of other confounding medications. Pregnant women taking antipsychotics, particularly atypicals, should be monitored for excessive weight gain and glucose intolerance, side effects that can present risks for both mother and infant.

Post-partum depression

Women are at higher risk of developing mood disorders during the post-partum period. The "post-partum blues," marked by sadness, irritability, and bouts of crying during the first 3 to 5 days after birth, is extremely common, occurring in up to 80% of women in the post-partum period. It is considered normal in the absence of marked impairment in functioning, or suicidal or homicidal ideation, and usually resolves within 10 days. About 10–15% of women go on to develop a full-blown post-partum depression (Gavin *et al.* 2005). Evidence suggests that women are at highest risk for a post-partum mood episode during the first 3 months after birth (Munk-Olsen *et al.* 2006), but clinically women often present much later. In the DSM-IV, post-partum depression is classified as a specifier of major depressive disorder (MDD), and as such, is diagnosed using the same criteria.

Women with a history of mood disorders should be carefully monitored during the post-partum period, as antenatal depression increases the risk for post-partum depression (Beck, 1996). Similarly, women with a history of post-partum depression are at significantly higher risk of recurrence, with rates as high as 50% (Kupfer and Frank, 1987). Mothers of preterm infants (Logsdon *et al.* 1997) and adolescent mothers (Troutman and Cutrona, 1990) are also at increased risk for developing PPD.

Post-partum depression is not only painful for the mother, it may also affect her ability to care for and bond with her infant. Infants of postnatally depressed mothers have been shown to have dysregulated patterns of attention and arousal, more frequent behavioral problems, and subtle impairments in cognitive function (Murray *et al.* 2003). In the most severe cases, PPD increases the risk of marital disruption and divorce, child abuse and neglect, and, rarely, maternal suicide or infanticide.

Treatment of post-partum depression

Evidence-based treatment options for the management of post-partum depression primarily consist of psychotherapy and medications. Ng *et al.* (2010) summarized the safety and efficacy of somatic treatments for the management of post-partum depression. Of nine investigations using antidepressants, seven investigated the effectiveness of SSRIs; sertraline (n = 3), paroxetine (n = 2), fluoxetine (n = 1), and various (n = 1); two included TCAs (nortriptyline and various); and one each investigated an SNRI (venlafaxine) and a norepinephrine reuptake inhibitor (bupropion). Study populations tended to be small. The effectiveness of antidepressant interventions was generally favorable and robust.

The beneficial effect of hormones has been demonstrated in two studies, one using transdermal estradiol and another using oral 17*B* estradiol. Although both studies demonstrated efficacy, both had significant limitations. In general, hormone therapy is avoided because of the potential side effects including thromboembolic events. Three clinical trials using up to 2.8 g of omega-3 fatty acids did not show substantial improvement in the symptoms of PPD.

Psychological approaches to the treatment of PPD such as cognitive behavior therapy, interpersonal psychotherapy, and psychodynamic psychotherapy have been described by Dennis and Hodnett (2007). All hold promise as effective treatment options for mothers with mild to moderate depression and mothers who may not want to take medication.

The number of high-quality research studies of somatic interventions for PPD is very limited and preclude any strong evidence-based recommendations. Guidelines include consideration of the most effective antidepressant used by the patient in the past and consideration of the mother's breastfeeding status.

Treatment of PPD in the breastfeeding mother raises the possible risk of infant drug exposure through breast milk. The benefits of breastfeeding for the infant and the mother are well documented. Data from a large number of studies reviewed by Berle and Spigset (2011) report that in the SSRI group, sertraline and

paroxetine are excreted in milk in low amounts that do not produce measurable concentrations in the infant plasma. These drugs have been associated with minimal clear-cut adverse effects in the infant. In contrast, the highest infant plasma levels have been reported for fluoxetine, citalopram, and venlafaxine. Adverse effects such as irritability, sleep and feeding problems, hypotonia, or colic have been reported with fluoxetine and citalopram. A single case of seizures was reported in a 6-month-old bupropion breastfed infant. Long-term neurobehavioral data for breastfed infants is not available.

Although all decisions must be on a case by case basis, paroxetine and sertraline are often recommended as first-line drugs. While concern has been expressed for fluoxetine, citalopram, and venlafaxine, if the mother has been previously treated with one of these agents, breastfeeding may generally be allowed using a risk–benefit analysis. For many other medications, there are few cases reported in the literature and so they are not recommended for first-line therapies, but should be considered in special cases.

Conventional treatment alternatives for nonremission

Electroconvulsive therapy

In a review of the literature, Anderson and Reti (2009) reported on 339 cases of ECT in pregnancy. The total number of fetal or neonatal abnormalities possibly due to ECT is 11, including: eight cases of transient fetal arrhythmias, one fetal death due to status epilepticus, one miscarriage in the first trimester, and one case of fetal interhemispheric infarction. Maternal adverse effects include premature contractions, preterm labor, vaginal bleeding, abdominal pain, pulmonary aspiration, and placental abruption. Of 39 reported cases of children between the ages of 2 weeks to 19 years, whose the mothers received a course of ECT, all were physically-normal, but two were described as mentally deficient. Both mothers received ECT in the second and third trimesters.

While ECT can be considered in pregnant women with severe mental illness, acute suicidal risk, catatonia, and psychosis, the treatment should take place in the labor and delivery suite in the presence of the obstetrician, psychiatrist, and anesthesiologist.

Newer treatment alternatives for nonremission

Transcranial magnetic stimulation (TMS)

A small, open-label pilot study found that 7 of 10 pregnant women with major depression responded to TMS, with no adverse pregnancy or fetal outcomes (Kim *et al.* 2011).

Vagal nerve stimulation (VNS)

A single case study found VNS to be safe during pregnancy in a woman receiving treatment throughout pregnancy, labor, and delivery (Husain *et al.* 2005).

Clinical pearls of therapeutic wisdom

Clinicians who prescribe a treatment are responsible for understanding and informing their patients of the risks and benefits of all treatment decisions, including the decision not to treat (Spinelli, 2012).

Studies that demonstrate adverse pregnancy outcomes often receive attention in the media. Law firms seek plaintiffs to bring lawsuits based on these publications (Spinelli, 2012). The potential for legal action is a common concern for physicians who fear a negative outcome. There is considerable evidence that the decision not to use antidepressant medication in a woman who is depressed or likely to have a recurrence during pregnancy may generate greater risks to the woman and her fetus than the risks of exposure to the medication (Spinelli, 2012). *Failing to provide treatment* may also result in a negative outcome and form the basis of legal action. Liability risk is minimized by careful documentation. The clinical decision-making and treatment plan should be documented by "thinking aloud on paper" (Wisner *et al.* 2000).

Future directions

While many studies yield important information, findings in birth defects studies are limited because of methodological shortcomings and inability to determine cause and effect. Lack of consistency across studies with respect to specific drugs and specific malformations makes it difficult to translate the findings into clinical practice. Methodological study problems include insufficient power, ascertainment, or classification of birth defects, inability to address potential confounding, and poor information on exposure such as recall bias. These limitations must guide the clinician's reading and interpretation of the literature.

Future studies should focus on specific antidepressants, with study designs that control for maternal disease and severity, co-morbidities, and other exposures. Additionally, long-term, follow-up studies are needed to clarify any developmental impact of *in utero* exposure to antidepressants.

It is incumbent on researchers to make clear the meaning and limitations of the research for other clinicians and the women whom they treat. Medical journals must be encouraged to provide comprehensive discussions of study limitations. Ultimately our informed clinical judgment about the overall risks and benefits, informed by a critical, detailed reading of the medical literature must be clearly communicated to everyone involved – patients, their families, and other physicians involved in the care of pregnant women (Spinelli, 2012).

References

Alwan, S., Reefhuis, J., Rasmussen, S.A. *et al.* (2007). Use of selective serotonin-reuptake inhibitors in pregnancy and the risk of birth defects. *New England Journal of Medicine*, 356, 2684–2692.

Alwan, S., Reefhuis, J., Botto, L.D. *et al.* (2010). National Birth Defects Prevention Study: Maternal use of bupropion and risk for congenital heart defects. *American Journal of Obstetrics and Gynecology*, 203, 52.e1–52.e6.

Alwan, S., Reefhuis, J., Rasmussen, S.A. *et al.* (2011). National Birth Defects Prevention Study: Patterns of antidepressant medication use among pregnant women in a United States population. *J Clin Pharmacology*, 51, 264–270.

Anderson, E.L. and Reti, I.M. (2009). ECT in pregnancy: a review of the literature from 1941 to 2007. *Psychosomatic Medicine*, 71, 235–242.

Beck, C.T. (1996). A meta-analysis of predictors of postpartum depression. *Nurse Researcher*, 45, 297–303.

Bennett, H.A., Einarson, A., Taddio, A. *et al.* (2004). Depression during pregnancy: Overview of clinical factors. *Clinical Drug Investigation*, 24, 157–179.

Berle, J.O. and Spigset, O. (2011). Antidepressant use during breastfeeding. *Current Women's Health Reviews*, 7, 28–34.

Broy P. and Bérard A. (2010). Gestational exposure to antidepressants and the risk of spontaneous abortion: A review. *Current Drug Delivery*, 7, 76–92.

Casper, R.C., Fleisher, B.E., Lee-Ancajas, J.C. *et al.* (2003). Follow-up of children of depressed mothers exposed or not exposed to antidepressant drugs during pregnancy. *Journal of Pediatrics*, 142, 402–408.

CDC (2008). Centers for Disease Control and Prevention: update on overall prevalence of major birth defects: Atlanta, Georgia, 1978–2005. *Morbidity and Mortality Weekly Report*, 57,1–5.

Chambers, C. (2009). Selective serotonin reuptake inhibitors and congenital malformations. *British Medical Journal*, 33, 703–704.

Chambers, C.D., Johnson, K.A., Dick, L.M. *et al.* (1996). Birth outcomes in pregnant women taking fluoxetine. *New England Journal of Medicine*, 335, 1010–1015.

Chun-Fai-Chan, B., Koren, G., Fayez, I. *et al.* (2005). Pregnancy outcome of women exposed to bupropion during pregnancy: A prospective comparative study. *American Journal of Obstetrics and Gynecology*, 192, 932–936.

Cole, J.A., Ephross, S.A., Cosmatos, I.S. *et al.* (2007). Paroxetine in the first trimester and the prevalence of congenital malformations. *Pharmacoepidemiology and Drug Safety*, 16, 1075–1085.

Croen, L.A., Grether, J.K., Yoshida, C.K. *et al.* (2011). Antidepressant use during pregnancy and childhood autism spectrum disorders. *Archives of General Psychiatry*, 68, 1104–1112.

Daniels, J.L., Forssen, U., Hultman, C.M. *et al.* (2008). Parental psychiatric disorders associated with autism spectrum disorders in the offspring. *Pediatrics*, 121, 1357–1362.

Davis, R.L., Rubanowise, D., McPhillips, H. *et al.* (2007). Risks of congenital malformations and perinatal events among infants exposed to antidepressant medications during pregnancy. *Pharmacoepidemiology and Drug Safety*, 16, 1086–1094.

Deave, T., Heron, J., Evans, J. *et al.* (2008). The impact of maternal depression in pregnancy on early child development. *International Journal of Obstetrics and Gynaecology*, 115, 1043–1051.

Dennis, C.L. and Hodnett, E. (2007). Psychosocial and psychological interventions for treating postpartum depression. *Cochrane Database of Systematic Reviews*, 17, CD006116.

Djulus, J., Koren, G., Einarson, A. *et al.* (2006). Exposure to Mirtazapine during pregnancy: A prospective, comparative study of birth outcomes. *Journal of Clinical Psychiatry*, 67, 1280–1284.

Eberhard-Gran, M., Eskild, A., and Opjordsmoen, S. (2005). Treating mood disorders during pregnancy: Safety considerations. *Drug Safety*, 28, 695–706.

Einarson, A. and Boskovic, R. (2009). Use and safety of antipsychotic drugs during pregnancy. *Journal of Psychiatric Practice*, 15, 183–192.

Einarson, A., Fatoye, B., Sarkar, M. *et al.* (2001). Pregnancy outcome following gestational exposure to venlafaxine: A multicenter prospective controlled study. *American Journal of Psychiatry*, 158, 1728–1730.

Einarson, A., Bonari, L., Voger-Lavigne, S. *et al.* (2003). A multicentre prospective controlled study to determine the safety of trazodone and nefazodone use during pregnancy. *Canadian Journal of Psychiatry*, 48, 106–110.

Einarson, A., Choi, J., Einarson, T.R. *et al.* (2009). Incidence of major malformations in infants following antidepressant exposure in pregnancy: Results of a large prospective cohort study. *Canadian Journal of Psychiatry*, 54, 242–246.

Einarson, T.R. and Einarson, A. (2005). Newer antidepressants in pregnancy and rates of major malformations: A meta-analysis of prospective comparative studies. *Pharmacoepidemiology and Drug Safety*, 14, 823–827.

Figueroa, R. (2010). Use of antidepressants during pregnancy and risk of attention-deficit/hyperactivity disorder in the offspring. *Journal of Devopmental and Behavioral Pediatrics*, 31, 641–648.

Gavin, N.I., Gaynes, B.N., Lohr, K.N. *et al.* (2005). Perinatal depression: a systematic review of prevalence and incidence. *Obstetrics and Gynecology*, 106, 1071–1083.

Gaynes, B.N., Gavin, N., Meltzer-Brody, S. *et al.* (2005). *Perinatal Depression: Prevalence, Screening Accuracy, and Screening Outcomes. Evidence Report/Technology Assessment No. 119. AHRQ Publication No. 05-E006-1.* Agency for Healthcare Research and Quality. US Department of Health and Human Services.

GlaxoSmithKlein (2006). Updated preliminary report on bupropion and other antidepressants including paroxetine in pregnancy, and the occurrence of cardiovascular and other major malformations.

Grote, N.K., Bridge, J.A., Gavin, A.R. *et al.* (2010). A meta-analysis of depression during pregnancy and the risk of preterm birth, low birth weight, and intrauterine growth restriction. *Archives of General Psychiatry*, 67, 1012–1024.

Heinonen, O.P., Slone, D., and Shapiro, S. (1999). *Birth Defects and Drugs in Pregnancy*. Littleton, MA: Publishing Sciences Group.

Horrigan, T.J., Schroeder, A.V., and Schaffer, R.M. (2000). The triad of substance abuse, violence, and depression are interrelated in pregnancy. *Journal of Substance Abuse*, 18, 55–58.

Husain, M.M., Stegman, D., and Trevino, K. (2005). Pregnancy and delivery while receiving vagus nerve stimulation for the treatment of major depression: a case report. *Annals of General Psychiatry*, 4, 16.

Jones, I.N. and Craddock, N. (2001). Familiality of the puerperal trigger in bipolar disorder: Results of a family study. *American Journal of Psychiatry*, 158, 913–917.

Källén, B.A. and Otterblad Olausson, P. (2003). Maternal drug use in early pregnancy and infant cardiovascular defect. *Reproductive Toxicology*, 17, 255–261.

Källén B.A. and Otterblad Olausson, P. (2007). Maternal use of selective serotonin re-uptake inhibitors in early pregnancy and infant congenital malformations. *Birth Defects Research A, Clinical and Molecular Teratology*, 79, 301–308.

Kelly, R.H., Danielsen, B., Golding, J. *et al.* (1999). Adequacy of prenatal care among women with psychiatric diagnoses giving birth in California in 1994 and 1995. *Psychiatric Services*, 50, 1584–1590.

Kieler, H., Artama, M., Engeland, A. *et al.* (2012). Selective serotonin reuptake inhibitors and risk of persistent pulmonary hypertension in the newborn: Population based cohort study from the five Nordic countries. *British Medical Journal*, 344, d8012.

Kim, D.R., Epperson, N., Paré, E. *et al.* (2011). An open label pilot study of transcranial magnetic stimulation for pregnant women with major depressive disorder. *Journal of Women's Health*, 20, 255–261.

Kulin, N.A., Pastuszak, A., Sage, S.A. *et al.* (1998). Pregnancy outcome following maternal use of the new selective serotonin reuptake inhibitors: A prospective controlled multicenter study. *Journal of the American Medical Association*, 279, 609–610.

Kupfer, D.J. and Frank, E. (1987). Relapse in recurrent unipolar depression. *American Journal of Psychiatry*, 144, 86–88.

Kurki, T., Hiilesmaa, V., Raitasalo, R. *et al.* (2000). Depression and anxiety in early pregnancy and risk for preeclampsia. *Obstetrics and Gynecology*, 95, 487–490.

Laine, K., Heikkinen, T., Ekblad, U., and Kero, P. (2003). Effects of exposure to selective serotonin reuptake inhibitors during pregnancy on serotonergic symptoms in newborns and cord blood monoamine and prolactin concentrations. *Archives of General Psychiatry*, 60, 720–726.

Lennestal, R. and Källén, B. (2007). Delivery outcome in relation to maternal use of some recently introduced antidepressants. *Journal of Clinical Psychopharmacology*, 27, 607–613.

Levinson-Castiel, R., Merlob, P., Linder, N. *et al.* (2006). Neonatal abstinence syndrome after in utero exposure to selective serotonin reuptake inhibitors in term infants. *Archives of Pediatric and Adolescent Medicine*, 160, 173–176.

Logsdon, M.C., Davis, D.W., Birkimer, J.C. *et al.* (1997). Predictors of depression in mothers of pre-term infants. *Journal of Social Behavior and Personality*, 12, 73–88.

Lorenzo, L., Byers, B., and Einarson, A. (2011). Antidepressant use in pregnancy. *Expert Opinion on Drug Safety*, 10, 883–889.

Louik, C., Lin, A.E., Werler, M.M. *et al.* (2007). First-trimester use of selective serotonin-reuptake inhibitors and the risk of birth defects. *New England Journal of Medicine*, 356, 2675–2683.

Malm, H., Klaukka, T., and Neuvonen, P.J. (2005). Risks associated with selective serotonin reuptake inhibitors in pregnancy. *Obstetrics and Gynecology*, 106, 1289–1296.

Malm, H., Artama, M., Gissler. M. *et al.* (2011). Serotonin reuptake inhibitors and risk for major congenital anomalies. *Obstetrics and Gynecology*, 118, 111–120.

Manber, R., Schnyer, R.N., Lyell, D. *et al.* (2010). Acupuncture for depression during pregnancy: A randomized controlled trial. *Obstetrics and Gynecology*, 115, 511–520.

McElhatton, P.R., Garbis, H.M., Eléfant, E. *et al.* (1996). The outcome of pregnancy in 689 women exposed to therapeutic doses of antidepressants: A collaborative study of the European Network of Teratology Information Services (ENTIS). *Reproductive Toxicology*, 10, 285–294.

Misri, S., Reebye, P., Kendrick, K. *et al.* (2006). Internalizing behaviors in 4-year-old children exposed in utero to psychotropic medications. *American Journal of Psychiatry*, 163, 1026–1032.

Moses-Kolko, E.L., Bogen, D., Perel, J. *et al.* (2005). Neonatal signs after late in utero exposure to serotonin reuptake inhibitors: Literature review and implications for clinical applications. *Journal of the American Medical Association*, 293, 2372–2383.

Munk-Olsen, T., Laursen, T.M., Pedersen, C.B. *et al.* (2006). New parents and mental disorders: A population-based register study. *Journal of American Medical Association*, 296, 2582–2589.

Murray, L., Cooper, P., and Hipwell, A. (2003). Mental health of parents caring for infants. *Archives of Women's Mental Health*, 6 Suppl 2, S71–S77.

Ng, R.C., Hirata, C.K., Yeung, W. *et al.* (2010). Pharmacologic treatment for postpartum depression: a systematic review. *Pharmacotherapy*, 30(9), 928–41.

Nulman, I., Rovet, J., Stewart, D.E. *et al.* (2002). Child development following exposure to tricyclic antidepressants or fluoxetine throughout fetal life: a prospective, controlled study. *American Journal of Psychiatry*, 159, 1889–1895.

Oberlander, T.F., Warburton, W., Misri, S. *et al.* (2006). Neonatal outcomes after prenatal exposure to selective serotonin reuptake inhibitor anti-depressants and maternal depression using population-based linked health data. *Archives of General Psychiatry*, 63, 898–906.

Oberlander, T.F., Warburton, W., Misri, S. *et al.* (2008). Effects of timing and duration of gestational exposure to serotonin reuptake inhibitor antidepressants: population-based study. *British Journal of Psychiatry*, 92, 338–343.

Occhiogrosso, M., Omran, S.S., and Altemus, M. (2012). Persistent pulmonary hypertension of the newborn and SSRIs: Lessons from clinical and translational studies. *American Journal of Psychiatry*, 169, 134–140.

O'Connor, T.G., Heron, J., Golding, J. et al. (2002). Maternal antenatal anxiety and children's behavioural/emotional problems at 4 years. *British Journal of Psychiatry*, 80, 502–508.

Pedersen, L.H., Henriksen, T.B., and Vestergaard, M. (2009). Selective serotonin reuptake inhibitors in pregnancy and congenital malformations: Population based cohort study. *British Medical Journal*, 339, b3569.

Pedersen, L.H., Henriksen, T.B., and Olsen J. (2010). Fetal exposure to antidepressants and normal milestone development at 6 and 19 months of age. *Pediatrics*, 125, 600–608.

Petersen, I., Gilbert, R.E., and Evans, S.J. (2011). Pregnancy as a major determinant for discontinuation of antidepressants: An analysis of data from The Health Improvement Network. *Clinical Psychiatry*, 72, 979–985.

Reimers, A., Helde, G., Bråthen, G., et al. (2011). Lamotrigine and its N2-glucuronide during pregnancy: the significance of renal clearance and estradiol. *Epilepsy Research*, Feb 26, epub ahead of print.

Reis, M. and Källén, B. (2010). Delivery outcome after maternal use of antidepressant drugs in pregnancy: An update using Swedish data. *Psychological Medicine*, 40, 1723–1733.

Shamsi, U., Hatcher, J., Shamsi, A. et al. (2010). A multicentre matched case control study of risk factors for preeclampsia in healthy women in Pakistan. *BMC Women's Health*, 10, 14.

Sit, D.K., Perel, J.M., Helsel, J.C. et al. (2008). Changes in antidepressant metabolism and dosing across pregnancy and early postpartum. *Journal of Clinical Psychiatry*, 69, 652–658.

Spinelli, M.G. (1997). Interpersonal psychotherapy for depressed antepartum women: A pilot study. *American Journal of Psychiatry*, 154, 1028–1030.

Spinelli, M.G. (2012). Antidepressant treatment during pregnancy. *American Journal of Psychiatry*, 169, 121–124.

Spinelli, M.G. and Endicott, J. (2003). Controlled clinical trial of interpersonal psychotherapy versus parenting education program for depressed pregnant women. *American Journal of Psychiatry*, 160, 555–562.

Su, K.P., Huang, S.Y., Chiu, T.H. et al. (2008). Omega-3 fatty acids for major depressive disorder during pregnancy: Results from a randomized, double-blind, placebo-controlled trial. *Journal of Clinical Psychiatry*, 69, 633–634.

Troutman, B. and Cutrona, C. (1990). Nonpsychotic postpartum depression among adolescents. *Journal of Abnormal Psychology*, 99, 69–78.

Udechuku, A., Nguyen, T., Hill, R. et al. (2010). Antidepressants in pregnancy: A systematic review. *Australian and New Zealand Journal of Psychiatry*, 44, 978–996.

Viguera, A.C., Whitfield, T., Baldessarini, R.J. et al. (2007). Risk of recurrence in women with bipolar disorder during pregnancy: Prospective study of mood stabilizer discontinuation. *American Journal of Psychiatry*, 164, 1817–1824.

Warburton, W., Hertzman, C., and Oberlander, T.F. (2010). A register study of the impact of stopping third trimester selective serotonin reuptake inhibitor exposure on neonatal health. *Acta Psychiatrica Scandanavica*, 121, 471–479.

Wichman, C.L., Moore, K.M., Lang, T.R. et al. (2009). Congenital heart disease associated with selective serotonin reuptake inhibitor use during pregnancy. *Mayo Clinic Proceedings*, 84, 23–27.

Wirz-Justice, A., Bader, A., Frisch, U. et al. (2011). A randomized, double-blind, placebo-controlled study of light therapy for antepartum depression. *Journal of Clinical Psychiatry*, 72, 986–993.

Wisner, K.L., Zarin, D.A., Holmboe, E.S. et al. (2000). Risk-benefit decision making for treatment of depression during pregnancy. *American Journal of Psychiatry*, 157, 1933–1940.

Wisner, K.L., Sit, D.K., Hanusa, B.H. et al. (2009). Major depression and antidepressant treatment: Impact on pregnancy and neonatal outcomes. *American Journal of Psychiatry*, 166, 557–566.

Wurst, K.E., Poole, C., Ephross, S.A. et al. (2010). First trimester paroxetine use and the prevalence of congenital, specifically cardiac, defects: A meta-analysis of epidemiological studies. *Birth Defects Research A, Clinical and Molecular Teratology*, 88, 159–170.

Yonkers, K.A., Wisner, K.L., Stowe, Z. et al. (2004). Management of bipolar disorder during pregnancy and the postpartum period. *American Journal of Psychiatry*, 161, 608–620.

Yonkers, K.A., Wisner, K.L., Stewart, D.E. et al. (2009). The management of depression during pregnancy: A report from the American Psychiatry Association and the American College of Obstetricians and Gynecologists. *Obstetrics and Gynecology*, 114, 703–713.

Chapter

16

Depression and the menstrual cycle

Benicio N. Frey, Luciano Minuzzi, Roberto Sassi, and Meir Steiner

Introduction

Hippocrates was the first to describe a syndrome addressing the relationship between depression and the menstrual cycle, "The blood of females is subject to intermittent 'agitations' and as a result the 'agitated blood' makes its way from the head to the uterus whence it is expelled." Trotula of Salerno, an eleventh-century female gynecologist, remarked in *The Diseases of Women*, "There are young women who are relieved when the menses are called forth" (Mason-Hohl, 1940). In modern times, a cluster of premenstrual symptoms has been variably referred to as premenstrual tension syndrome (Frank, 1931), premenstrual syndrome (Greene and Dalton, 1953, Endicott, 2000), or, more recently, premenstrual dysphoric disorder (PMDD) (American Psychiatric Association, 2000).

There are several ways by which hormonal fluctuations associated with the menstrual cycle can induce changes in mood and behavior, and in this chapter we will discuss primarily the symptoms that occur repeatedly in association with the menstrual cycle and during the menopause transition.

Premenstrual syndrome and premenstrual dysphoric disorder

Premenstrual syndrome (PMS) is characterized by the presence of psychological and somatic symptoms that occur during the luteal phase of the menstrual cycle and remit during the week following the onset of menses. Premenstrual symptoms typically peak on the day before or the day of onset of menses and they may still be significant in the first 2–3 days of bleeding. Psychological symptoms associated with PMS include irritability or anger, mood lability, low/depressed mood, anxiety, and tension, whereas somatic symptoms may include breast tenderness, bloating, cramping, and fatigue. While up to 80% of women experience at least one of these symptoms during the premenstrual period, PMS is a relatively common condition that affects about 15–30% of women. The most severe form of PMS, namely premenstrual dysphoric disorder (PMDD), affects between 3–8% of women and is associated with a marked negative impact on work, social, and/or interpersonal functioning. Using the global burden of disability model, it has been estimated that women with PMDD experience 3.8 years of disability during their reproductive years (Halbreich *et al.* 2003). The prevalence of PMS and PMDD vary depending on the diagnostic tools/questionnaires used to quantify the premenstrual symptoms and on the population studied. It has been generally accepted that retrospective assessments tend to overestimate the frequency and severity of PMS symptoms. Current DSM-IV criteria require a prospective evaluation of at least two menstrual cycles in order to determine a diagnosis of PMDD. A large community-based epidemiological study found a 12-month prevalence of 5.8% for PMDD and 18.6% of "sub-threshold PMDD" (moderate to severe PMS) (Wittchen *et al.* 2002). Similar prevalence rates were also found in a large probability sample in both adults and adolescent females (Steiner *et al.* 2003, 2011). This is consistent with three studies that evaluated the prevalence of PMDD prospectively, finding prevalence rates ranging from 4.6 to 6.4% (Rivera-Tovar and Frank, 1990, Sternfeld *et al.* 2002, Cohen *et al.* 2002b).

PMDD is currently under review for possible inclusion as a new diagnostic category in DSM-5. These revised diagnostic criteria are being informed by a large recent secondary analysis of relevant datasets (Hartlage *et al.* 2012). The panel of experts assessing

Clinical Handbook for the Management of Mood Disorders, ed. J. John Mann, Patrick J. McGrath, and Steven P. Roose.
Published by Cambridge University Press. © Cambridge University Press 2013.

the validity of PMDD has confirmed that there is sufficient empirical evidence for its inclusion as a distinct diagnosis (Epperson et al. 2012). This is further supported by a consensus on diagnostic criteria recently published by the International Society for Premenstrual Disorders (ISPMD) (O'Brien et al. 2011). One of the important factors in assessing diagnostic validity is the presence of familial risk, and more specifically, heritability. The genetic heritability of premenstrual symptoms is estimated between 30–80% (reviewed in Epperson et al. 2012). In a twin registry study, the best-fitting model revealed a 56% heritability rate for premenstrual symptoms and found no impact of family environmental factors (Kendler et al. 1992). However, a number of studies have found a strong association between PMS/PMDD and history of previous trauma (Golding et al. 2000, Perkonigg et al. 2004). In addition, two studies suggested that PMDD is more prevalent in women with seasonal affective disorders (Maskall et al. 1997, Praschak-Rieder et al. 2001). To our knowledge, no studies looking at psychopathology in the offspring of women with PMDD have been reported, limiting our understanding of the familial patterns of segregation of PMDD and other Axis I pathologies.

Several studies have refuted the hypothesis that PMS/PMDD is associated with abnormalities in circulating ovarian hormones. Rather, women with PMS/PMDD are more prone to develop premenstrual emotional and physical symptoms in response to normal late luteal phase hormonal fluctuation (Rubinow and Schmidt, 2006). Direct evidence of the role of estrogen and progesterone in the etiology of premenstrual symptoms come from a seminal study by Schmidt et al. (1998) showing that suppression of ovarian function with the GnRH agonist leuprolide acetate alleviates premenstrual symptoms. Reintroduction of estradiol or progesterone was associated with re-emergence of premenstrual symptoms in women with history of PMS, but not in women with no PMS. This is consistent with a number of studies showing that PMS/PMDD tend to resolve after natural, surgical, or chemical menopause.

Women with PMDD are more likely to be diagnosed with co-morbid Axis I disorders than women without PMDD. In particular, women with PMDD exhibit an elevated risk for co-morbid bipolar and major depressive disorder, dysthymia, PTSD, and social phobia (Wittchen et al. 2002). Although still understudied, there is evidence suggesting that up to

two-thirds of women with major depression or bipolar disorder report premenstrual exacerbation (PME) of mood symptoms (Dias et al. 2011). A prospective, community-based study found that among 900 women who suffered with "depressive disorders," including major depression, dysthymia, or sub-clinical depression, 58% reported premenstrual worsening of at least one depressive symptom (Hartlage et al. 2004). In this study, the most common depressive symptoms that exacerbated premenstrually were insomnia/hypersomnia, changes in appetite, fatigue, and worthlessness/guilt. Co-morbidity is not limited to mental disorders only. PME is also noted in many medical conditions, including migraine, asthma, epilepsy, irritable bowel syndrome, autoimmune disorders, and pain (Steiner et al. 2006a). Thus, clinical changes that occur during the premenstrual period are not specific to the diagnosis of PMDD, and other mental and physical pathologies need to be assessed in women with premenstrual exacerbation of symptoms.

Initial management of PMDD

Assessing the clinical severity

The initial step, before any therapeutic approaches can be implemented, is the confirmation of the diagnosis and the assessment of clinical severity. The ICD-10 diagnosis of PMS requires only one premenstrual symptom (World Health Organization, 2004), while the more strict DSM PMDD criteria currently require at least 5 out of 11 symptoms (American Psychiatric Association, 2000). Moreover, at least one symptom has to be from the four "core" symptoms of the disorder, i.e. irritability, affective lability, anxiety or tension, and depressed mood or dysphoria. However, neither definition of PMS/PMDD allows for a measure of the severity of the illness. Prospective daily charting for at least two consecutive symptomatic cycles can be used to confirm the diagnosis and to measure clinical severity, and is still considered the "gold standard" in PMDD diagnosis. At least 65 instruments have been identified that were developed specifically to measure premenstrual symptoms (Budeiri et al. 1994). The ones most commonly used are: Prospective Record of the Impact and Severity of Menstruation (PRISM), Calendar of Premenstrual Experiences (COPE), Daily Diary for Premenstrual Syndrome (DPS), Visual Analogue Scale (VAS) for Premenstrual Mood Symptoms, and Daily Record of Severity of Problems (DRSP). The DRSP is in line with DSM-IV diagnostic criteria for PMDD and provides sensitive, reliable, and valid measures of PMDD symptoms and impairment (Endicott et al. 2006). DRSP scores have moderate to high correlations with other measures of severity of illness, and the summary scores are sensitive to change and treatment differences. It has been approved by the FDA and by the ISPMD to be used in clinical studies.

However, the requirement to prospectively chart symptoms daily for a minimum of two symptomatic cycles is impractical and unrealistic in a busy primary care practice. Based on clinical experience of the reluctance of patients, as well as feedback from primary health care providers to initiate treatment only after completion of daily charting for two symptomatic cycles, Steiner et al. developed adult (2003) and adolescent (2011) versions of a simple, user-friendly screening tool, the Premenstrual Symptoms Screening Tool (PSST). The PSST includes a list of symptoms and a measure of impairment in line with the DSM-IV diagnostic criteria for PMDD. The PSST is a practical tool that helps clinicians to screen women at risk for PMDD in a fast and reliable way and quickly evaluate the degree of symptom severity.

Antidepressants

Antidepressant medications with primary serotonergic action, such as the selective serotonin reuptake inhibitors (SSRIs), have become the mainstay of pharmacological treatment of PMDD, with proven safety and efficacy (Steiner et al. 2006b, Pearlstein and Steiner, 2008, Vigod, 2009). Many randomized, controlled trials have demonstrated efficacy of medications such as fluoxetine (Stone et al. 1991, Menkes et al. 1992, Wood, 1992, Steiner et al. 1995, Ozeren et al. 1997, Pearlstein et al. 1997, Su et al. 1997, Steiner et al. 2001, Cohen et al. 2002a, Miner et al. 2002), sertraline (Yonkers et al. 1997, Young et al. 1998, Freeman et al. 1999, Jermain et al. 1999, Halbreich et al. 2002, Freeman et al. 2004a, Kornstein et al. 2006), and paroxetine (Eriksson et al. 1995, Cohen et al. 2004b, Pearlstein et al. 2005b, Steiner et al. 2005, Landén et al. 2007). There is less data available for citalopram (Wikander et al. 1998), escitalopram (Eriksson et al. 2008), fluvoxamine (Veeninga et al. 1990, Freeman et al. 1996), and clomipramine (Sundblad et al. 1992, 1993), though. Nonetheless, the efficacy of serotonergic medications has been confirmed in at least two different metaanalyses (Shah et al. 2008, Brown et al. 2009).

There is also good evidence that the serotonin-norepinephrine reuptake inhibitors (SNRIs), venlafaxine (Freeman et al. 2001, Cohen et al. 2004a) and duloxetine (Mazza et al. 2008, Ramos et al. 2009) are also efficacious in the treatment of PMDD. Interestingly, the antidepressant bupropion, whose mechanism of action is less likely to involve serotonin, does not seem to produce a significant improvement in PMDD symptoms (Pearlstein et al. 1997). However, only approximately 60% of patients with PMDD respond to treatment with SSRIs (Dimmock et al. 2000); thus, it is unlikely that isolated premenstrual serotonin deficiency is the only etiological variable in all PMDD patients.

Notably, the effects of antidepressant agents in PMDD seem to occur much earlier (within a few days) as compared to the typical 2 or more weeks observed in individuals with major depression (Landén et al. 2009, Steinberg et al. 2012). Therefore, antidepressant agents can often be used intermittently, during the late luteal phase only (Steiner et al. 2005). This short-term use of medications has the advantage of fewer side effects, as well as no significant discontinuation symptoms, likely due to the lack of sustained use (Vigod et al. 2010). There is evidence that the length of treatment, and not the dosing method, is what correlates better with recurrence of symptoms: relapse rates are much higher after short-term treatment (4 months) compared with long-term treatment (12 months) (Freeman et al. 2009a).

Vignette

Mrs. P is a 29-year-old, happily married woman with two children, aged 5 and 3. She is gainfully employed as a full-time outpatient nurse. Menarche at the age of 13 and her menstrual cycles were always and are still regular. She has had mild premenstrual symptoms for as long as she can remember, and prior to having children she used an oral contraceptive pill which did not affect these symptoms. As of late, the premenstrual symptoms became more bothersome with severe irritability, tearfulness, dysphoria, difficulty concentrating, feeling overwhelmed, bloating, breast tenderness, and insomnia. These symptoms have mostly affected her relationships with her family, and co-workers have also noted change in her behavior. Normally symptoms would start 5–7 days prior to and last 1–2 days into menses. At all other times she felt perfectly normal. She has no other past or current psychiatric issues and is no longer on the pill since her husband has a vasectomy. She scored moderate to severe symptoms on the PSST and prospective charting on the DRSP confirmed the on–off nature of her complaints. Despite the fact that Mrs. P is adhering to a healthy diet, exercises regularly, and has tried over-the-counter treatment with calcium and vitamin B6, her symptoms have not subsided. Treatment with intermittent dosing (late luteal phase only) of s-citalopram 10 mg QAM, brought an almost immediate relief of symptoms. She has now maintained this regimen for over 2 years and continues to be symptom free.

Hormonal strategies

Given that women with PMDD are more sensitive to the normal hormonal fluctuations of the menstrual cycle, several trials have been conducted to examine whether manipulation of the female sex hormones could lead to an effective treatment of PMDD. The theoretical goal of such strategies is to suppress the periodic hormonal fluctuations associated with the normal menstrual cycle, and therefore avoid the mood changes in PMDD (Pearlstein and Steiner, 2000).

Several ovulation-suppression treatments have not shown to be fully effective in treating PMDD, however, and they often carry significant side effects (Vigod et al. 2010). Combined oral contraceptives containing progestins derived from 19-nortestosterone do not seem to be helpful in PMDD, although these pills do suppress ovulation, since these progestins may produce side effects that are similar to PMDD, including irritability and water retention (Rapkin, 2003). On the other hand, newer oral contraceptives that contain drospirenone, a spironolactone derivative with mild diuretic properties, along with low-dose estrogen, seem to have better efficacy on PMDD (Pearlstein et al. 2005a, Yonkers et al. 2005). Several randomized, controlled trials have contrasted the efficacy of contraceptives containing ethinyl estradiol and drospirenone with placebo and with other contraceptives for the treatment of PMDD, and according to a recent Cochrane meta-analysis the drospirenone-containing pills seem to be efficacious in PMDD (Lopez et al. 2012). However, the long-term clinical usefulness of these data is still unclear, since most trials had a robust placebo response, and were limited to only three cycles. Moreover, little evidence was available in treating women with less severe symptoms of PMDD, direct comparisons with other oral contraceptives were inconclusive, and few studies compared intermittent vs. continuous contraceptive use (Freeman et al. 2012). Nevertheless, for women who are seeking contraception, drospirenone-containing oral contraceptives may be a reasonable choice for patients suffering with PMDD. Like any other oral combined contraceptives, though, this medication increases the risk for deep vein thrombosis and pulmonary embolism, in particular among women with other thrombotic risk factors. Progesterone, which in the past has been claimed to be beneficial in treating PMS, has recently been reviewed by the Cochrane Collaboration. The trials did not show that progesterone is an effective treatment for PMS nor that it is not (Ford et al. 2012).

Another hormonal approach that produces suppression of ovarian activity is the use of the GnRH agonist leuprolide acetate. This "medical oophorectomy" does lead to significant improvement in 60–70% of women with PMDD (Mortola et al. 1991, Mezrow et al. 1994, Freeman et al. 1997, Schmidt et al. 1998, Pincus et al. 2011), which is a higher efficacy rate than observed in most SSRI studies. Still, some women do not respond to such an approach, and the side effects associated with this medication, including menopausal-like hypoestrogenism and osteoporosis, are intolerable or undesirable to many patients (Mitwally et al. 2002, Vigod et al. 2010). Danazol, a synthetic steroid, has been studied as a treatment for PMS and PMDD (Sarno et al. 1987, Halbreich et al. 1991, Hahn et al. 1995, O'Brien and Abukhalil, 1999), with partial efficacy, in particular for the physical symptoms, e.g., mastalgia (O'Brien and Abukhalil, 1999). Danazol is associated with multiple side effects, such as weight gain, mood changes, and acne, when given in doses high enough to inhibit ovulation (600–800 mg/d). Lower doses (200 mg/d) are better tolerated, but do not prevent ovulation, and can cause virilization of the fetus if conception occurs (Vigod et al. 2010). Last, bilateral oophorectomy has been successfully used as a treatment of severe and treatment-resistant PMDD (Cronje et al. 2004, Reid, 2012), but the irreversible and extreme nature of this approach severely limits its clinical utility.

Nonpharmacological interventions

Once the diagnosis is made and the degree of symptom severity ("on–offness") is established, treatment can then be implemented (Steiner and Wilkins, 1996). Mild cases, or cases that fall short of the strict DSM criteria for PMDD, but still lead to functional difficulties, can be treated with nonpharmacological interventions. Relaxation techniques (Goodale et al. 1990, Morse et al. 1991) and group psychoeducation and support (Walton and Youngkin, 1987, Seideman, 1990, Morse, 1999) have been effective in partially reducing premenstrual symptoms, although with minimal impact on overall depressive, anxiety, and physical symptoms. Cognitive behaviour therapy (CBT) has been studied for both PMS and PMDD, given that it is the therapy modality with best evidence in managing other disorders that share symptoms with PMDD, such as anxiety, depression, and pain. However, a systematic review of the literature published in 2009 showed disappointing results (Lustyk *et al.* 2009): although the studies reviewed had discrepant methodologies, the overall impression was that CBT did not produce a significant improvement in PMDD, and was clearly inferior to pharmacotherapy, and in some cases even to basic behavioral interventions such as relaxation. Other forms of therapy that include acceptance strategies and mindfulness hold some promise, but no data are available yet.

Complementary and alternative approaches

Complementary and alternative treatments, including dietary modifications, have been explored as potential strategies in women who either prefer to not use pharmacological approaches or have only partial response to standard treatments (Pearlstein and Steiner, 2008). Daily calcium supplementation of 1000 mg has been examined in randomized, double-blind trials, and there is evidence of significant improvement in symptoms, in particular negative affect, water retention, and pain (Thys-Jacob *et al.* 1989, Ghanbari *et al.* 2009). A higher dietary intake of calcium and vitamin D also seem to reduce the overall risk of developing PMS among healthy women (Bertone-Johnson *et al.* 2005). Vitamin B6 also has shown significant evidence of improvement in PMS symptoms: Wyatt *et al.* (1999) performed a systematic review of nine published trials on vitamin B6 supplementation up to 100 mg/d, and reported that although the quality of the trials varied significantly and only one of the nine trials had sufficient power to detect a clinically significant effect, vitamin B6 was overall superior to placebo in reducing premenstrual symptoms. Importantly, both vitamin B6 and calcium are considered "low-risk" interventions due to their minimal side effect risk, and can be used in combination with other treatments, or intermittently.

Small trials suggest a role for saffron, Qi therapy, massage, reflexology, gingko biloba, chiropractic manipulation, biofeedback, and bright light therapy in ameliorating PMDD symptoms (Jang and Lee, 2004, Krasnik *et al.* 2005, Agha-Hosseini *et al.* 2008, Pearlstein and Steiner, 2008, Whelan *et al.* 2009, Vigod *et al.* 2010, Dante and Facchinetti, 2011). Four trials were conducted with chasteberry (*Vitex agnus castus*), which showed superior results in treating PMS when compared to placebo (Dante and Facchinetti, 2011). Complex carbohydrate supplementation, believed to increase the availability of tryptophan levels and thus increase serotonin synthesis, has produced positive results in at least two studies (Sayegh *et al.* 1995, Freeman *et al.* 2002). On the other hand, negative results were seen with St. John's Wort (*Hypericum perforatum*), evening primrose oil, and magnesium oxide (Whelan *et al.* 2009, Dante and Facchinetti, 2011).

Overall, in mild cases of PMDD, it is reasonable to initiate treatment with nonpharmacological strategies, in particular if choosing the ones with best clinical evidence. This approach can be tried as well for women who refuse pharmacological interventions. However, some women may not respond to such approaches, or their symptoms may be too severe and in need of more immediate treatment. In these cases, psychopharmacological interventions such as SSRIs/SNRIs or hormonal manipulations may be necessary. Alternative approaches can also be used in cases where the traditional pharmacological treatments were only partially effective; such add-on strategies are considered safe, although studies are still lacking.

Maintenance treatment

Most clinical trials on the treatment of PMS/PMDD were focused on short-term outcomes, with a typical follow-up of 3 months. Anecdotal evidence from case reports and open-label trials suggested that PMDD symptoms tended to return rapidly after treatment discontinuation (Elks 1993, Freeman *et al.* 2004c, Pearlstein and Stone, 1994). A clear characterization of an adequate maintenance treatment of PMDD is of crucial clinical relevance: given the costs and potential side effects of the pharmacological treatment options, it is necessary to know how long a medication should be continued after response is achieved, and what are the risks of relapse after discontinuation. To our knowledge, however, only one study has addressed these questions in a controlled manner: this 18-month study followed 174 patients with PMS/PMDD randomized to a double-blind switch to placebo after 4 or 12 months of sertraline treatment, and found that relapse rates were higher in women exposed to a shorter treatment, those with more severe symptoms at baseline, and those who did not achieve remission (Freeman *et al.* 2009a). Long-term maintenance and discontinuation studies are sorely needed in PMS/PMDD.

Vignette

Miss Q is a 34-year-old single librarian. She has a history of early-onset dysthymia and has had three episodes of major depression – the first at age 23 required hospitalization. Menarche at age 14 with mostly regular cycles. She has had several trials of different oral contraceptives, but was unable to tolerate them, in particular because they aggravated her symptoms of depression. Over the years, she has been treated with a variety of antidepressants with minimal success. Currently, she is being treated with sertraline 150 mg and has been in remission for the past 2 years. She has noted that as of late, she is experiencing a reoccurrence of symptoms, especially irritability, anxiety, and low mood for a few days on a regular, monthly basis. She decided to keep a diary and noticed that the symptoms are limited to her late luteal phase. On the advice of her psychiatrist, she increased the dose of sertraline by 25 mg during the last week of each cycle, which proved helpful in alleviating the premenstrual exacerbation of symptoms.

Depression and menopause transition

Menopause transition (MT) is the late period of a woman's reproductive life characterized by progressive irregularities in the menstrual cycle that will culminate with the final menstrual period (menopause). Prospective studies have consistently shown that during MT women are at higher risk to develop depressive symptoms and/or to meet criteria for major depressive disorder (MDD). A long-term prospective study – The Penn Ovarian Aging Study (Freeman *et al.* 2004b) – followed 231 women with no previous history of depression for 8 years. Women at MT were four times more likely to have depressive symptoms and twice as likely to develop MDD as premenopausal women. The Harvard Study of Moods and Cycles followed 460 women with no previous history of depression for 6–8 years. Perimenopausal women were nearly twice as likely to develop depressive symptoms compared to those who remained premenopausal (Cohen *et al.* 2006). The Massachusetts Women's Health Study

followed 2356 middle-aged women for 5 years and found an increased risk for MDD in perimenopausal women, especially in those with menopause-related vasomotor symptoms (Avis *et al.* 1994). Two large studies, the Study of Women's Health Across the Nation (3302 women) and the Seattle Midlife Women's Health Study (508 women), both revealed a heightened risk for MDD during the MT, with the presence of hot flashes being an independent risk factor (Bromberger *et al.* 2007, Woods *et al.* 2008, Bromberger and Kravitz, 2011). Other factors have been identified as being associated with depression during the menopausal transition, including age, ethnicity (higher risk in African American, lower risk in Asian populations), low education, family history of depression, post-partum blues or depression, high body mass index, use of hormone therapy or antidepressants, cigarette smoking, stressful life events, and presence of vasomotor symptoms (Avis *et al.* 1994, Maartens *et al.* 2002, Freeman *et al.* 2004b, Bromberger *et al.* 2007, Woods *et al.* 2008, Freeman *et al.* 2009b, Bromberger and Kravitz, 2011).

Initial management of depression during the menopause transition

Antidepressants

Selective serotonin reuptake inhibitors (SSRIs) and serotonin–norepinephrine reuptake inhibitors (SNRIs) are efficacious for the treatment of MDD (Soares *et al.* 2003, Ushiroyama *et al.* 2004, Joffe *et al.* 2007) and vasomotor symptoms (Stearns *et al.* 2003, Evans *et al.* 2005, Speroff *et al.* 2008) in MT and/or postmenopause according to several open trials and randomized controlled trials (RCTs). Monotherapy with citalopram and escitalopram produce high remission rates of depressive symptoms (86.6% and 75%, respectively), and also a significant improvement in menopause-related symptoms, e.g., hot flashes, night sweats, and somatic complaints in two open-trial studies (Soares *et al.* 2003, 2006). The SNRI desvenlafaxine produced higher response (58.6%) and remission (38.2%) rates compared to placebo in an 8-week RCT in perimenopausal and postmenopausal women with MDD (Kornstein *et al.* 2010). A reanalysis of a pooled dataset of eight RCTs of antidepressants in MDD patients (Thase *et al.* 2005) showed higher remission rates with the SNRI venlafaxine (48%) compared to SSRIs (28%) among depressed women aged >50 years who were not receiving estrogen therapies. However, these results need to be confirmed in prospective

225

studies looking at response/remission rates with SSRI vs. SNRI in peri/postmenopausal women with depression. Interestingly, depressed women receiving estrogen-based therapies presented better SSRI response, leading to a significant reduction in the difference between the response of SNRI compared to SSRI groups. These results might indicate that premenopausal women may benefit from the priming/synergistic effects of estrogens while on SSRIs. Conversely, it is possible that in the context of very low levels of circulating estrogen during postmenopausal years, women would not sustain the same response to SSRIs and could have a more robust response to antidepressants that act preferably on noradrenergic neurotransmission. In the same context, mirtazapine and citalopram were tested as adjunctive treatments to estrogen therapy in depressed peri/postmenopausal women and showed high remission rates (Joffe *et al.* 2001, Soares *et al.* 2003).

Hormone therapy

Two randomized, placebo-controlled trials have investigated the antidepressant effects of estrogen during MT. Six to twelve weeks of treatment with transdermal 17β-estradiol 50–100 μg was used for the treatment of depression in perimenopausal women, with remission rates of 68–80% compared to 20–22% with placebo (Schmidt *et al.* 2000, Soares *et al.* 2001). However, a study with transdermal estradiol 100 μg for 8 weeks did not show efficacy for the treatment of MDD in postmenopausal women (Morrison *et al.* 2004). Together, these studies suggest that the MT might not only be a critical window of risk for depression, but also a window of opportunity for the use of hormonal strategies in the management of depression in this population at risk (Soares, 2008). It should be noted that these hormonal agents are contraindicated in women with history or suspected estrogen-dependent neoplasia, endometrial hyperplasia, thromboembolism or thrombophlebitis, liver dysfunction, genital bleeding, stroke, myocardial infarction, coronary heart disease, porphyria, or ophthalmic vascular disease.

Vignette

Mrs. S is a 49-year-old married woman who works as a clerk. She has a previous history of mild to moderate premenstrual symptoms that never required medical attention. Her current depressive episode started 3 years ago with low mood, loss of interest in things that normally would give her pleasure, fatigue, insomnia, decreased appetite, and feelings of worthlessness, along with moderate headaches. After treatment with a selective serotonin reuptake inhibitor (SSRI), she remained euthymic and stable until about 8 months ago, when she noticed menstrual cycle irregularities. After maximizing the dose of SSRI, she still exhibited significant depressive symptoms accompanied by mood swings, hot flashes, and night sweats, which affected her sleep quality and overall daily functioning. After 10 weeks of combined use of estradiol (transdermal E2 100 μg/d) and SSRI, Mrs. S reported that both depressive and vasomotor symptoms were alleviated. She was also prescribed continuous progesterone (100 mg/d) for endometrial protection, and she remained asymptomatic.

Atypical antipsychotics

An 8-week open trial investigated the effectiveness of the atypical antipsychotic quetiapine XR in the treatment of depression and menopause-related symptoms. Quetiapine XR, in a dose range of 150–300 mg/d, was efficacious in treatment of depression and alleviation of menopause-related symptoms in peri/postmenopausal women (Soares *et al.* 2010).

Treatment alternatives for nonremission

Two studies have showed the efficacy of botanical agents in depressive symptoms during MT. A 12-week open trial with St. John's Wort (*Hypericum perforatum*) evaluated 111 women (aged between 43–65 years old) with climacteric symptoms, in which participants without depression showed significant improvement of psychological and somatic symptoms (Grube *et al.* 1999). A RCT investigated the efficacy of a combination of black cohosh and St. John's Wort in 301 women with climacteric complaints but no formal diagnosis of depression and showed a 41.8% improvement in depressive symptoms from baseline to 16 weeks (Uebelhack *et al.* 2006).

A recent open trial investigated the efficacy of omega-3 fatty acids in 20 perimenopausal women with MDD. After 8 weeks of omega-3 fatty acid capsules (eicosapentaenoic acid and docosahexaenoic acid, 2 g/d), 70% of the patients presented a decrease of ≥50% in MADRS scores, with remission rates of 45% (Freeman *et al.* 2011).

To date, no studies have evaluated the efficacy of psychotherapy treatment for depression in the specific population of perimenopausal women.

In summary, available evidence indicates that transdermal estrogen, SSRIs, SNRIs, and quetiapine XR are effective options in the treatment of MDD during MT. Antidepressants remain the first choice for the management of depression in any given age/reproductive staging group. More systematic data on botanical agents and other nonhormonal treatment strategies for depression in MT women are needed to better evaluate the benefits of these agents in this population.

Future directions

The correlation between mood symptoms and the female reproductive cycle has been well documented clinically, but its pathophysiological underpinnings are not fully understood. Although initial speculations suggested that women with depressive symptoms during the premenstrual period and/or menopausal transition would have abnormal hormonal fluctuations during these vulnerable periods, the data so far has not confirmed this hypothesis: rather, it seems that these women are vulnerable to normal changes in the hormonal milieu. The theoretical framework that hormonal manipulations during these windows of vulnerability should be enough to address these symptoms has only been partially effective, given that hormonal treatments for PMDD and depression in the menopausal transition do not seem to be as effective as expected, and may cause minor side effects. On the other hand, treatments that do not directly target hormonal levels, in particular SSRI and SNRI antidepressants, have shown better efficacy and tolerability. These findings may be explained by potential biological interactions between the sex hormones and the monoamine systems. Indeed, the putative multiple layers of biological connectivity between estrogen, progesterone, and serotonin signaling pathways, for instance, are being actively explored in a variety of approaches, from animal models to imaging studies (Lokuge *et al.* 2011, Benmansour *et al.* 2012). A more thorough understanding of these complex interactions might eventually guide our treatment decisions for these vulnerable women.

Currently, our treatment approaches are primarily based on severity of initial presentation. For instance, in mild cases of PMDD or depression during the menopausal transition, it is reasonable to initiate treatment with nonpharmacological strategies. However, some women may not respond to such interventions, or their symptoms may be too severe and in need of more immediate treatment. In these cases, psychopharmacological interventions such as SSRIs/SNRIs or hormonal manipulations may be necessary. Still, there is a dearth of longitudinal maintenance and discontinuation studies, as well as clinical trials with specific clinical populations, such as women with co-morbid disorders or partial-responders. Future studies should address these crucial clinical questions, and enrich our ability to offer evidence-based treatments to women with depression associated with the reproductive cycle.

References

Agha-Hosseini, M., Kashani, L., Aleyaseen, A. *et al.* (2008). Crocus sativus L. (saffron) in the treatment of premenstrual syndrome: a double-blind, randomised and placebo-controlled trial. *BJOG: An International Journal of Obstetrics and Gynaecology*, 115, 515–519.

American Psychiatric Association (APA) (2000). *Diagnostic and Statistical Manual of Mental Disorders, Fourth Edition, Text Revision*. Washington, DC: American Psychiatric Association.

Avis, N.E., Brambilla, D., McKinlay, S.M., and Vass, K. (1994). A longitudinal analysis of the association between menopause and depression. Results from the Massachusetts Women's Health Study. *Annals of Epidemiology*, 4, 214–220.

Benmansour, S., Weaver, R.S., Barton, A.K. *et al.* (2012). Comparison of the effects of estradiol and progesterone on serotonergic function. *Biological Psychiatry*, 71, 633–641.

Bertone-Johnson, E.R., Hankinson, S.E., Bendich, A. *et al.* (2005). Calcium and vitamin D intake and risk of incident premenstrual syndrome. *Archives of Internal Medicine*, 165, 1246–1252.

Bromberger, J.T. and Kravitz, H.M. (2011). Mood and menopause: Findings from the Study of Women's Health Across the Nation (SWAN) over 10 years. *Obstetrics and Gynecology Clinics of North America*, 38, 609–625.

Bromberger, J.T., Matthews, K.A., Schott, L.L. *et al.* (2007). Depressive symptoms during the menopausal transition: the Study of Women's Health Across the Nation (SWAN). *Journal of Affective Disorders*, 103, 267–272.

Brown, J., O'Brien, P.M.S., Marjoribanks, J., and Wyatt, K. (2009). Selective serotonin reuptake inhibitors for premenstrual syndrome. *Cochrane Database of Systematic Reviews*, 2, CD001396.

Budeiri, D.J., Li Wan Po, A., and Dornan, J.C. (1994). Clinical trials of treatments for premenstrual syndrome: entry criteria and scales for measuring treatment outcomes. *British Journal of Obstetrics and Gynaecology*, 101, 689–695.

Cohen, L.S., Miner, C., Brown, E. *et al.* (2002a). Premenstrual daily fluoxetine for premenstrual dysphoric disorder: A placebo-controlled, clinical trial using computerized diaries. *Obstetrics and Gynecology*, 100, 435–444.

Cohen, L.S., Soares, C.N., Otto, M.W. *et al.* (2002b). Prevalence and predictors of premenstrual dysphoric disorder (PMDD) in older premenopausal women. The Harvard Study of Moods and Cycles. *Journal of Affective Disorders*, 70, 125–132.

Cohen, L.S., Soares, C.N., Lyster, A. *et al.* (2004a). Efficacy and tolerability of premenstrual use of venlafaxine (flexible dose) in the treatment of premenstrual dysphoric disorder. *Journal of Clinical Psychopharmacology*, 24, 540–543.

Cohen, L.S., Soares, C.N., Yonkers, K.A. *et al.* (2004b). Paroxetine controlled release for premenstrual dysphoric disorder: A double-blind, placebo-controlled trial. *Psychosomatic Medicine*, 66, 707–713.

Cohen, L.S., Soares, C.N., Vitonis, A.F. *et al.* (2006). Risk for new onset of depression during the menopausal transition: The Harvard Study of Moods and Cycles. *Archives of General Psychiatry*, 63, 385–390.

Cronje, W.H., Vashisht, A., and Studd, J.W.W. (2004). Hysterectomy and bilateral oophorectomy for severe premenstrual syndrome. *Human Reproduction*, 19, 2152–2155.

Dante, G. and Facchinetti, F. (2011). Herbal treatments for alleviating premenstrual symptoms: A systematic review. *Journal of Psychosomatic Obstetrics and Gynaecology*, 32, 42–51.

Dias, R.S., Lafer, B., Russo, C. *et al.* (2011). Longitudinal follow-up of bipolar disorder in women with premenstrual exacerbation: Findings from STEP-BD. *American Journal of Psychiatry*, 168, 386–394.

Dimmock, P.W., Wyatt, K.M., Jones, P.W., and O'Brien, P. M. (2000). Efficacy of selective serotonin-reuptake inhibitors in premenstrual syndrome: A systematic review. *The Lancet*, 356, 1131–1136.

Elks, M.L. (1993). Open trial of fluoxetine therapy for premenstrual syndrome. *Southern Medical Journal*, 86, 503–507.

Endicott, J. (2000). History, evolution, and diagnosis of premenstrual dysphoric disorder. *Journal of Clinical Psychiatry*, 61 Suppl 12, 5–8.

Endicott, J., Nee, J., and Harrison, W. (2006). Daily Record of Severity of Problems (DRSP): Reliability and validity. *Archives of Women's Mental Health*, 9, 41–49.

Epperson, C.N., Steiner, M., Hartlage, S.A. *et al.* (2012). Premenstrual dysphoric disorder: Evidence for a new category for DSM-5. *American Journal of Psychiatry*, 169, 465–475.

Eriksson, E., Hedberg, M.A., Andersch, B., and Sundblad, C. (1995). The serotonin reuptake inhibitor paroxetine is superior to the noradrenaline reuptake inhibitor maprotiline in the treatment of premenstrual syndrome. *Neuropsychopharmacology*, 12, 167–176.

Eriksson, E., Ekman, A., Sinclair, S. *et al.* (2008). Escitalopram administered in the luteal phase exerts a marked and dose-dependent effect in premenstrual dysphoric disorder. *Journal of Clinical Psychopharmacology*, 28, 195–202.

Evans, M.L., Pritts, E., Vittinghoff, E. *et al.* (2005). Management of postmenopausal hot flushes with venlafaxine hydrochloride: A randomized, controlled trial. *Obstetrics and Gynecology*, 105, 161–166.

Ford, O., Lethaby, A., Roberts, H., and Mol, B.W. (2012). Progesterone for premenstrual syndrome. *Cochrane Database of Systematic Reviews*, 3, CD003415.

Frank R.T. (1931). The hormonal causes of premenstrual tension. *Archives of Neurological Psychiatry*, 26, 1053–1057.

Freeman, E.W., Rickels, K., and Sondheimer, S.J. (1996). Fluvoxamine for premenstrual dysphoric disorder: A pilot study. *Journal of Clinical Psychiatry*, 57 Suppl 8, 56–60.

Freeman, E.W., Sondheimer, S.J., and Rickels, K. (1997). Gonadotropin-releasing hormone agonist in the treatment of premenstrual symptoms with and without ongoing dysphoria: A controlled study. *Psychopharmacology Bulletin*, 33, 303–309.

Freeman, E.W., Rickels, K., Sondheimer, S.J., and Polansky, M. (1999). Differential response to antidepressants in women with premenstrual syndrome/premenstrual dysphoric disorder: A randomized controlled trial. *Archives of General Psychiatry*, 56, 932–939.

Freeman, E.W., Stout, A.L., Endicoft, J., and Spiers, P. (2002). Treatment of premenstrual syndrome with a carbohydrate-rich beverage. *International Journal of Gynecology and Obstetrics*, 77, 253–254.

Freeman, E.W., Rickels, K., Yonkers, K.A. *et al.* (2001). Venlafaxine in the treatment of premenstrual dysphoric disorder. *Obstetrics and Gynecology*, 98, 737–744.

Freeman, E.W., Rickels, K., Sondheimer, S.J. *et al.* (2004a). Continuous or intermittent dosing with sertraline for patients with severe premenstrual syndrome or premenstrual dysphoric disorder. *The American Journal of Psychiatry*, 161, 343–351.

Freeman, E.W., Sammel, M.D., Liu, L. *et al.* (2004b). Hormones and menopausal status as predictors of depression in women in transition to menopause. *Archives of General Psychiatry*, 61, 62–70.

Freeman, E.W., Sondheimer, S.J., Rickels, K., and Martin, P.G. (2004c). A pilot naturalistic follow-up of extended sertraline treatment for severe premenstrual syndrome. *Journal of Clinical Psychopharmacology*, 24, 351–353.

Freeman, E.W, Rickels, K., Sammel, M.D. *et al.* (2009a). Time to relapse after short- or long-term treatment of severe premenstrual syndrome with sertraline. *Archives of General Psychiatry*, 66, 537–544.

Freeman, E.W., Sammel, M.D., and Lin, H. (2009b). Temporal associations of hot flashes and depression in the transition to menopause. *Menopause*, 16, 728–734.

Freeman, M.P., Hibbeln, J.R., Silver, M. *et al.* (2011). Omega-3 fatty acids for major depressive disorder associated with the menopausal transition: a preliminary open trial. *Menopause*, 18, 279–284.

Freeman, E.W., Halbreich, U., Grubb, G.S. *et al.* (2012). An overview of four studies of a continuous oral contraceptive (levonorgestrel 90 mcg/ethinyl estradiol 20 mcg) on premenstrual dysphoric disorder and premenstrual syndrome. *Contraception*, 85, 437–445.

Ghanbari, Z., Haghollahi, F., Shariat, M. *et al.* (2009). Effects of calcium supplement therapy in women with premenstrual syndrome. *Taiwanese Journal of Obstetrics and Gynecology*, 48, 124–129.

Golding, J.M., Taylor, D.L., Menard, L., and King, M.J. (2000). Prevalence of sexual abuse history in a sample of women seeking treatment for premenstrual syndrome. *Journal of Psychosomatic Obstetrics and Gynaecology*, 21, 69–80.

Goodale, I.L., Domar, A.D., and Benson, H. (1990). Alleviation of premenstrual syndrome symptoms with the relaxation response. *Obstetrics and Gynecology*, 75, 649–655.

Greene, R. and Dalton, K. (1953). The premenstrual syndrome. *British Medical Journal*, 1, 1007–1014.

Grube, B., Walper, A., and Wheatley, D. (1999). St. John's Wort extract: Efficacy for menopausal symptoms of psychological origin. *Advances in Therapy*, 16, 177–186.

Hahn, P.M., Van Vugt, D.A., and Reid, R.L. (1995). A randomized, placebo-controlled, crossover trial of danazol for the treatment of premenstrual syndrome. *Psychoneuroendocrinology*, 20(2), 193–209.

Halbreich, U., Rojansky, N., and Palter, S. (1991). Elimination of ovulation and menstrual cyclicity (with danazol) improves dysphoric premenstrual syndromes. *Fertility and Sterility*, 56, 1066–1069.

Halbreich, U., Borenstein, J., Pearlstein, T., and Kahn, L.S. (2003). The prevalence, impairment, impact, and burden of premenstrual dysphoric disorder (PMS/PMDD). *Psychoneuroendocrinology*, 28 Suppl 3, 1–23.

Halbreich, U., Bergeron, R., Yonkers, K.A. *et al.* (2002). Efficacy of intermittent, luteal phase sertraline treatment of premenstrual dysphoric disorder. *Obstetrics and Gynecology*, 100, 1219–1229.

Hartlage, S.A., Brandenburg, D.L., and Kravitz, H.M. (2004). Premenstrual exacerbation of depressive disorders in a community-based sample in the United States. *Psychosomatic Medicine*, 66, 698–706.

Hartlage, S.A., Freels, S., Gotman, N., and Yonkers, K. (2012). Criteria for premenstrual dysphoric disorder: Secondary analyses of relevant data sets. *Archives of General Psychiatry*, 69, 300–305.

Jang, H.-S. and Lee, M.S. (2004). Effects of qi therapy (external qigong) on premenstrual syndrome: A randomized placebo-controlled study. *Journal of Alternative and Complementary Medicine*, 10, 456–462.

Jermain, D.M., Preece, C.K., Sykes, R.L. *et al.* (1999). Luteal phase sertraline treatment for premenstrual dysphoric disorder: Results of a double-blind, placebo-controlled, crossover study. *Archives of Family Medicine*, 8, 328–332.

Joffe, H., Groninger, H., Soares, C. *et al.* (2001). An open trial of mirtazapine in menopausal women with depression unresponsive to estrogen replacement therapy. *Journal of Women's Health and Gender-Based Medicine*, 10, 999–1004.

Joffe, H., Soares, C.N., Petrillo, L.F. *et al.* (2007). Treatment of depression and menopause-related symptoms with the serotonin–norepinephrine reuptake inhibitor duloxetine. *Journal of Clinical Psychiatry*, 68, 943–950.

Kendler, K.S., Silberg, J.L., Neale, M.C. *et al.* (1992). Genetic and environmental factors in the aetiology of menstrual, premenstrual and neurotic symptoms: A population-based twin study. *Psychological Medicine*, 22, 85–100.

Kornstein, S.G, Pearlstein, T.B., Fayyad, R. *et al.* (2006). Low-dose sertraline in the treatment of moderate-to-severe premenstrual syndrome: Efficacy of 3 dosing strategies. *Journal of Clinical Psychiatry*, 67, 1624–1632.

Kornstein, S.G., Qin, J., Reddy, S. *et al.* (2010). Short-term efficacy and safety of desvenlafaxine in a randomized, placebo-controlled study of perimenopausal and postmenopausal women with major depressive disorder. *Journal of Clinical Psychiatry*, 71, 1088–1096.

Kraemer, G.R. and Kraemer, R.R. (1998). Premenstrual syndrome: Diagnosis and treatment experiences. *Journal of Women"s Health*, 7, 893–907.

Krasnik, C., Montori, V.M., Guyatt, G.H. *et al.* (2005). The effect of bright light therapy on depression associated with premenstrual dysphoric disorder. *American Journal of Obstetrics and Gynecology*, 193, 658–661.

Landén, M., Nissbrandt, H., Allgulander, C. *et al.* (2007). Placebo-controlled trial comparing intermittent and continuous paroxetine in premenstrual dysphoric disorder. *Neuropsychopharmacology*, 32, 153–161.

Landén, M., Erlandsson, H., Bengtsson, F. *et al.* (2009). Short onset of action of a serotonin reuptake inhibitor when used to reduce premenstrual irritability. *Neuropsychopharmacology*, 34, 585–592.

Lokuge, S., Frey, B.N., Foster, J.A. *et al.* (2011). Depression in women: windows of vulnerability and new insights into the link between estrogen and serotonin. *Journal of Clinical Psychiatry*, 72, e1563–e1569.

Lopez, L.M., Kaptein, A.A., and Helmerhorst, F.M. (2012). Oral contraceptives containing drospirenone for premenstrual syndrome. *Cochrane Database of Systematic Reviews*, 2, CD006586.

Lustyk, M.K.B., Gerrish, W.G., Shaver, S., and Keys, S.L. (2009). Cognitive-behavioral therapy for premenstrual syndrome and premenstrual dysphoric disorder: A systematic review. *Archives of Women's Mental Health*, 12, 85–96.

Maartens, L.W., Knottnerus, J.A., and Pop, V.J. (2002). Menopausal transition and increased depressive symptomatology: A community based prospective study. *Maturitas*, 42, 195–200.

Maskall, D.D., Lam, R.W., Misri, S. *et al.* (1997). Seasonality of symptoms in women with late luteal phase dysphoric disorder. *The American Journal of Psychiatry*, 154, 1436–1441.

Mason-Hohl, E. (1940). *The Diseases of Women, by Trotula of Salerno: A Translation of Passionibus Mulierum Curandorum by Elizabeth Mason-Hohl, MD*. Los Angeles, CA: Ward Ritchie Press.

Mazza, M., Harnic, D., Catalano, V. *et al.* (2008). Duloxetine for premenstrual dysphoric disorder: A pilot study. *Expert Opinion on Pharmacotherapy*, 9, 517–521.

Menkes, D.B., Taghavi, E., Mason, P.A. *et al.* (1992). Fluoxetine treatment of severe premenstrual syndrome. *British Medical Journal*, 305, 346–347.

Mezrow, G., Shoupe, D., Spicer, D. *et al.* (1994). Depot leuprolide acetate with estrogen and progestin add-back for long-term treatment of premenstrual syndrome. *Fertility and Sterility*, 62, 932–937.

Miner, C., Brown, E., McCray, S. *et al.* (2002). Weekly luteal-phase dosing with enteric-coated fluoxetine 90 mg in premenstrual dysphoric disorder: A randomized, double-blind, placebo-controlled clinical trial. *Clinical Therapeutics*, 24, 417–433.

Mitwally, M.F., Kahn, L.S., and Halbreich, U. (2002). Pharmacotherapy of premenstrual syndromes and premenstrual dysphoric disorder: Current practices. *Expert Opinion on Pharmacotherapy*, 3, 1577–1590.

Morrison, M.F., Kallan, M.J., Have, T.T. *et al.* (2004). Lack of efficacy of estradiol for depression in postmenopausal women: A randomized, controlled trial. *Biological Psychiatry*, 55, 406–412.

Morse, C.A., Dennerstein, L., Farrell, E., and Varnavides, K. (1991). A comparison of hormone therapy, coping skills training, and relaxation for the relief of premenstrual syndrome. *Journal of Behavioral Medicine*, 14, 469–489.

Morse, G. (1999). Positively reframing perceptions of the menstrual cycle among women with premenstrual syndrome. *Journal of Obstetric, Gynecologic, and Neonatal Nursing*, 28, 165–174.

Mortola, J.F., Girton, L., and Fischer, U. (1991). Successful treatment of severe premenstrual syndrome by combined use of gonadotropin-releasing hormone agonist and estrogen/progestin. *Journal of Clinical Endocrinology and Metabolism*, 72, 252A–252F.

O'Brien, P.M. and Abukhalil, I.E. (1999). Randomized controlled trial of the management of premenstrual syndrome and premenstrual mastalgia using luteal phase-only danazol. *American Journal of Obstetrics and Gynecology*, 180, 18–23.

O'Brien, P.M.S., Bäckström, T., Brown, C. *et al.* (2011). Towards a consensus on diagnostic criteria, measurement and trial design of the premenstrual disorders: The ISPMD Montreal Consensus. *Archives of Women's Mental Health*, 14, 13–21.

Özeren, S., Çorakçi, A., İzzet, Y. *et al.* (1997). Fluoxetine in the treatment of premenstrual syndrome. *European Journal of Obstetrics, Gynecology, and Reproductive Biology*, 73, 167–170.

Pearlstein, T. and Steiner, M. (2000). Non-antidepressant treatment of premenstrual syndrome. *Journal of Clinical Psychiatry*, 61 Suppl 12, 22–27.

Pearlstein, T. and Steiner, M. (2008). Premenstrual dysphoric disorder: Burden of illness and treatment update. *Journal of Psychiatry and Neuroscience*, 33, 291–301.

Pearlstein, T.B. and Stone, A.B. (1994). Long-term fluoxetine treatment of late luteal phase dysphoric disorder. *Journal of Clinical Psychiatry*, 55, 332–335.

Pearlstein, T.B., Bachmann, G.A., Zacur, H.A., and Yonkers, K.A. (2005a). Treatment of premenstrual dysphoric disorder with a new drospirenone-containing oral contraceptive formulation. *Contraception*, 72, 414–421.

Pearlstein, T.B., Bellew, K.M., Endicott, J., and Steiner, M. (2005b). Paroxetine controlled release for premenstrual dysphoric disorder: remission analysis following a randomized, double-blind, placebo-controlled trial. *Primary Care Companion to the Journal of Clinical Psychiatry*, 7, 53–60.

Pearlstein, T.B., Stone, A.B., Lund, S.A. *et al.* (1997). Comparison of fluoxetine, bupropion, and placebo in the treatment of premenstrual dysphoric disorder. *Journal of Clinical Psychopharmacology*, 17, 261–266.

Perkonigg, A., Yonkers, K.A., Pfister, H. *et al.* (2004). Risk factors for premenstrual dysphoric disorder in a community sample of young women: The role of traumatic events and posttraumatic stress disorder. *Journal of Clinical Psychiatry*, 65, 1314–1322.

Pincus, S.M., Alam, S., Rubinow, D.R. *et al.* (2011). Predicting response to leuprolide of women with premenstrual dysphoric disorder by daily mood rating dynamics. *Journal of Psychiatric Research*, 45, 386–394.

Praschak-Rieder, N., Willeit, M., Neumeister, A. *et al.* (2001). Prevalence of premenstrual dysphoric disorder in female patients with seasonal affective disorder. *Journal of Affective Disorders*, 63, 239–242.

Ramos, M.G., Hara, C., and Rocha, F.L. (2009). Duloxetine treatment for women with premenstrual dysphoric disorder: A single-blind trial. *The International Journal of Neuropsychopharmacology*, 12, 1081–1088.

Rapkin, A. (2003). A review of treatment of premenstrual syndrome and premenstrual dysphoric disorder. *Psychoneuroendocrinology*, 28 Suppl 3, 39–53.

Rasgon, N., Serra, M., Biggio, G., Pisu, M.G. *et al.* (2001). Neuroactive steroid-serotonergic interaction: responses to an intravenous L-tryptophan challenge in women with premenstrual syndrome. *European Journal of Endocrinology*, 145, 25–33.

Reid, R.L. (2012). When should surgical treatment be considered for premenstrual dysphoric disorder. *Menopause International*, 18, 77–81.

Rivera-Tovar, A.D. and Frank, E. (1990). Late luteal phase dysphoric disorder in young women. *The American Journal of Psychiatry*, 147, 1634–1636.

Rubinow, D.R. and Schmidt, P.J. (2006). Gonadal steroid regulation of mood: The lessons of premenstrual syndrome. *Frontiers in Neuroendocrinology*, 27, 210–216.

Sarno, A.P., Miller, E.J., and Lundblad, E.G. (1987). Premenstrual syndrome: beneficial effects of periodic, low-dose danazol. *Obstetrics and Gynecology*, 70, 33–36.

Sayegh, R., Shiff, I., Wurtman, J. *et al.* (1995). The effect of a carbohydrate-rich beverage on mood, appetite, and cognitive function in women with premenstrual syndrome. *Obstetrics and Gynecology*, 86, 520–528.

Schmidt, P.J., Nieman, L.K., Danaceau, M.A. *et al.* (1998). Differential behavioral effects of gonadal steroids in women with and in those without premenstrual syndrome. *The New England Journal of Medicine*, 338, 209–216.

Schmidt, P.J., Nieman, L., Danaceau, M.A. *et al.* (2000). Estrogen replacement in perimenopause-related depression: A preliminary report. *American Journal of Obstetrics and Gynecology*, 183, 414–420.

Seideman, R.Y. (1990). Effects of a premenstrual syndrome education program on premenstrual symptomatology. *Health Care for Women International*, 11, 491–501.

Shah, N.R., Jones, J.B., Aperi, J. *et al.* (2008). Selective serotonin reuptake inhibitors for premenstrual syndrome and premenstrual dysphoric disorder: a meta-analysis. *Obstetrics and Gynecology*, 111, 1175–1182.

Singh, B.B., Berman, B.M., Simpson, R.L., and Annechild, A. (1998). Incidence of premenstrual syndrome and remedy usage: A national probability sample study. *Alternative Therapies in Health and Medicine*, 4, 75–79.

Soares, C.N. (2008). Depression during the menopausal transition: Window of vulnerability or continuum of risk? *Menopause*, 15, 207–209.

Soares, C.N., Almeida, O.P., Joffe, H., and Cohen, L.S. (2001). Efficacy of estradiol for the treatment of depressive disorders in perimenopausal women: A double-blind, randomized, placebo-controlled trial. *Archives of General Psychiatry*, 58, 529–534.

Soares, C.N., Frey, B.N., Haber, E., and Steiner, M. (2010). A pilot, 8-week, placebo lead-in trial of quetiapine extended release for depression in midlife women: Impact on mood and menopuase-related symptoms. *Journal of Clinical Psychopharmacology*, 30, 612–615.

Soares, C.N., Poitras, J.R., Prouty, J. *et al.* (2003). Efficacy of citalopram as a monotherapy or as an adjunctive treatment to estrogen therapy for perimenopausal and postmenopausal women with depression and vasomotor symptoms. *Journal of Clinical Psychiatry*, 64, 473–479.

Soares, C.N., Arsenio, H., Joffe, H. *et al.* (2006). Escitalopram versus ethinyl estradiol and norethindrone acetate for symptomatic peri- and postmenopausal women: Impact on depression, vasomotor symptoms, sleep, and quality of life. *Menopause*, 13, 780–786.

Speroff, L., Gass, M., Constantine, G. *et al.* (2008). Efficacy and tolerability of desvenlafaxine succinate treatment for menopausal vasomotor symptoms: A randomized controlled trial. *Obstetrics and Gynecology*, 111, 77–87.

Stearns, V., Beebe, K.L., Iyengar, M., and Dube, E. (2003). Paroxetine controlled release in the treatment of menopausal hot flashes: A randomized controlled trial. *The Journal of the American Medical Association*, 289, 2827–2834.

Steinberg, E.M., Cardoso, G.M.P., Martinez, P.E. *et al.* (2012). Rapid response to fluoxetine in women with premenstrual dysphoric disorder. *Depression and Anxiety*, 29, 531–540.

Steiner, M. and Wilkins, A. (1996). Diagnosis and assessment of premenstrual dysphoria. *Psychiatric Annals*, 26, 571–575.

Steiner, M., Macdougall, M., and Brown, E. (2003). The premenstrual symptoms screening tool (PSST) for clinicians. *Archives of Women's Mental Health*, 6, 203–209.

Steiner, M., Steinberg, M., Stewart, D. *et al.* (1995). Fluoxetine in the treatment of premenstrual dysphoria. *The New England Journal of Medicine*, 332, 1529–1534.

Steiner, M., Romano, S.J., Babcock, S. *et al.* (2001). The efficacy of fluoxetine in improving physical symptoms associated with premenstrual dysphoric disorder. *BJOG: An International Journal of Obstetrics and Gynaecology*, 108, 462–468.

Steiner, M., Hirschberg, A.L., Bergeron, R. *et al.* (2005). Luteal phase dosing with paroxetine controlled release (CR) in the treatment of premenstrual dysphoric disorder. *American Journal of Obstetrics and Gynecology*, 193, 352–360.

Steiner, M., Peer, M., and Soares, C.N. (2006a). Comorbidity and premenstrual syndrome: Recognition and treatment approaches. *Gynaecology Forum*, 11, 13–16.

Steiner, M., Pearlstein, T., Cohen, L.S. *et al.* (2006b). Expert guidelines for the treatment of severe PMS, PMDD, and comorbidities: the role of SSRIs. *Journal of Women's Health*, 15, 57–69.

Steiner, M., Peer, M., Pavlova, E. *et al.* (2011). The Premenstrual symptoms screening tool revised for adolescents (PSST-A): Prevalence of severe PMS and premenstrual dysphoric disorder in adolescents. *Archives of Women's Mental Health*, 14, 77–81.

Sternfeld, B., Swindle, R., Chawla, A. *et al.* (2002). Severity of premenstrual symptoms in a health maintenance organization population. *Obstetrics and Gynecology*, 99, 1014–1024.

Stone, A.B., Pearlstein, T.B., and Brown, W.A. (1991). Fluoxetine in the treatment of late luteal phase dysphoric disorder. *Journal of Clinical Psychiatry*, 52, 290–293.

Su, T.P., Schmidt, P.J., Danaceau, M.A. *et al.* (1997). Fluoxetine in the treatment of premenstrual dysphoria. *Neuropsychopharmacology*, 16, 346–356.

Sundblad, C., Hedberg, M.A., and Eriksson, E. (1993). Clomipramine administered during the luteal phase reduces the symptoms of premenstrual syndrome: A placebo-controlled trial. *Neuropsychopharmacology*, 9, 133–145.

Sundblad, C., Modigh, K., Andersch, B., and Eriksson, E. (1992). Clomipramine effectively reduces premenstrual irritability and dysphoria: A placebo-controlled trial. *Acta Psychiatrica Scandinavica*, 85, 39–47.

Thase, M.E., Entsuah, R., Cantillon, M. *et al.* (2005). Relative antidepressant efficacy of venlafaxine and SSRIs: Sex-age interactions. *Journal of Women's Health*, 14, 609–616.

Thys-Jacobs, S., Ceccarelli, S., Bierman, A. *et al.* (1989). Calcium supplementation in premenstrual syndrome: A randomized crossover trial. *Journal of General Internal Medicine*, 4, 183–189.

Uebelhack, R., Blohmer, J., Graubaum, H. *et al.* (2006). Black cohosh and St. John's Wort for climacteric complaints: a randomized trial. *Obstetrics and Gynecology*, 107, 247–255.

Ushiroyama, T., Ikeda, A., and Ueki, M. (2004). Evaluation of double-blind comparison of fluvoxamine and paroxetine in the treatment of depressed outpatients in menopause transition. *Journal of Medicine*, 35, 151–162.

Veeninga, A.T., Westenberg, H.G., and Weusten, J.T. (1990). Fluvoxamine in the treatment of menstrually related mood disorders. *Psychopharmacology*, 102, 414–416.

Vigod, S.N., Ross, L.E., and Steiner, M. (2009). Understanding and treating premenstrual dysphoric disorder: An update for the women's health practitioner. *Obstetrics and Gynecology Clinics of North America*, 36, 907–24, xii.

Vigod, S.N., Frey, B.N., Soares, C.N., and Steiner, M. (2010). Approach to premenstrual dysphoria for the mental health practitioner. *The Psychiatric Clinics of North America*, 33, 257–272.

Walton, J. and Youngkin, E. (1987). The effect of a support group on self-esteem of women with premenstrual syndrome. *Journal of Obstetric, Gynecologic, and Neonatal Nursing*, 16, 174–178.

Whelan, A.M., Jurgens, T.M., and Naylor, H. (2009). Herbs, vitamins and minerals in the treatment of premenstrual syndrome: A systematic review. *Canadian Journal of Clinical Pharmacology*, 16, e407–e429.

Wikander, I., Sundblad, C., Andersch, B. *et al.* (1998). Citalopram in premenstrual dysphoria: Is intermittent treatment during luteal phases more effective than continuous medication throughout the menstrual cycle? *Journal of Clinical Psychopharmacology*, 18, 390–398.

Wittchen, H.U., Becker, E., Lieb, R., and Krause, P. (2002). Prevalence, incidence and stability of premenstrual dysphoric disorder in the community. *Psychological Medicine*, 32, 119–132.

Woods, N.F., Smith-DiJulio, K., Pervical, D.B. *et al.* (2008). Depressed mood during the menopausal transition and early postmenopause: Observations from the Seattle Midlife Women's Health Study. *Menopause*, 15, 223–232.

Wood, S.H., Mortola, J.F., Chan, Y.F. *et al.* (1992). Treatment of premenstrual syndrome with fluoxetine: A double-blind, placebo-controlled, crossover study. *Obstetrics and Gynecology*, 80, 339–344.

World Health Organization (WHO) (2004). *International Statistical Classification of Diseases and Health-Related Problems*. Geneva: World Health Organization.

Wyatt, K.M., Dimmock, P.W., Jones, P.W., and Shaughn O'Brien, P.M. (1999). Efficacy of vitamin B-6 in the treatment of premenstrual syndrome: Systematic review. *British Medical Journal*, 318, 1375–1381.

Yonkers, K.A., Halbreich, U., Freeman, E. *et al.* (1997). Symptomatic improvement of premenstrual dysphoric disorder with sertraline treatment: A randomized controlled trial. Sertraline Premenstrual Dysphoric Collaborative Study Group. *The Journal of the American Medical Association*, 278, 983–988.

Yonkers, K.A., Brown, C., Pearlstein, T.B. *et al.* (2005). Efficacy of a new low-dose oral contraceptive with drospirenone in premenstrual dysphoric disorder. *Obstetrics and Gynecology*, 106, 492–501.

Young, S.A., Hurt, P.H., Benedek, D.M., and Howard, R.S. (1998). Treatment of premenstrual dysphoric disorder with sertraline during the luteal phase: A randomized, double-blind, placebo-controlled crossover trial. *Journal of Clinical Psychiatry*, 59, 76–80.

Depression in the context of alcoholism and other substance-use disorders

Edward V. Nunes, Jr and Frances R. Levin

Introduction

Depressive disorders and alcohol or other substance-use disorders commonly co-occur. Multiple community-based surveys have shown that the presence of major depression or dysthymia at least doubles the odds of an alcohol or other drug-use disorder (Grant, 1995, Grant and Harford, 1995). Between 20% and 50% of patients presenting for treatment of an alcohol or drug problem may manifest major depression (Hasin *et al.* 2004). Conversely, substance-use problems are also common among patients presenting for treatment of depression, particularly when one includes nicotine dependence. Depression has a negative prognostic effect on substance-use disorders, being associated with increased severity and worse treatment response (Rounsaville *et al.* 1986, 1987, Greenfield *et al.* 1998, Hasin *et al.* 2002, 2004). Alcoholism among depressed patients is associated with greater severity of depression – earlier onset, more episodes of major depression, and increased suicide risk (Murphy *et al.* 1992, Sher *et al.* 2008). Thus, it is important for clinicians to be alert to this co-morbidity and be prepared to account for it in diagnostic assessment and treatment planning.

Initial management

Diagnosis of depression in the setting of substance-use disorder

Relationships between substance use and mood syndromes

In approaching a patient with depression and substance abuse, it is important to appreciate the variety and complexity of possible relationships between the two syndromes. Table 17.1 summarizes these potential relationships (with examples). First, it is important to recognize that depression and related symptoms (anhedonia, anxiety, fatigue, sleep and appetite disturbances, etc.) may be caused by chronic substance use. These symptoms may be part of intoxication or withdrawal syndromes, or what DSM-IV calls "substance-induced depression."

Second, a depressive disorder may co-occur with substance abuse for a variety of reasons. Substance abuse may emerge as an effort to "self-medicate" depressive symptoms. Substance and mood disorders may occur together because of common risk factors such as common genetic factors, stress, trauma, or other psychiatric disorders. Both disorders are common in the population, so some co-morbidity will occur by chance. Mood and substance abuse may interact in different ways over the course of illness. For example, mood symptoms may become conditioned cues or "triggers" prompting substance use.

DSM-IV independent and substance-induced depression

DSM-IV (American Psychiatric Association, 1994) advanced the field by distinguishing three categories of depression in the presence of substance abuse: (1) depressive symptoms that represent usual effects of substance use, (2) "independent" depressive disorder, and (3) "substance-induced" depression.

Depressive symptoms that are usual effects of substances

A review of the DSM-IV syndromes of alcohol and drug intoxication and withdrawal will show many symptoms that overlap with symptoms of major depression or dysthymia, including disturbances of mood, sleep, appetite, and energy (Nunes and Weiss, 2009). These symptoms should resolve quickly in the absence of repeated substance use – on the order of

Clinical Handbook for the Management of Mood Disorders, ed. J. John Mann, Patrick J. McGrath, and Steven P. Roose. Published by Cambridge University Press. © Cambridge University Press 2013.

Table 17.1 Possible relationships between depression and substance abuse

Relationship	Patterns and examples
Substance abuse causes depression	• Intoxication or withdrawal effects – e.g., a patient experiences insomnia, fatigue, and depressed mood in the 24 hours after an episode of cocaine use. • DSM-IV substance-induced depression – e.g., an alcoholic patient enters residential treatment with a full major depressive syndrome, which gradually resolves over 2 weeks of enforced abstinence. • Substance abuse triggers depression, which then takes on a life of its own – e.g., an opioid-dependent patient, abstinent for 3 years, relapses and develops major depression; he completes detoxification and enters residential treatment, but the depression persists.
Depression causes substance abuse	• Self-medication – e.g., a woman develops major depression with anxiety and insomnia; she begins to drink heavily every evening to calm down and get to sleep; she is unable to reduce her drinking despite several attempts. • Depression triggers the onset of a substance-use disorder, which then takes on a life of its own – e.g., the patient in the previous example starts an antidepressant medication; the depression remits, but the drinking is unchanged, disrupting her work performance and social life.
Depression and substance abuse co-occur because of shared risk factors	• Common genetic factors, stress, trauma, other psychiatric disorders such as ADHD or antisocial personality – e.g., a man is involved in a serious auto accident and is badly injured; he develops a major depression and dependence on narcotic analgesics.
Depression and substance abuse are independent disorders	• Both sets of disorders are common in the population; assortative mating may contribute – e.g., a woman presents with major depression and alcohol dependence; her father has a history of drinking problems; her mother sounds depressed and takes an antidepressant.
Depression and substance abuse become inter-related over time	• Dysphoric mood becomes a conditioned cue triggering substance use – e.g., a woman with atypical depression and rejection sensitivity binge drinks when she feels slighted by friends or co-workers. • Depression and substance abuse combine to increase overall severity and treatment resistance – e.g., a man with major depression begins staying up late using cocaine and missing work; he loses his job; the depression gets worse and cocaine use continues; he enters treatment but has poor treatment adherence and fails to improve.

hours for intoxication syndromes to a few days for withdrawal syndromes (American Psychiatric Association, 1994).

Independent depression syndrome

This describes a patient who meets criteria for major depression or dysthymia, and it is clear in the history that the depression is independent of effects of substances. Evidence for this includes that the depression long antedates substance abuse or emerges or persists during a period of at least 1 month's abstinence. The period of one month is based on evidence that most mood symptoms among substance-dependent patients resolve within a month or less of enforced abstinence on an inpatient unit (Nunes and Raby, 2005).

Substance-induced depression

DSM-IV introduced this category to recognize the existence of syndromes of depression that cannot be established to be independent, according to the criteria above, but that nonetheless appear to "exceed the usual effects of substance intoxication or withdrawal" and "require clinical attention" (American Psychiatric Association, 1994). Substance-use problems are often of early onset and chronic, making it difficult to find episodes of abstinence in the history, during which to assess depression. Thus, a depression syndrome may have only occurred during periods of active substance use, but the symptoms exceed what would be expected from substance effects.

Longitudinal observation in a clinical sample of mixed alcohol- and drug-dependent patients has shown that both independent depression and substance-induced depression, diagnosed with the PRISM interview, have adverse prognostic effects on the outcome of substance use, such as less likelihood of remission, greater risk of relapse after a period of abstinence, and increased suicidal ideation (Aharonovich *et al.* 2002, Hasin *et al.* 2002).

Two-thirds of depressions that are diagnosed as "substance-induced" in the current episode convert to "independent" over a 1-year follow-up – that is, they are observed to persist during a period of at least 1 month of abstinence (Nunes *et al.* 2006). Taken together, these data suggest that a current major depression syndrome that is convincing by clinical history (exceeding transient intoxication or withdrawal effects) should be, as DSM-IV suggests, taken seriously and addressed in the treatment plan.

Clinical history

The goal of the clinical history is to distinguish mood symptoms that are caused by substance use from bona fide depressive syndromes as best as possible, and to try to understand the relationship between the disorders for a given patient.

Here a "parallel history" is useful. First the history of substance-use problems over the patient's lifetime is reviewed, eliciting age at onset of use of various substances, onsets of abuse or dependence diagnoses, and subsequent periods of abstinence or remission. Next the history of depression is reviewed and compared to the substance-use history. Depression syndromes that occurred prior to the lifetime onset of substance-use problems or during periods of abstinence suggest a true depressive disorder that is independent of the substance-use problems. It has been shown that these historical landmarks and distinctions can be assessed reliably (Nunes *et al.* 1996, Hasin *et al.* 2006).

When a depression syndrome and substance-use problems occur together, it is useful to examine each of the depressive symptoms to assess whether the symptom appears consistent with intoxication or withdrawal effects of the substances involved or whether it exceeds the expected effects of the substances. For example, if a patient uses cocaine twice per week and only experiences insomnia on the days when cocaine was used, this would seem consistent with a usual effect of cocaine intoxication. However, if the insomnia occurs every night, even when cocaine was not used, this could be more consistent with a substance-independent depressive syndrome.

The PRISM interview is a semistructured clinical interview (Hasin *et al.* 2006), which guides the interviewer in distinguishing usual effects of substances, DSM-IV substance-induced depression, or independent depression. Training on this interview may be helpful to clinicians in learning how to approach diagnosis of depression in substance-abusing populations.

Identifying other co-occurring disorders

A number of other psychiatric disorders – e.g., bipolar disorder, ADHD, PTSD, and some other anxiety disorders, antisocial and borderline personality – co-occur with substance-use disorders and may account for some of the association between depression and substance abuse (Compton *et al.* 2007, Hasin *et al.* 2007). These disorders often have specific treatment implications. They may also be easier to distinguish from substance-induced symptoms. For example, cardinal symptoms of the anxiety disorders (e.g., reactions to reminders of a traumatic event in PTSD, fear of public speaking in social phobia, or fear of bridges in agoraphobia) are not typical effects of substances.

Neuropsychological deficits

Subtle deficits in attention, memory, and executive functioning are common among substance-dependent patients (Bates *et al.* 2002, Aharonovich *et al.* 2006), as well as problems with impulse control, emotional regulation, and irritability (Tarter *et al.* 2003). These sorts of deficits can make it difficult for substance-dependent patients to stay organized, cope with stress, and adhere to treatment recommendations.

Co-occurring medical disorders

Chronic medical disorders, especially those producing chronic pain, also need to be considered. Substance-dependent patients often have histories of traumatic injuries that may lead to chronic musculo-skeletal pain. Pain can promote depression and can also promote opioid or other drug dependence. Appropriate pain management and physical rehabilitation would be an important component of the management of such patients.

Past history of treatment response

It is generally helpful to ascertain the results of past treatment efforts, as this can be a good guide to current treatment planning. Has the patient had past courses of treatment for the substance-use problem? Did successful treatment of the substance-use problem result in resolution of depression? Have there been past trials of treatments for depression, and what were the results?

Table 17.2 FDA-approved medications for treatment of substance-use disorders

Substance-use disorder	Medication	Mechanism and principal effects
Nicotine	Nicotine replacement products (e.g., patch, gum)	Agonist replacement; reduces nicotine withdrawal
	Bupropion	Reduces post-quit dysphoria and craving
	Varenicline	High affinity, partial agonist; reduces withdrawal and blocks effects of nicotine
Alcohol	Disulfiram	Produces toxicity if the patient drinks alcohol
	Naltrexone	Partial blockade of alcohol effects for some individuals
	Acamprosate	Glutamatergic mechanism; modest effect on preventing relapse
Opioid	Methadone	Agonist replacement – full agonist; reduces withdrawal during detoxification or effective for long-term maintenance
	Buprenorphine–naloxone sub-lingual tablets, buprenorphine sub-lingual tablets and film	Agonist replacement – high affinity, partial agonist; reduces withdrawal or effective for long-term maintenance
	Naltrexone, oral and long-acting injection	Antagonist; blocks effects of opioids

Evaluation and treatment of the substance-use disorder

Assessment of substance use

It is important to ask about substance use during routine psychiatric assessment. Patients may not be forthcoming about substance abuse due to stigma, or may be unaware that their level of substance use is problematic or that is may cause or worsen mood problems. A variety of brief screening instruments have also been developed that can complement clinical history (Zgierska and Fleming, 2009). If a patient screens positive for substance use, then the diagnostic criteria for substance abuse or dependence diagnoses (American Psychiatric Association, 1994) can be queried.

It is important to recognize that even what seem like modest levels of substance use may produce mood symptoms or otherwise contribute to the severity of depression. A common example is that even two or three alcoholic drinks consumed in the evening may promote middle or terminal insomnia, because of rebound arousal as the blood alcohol level drops.

Substance type, severity, and choice of treatment setting

It is important to evaluate the type and level of care that a patient is receiving or should be receiving for substance-use problems. If the substance-use problem is poorly controlled, this will make treatment of co-occurring depression or other psychiatric disorders more difficult. If the substance-use problem improves or resolves, mood symptoms may improve as well.

The American Society of Addiction Medicine Patient Placement Criteria (ASAM-PPT) (Mee-Lee and Gastfriend, 2008) are widely accepted and provide a useful guide. The ASAM-PPT recommend evaluating the patient along six dimensions of severity: (1) potential severity of intoxication and withdrawal, (2) biomedical problems, (3) emotional–behavioral problems (including severity of co-occurring psychiatric disorders), (4) treatment acceptance vs. resistance, (5) relapse risk and potential severity, and (6) recovery environment. Severe substance dependence may require residential or intensive outpatient treatment. However, most mild to moderate cases may be managed in routine outpatient settings such as the office or psychiatric clinic, with referral to specialized substance-abuse treatment as needed (Sharon *et al.* 2003).

Medication treatments for substance-use disorders

Nicotine, alcohol, and opioid dependence have effective, FDA-approved medications (Raby *et al.* 2008), summarized in Table 17.2. Opioid dependence is particularly persistent and can be difficult to control without appropriate medication. With the exception of methadone, which can only be legally prescribed for treatment of opioid dependence in specially licensed clinics, the medications listed in Table 17.2 can generally be used in routine, office-based practice. Overall, these medications are underutilized. Primary care clinicians, including general psychiatrists, are encouraged to become comfortable prescribing them.

Evidence-based outpatient counseling methods

Advice from a physician and motivational interviewing/motivational enhancement therapy (Miller and Rollnick, 2002) are brief interventions that are effective in addressing substance-use problems and compatible with routine psychiatric practice. Patients can be referred for other evidence-based practices, such as cognitive–behavioral relapse prevention (Carroll *et al.* 1994, Rawson *et al.* 2002), or to self-help groups such as Alcoholics Anonymous. High placebo response rates in controlled trials of antidepressant medications, reviewed below, suggest counseling alone may be effective in improving both substance and mood problems for some patients with dual diagnosis (Nunes and Levin, 2004). Thus, for outpatients with moderate levels of substance use and depression severity, a good first step may be to offer an evidence-based outpatient treatment for substance-use problems. For those who do not improve, an antidepressant may then be considered.

Inpatient treatment

Hospitalization enforces abstinence and will thus facilitate the differentiation of substance-induced from independent depressive symptoms. Some of the strongest evidence for the effectiveness of antidepressant medications among depressed alcoholics comes from studies in which the diagnosis of depression was confirmed after at least a week of abstinence on an inpatient unit (Cornelius *et al.* 1997, Roy, 1998). Thus, particularly for patients with more severe substance-use problems, an initial hospitalization for intensive treatment of the substance-use problem may be a good path to take, followed by initiation of antidepressant treatment if the depression does not quickly resolve in the week after admission.

Antidepressant medication treatment
Efficacy

A number of placebo-controlled trials have evaluated the efficacy of antidepressant medications for the treatment of patients presenting with co-occurring depressive disorders, and alcohol- or other drug-use disorders. These studies have been summarized in several meta-analyses and reviews (Nunes and Levin, 2004, Nunes *et al.* 2004, Pettinati, 2004, Torrens *et al.* 2005, Nunes and Levin, 2008, Hobbs *et al.* 2011, Iovieno *et al.* 2011).

The first point about this literature is that a number of trials have examined antidepressant medications for substance-use disorders in the absence of depression or with depressive symptoms, but without a diagnosed depressive disorder. These studies show little evidence of efficacy of antidepressants (Nunes *et al.* 2004, Torrens *et al.* 2005). This suggests the importance of a clinical history to establish the presence of a depressive disorder.

Among those studies that diagnosed a depressive disorder (major depression, dysthymia) by clinical history and/or structured interview, roughly half showed significant beneficial effects of antidepressant medication for mood outcome, while the other half were negative. The magnitude of the overall effect, estimated from one meta-analysis (Nunes and Levin, 2004), is similar to that found among routine outpatient antidepressant trials (Walsh *et al.* 2002). Medication tended to improve substance-use outcomes in those trials with robust antidepressant effects. This is consistent with the idea that improvement in depression in turn mediates improvement in substance-use (Nunes and Levin, 2004). Overall, the findings suggest that among substance-dependent patients with a carefully diagnosed depressive disorder, antidepressant medication may be effective and should be considered as part of a larger treatment plan for patients with both disorders.

Determinants of antidepressant medication effectiveness

A moderator analysis was conducted to examine features of the clinical trials that might explain differences between positive and negative studies and provide clues to guide practice (Nunes and Levin, 2004). The findings are summarized in Table 17.3, along with their clinical implications. Most striking is the role of placebo response, similar to what is found in antidepressant trials in major depressive disorder without substance abuse. Studies published since this meta-analysis have tended to conform to the same pattern – high placebo response associated with lack of effect (e.g., Gual *et al.* 2003, Kranzler *et al.* 2006, Cornelius *et al.* 2009) and low to moderate placebo response tending to be associated with some evidence of beneficial effects (Hernandez-Avila *et al.* 2004, McDowell *et al.* 2005, Riggs *et al.* 2007). Among studies with low placebo response, medium to large effects of medication were observed on both mood and substance-use

Table 17.3 Factors that predict response to antidepressant medication and clinical implications based on meta-analysis of clinical trials among patients with co-occurring depression and substance-use disorder (Nunes and Levin, 2004, 2008)

Factors predicting response to antidepressants	Clinical implications
Low placebo response *Diagnosis of depression after at least a week of abstinence*	• Begin by advising abstinence or initiating specific treatment for the substance-use disorder if indicated. • If substance dependence is severe or resistant consider hospitalization for detoxification. • For alcohol dependence, consider disulfiram, naltrexone, or acamprosate. • Opioid dependence should be stabilized on methadone maintenance, buprenorphine maintenance, or naltrexone. • Depression may resolve with abstinence or substantial reduction in substance use. • Depression that persists for at least a week after abstinence is achieved should be considered for specific antidepressant treatment – how long to wait after abstinence is achieved is up to clinical judgment; DSM-IV suggests 1 month, but this may be too long. • If patient cannot achieve abstinence, then clinical judgment may dictate treating the depression depending upon its history (evidence of past episodes of independent depression) and severity.
Absence of concurrent manual-guided psychosocial intervention for substance-use disorder	• Consider beginning treatment with a psychosocial/behavioral treatment for substance abuse or depression. • Clinical trials in which a manual-guided intervention was offered to all patients demonstrated high placebo response and little evidence of efficacy of medication over placebo. • Cognitive behavioral and other psychotherapeutic techniques are effective for depression and do not involve concerns about side effects or interactions with alcohol or drugs.
Class of antidepressant medication	• Choose an SSRI as first-line treatment due to good safety and tolerability. • Consider a noradrenergic antidepressant if SSRI trial fails. • There are more positive clinical trials for tricyclic antidepressants and other medications with noradrenergic or mixed mechanisms, and fewer positive trials with SSRIs, though many SSRI trials also had high placebo response.
Alcohol-dependent patients vs. drug-dependent patients	• There are more trials and more positive trials supporting efficacy of antidepressants among depressed alcoholics. • Fewer trials and fewer positive trials among drug-dependent patients with depression. • Among drug-dependent patients, proceed with more emphasis on treatment of the drug problem. Opioid dependence should be stabilized on methadone or buprenorphine maintenance, or naltrexone.

outcome. In contrast, many studies had high placebo response, and most of these were negative. Studies with low placebo response and larger effects were characterized by a period of enforced abstinence (on inpatient units in several studies) prior to confirming the diagnosis of depression, and tricyclic or other mixed mechanism antidepressants. Studies with high placebo response and no medication effect were characterized by diagnosis of depression during active substance use, delivery of evidence-based, manual-guided therapies for substance abuse to all patients in the trials, and SSRI antidepressants.

Clinical implications (Table 17.3) include the potential advantage of establishing abstinence before diagnosing depression (as in the inpatient studies) and potential good treatment response to manual-guided treatments for substance-use disorders. This suggests a clinical model in which treatment for the substance-use problem is initiated and response of depression monitored. Many patients may respond to substance-abuse treatment alone, and for the rest, antidepressant medication should be started.

It is not clear how much to make of the poor performance of SSRIs, since most of the SSRI trials had high placebo response rates. However, SSRIs have been found in several trials to worsen alcohol-use outcomes among alcoholics of the early-onset type (Kranzler *et al.* 1996, Pettinati *et al.* 2000, Brady *et al.* 2005). SSRIs may still be considered a first-line treatment among depressed substance abusers due to their good tolerability and safety, but a non-SSRI antidepressant might be considered if an SSRI trial fails.

Populations

More of the controlled trials involved alcohol-dependent patients than drug-dependent patients. Hence, the conclusions are more firm for alcohol-dependent patients, and more research is needed for those with drug dependence. Only two of these trials involved adolescents, yielding mixed evidence on efficacy (Riggs *et al.* 2007, Cornelius *et al.* 2009).

Safety

Reports of adverse events from these clinical trials suggest that treating substance-dependent patients with antidepressant medications is relatively safe. However, infrequent serious adverse events have been reported, such as seizures among patients in tricyclic trials (Nunes *et al.* 1995, 1998). Alcohol and other drugs, particularly when taken in large amounts, have the potential to produce sedation and disinhibition, which may be worsened by combination with other CNS-active medications. Most of the clinical trials cited above involved outpatients with predominantly moderate levels of substance abuse or already under treatment (e.g., methadone maintenance). Hence, with more severe levels of substance abuse, caution is warranted. In an open-label trial of citalopram in over 2000 patients in primary care with major depression, serious adverse events (SAEs) were rare (1.5%), even among patients with combined major depression and alcohol- or drug-use disorders (3.3%) (Davis *et al.* 2010). This suggests that for the average outpatient with substance-use disorders of mild to moderate severity, the toxicity of second-generation antidepressants is low.

Nicotine dependence

Clinical trials of medications for nicotine dependence have generally excluded patients with current major depression on the assumption that major depression should be independently treated. It is interesting that several antidepressant medications with noradrenergic mechanisms, namely bupropion and nortriptyline, are effective in helping patients quit smoking.

This effect seems to hold whether or not there is a past history of major depression (Hall *et al.* 1998, Cox *et al.* 2004). The effect of nortriptyline is mediated by its ability to reduce dysphoria emerging after quitting smoking (Hall *et al.* 1998). A history of major depression is common among nicotine-dependent patients

and reduces the likelihood of successfully quitting (Glassman *et al.* 1990). Further, persistent and sometimes quite severe major depression has been shown to emerge after quitting smoking, as if chronic smoking were functioning as an antidepressant (Stage *et al.* 1996). These findings suggest the complexity of the relationship between depression and nicotine dependence. Clinically, for patients wishing to quit smoking cigarettes, it would seem prudent to treat a depressive disorder before a quit attempt is undertaken. Bupropion or nortriptyline should be considered, as they may both treat the depression and facilitate abstinence. Clinical trials of SSRIs for smoking cessation have been negative (Hughes *et al.* 2007).

Varenicline, the high affinity, partial nicotine receptor agonist, is arguably the most powerful medication treatment for nicotine dependence. However, risks include neuropsychiatric side effects such as irritability and other mood symptoms (Ebbert *et al.* 2010). Thus, in a depressed smoker it would seem prudent to first try an antidepressant, get the depression under control, and then consider varenicline as a second-line treatment if smoking persists.

Maintenance treatment

Few studies have examined the long-term treatment of co-occurring depression and substance-use disorders systematically. However, both depression and substance-use disorders often follow a chronic, relapsing course. Thus, it would make sense that an effective treatment strategy, once achieved, should be discontinued with caution.

Long-term continuation of antidepressant medication

It has been shown in longitudinal, observational studies that depression is associated with worse outcomes of substance-use problems (Rounsaville *et al.* 1986, 1987), and that, in particular, depression occurring during periods of abstinence over a long-term follow-up increased the risk of relapse to substance abuse (Hasin *et al.* 2002). One small trial among alcohol-dependent patients with depression showed that continuation of imipramine was associated with maintenance of improvement, while discontinuation was associated with relapse of both depression and drinking (Nunes *et al.* 1993).

Continuation of medications for substance-use disorders

In the treatment of opioid dependence, discontinuation of agonist replacement therapy (methadone or buprenorphine maintenance) results in very high rates of relapse, over 90% in one large study (Weiss *et al.* 2011). The stress associated with relapse would have the potential, in turn, to promote depression in vulnerable individuals. Thus, tapering of agonist replacement for opioid dependence should generally be discouraged or undertaken only with great caution in a select few.

Treatment alternatives for nonremission

There is little systematic evidence with respect to treatment alternatives when an initial treatment trial fails for a patient with co-occurring depression and substance-use problems. Certainly, if a patient enters substance-use treatment and achieves abstinence, but remains depressed, the depression should be directly treated. Given that there are a variety of medication and behavioral treatments available for substance-use disorders, as well as for depression, the general principle applies that if one treatment regimen is failing, an alternative should be tried. For substance abuse that is persistent and severe, a higher level of care should be considered (Mee-Lee and Gastfriend, 2008).

Combination of antidepressant medication with medications for the substance-use problem should be considered in treatment-resistant patients. A recent trial showed that for patients with co-occurring major depression and alcohol dependence, the combination of sertraline with naltrexone produced superior outcome to either treatment alone or placebo (Pettinati *et al.* 2010).

Conclusions and "clinical pearls of therapeutic wisdom"

This chapter has reviewed diagnostic and longitudinal studies, clinical trials, and clinical experience to develop recommendations for the diagnosis and treatment of co-occurring depression and substance-use disorders. The recommendations can be summarized as follows:

- *Parallel history*. Take a longitudinal, parallel history of mood and substance symptoms over the patient's lifetime in an effort to understand the temporal and causal relationships between the disorders. Information from family members or from previous treatment episodes is helpful.

- *Distinguish usual effects of substances and apply DSM-IV criteria for substance-induced and independent depression*. In the history, try to distinguish depression symptoms that are transient, expected effects of substances (see DSM-IV intoxication and withdrawal syndromes) from depression symptoms that exceed what would be expected from the effects of substances and would qualify toward a DSM-IV diagnosis of either substance-induced or independent depression.

- *Pay attention to DSM-IV substance-induced depression*. DSM-IV defines substance-induced depression as a depression syndrome that cannot be established as independent, yet exceeds the expected effects of substances. This syndrome has adverse prognostic effects, may persist into abstinence in the future, and warrants clinical attention.

- *Look for other co-occurring psychiatric disorders*. "Where there's smoke, there's fire." When a patient presents with co-occurring depression and substance abuse, other disorders are likely. Look for bipolar disorder, ADHD, PTSD, other anxiety disorders (social phobia, agoraphobia, panic disorder), or personality disorder (borderline or antisocial).

- *Look for medical problems*. Co-morbidity is associated with increased severity, which may extend to medical problems, such as sexually transmitted diseases, viral hepatitis, adverse effects of substance abuse (e.g., smoking-related disorders, alcoholic liver disease), and chronic pain.

- *Treat both substance use and depression*. Keep both on the problem list and the treatment plan. Antidepressant medications appear effective and relatively safe in carefully diagnosed depressed patients with substance-use disorders. Concurrent treatment of the substance-use problem is also important and may in and of itself contribute to improvement of depression.

- *Learn and use the medication treatments for substance-use disorders*. There are a number of effective medications (see Table 17.2), which are underutilized.

- *Become familiar with the behavioral treatments for substance-use disorders.* Become comfortable delivering the basic ones (e.g., brief advice, motivational interviewing) and know where to refer for more involved and more intensive treatments.
- *Resist discouragement in the face of treatment resistance, relapse, and nonadherence.* Both depression and substance-use disorders are chronic, relapsing disorders, and may be treatment-resistant. Treatment adherence may be a challenge. Patience and persistence are needed.

Future directions

Given the variable evidence on effectiveness of SSRIs among depressed substance-dependent patients, research on other new-generation antidepressants with noradrenergic or mixed mechanisms of action would be valuable. More research on combinations, such as sertraline and naltrexone (Pettinati *et al.* 2010), should be considered. Behavioral treatments also have been successful for both depression and substance-use problems, but few controlled trials have examined behavioral treatments targeting patients with both disorders.

More research on the underlying mechanisms of co-occurring depression and substance-use problems is also called for. Addiction is, in one respect, a disorder of the brain reward system, and anhedonia is a cardinal symptom of depression. Thus, the co-occurrence may hold clues to the pathophysiology of both sets of disorders.

Finally, at a practical level, there are serious barriers to the delivery of effective care to patients with co-occurring disorders. The treatment systems for mental disorders and substance-use disorders have been historically separate, such that clinicians working with mood disorders have had limited knowledge of the evaluation and treatment of substance-use disorders, and vice versa. Further, evidence-based treatments, such as medications for substance-use disorders, do not get used. More work is needed both on education and training of the workforces and on the development of systems of care to most effectively manage co-occurring disorders in a co-ordinated fashion.

Acknowledgments

NIDA grant K24 DA022412 (Dr. Nunes) and NIDA grant K24 DA029647 (Dr. Levin).

References

Aharonovich, E., Liu, X., Nunes, E., and Hasin, D.S. (2002). Suicide attempts in substance abusers: Effects of major depression in relation to substance use disorders. *American Journal of Psychiatry*, 159, 1600–1602.

Aharonovich, E., Hasin, D.S., Brooks, A.C. *et al.* (2006). Cognitive deficits predict low treatment retention in cocaine-dependent patients. *Drug and Alcohol Dependence*, 81, 313–322.

American Psychiatric Association (1994). *Diagnostic and Statistical Manual of Mental Disorders, Fourth Edition*. Washington, DC: American Psychiatric Publishing.

Bates, M.E., Bowden, S.C., and Barry, D. (2002). Neurocognitive impairment associated with alcohol use disorders: Implications for treatment. *Experimental and Clinical Psychopharmacology*, 10, 193–212.

Brady, K.T., Sonne, S., Anton, R.F. *et al.* (2005). Sertraline in the treatment of co-occurring alcohol dependence and posttraumatic stress disorder. *Alcoholism: Clinical and Experimental Research*, 29, 395–401.

Carroll, K.M., Rounsaville, B.J., Nich, C. *et al.* (1994). One-year follow-up of psychotherapy and pharmacotherapy for cocaine dependence: Delayed emergence of psychotherapy effects. *Archives of General Psychiatry*, 51, 989–997.

Compton, W.M., Thomas, Y.F., Stinson, F.S., and Grant, B.F. (2007). Prevalence, correlates, disability, and comorbidity of DSM-IV drug abuse and dependence in the United States: Results from the National Epidemiologic Survey on Alcohol and Related Conditions. *Archives of General Psychiatry*, 64, 566–576.

Cornelius, J.R., Salloum, I.M., Ehler, J.G. *et al.* (1997). Fluoxetine in depressed alcoholics: A double–blind, placebo–controlled trial. *Archives of General Psychiatry*, 54, 700–705.

Cornelius, J.R., Bukstein, O.G., Wood, D.S. *et al.* (2009). Double-blind placebo-controlled trial of fluoxetine in adolescents with comorbid major depression and an alcohol use disorder. *Addictive Behaviors*, 34, 905–909.

Cox, L.S., Patten, C.A., Niaura, R.S. *et al.* (2004). Efficacy of bupropion for relapse prevention in smokers with and without a past history of major depression. *Journal of General Internal Medicine*, 19, 828–834.

Davis, L.L., Wisniewski, S.R., Howland, R.H. *et al.* (2010). Does comorbid substance use disorder impair recovery from major depression with SSRI treatment? An analysis of the STAR*D level one treatment outcomes. *Drug and Alcohol Dependence*, 107, 161–170.

Ebbert, J.O., Wyatt, K.D., Hays, J.T., Klee, E.W., and Hurt, R.D. (2010). Varenicline for smoking cessation: Efficacy, safety, and treatment recommendations. *Journal of Patient Preference and Adherence*, 4, 355–362.

Glassman, A.H., Helzer, J.E., Covey, L.S. *et al.* (1990). Smoking, smoking cessation, and major depression. *Journal of the American Medical Association*, 264, 1546–1549.

Grant, B. (1995). Comorbidity between DSM-IV drug use disorders and major depression: Results of a national survey. *Journal of Substance Abuse*, 7, 481–497.

Grant, B.F. and Harford, T.C. (1995). Comorbidity between DSM-IV alcohol use disorders and major depression: Results of a national survey. *Drug and Alcohol Dependence*, 39, 197–206.

Greenfield, S.F., Weiss, R.D., Muenz, L.R. *et al.* (1998). The effect of depression on return to drinking: A prospective study. *Archives of General Psychiatry*, 55, 259–265.

Gual, A., Balcells, M., Torres, M. *et al.* (2003). Sertraline for the prevention of relapse in detoxicated alcohol-dependent patients with a comorbid depressive disorder: A randomized controlled trial. *Alcohol and Alcoholism*, 38, 619–625.

Hall, S.M., Reus, V.I., Muñoz, R.F. *et al.* (1998). Nortriptyline and cognitive-behavioral therapy in the treatment of cigarette smoking. *Archives of General Psychiatry*, 55, 683–690.

Hasin, D., Nunes E., and Meydan J. (2004). Comorbidity of alcohol, drug and psychiatric disorders: epidemiology. In Kranzler, H.R. and Tinsley, J.A., eds., *Dual Diagnosis and Treatment: Substance Abuse and Comorbid Disorders, Second Edition*. New York: Marcel Dekker, 1–34.

Hasin, D., Liu, X., Nunes, E. *et al.* (2002). Effects of major depression on remission and relapse of substance dependence. *Archives of General Psychiatry*, 59, 375–380.

Hasin, D., Samet, S., Nunes, E. *et al.* (2006). Diagnosis of comorbid psychiatric disorders in substance users assessed with the Psychiatric Research Interview for Substance and Mental Disorders for DSM-IV. *American Journal of Psychiatry*, 163, 689–696.

Hasin, D.S., Stinson, F.S., Ogburn, E., and Grant, B.F. (2007). Prevalence, correlates, disability, and comorbidity of DSM-IV alcohol abuse and dependence in the United States: results from the National Epidemiologic Survey on Alcohol and Related Conditions. *Archives of General Psychiatry*, 64, 830–842.

Hernandez-Avila, C.A., Modesto-Lowe, V., Feinn, R., and Kranzler, H.R. (2004). Nefazodone treatment of comorbid alcohol dependence and major depression. *Alcoholism: Clinical and Experimental Research*, 28, 433–440.

Hobbs, J.D., Kushner, M.G., Lee, S.S., Reardon, S.M., and Maurer, E.W. (2011). Meta-analysis of supplemental treatment for depressive and anxiety disorders in patients being treated for alcohol dependence. *American Journal on Addictions*, 20, 319–329.

Hughes, J.R., Stead, L.F., and Lancaster, T. (2007). Antidepressants for smoking cessation. *Cochrane Database of Systematic Reviews*, 1, CD000031.

Iovieno, N., Tedeschini, E., Bentley, K.H., Evins, A.E., and Papakostas, G.I. (2011). Antidepressants for major depressive disorder and dysthymic disorder in patients with comorbid alcohol use disorders: a meta-analysis of placebo-controlled randomized trials. *Journal of Clinical Psychiatry*, 72, 1144–1151.

Kranzler, H.R., Burleson, J.A., Brown, J., and Babor, T.F. (1996). Fluoxetine treatment seems to reduce the beneficial effects of cognitive-behavioral therapy in type B alcoholics. *Alcoholism: Clinical and Experimental Research*, 20, 1534–1141.

Kranzler, H.R., Mueller, T., Cornelius, J. *et al.* (2006). Sertraline treatment of co-occurring alcohol dependence and major depression. *Journal of Clinical Psychopharmacology*, 26, 13–20.

McDowell, D., Nunes, E.V., Seracini, A.M. *et al.* (2005). Desipramine treatment of cocaine-dependent patients with depression: A placebo-controlled trial. *Drug and Alcohol Dependence*, 80, 209–221.

Mee-Lee, D. and Gastfriend, D.R. (2008). Patient placement criteria. In Galanter, M. and Kleber, H.D., eds., *American Psychiatric Publishing Textbook of Substance Abuse Treatment, Fourth Edition*. Washington, DC: American Psychiatric Publishing, Inc., 79–92.

Miller, W.R. and Rollnick, S. (2002). *Motivational Interviewing: Preparing People for Change, Second Edition*. New York: Guilford Press.

Murphy, G., Wetzel, R., Robins, E., and McEvoy, L. (1992). Multiple risk factors predict suicide in alcoholism. *Archives of General Psychiatry*, 49, 459–463.

Nunes, E.V. and Levin, F.R. (2004). Treatment of depression in patients with alcohol or other drug dependence: a meta-analysis. *Journal of the American Medical Association*, 291, 1887–1896.

Nunes, E.V. and Raby, W.N. (2005). Comorbidity of depression and substance abuse. In Licinio, J. and Wong, M., eds., *Biology of Depression: From Novel Insights to Therapeutic Strategies*. Weinheim: Wiley-VCH Verlag GmbH and Co. KGaA, 341–364.

Nunes, E.V. and Levin, F.R. (2008). Treatment of co-occurring depression and substance dependence: using meta-analysis to guide clinical recommendations. *Psychiatric Annals*, 38(11), nihpa 128505.

Nunes, E.V. and Weiss, R.D. (2009). Co-occurring addiction and affective disorders. In Ries, R.K., Fiellin, D.A., Miller, S.C., and Saitz, R., eds., *Principles of Addiction Medicine, Fourth Edition*. Philadelphia: Lippincott Williams and Wilkins, 1151–1181.

Nunes, E.V., Sullivan, M.A., and Levin, F.R. (2004). Treatment of depression in patients with opiate dependence. *Biological Psychiatry*, 56, 793–802.

Nunes, E.V., Liu, X., Samet, S., Matseoane, K., and Hasin, D. (2006). Independent versus substance-induced major depressive disorder in substance-dependent patients: Observational study of course during follow-up. *Journal of Clinical Psychiatry*, 67, 1561–1567.

Nunes, E.V., McGrath, P.J., Quitkin, F.M. *et al.* (1993). Imipramine treatment of alcoholism with comorbid depression. *American Journal of Psychiatry*, 150, 963–965.

Nunes, E.V., McGrath, P.J., Quitkin, F.M. *et al.* (1995). Imipramine treatment of cocaine abuse: Possible boundaries of efficacy. *Drug and Alcohol Dependence*, 39, 185–195.

Nunes, E.V., Goehl, L., Seracini, A. *et al.* (1996). A modification of the structured clinical interview for DSM-III-R to evaluate methadone patients: Test-retest reliability. *American Journal on Addictions*, 5, 241–248.

Nunes, E.V., Quitkin, F.M., Donovan, S.J. *et al.* (1998). Imipramine treatment of opiate–dependent patients with depressive disorders: A placebo–controlled trial. *Archives of General Psychiatry*, 55, 153–160.

Pettinati, H.M. (2004). Antidepressant treatment of co-occurring depression and alcohol dependence. *Biological Psychiatry*, 56, 785–792.

Pettinati, H.M., Volpicelli, J.R., Kranzler, H.R. *et al.* (2000). Sertraline treatment for alcohol dependence: Interactive effects of medication and alcoholic subtype. *Alcoholism: Clinical and Experimental Research*, 24, 1041–1049.

Pettinati, H.M., Oslin, D.W., Kampman, K.M. *et al.* (2010). A double-blind, placebo-controlled trial combining sertraline and naltrexone for treating co-occurring depression and alcohol dependence. *American Journal of Psychiatry*, 167, 668–675.

Raby, W.N., Levin, F.R., and Nunes, E.V. (2008). Pharmacological treatment of substance abuse disorders. In Tasman, A., Kay, J., Lieberman, J.A., First, M.B., and Maj, M., eds., *Psychiatry, Third Edition*. Chichester, England: John Wiley & Sons, Ltd., 2390–2416.

Rawson, R.A., Huber, A., McCann, M. *et al.* (2002). A comparison of contingency management and cognitive-behavioral approaches during methadone maintenance treatment for cocaine dependence. *Archives of General Psychiatry*, 59, 817–824.

Riggs, P.D., Mikulich-Gilbertson, S.K., Davies, R.D. *et al.* (2007). A randomized controlled trial of fluoxetine and cognitive behavioral therapy in adolescents with major depression, behavior problems, and substance use

disorders. *Archives of Pediatrics and Adolescent Medicine*, 161, 1026–1034.

Rounsaville, B.J., Kosten, T.R., Weissman, M.M., and Kleber, H.D. (1986). Prognostic significance of psychopathology in treated opiate addicts: A 2.5 year follow–up study. *Archives of General Psychiatry*, 43, 739–745.

Rounsaville, B.J., Dolinsky, Z.S., Babor, T.F., and Meyer, R.E. (1987). Psychopathology as a predictor of treatment outcome in alcoholics. *Archives of General Psychiatry*, 44, 505–513.

Roy, A. (1998). Placebo–controlled study of sertraline in depressed recently abstinent alcoholics. *Biological Psychiatry*, 44, 633–637.

Sharon, E., Krebs, C., Turner, W. *et al.* (2003). Predictive validity of the ASAM Patient Placement Criteria for hospital utilization. *Journal of Addictive Diseases*, 22 Suppl 1, 79–93.

Sher, L., Stanley, B.H., Harkavy-Friedman, J.M. *et al.* (2008). Depressed patients with co-occurring alcohol use disorders: A unique patient population. *Journal of Clinical Psychiatry*, 69, 907–915.

Stage, K.B., Glassman, A.H., and Covey, L.S. (1996). Depression after smoking cessation: Case reports. *Journal of Clinical Psychiatry*, 57, 467–469.

Tarter, R.E., Kirisci, L., Mezzich, A. *et al.* (2003). Neurobehavioral disinhibition in childhood predicts early age at onset of substance use disorder. *American Journal of Psychiatry*, 160, 1078–1085.

Torrens, M., Fonseca, F., Mateu, G., and Farre, M. (2005). Efficacy of antidepressants in substance use disorders with and without comorbid depression: A systematic review and meta-analysis. *Drug and Alcohol Dependence*, 78, 1–22.

Walsh, B.T., Seidman, S.N., Sysko, R., and Gould, M. (2002). Placebo response in studies of major depression; Variable, substantial, and growing. *Journal of the American Medical Association*, 287, 1840–1847.

Weiss, R.D., Potter, J.S., Fiellin, D.A. *et al.* (2011). Adjunctive counseling during brief and extended buprenorphine–naloxone treatment for prescription opioid dependence: A 2-phase randomized controlled trial. *Archives of General Psychiatry*, 68, 1238–1246.

Zgierska, A. and Fleming, M.F. (2009). Screening and brief intervention. In Ries, R.K., Fiellin, D.A., Miller, S.C., and Saitz, R., eds., *Principles of Addiction Medicine, Fourth Edition*. Philadelphia, PA: Lippincott Williams and Wilkins, 267–278.

Chapter

18

Complementary and alternative treatments for mood disorders

Drew Ramsey, M. Elizabeth Sublette, and Philip R. Muskin

Patients with mood disorders are increasingly interested in complementary and alternative medicine (CAM) treatments; in the USA, consumers are more likely to use CAM treatments than traditional antidepressants or psychotherapy (Kessler *et al.* 2001). In one study of severely depressed patients, 53.6% reported using a CAM treatment within the previous year (Kessler *et al.* 2001). Patients may use CAM out of concern about risks of conventional pharmacologic treatments, perception of better efficacy, belief that naturalistic treatments are safer, convenience of bypassing a physician, and/or lower cost.

Given this environment, familiarity with CAM is essential for the psychiatric clinician. A careful history of CAM usage is necessary, as patients often combine CAM with traditional medications. Physicians must closely evaluate the appropriateness of specific CAM treatments on an individual basis, being aware of potential drug interactions. For some CAM treatments, there is evidence of effectiveness, although for many CAM agents there is variable and inconclusive efficacy data and lack of quality control. The clinician who is knowledgeable can better educate patients about safety and efficacy with regard to use of both traditional and nontraditional treatments. Patients should be explicitly informed whenever particular treatments are not FDA approved. This chapter reviews the evidence concerning frequently used CAM treatments and provides clinicians with basic information needed to integrate CAM interventions into clinical practice.

Omega-3 fatty acids

Omega-3 (or n-3) polyunsaturated fatty acids are essential nutrients because the body cannot manufacture them. There are three clinically relevant

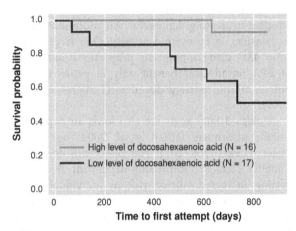

Figure 18.1 Kaplan–Meier survival analysis of suicide attempt outcome by docosahexaenoic acid percentages of total phospholipid fatty acid status categorized by a median split of percentage of plasma phospholipid levels. Reprinted with permission from the *Americal Journal of Psychiatry*, (Copyright 2006), American Psychiatric Association

forms, alpha-linolenic acid (ALA), eicosapentaenoic acid (EPA), and docosahexaenoic acid (DHA). DHA crosses the blood–brain barrier, and it is the predominant brain omega-3 fatty acid.

Seafood is the main food source of EPA and DHA. People in countries with low *per capita* fish intake (like the USA) have an estimated 20-fold reduction in levels of omega-3 fatty acids, relative to the competing omega-6 fatty acids, compared with pre-industrial times (Simopoulos, 2006). This is due to modern food production practices, such as use of high omega-6 cooking oils and the content of animal feed.

Review of the evidence

Meta-analysis results indicate that omega-3 fatty acid levels are lower in major depression than in normal

Clinical Handbook for the Management of Mood Disorders, ed. J. John Mann, Patrick J. McGrath, and Steven P. Roose.
Published by Cambridge University Press. © Cambridge University Press 2013.

controls (Lin *et al.* 2010). In randomized, placebo-controlled clinical trials (RCTs), omega-3 fatty acid supplements were effective in adults and children with diagnosed depressive disorders in studies using fish oil formulations enriched in EPA relative to DHA (Martins, 2009, Sublette *et al.* 2011), although a publication bias exists in favor of positive studies. In contrast, RCTs with high proportions of DHA were ineffective, a counterintuitive finding since DHA levels are greater than EPA levels in the brain. There is no evidence that ALA (found in flaxseed-based supplements) is effective in treating depression. An additional factor to consider is co-morbid anxiety. One large study (n = 432) using appropriate proportions and doses of EPA found clear benefit only in patients without co-morbid anxiety disorders (Lespérance *et al.* 2011).

Omega-3 fatty acids are also lower in depressed suicide attempters (Huan *et al.* 2004) and completers (Lewis *et al.* 2011) compared with depressed nonattempters, a concentration-dependent effect, suggesting increased suicide risk in individuals with extremely low omega-3 levels. One prospective study has shown that DHA levels are significant predictors of future suicide attempt (Sublette *et al.* 2006) (see Figure 18.1). In studies of self-harming individuals, omega-3 fatty acid supplementation has been shown to reduce suicidal ideation (Hallahan *et al.* 2007) and aggression (Zanarini and Frankenburg, 2003), which may be risk factors for suicide.

Comparing omega-3 fatty acid treatment to conventional antidepressants in major depression RCTs, reveals parallel response times for separating from placebo: 2 weeks (Nemets *et al.* 2002), 4 weeks (Peet and Horrobin, 2002, Su *et al.* 2003), and 8 weeks (Nemets *et al.* 2006).

One published double-blind study (N = 48) directly compared fluoxetine and EPA (Jazayeri *et al.* 2008) and found equivalent response rates with either agent after 8 weeks and a superior response with a combination of both: decreases in Hamilton Depression scores of 50, 56 and 81% (fluoxetine, EPA, fluoxetine + EPA, respectively).

Thus, evidence to date suggests that omega-3 fatty acid deficiency is associated with depression and with suicide risk, and that EPA-rich formulations may be effective in major depressive episodes as monotherapy or as augmentation of traditional antidepressants.

Side effects and drug interactions

Omega-3 fatty acids are generally well tolerated. The most common side effect is gastrointestinal upset, mitigated by ingestion with food. There is a hypothetical risk of increased bleeding due to inhibition of platelet function. However, clinical experience – including in patients with cardiovascular illness, dialysis patients, and pregnant women – has been "virtually unanimous" (Harris, 2007) that omega-3 fatty acids do not increase risk of bleeding. Nevertheless, a prudent approach to depressed patients on anticoagulant therapy would be to include a cardiologist or hematologist in the decision to use omega-3 fatty acids. There are no other known drug interactions with fish oil. Patients should be queried about possible fish/shellfish allergies.

Use in clinical practice

The FDA considers omega-3 fatty acids a safe dietary supplement, provided that daily intakes of EPA and DHA do not exceed 3 g per day from all sources. Several clinical trials have used higher amounts without significant adverse events (Stoll *et al.* 1999, Peet and Horrobin, 2002, Su *et al.* 2003, Keck *et al.* 2006), but there is no evidence that doses greater than 2 g per day of EPA are effective in depression. Eating fish carries an increased risk of excessive consumption of mercury and heavy metals that is avoided by the use of purified fish oil supplements.

Preparations containing EPA and DHA are FDA-approved for treatment of hypertriglyceridemia and have a qualified health claim for reducing risk of coronary heart disease. Based on meta-analytic data (Martins, 2009, Sublette *et al.* 2011), consumers should look for products with the EPA component at around or above 60% (EPA/(EPA + DHA)) and a net dose of EPA (i.e., EPA – DHA) of 200–2200 mg/d. (Note: milligram amounts on supplement labeling are *per serving*, not per capsule.)

Fish oil is available as gel caps or as liquid, and may be more palatable if kept in the refrigerator. Avoid products exhibiting a fishy taste or smell, which suggests oxidation. The presence of an antioxidant such as vitamin E is important for stability.

Consideration

Omega-3 fatty acids are not presently FDA-approved for treatment of depression, and the evidence for their effectiveness is limited. Given their excellent safety profile, however, there is little risk and considerable potential benefit in using them as an augmenting agent (Freeman *et al.* 2006), particularly in the absence of a co-morbid anxiety disorder. A trial of omega-3 fatty acids as monotherapy may be a viable option for patients who decline conventional medications, including pregnant or nursing mothers, as omega-3 fatty acids have beneficial effects on the developing fetal brain. Benefits to cardiovascular and inflammatory status are particularly relevant to depressed patients, as they have a higher co-morbidity of cardiovascular and immune disorders (Dinan, 2009).

St. John's wort

St. John's wort (*Hypericum perforatum*, SJW) is a flowering plant found in Europe and Asia and used as a medicinal compound since ancient times. Extracts of SJW contain multiple psychopharmacologically active compounds, notably hypericin, hyperforin, and bioactive flavanoids (Barnes *et al.* 2001). This diversity of phytochemicals results in complex mechanisms of action that have been partially characterized in preclinical studies. SJW inhibits reuptake of multiple neurotransmitters including dopamine, L-glutamate, gamma-aminobutyric acid (GABA), and norepinephrine (Barnes *et al.* 2001). Hypericin and SJW flavonoids both appear to protect the brain from stress-induced effects on gene transcription (Butterweck *et al.* 2001, 2004). Other constituents of SJW exhibit anti-inflammatory activity (Huang *et al.* 2011) that may contribute to its antidepressant effect.

Review of the evidence

SJW has been extensively studied as a monotherapy for the treatment of depression. A 2008 Cochrane review found a total of 29 randomized, controlled trials involving 5498 patients with major depression and concluded that SJW has the same efficacy as conventional antidepressants, but with fewer side effects (Linde *et al.* 2008). The SJW formulation WS5570 was superior to placebo in a 6-week trial of 332 patients (70%, 61% response; 33%, 40% remission, 600 mg/d and 1200 mg/d, respectively) (Kasper *et al.* 2006), while a multi-center placebo-controlled trial of 900–1200 mg/d with 200 patients did not support the use of SJW (Shelton *et al.* 2001). In two additional RCTs neither SJW nor treatment comparators, sertraline and citalopram, demonstrated superior efficacy over placebo (Group, 2002, Rapaport *et al.* 2011).

While generally considered more appropriate for mild to moderate depression, a 6-week, multi-center trial of 251 outpatients with more severe major depression treated with either higher doses of standardized SJW preparation (900–1800 mg/d) or paroxetine (20–40 mg/d) found SJW was at least as efficacious as paroxetine (70 vs. 50% response, 50 vs. 35% remission, respectively) and better tolerated (Szegedi *et al.* 2005).

Little data exist regarding pediatric populations; however, SJW is labeled for the treatment of adolescent depression in Germany, where it is prescribed more commonly than SSRI or TCA antidepressants (Fegert *et al.* 2006). An open-label, 8-week trial of 33 juveniles (mean age 10.5 years) of SJW 450–900 mg/d found response in 25 participants (Findling *et al.* 2003) and another open-label trial with 26 depressed adolescents found improvement in patients who completed an 8-week course, although dropout was high (Simeon *et al.* 2005).

Side effects and drug interactions

Post-marketing surveillance surveys of 34 804 patients found a low incidence of side effects and adverse events, ranging from 0 to 6% (Schulz, 2006). The most common side effects with SJW included gastrointestinal upset, photosensitivity, and mild agitation.

SJW interacts with medications via induction of cytochrome P450 3A4 and 1A2, along with inhibition of P-glycoprotein in the intestinal wall. It can lower the blood levels of several other psychotropics such as alprazolam, amitriptyline, and methadone SJW can cause serotonin syndrome if used in combination with SSRIs or buspirone (Izzo, 2004). Known drug interactions via activation of cytochrome 450 3A4 include interference with oral contraceptives, antiretrovirals (e.g., indinavir, nevirapine), chemotherapy (e.g., irinotecan, imatinib), and immunosuppressants (e.g., cyclosporin) (Borrelli and Izzo, 2009). Prior to surgery, SJW should be discontinued due to potential interactions with general anesthesia (Rowe and Baker, 2009).

Use in clinical practice

The multiple formulations and preparations available to patients complicate the use of SJW. Clinical trials that showed efficacy in mild to moderate depression generally administered 600 to 1200 mg per day, although higher doses were efficacious for some patients (Brown *et al.* 2009); the maximum dose used was 1800 mg/d (Carpenter, 2011). As a general guideline, formulations should contain a standardized concentration of hypericin of at least 0.3%. The WS5570 formulation used in German trials is available in the USA. For information on other specific compounds, clinicians may consult an independent testing source such as consumerlabs.org.

Consideration

Although SJW is not FDA-approved for treatment of depression, the evidence suggests that it is as effective as other conventional antidepressants and better tolerated. Drug interactions dictate avoidance of SJW in patients with HIV, cancer, or transplants; and in women using oral contraceptives. Caution should be used in combining SJW with other serotonergic medicines, such as SSRIs or triptans, due to reports of serotonin syndrome. Like traditional antidepressants, SJW can induce mania in susceptible patients (Nierenberg *et al.* 1999).

Methylators

Three agents that have been implicated in depression are functionally linked through participation in the transmethylation cycle (See Figure 18.2): *S-adenosyl-L-methionine* (SAMe) and *L-methylfolate* carry 1-carbon methyl groups back and forth between homocysteine and methionine, with *cobalamin (vitamin B12)* as an essential co-factor. Abnormalities in the cycle can result in high homocysteine levels, which are associated with depression, although a causal link has not been shown. As transmethylation also extends to other vital substrates including DNA, phospholipids, and proteins, low levels of SAMe and L-methylfolate may impact depression by downregulating the synthesis of monoamines, although this has never been shown.

SAMe

S-adenosyl-methionine (SAMe) is the most diversely physiological, reactive, endogenous methyl donor in the brain, contributing 1-carbon groups to proteins, myelin, DNA, and catecholamine neurotransmitters (Coppen and Bolander-Gouaille, 2005). It is available by prescription in Europe and OTC in the USA. Low levels of SAMe have been found in the CSF of depressed patients (Bottiglieri *et al.* 1990). Due to

initial difficulty creating an oral form stable to first-pass metabolism, SAMe was initially studied as an intravenous agent, though stable oral forms are now available.

Review of the evidence

SAMe administration in oral, intravenous, and intramuscular forms can be efficacious for depression. While the data are limited by small sample sizes, various routes of administration, and methodological concerns, effect sizes were large in positive trials (Carpenter, 2011). In trials of up to 8 weeks, SAMe showed similar efficacy to TCA antidepressants and was an effective augmentation in patients nonresponsive to SRIs and SNRIs (Papakostas *et al.* 2010). In a recent placebo-controlled trial of SSRI nonresponders, augmentation with 800 mg of SAMe twice a day led to 46.1% and 35.8% response and remission rates, respectively (Fleisch *et al.* 2010), yielding a number needed to treat of 3 and 4. Two meta-analyses of SAMe clinical trials found superiority over placebo (Freeman *et al.* 2010). There is no long-term efficacy data.

Use in practice

SAMe is orally dosed in clinical trials as 800–1600 mg/d. It is generally well-tolerated; mild activation, anxiety, headaches, insomnia, and GI distress have been reported. Clinicians should be aware of the possible induction of mania.

Consideration

SAMe should be considered for the treatment of mild to moderate depression, though data currently do not support its use as a first-line agent. Preliminary evidence suggests that augmentation of SSRIs or SNRIs with SAMe can be helpful in treatment-refractory patients.

Vitamin B12

Vitamin B12, or cobalamin, is an essential co-factor for transmethylation. B12 is produced by bacteria and is high in meat, dairy products, seafood, and eggs. Supplements and fortified cereals generally contain cyanocobalamin, the most common synthetic form. B12 is a large molecule that requires the protein intrinsic factor, produced from parietal cells in the stomach, for its absorption. Thus, main risk factors of vitamin B12 deficiency are deficient intake and gastrointestinal conditions disrupting B12 absorption. In

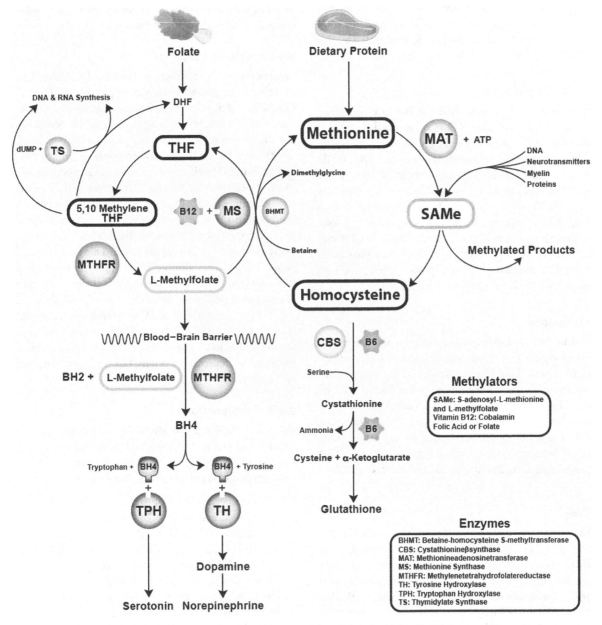

Figure 18.2 The methylation cycle. Via the transfer of methyl groups, the methylation cycle functionally links neurotransmitter and phospholipid synthesis, innate brain antioxidant production (glutathione), and homocystiene status. Both preclinical and clinical data suggest that SAMe, vitamin B12, and forms of folate (folic acid, L-methylfolate) have complimentary clinical applications in the treatment of mood disorders

a recent cross-sectional study of 689 men (Gilsing *et al.* 2010), 52% of vegans and 7% of vegetarians were B12 deficient. Achlorhydria, which is frequently seen in the elderly and also caused iatrogenically by proton-pump inhibitors such as omeprazole, interferes with B12 absorption from food, but not from supplements.

While macrocytic anemia has been the hallmark of B12 deficiency, it is a late stage, and more than a quarter of patients with B12 deficiency exhibit neuropsychiatric symptoms without hematological findings (Lindenbaum *et al.* 1988). Deficiency can be masked by folic acid supplementation, delaying the macrocytic anemia, but not the neuropsychiatric manifestations. About 10% of people with "low normal" levels of 200–400 pg/ml have B12 deficiency, as demonstrated by elevated homocysteine and methylmalonic acid.

Review of the evidence

Up to one-third of depressed patients are functionally deficient in vitamin B12 (Coppen and Bolander-Gouaille, 2005). B12 deficiency diminishes response to traditional antidepressants (Kate *et al.* 2010), while higher vitamin B12 levels are associated with better treatment outcomes in major depression (Hintikka *et al.* 2003). Deficiency has been associated with a number of symptoms, including depression, irritability, agitation, and psychosis (Lindenbaum *et al.* 1988, Bar-Shai *et al.* 2011). B12 deficiency was associated with a 70% increased risk of depression in a large survey of the elderly (Tiemeier *et al.* 2002).

Consideration

Vitamin B12 should be assessed in patients with mood disorders, and, if low, homocysteine and methylmalonic acid should be measured. At highest risk are patients with any GI condition, those taking proton-pump inhibitors, elderly patients, and those on vegetarian or vegan diets. While monthly IM injections of B12 were formerly recommended for repletion, these are no more advantageous than high dose 1–2 mg oral or sub-lingual treatment (Vidal-Alaball *et al.* 2005).

Folate

Folate is an essential B vitamin with multiple derivatives (see Figure 18.2), including the natural form *dihydrofolate* in foods such as legumes and leafy greens, and synthetic forms in supplements, and fortified in foods such as cereals and flour in the US since 1989 to reduce the incidence of neural tube defects. Commercially available synthetic forms are *folic acid, folinic acid* (or leucovorin), and *methylfolate* (of which L-methylfolate is the active enantiomer). L-methylfolate is available as an OTC supplement and prescription medications (Deplin). Both dihydrofolate and folic acid are inactive until metabolized via a pathway that includes two reducing enzymes, dihydrofolate reductase (DHFR) and methylenetetrahydrofolate reductase (MTHFR). Folinic acid bypasses DHFR, and L-methylfolate bypasses both enzymes, crossing the blood–brain barrier and serving as a requisite co-factor in the synthesis of serotonin, norepinephrine, and dopamine.

Review of the evidence

Folate deficiencies are common in mood disorders and correlate with illness severity (Coppen and Bolander-Gouaille, 2005). Open trials were positive for folinic acid (15–30 mg/d) as augmentation of SSRIs in treatment-refractory depressed patients (Alpert *et al.* 2002), and for methyltetrahydrofolate as monotherapy at 50 mg/d in elderly depressed subjects (Guaraldi *et al.* 1993) and at 90 mg/d in depressed subjects with chronic ethanol dependence (Di Palma, 1994). A double-blind trial of methylfolate 50 mg/d compared to trazodone 100 mg/d after a placebo lead-in found a decrease in depression scores at 4 and 8 weeks (Passeri *et al.* 1993). Two double-blind, placebo-controlled trials both sponsored by the manufacturer of Deplin (L-methylfolate) were positive for methylfolate 15 mg/d for 6 months added to standard treatment (Godfrey *et al.* 1990, Procter, 1991), while folic acid 0.5 mg added to 20 mg of fluoxetine improved clinical response in depressed women, but not men (Coppen and Bailey, 2000).

Use in clinical practice

Folate supplements are available in multiple formulations and strengths (Fava and Mischoulon, 2009). Folic acid is the most commonly used; however, L-methylfolate is preferable for three reasons:

1. *Pharmacogenomics*: Approximately 10% of Caucasians are homozygous for a polymorphism in the gene coding for the MTHFR enzyme, MTHFR C677T, that produces a less active form of the reductase, resulting in decreased bioavailability of folate to the brain. The T/T genotype is associated with major depression and bipolar disorder (Gilbody *et al.* 2007). L-methylfolate can directly cross the blood–brain barrier, bypassing the MTHFR reductase completely.

2. *Pharmacodynamics*: Certain medications, notably lamotrigine and methotrexate, inhibit DHFR, the enzyme that metabolizes folic acid. In fact, methotrexate is used as a cancer treatment precisely for its ability to reduce folate-stimulated tumor growth through DHFR inhibition, and folinic acid (as leucovorin) is given to rescue other tissues from the lack of folate.

3. Conversely, long-term supplementation with the folic acid form has been linked to an increased risk of cancer (Figueiredo *et al.* 2009, Baggott *et al.* 2011). L-methylfolate is available as a supplement or as a prescription medication (Deplin) in 7.5 mg or 10 mg strengths.

Consideration

Clinicians should rule out folate deficiency in patients with mood disorders, and patients with mood vulnerability should be encouraged to consume foods rich in natural folates. While long-term supplementation with folic acid carries some risk, shorter-term supplementation can be an effective augmentation strategy. Though industry-sponsored clinical trials support the use of L-methylfolate (Deplin) and there is mechanistic appeal, comparison trials with other forms of folate have not been performed.

Rhodiola rosea

Rhodiola rosea is a plant native to the Arctic regions of Europe, Asia, and North America. Extracts from its roots have been used as medicine for centuries. Also known as Golden Root, Arctic Root, or Rosen root, rhodiola is referenced in medical texts from the eighteenth century as a treatment for "hysteria," "strengthening of the head," to "enhance the intellects," and "restore weak nerves," related to its stimulating effects (Panossian *et al.* 2010).

Mechanism of action

Rhodiola is considered an adaptogen, a molecule that influences the stress response. Its reported ability to promote mental alertness, concentration, and reduce fatigue indicate possible utility as an augmentation strategy in mood disorders. Extracts contain numerous bioactive compounds involved in its mechanism of action including inhibitors of monoamineoxidase A and B (van Diermen *et al.* 2009).

Review of the evidence

The herb primarily relates to mood disorders for its use as a mild stimulant with possible neuroprotective effects. Only one trial has explored its use as antidepressant monotherapy and in this 6-week RTC the standardized extract, SR-5 340–680 mg/d was found to be superior to placebo in reducing both HAM-D and BDI scores (Darbinyan *et al.* 2007). A trial assessing the effect of 576 mg/d of SR-5 vs. placebo on stress-related fatigue found increased concentration and a modification of cortisol response in the treatment group (Olsson *et al.* 2009).

Use in practice

Overall, Rhodiola is well tolerated with rare side effects of irritability, insomnia, headache, and restlessness. Rhodiola is dosed at 200 to 600 mg per day. Though little is known about drug interactions, given Rhodiola's MAOI activity, caution should be exercised before combining Rhodiola with traditional MAO inhibitors or other stimulants. Rhodiola may also inhibit CYP3A4 enzymes and influence P-glycoprotein (Hellum *et al.* 2010).

Considerations

Currently, evidence does not support the use of Rhodiola as a primary treatment for depression, yet given the frequent complaints of fatigue and lack of concentration in mood disorder patients, it may provide an alternative to traditional stimulants. Clinicians should be cautious for interactions with drugs metabolized by CYP3A4 and aware of this herb's MAOI activity.

Acupuncture

Acupuncture has a long history of use in Chinese and Japanese medicine. The practice involves the insertion of fine needles into specific spots on the body to alleviate pain and to treat various physical, mental, and emotional conditions. There are a variety of styles of acupuncture ranging from those based on traditional Chinese principles, to medical acupuncture, which is based on the principles of neurophysiology and anatomy (Smith *et al.* 2010).

Review of the evidence

The most comprehensive review of acupuncture for depression to date is a recent meta-analysis in the Cochrane Database (Smith *et al.* 2010) assessing acupuncture with respect to a variety of comparators. The study, which included 30 RCTs with 2812 participants, found inadequate evidence for a beneficial effect of acupuncture compared with wait-list control or sham acupuncture control. However, two trials found benefit for acupuncture as an augmentation compared with medication alone, and three trials found that a sub-group of patients exhibited improvement in depression compared with SSRIs. An important note is that most trials were conducted with a high risk of bias, and therefore more controlled trials are needed.

Side effects and patient dosing

Acupuncture is a well-tolerated intervention when performed by an adequately trained practitioner. Adverse side effects include syncope, skin irritation, transient bleeding, and bruising at needle insertion site. The usual duration of the treatment is 4–8 weeks. The number of needles inserted at sessions varies (Ravindran *et al.* 2009).

Consideration

Acupuncture may be useful for some depressed individuals who wish to complement their treatment, although there is no substantial evidence of efficacy as a treatment for depression.

Yoga

Yoga is an ancient Indian system with many schools (i.e., Hatha, Iyengar, Bikram, Vinyasa, Kundalini), which incorporate breath control (pranayama), meditation (dhyana), and physical postures (asanas). There has been an increased scientific interest in yoga as a mental health intervention for mood disorders and some encouraging evidence, though the variety of techniques and methodological issues complicate interpretation of positive findings (Pilkington *et al.* 2005).

Review of the evidence

A 2010 review of Hatha yoga for depression revealed eight trials in the literature, along with support for a variety of yoga-based "mindfulness"-promoting techniques (Uebelacker *et al.* 2010). Sudarshan Kriya Yoga (SKY) was inferior to ECT, but equivalent to imipramine in a small sample of depressed, melancholic inpatients (Janakiramaiah *et al.* 2000). SKY reportedly decreased depression, anxiety, and influence physiological markers of stress such as decreasing salivary cortisol in breast cancer patients compared with a supportive therapy (Vadiraja *et al.* 2009).

Practicing yoga three times a week for 24 weeks improved sleep, and decreased depression and daytime dysfunction in elderly patients in assisted-living

facilities (Chen *et al.* 2010). Increases in GABA were found by magnetic resonance spectroscopy after yoga practice and correlated with improved mood compared to a control intervention of walking (Streeter *et al.* 2010). Currently, there are no clinical trials with a control group to measure the specific benefit.

Consideration

While no specific evidence supports yoga as a primary treatment of mood disorders, there is preliminary evidence of its ability to modulate the stress response and improve mood. Yoga may be an effective augmentation strategy in mood disorder patients with sleep disturbances and assist in the prevention of mood symptoms in patients with cancer.

Nutrition counseling

Given the realities of patient compliance with many mental health interventions, dietary counseling offers a unique opportunity to promote health. Dietary patterns are increasingly linked to the relative risk of developing a mood disorder. A Western diet of "processed or fried foods, refined grains, sugary products, and beer" increased the relative risk of developing depression over 5 years when compared to individuals who ate a "traditional" diet consisting of meat, fish, whole grains, vegetables, and fruit (Jacka *et al.* 2010). Consumption of *trans* fats and omega-6 fatty acids are linked to an increased risk of depression, while adherence to a Mediterranean diet of monounsaturated and omega-3 fats is protective (Wolfe *et al.* 2009, Sanchez-Villegas *et al.* 2011).

Consideration

Emphasizing intake of whole foods rich in omega-3 fatty acids, magnesium, iron, folates, and B vitamins can play a role in the comprehensive treatment of mood disorders, given recent evidence linking dietary patterns to the risk of depression; however, no dietary intervention studies have been performed to date.

Other CAM treatments

The literature on herbal treatments for psychiatric disorders is rapidly expanding. The pharmacology of numerous plant compounds was recently reviewed (Sarris *et al.* 2011b). While the majority of CAM literature has focused on depression, a recent review suggests a role for several agents in the management of bipolar disorder (Sarris *et al.* 2011a).

Tryptophan/5-hydroxytryptophan (5HTP)

The augmentation and depletion of L-tryptophan/5HTP have been studied to further elucidate serotonin's role in mood regulation. As tryptophan competes with other large, neutral amino acids (LNAAs) for transport into the brain, increasing the ratio of tryptophan to LNAAs affects serotonin synthesis. Both are currently available as supplements, although L-tryptophan was banned from 1991–2004 after an outbreak of eosinophilia myalgia syndrome (EMS) that affected more than 1500 people, with more than 30 fatalities, which was eventually traced to a contaminant. Since 2005, via the FDA's passive surveillance system there have been two possible cases of EMS, two reports of myalgias, and one confirmed case of EMS (Allen *et al.* 2011). A review of human trials revealed variable effects of supplementation on mood, cognition, and sleep (Silber and Schmitt, 2010), and currently there is no clear role for the use of tryptophan/5HTP in the treatment of mood disorders.

Vitamin D

Vitamin D deficiency and insufficiency (<30 ng/l) are linked to depressive symptoms, particularly in individuals with a history of a diagnosed depressive disorder (Hoang *et al.* 2011). Receptors are widely distributed throughout the brain (Berk *et al.* 2007). While seasonal variations in sunlight exposure implicate vitamin D as a contributor to seasonal affective disorder (SAD), a causal role has not been established (Parker and Brotchie, 2011). Low vitamin D levels are associated with low mood and worse cognition in the elderly (Wilkins *et al.* 2006), higher BDI depression scores in a sample of overweight and obese individuals (Jorde *et al.* 2008), and lower levels of D3 during childhood is associated with increased depressive symptoms during adolescence (Tolppanen *et al.* 2011), However, a 1-year intervention of weekly 20 000 IU or 40 000 IU of vitamin D3 in obese and overweight individuals did not find a significant difference in BDI scores compared with placebo (Jorde *et al.* 2008). Additionally, in a 5-year intervention study of elderly women, yearly high-dose vitamin D3 (500 000 IU) did eliminate deficiency, but did not separate from placebo in a number of mental health outcomes (Sanders *et al.*

2011). Psychiatrists should consider educating patients about vitamin D. Deficiencies are most common in the winter, in the elderly, in patients with low sunlight exposure (shift workers, medical professionals), and in individuals with pigmented skin (deficiency rates of up to 90%). While low levels of vitamin D are linked to depression, as of yet, no evidence supports supplementation as an effective preventive or treatment strategy of mood disorders.

DHEA

The hormone dehydropiandrosterone (DHEA) produced by the adrenal glands is the precursor to testosterone and estrogen. Some small clinical studies support the use of DHEA for major depressive disorder as both monotherapy and augmentation strategy (Wolkowitz *et al.* 1999, Schmidt *et al.* 2005). For dysthymia and sub-syndromal depression, DHEA monotherapy was more effective than placebo (Bloch *et al.* 1999) and a well-tolerated, efficacious treatment in HIV patients (Rabkin *et al.* 2006). In studies of depression, dosages of DHEA varied greatly from 25 to 450 mg/d. Safety data suggests potential adverse effects of DHEA on blood clotting and liver damage, and the induction of mania in vulnerable individuals (Ravindran *et al.* 2009). Therefore, no significant data support the use of DHEA in the treatment of mood disorders.

Crocus sativus

The flowers and stigma of the saffron flower (*Crocus sativus*) have demonstrated antidepressant effects in both preclinical data and small RTCs compared to placebo, imipramine, and fluoxetine (Akhondzadeh *et al.* 2004, Akhondzadeh Basti *et al.* 2007).

Conclusions

CAM treatments are preferred by patients with mood disorders; however, the evidence supporting their role is generally limited. Clinicians should carefully weigh the relative merits of choosing CAM over traditional treatments. Among the CAM treatments, evidence supports the use of SJW as a monotherapy, and omega-3, SAMe, and several methylators as augmentation strategies in the treatment of depression. Little evidence is available concerning the role of CAM in the treatment of bipolar disorder.

Methodological flaws are a consistent critique of CAM, and larger, longer-term studies are needed to assess CAM efficacy. Interventions such as yoga, acupuncture, and improved nutrition are inherently difficult to blind, complicating their assessment. Clinical experience suggests CAM may be helpful in engaging patients and useful in the treatment of carefully selected patients.

References

Akhondzadeh, S., Fallah-Pour, H., Afkham, K., Jamshidi, A.H., and Khalighi-Cigaroudi, F. (2004). Comparison of *Crocus sativus* L. and imipramine in the treatment of mild to moderate depression: A pilot double-blind randomized trial [ISRCTN45683816]. *BMC Complementary and Alternative Medicine*, 4, 12.

Akhondzadeh Basti, A., Moshiri, E., Noorbala, A.A. *et al.* (2007). Comparison of petal of *Crocus sativus* L. and fluoxetine in the treatment of depressed outpatients: A pilot double-blind randomized trial. *Progress in Neuropsychopharmacology and Biological Psychiatry*, 31, 439–442.

Allen, J.A., Peterson, A., Sufit, R. *et al.* (2011). Post-epidemic eosinophilia-myalgia syndrome associated with L-tryptophan. *Arthritis and Rheumatism*, 63, 3633–3639.

Alpert, J.E., Mischoulon, D., Rubenstein, G.E., Bottonari, K., Nierenberg, A.A., and Fava, M. (2002). Folinic acid (Leucovorin) as an adjunctive treatment for SSRI-refractory depression. *Annals of Clinical Psychiatry*, 14, 33–38.

Baggott, J.E., Oster, R.A., and Tamura, T. (2011). Meta-analysis of cancer risk in folic acid supplementation trials. *Cancer Epidemiology*, 36, 78–81.

Barnes, J., Anderson, L.A., and Phillipson, J.D. (2001). St John's wort (Hypericum perforatum L.): A review of its chemistry, pharmacology and clinical properties. *Journal of Pharmacy and Pharmacology*, 53, 583–600.

Bar-Shai, M., Gott, D., and Marmor, S. (2011). Acute psychotic depression as a sole manifestation of vitamin B12 deficiency. *Psychosomatics*, 52, 384–386.

Berk, M., Sanders, K.M., Pasco, J.A. *et al.* (2007). Vitamin D deficiency may play a role in depression. *Medical Hypotheses*, 69, 1316–1319.

Bloch, M., Schmidt, P.J., Danaceau, M.A., Adams, L.F., and Rubinow, D.R. (1999). Dehydroepiandrosterone treatment of midlife dysthymia. *Biological Psychiatry*, 45, 1533–1541.

Borrelli, F. and Izzo, A.A. (2009). Herb-drug interactions with St John's wort (*Hypericum perforatum*): An update on clinical observations. *AAPS Journal*, 11, 710–727.

Bottiglieri, T., Godfrey, P., Flynn, T. *et al.* (1990). Cerebrospinal fluid S-adenosylmethionine in depression and dementia: effects of treatment with parenteral and oral S-adenosylmethionine. *Journal of Neurology, Neurosurgery and Psychiatry*, 53, 1096–1098.

Brown, R.P., Gerbarg, P.L., and Muskin, P.R. (2009). *How to Use Herbs, Nutrients and Yoga in Mental Health Care.* New York, W.W. Norton.

Butterweck, V., Winterhoff, H., and Herkenham, M. (2001). St John's wort, hypericin, and imipramine: A comparative analysis of mRNA levels in brain areas involved in HPA axis control following short-term and long-term administration in normal and stressed rats. *Molecular Psychiatry*, 6, 547–564.

Butterweck, V., Hegger, M., and Winterhoff, H. (2004). Flavonoids of St. John's Wort reduce HPA axis function in the rat. *Planta Medica*, 70, 1008–1011.

Carpenter, D.J. (2011). St. John's wort and S-adenosyl-methionine as "natural" alternatives to conventional antidepressants in the era of the suicidality boxed warning: what is the evidence for clinically relevant benefit? *Alternative Medical Reviews*, 16, 17–39.

Chen, K.M., Chen, M.H., Lin, M.H. *et al.* (2010). Effects of yoga on sleep quality and depression in elders in assisted living facilities. *Journal of Nursing Research*, 18, 53–61.

Coppen, A. and Bailey, J. (2000). Enhancement of the antidepressant action of fluoxetine by folic acid: A randomised, placebo controlled trial. *Journal of Affective Disorders*, 60, 121–130.

Coppen, A. and Bolander-Gouaille, C. (2005). Treatment of depression: time to consider folic acid and vitamin B12. *Journal of Psychopharmacology*, 19, 59–65.

Darbinyan, V., Aslanyan, G., Amroyan, E. *et al.* (2007). Clinical trial of Rhodiola rosea L. extract SHR-5 in the treatment of mild to moderate depression. *Nordic Journal of Psychiatry*, 61, 343–348.

Dinan, T.G. (2009). Inflammatory markers in depression. *Current Opinion in Psychiatry*, 22, 32–36.

Di Palma, C., Urani, R., Agricola, R. *et al.* (1994). Is methylfolate effective in relieving major depression in ceronic alcoholics? A hypothesis of treatment. *Current Therapeutic Research*, 55, 559–568.

Fava, M. and Mischoulon, D. (2009). Folate in depression: Efficacy, safety, differences in formulations, and clinical issues. *Journal of Clinical Psychiatry*, 70 Suppl 5, 12–17.

Fegert, J.M., Kölch, M., Zito, J.M., Glaeske, G., and Janhsen, K. (2006). Antidepressant use in children and adolescents in Germany. *Journal of Child and Adolescent Psychopharmacology*, 16, 197–206.

Figueiredo, J.C., Grau, M.V., Haile, R.W. *et al.* (2009). Folic acid and risk of prostate cancer: Results from a randomized clinical trial. *Journal of the National Cancer Institute*, 101, 432–435.

Findling, R.L., McNamara, N.K., O'Riordan, M.A. *et al.* (2003). An open-label pilot study of St. John's wort in juvenile depression. *Journal of the American Academy of Child and Adolescent Psychiatry*, 42, 908–914.

Fleisch, S.B., Travis, M.J., and Ryan, N.D. (2010). Discrepancy in response and remission rates for SAMe-treated patients in a double-blind, randomized clinical trial. *American Journal of Psychiatry*, 167, 1533; author reply 1533.

Freeman, M.P., Hibbeln, J.R., Wisner, K.L. *et al.* (2006). Omega-3 fatty acids: evidence basis for treatment and future research in psychiatry. *Journal of Clinical Psychiatry*, 67, 1954–1967.

Freeman, M.P., Fava, M., Lake, J. *et al.* (2010). Complementary and alternative medicine in major depressive disorder: The American Psychiatric Association Task Force report. *Journal of Clinical Psychiatry*, 71, 669–681.

Gilbody, S., Lewis, S., and Lightfoot, T. (2007). Methylenetetrahydrofolate reductase (MTHFR) genetic polymorphisms and psychiatric disorders: A HuGE review. *American Journal of Epidemiology*, 165, 1–13.

Gilsing, A.M., Crowe, F.L., Lloyd-Wright, Z. *et al.* (2010). Serum concentrations of vitamin B12 and folate in British male omnivores, vegetarians and vegans: Results from a cross-sectional analysis of the EPIC-Oxford cohort study. *European Journal of Clinical Nutrition*, 64, 933–939.

Godfrey, P.S., Toone, B.K., Carney, M.W. *et al.* (1990). Enhancement of recovery from psychiatric illness by methylfolate. *Lancet*, 336, 392–395.

Group, Hypericum Depression Trial Study (2002). Effect of *Hypericum perforatum* (St John's wort) in major depressive disorder: A randomized controlled trial. *Journal of the American Medical Association*, 287, 1807–1814.

Guaraldi, G.P., Fava, M., Mazzi, F., and La Greca, P. (1993). An open trial of methyltetrahydrofolate in elderly depressed patients. *Annals of Clinical Psychiatry*, 5, 101–105.

Hallahan, B., Hibbeln, J.R., Davis, J.M., and Garland, M.R. (2007). Omega-3 fatty acid supplementation in patients with recurrent self-harm. Single-centre double-blind randomised controlled trial. *British Journal of Psychiatry*, 190, 118–122.

Harris, W.S. (2007). Expert opinion: omega-3 fatty acids and bleeding-cause for concern? *American Journal of Cardiology*, 99, 44C–46C.

Hellum, B.H., Tosse, A., Hoybakk, K. *et al.* (2010). Potent in vitro inhibition of CYP3A4 and P-glycoprotein by *Rhodiola rosea*. *Planta Medica*, 76, 331–338.

Hintikka, J., Tolmunen, T., Tanskanen, A., and Viinamäki, H. (2003). High vitamin B12 level and good treatment outcome may be associated in major depressive disorder. *BMC Psychiatry*, 3, 17.

Hoang, M.T., Defina, L.F., Willis, B.L. *et al.* (2011). Association between low serum 25-hydroxyvitamin D and depression in a large sample of healthy adults: The Cooper Center longitudinal study. *Mayo Clinic Proceedings*, 86, 1050–1055.

Huan, M., Hamazaki, K., Sun, Y. *et al.* (2004). Suicide attempt and n-3 fatty acid levels in red blood cells: A case control study in China. *Biological Psychiatry*, 56, 490–496.

Huang, N., Rizshsky, L., Hauck, C. *et al.* (2011). Identification of anti-inflammatory constituents in *Hypericum perforatum* and *Hypericum gentianoides* extracts using RAW 264.7 mouse macrophages. *Phytochemistry*, 72, 2015–2023.

Izzo, A.A. (2004). Drug interactions with St. John's Wort (*Hypericum perforatum*): A review of the clinical evidence. *International Journal of Clinical Pharmacology and Therapeutics*, 42, 139–148.

Jacka, F.N., Pasco, J.A., Mykletun, A. *et al.* (2010). Association of Western and traditional diets with depression and anxiety in women. *American Journal of Psychiatry*, 167, 305–311.

Janakiramaiah, N., Gangadhar, B.N., Naga Venkatesha Murthy, P. J. *et al.* (2000). Antidepressant efficacy of Sudarshan Kriya Yoga (SKY) in melancholia: A randomized comparison with electroconvulsive therapy (ECT) and imipramine. *Journal of Affective Disorders*, 57, 255–259.

Jazayeri, S., Tehrani-Doost, M., Keshavarz, S.A. *et al.* (2008). Comparison of therapeutic effects of omega-3 fatty acid eicosapentaenoic acid and fluoxetine, separately and in combination, in major depressive disorder. *Australian and New Zealand Journal of Psychiatry*, 42, 192–198.

Jorde, R., Sneve, M., Figenschau, Y., Svartberg, J., and Waterloo, K. (2008). Effects of vitamin D supplementation on symptoms of depression in overweight and obese subjects: Randomized double blind trial. *Journal of Internal Medicine*, 264, 599–609.

Kasper, S., Anghelescu, I.G., Szegedi, A., Dienel, A., and Kieser, M. (2006). Superior efficacy of St John's wort extract WS 5570 compared to placebo in patients with major depression: A randomized, double-blind, placebo-controlled, multi-center trial [ISRCTN77277298]. *BMC Medicine*, 4, 14.

Kate, N., Grover, S., and Agarwal, M. (2010). Does B12 deficiency lead to lack of treatment response to conventional antidepressants? *Psychiatry (Edgmont)*, 7, 42–44.

Keck, P.E., Jr., Mintz, J., McElroy, S.L. *et al.* (2006). Double-blind, randomized, placebo-controlled trials of ethyl-eicosapentanoate in the treatment of bipolar depression and rapid cycling bipolar disorder. *Biological Psychiatry*, 60, 1020–1022.

Kessler, R.C., Soukup, J., Davis, R.B. *et al.* (2001). The use of complementary and alternative therapies to treat anxiety and depression in the United States. *American Journal of Psychiatry*, 158, 289–294.

Lespérance, F., Frasure-Smith, N., St-André, E. *et al.* (2011). The efficacy of omega-3 supplementation for major depression: A randomized controlled trial. *Journal of Clinical Psychiatry*, 72, 1054–1062.

Lewis, M.D., Hibbeln, J.R., Johnson, J.E. *et al.* (2011). Suicide deaths of active-duty US military and omega-3 fatty-acid status: A case-control comparison. *Journal of Clinical Psychiatry*, 72, 1585–1590.

Lin, P.Y., Huang, S.Y., and Su, K.P. (2010). A meta-analytic review of polyunsaturated fatty acid compositions in patients with depression. *Biological Psychiatry*, 68, 140–147.

Linde, K., Berner, M.M., and Kriston, L. (2008). St John's wort for major depression. *Cochrane Database of Systematic Reviews*, 4, CD000448.

Lindenbaum, J., Healton, E.B., Savage, D.G. *et al.* (1988). Neuropsychiatric disorders caused by cobalamin deficiency in the absence of anemia or macrocytosis. *New England Journal of Medicine*, 318, 1720–1728.

Martins, J.G. (2009). EPA but not DHA appears to be responsible for the efficacy of omega-3 long chain polyunsaturated fatty acid supplementation in depression: Evidence from a meta-analysis of randomized controlled trials. *Journal of the American College of Nutrition*, 28, 525–542.

Nierenberg, A.A., Burt, T., Matthews, J., and Weiss, A.P. (1999). Mania associated with St. John's wort. *Biological Psychiatry*, 46, 1707–1708.

Nemets, B., Stahl, Z., and Belmaker, R. (2002). Addition of omega-3 fatty acid to maintenance medication treatment for recurrent unipolar depressive disorder. *American Journal of Psychiatry*, 159, 477–479.

Nemets, H., Nemets, B., Apter, A., Bracha, Z., and Belmaker, R.H. (2006). Omega-3 treatment of childhood depression: A controlled, double-blind pilot study. *American Journal of Psychiatry*, 163, 1098–1100.

Olsson, E.M., Von Schéele, B., and Panossian, A.G. (2009). A randomised, double-blind, placebo-controlled, parallel-group study of the standardised extract SHR-5 of the roots of Rhodiola rosea in the treatment of subjects with stress-related fatigue. *Planta Medica*, 75, 105–112.

Panossian, A., Wikman, G., and Sarris, J. (2010). Rosen root (*Rhodiola rosea*): traditional use, chemical composition, pharmacology and clinical efficacy. *Phytomedicine*, 17, 481–493.

Papakostas, G.I., Mischoulon, D., Shyu, I., Alpert, J.E., and Fava, M. (2010). S-adenosylmethionine (SAMe) augmentation of serotonin reuptake inhibitors for antidepressant nonresponders with major depressive disorder: A double-blind, randomized clinical trial. *American Journal of Psychiatry*, 167, 942–948.

Parker, G. and Brotchie, H. (2011). 'D' for depression: Any role for vitamin D? 'Food for Thought' II. *Acta Psychiatrica Scandinavica*, 124, 243–249.

Passeri, M., Cucinotta, D., Abate, G. *et al.* (1993). Oral 5′-methyltetrahydrofolic acid in senile organic mental disorders with depression: Results of a double-blind multicenter study. *Aging (Milano)*, 5, 63–71.

Peet, M. and Horrobin, D. (2002). A dose-ranging study of the effects of ethyl-eicosapentaenoate in patients with ongoing depression despite apparently adequate treatment with standard drugs. *Archives of General Psychiatry*, 59, 913–919.

Pilkington, K., Kirkwood, G., Rampes, H., and Richardson, J. (2005). Yoga for depression: The research evidence. *Journal of Affective Disorders*, 89, 13–24.

Procter, A. (1991). Enhancement of recovery from psychiatric illness by methylfolate. *British Journal of Psychiatry*, 159, 271–272.

Rabkin, J.G., McElhiney, M.C., Rabkin, R., McGrath, P.J., and Ferrando, S.J. (2006). Placebo-controlled trial of dehydroepiandrosterone (DHEA) for treatment of nonmajor depression in patients with HIV/AIDS. *American Journal of Psychiatry*, 163, 59–66.

Rapaport, M.H., Nierenberg, A.A., Howland, R. *et al.* (2011). The treatment of minor depression with St. John's Wort or citalopram: Failure to show benefit over placebo. *Journal of Psychiatric Research*, 45, 931–941.

Ravindran, A.V., Lam, R.W., Filteau, M.J. *et al.* (2009). Canadian Network for Mood and Anxiety Treatments (CANMAT) clinical guidelines for the management of major depressive disorder in adults. V. Complementary and alternative medicine treatments. *Journal of Affective Disorders*, 117 Suppl 1, S54–S64.

Rowe, D.J. and Baker, A.C. (2009). Perioperative risks and benefits of herbal supplements in aesthetic surgery. *Aesthetic Surgery Journal*, 29, 150–157.

Sanchez-Villegas, A., Verberne, L., deIrala, J. *et al.* (2011). Dietary fat intake and the risk of depression: The SUN Project. *PLoS One*, 6, e16268.

Sanders, K.M., Stuart, A.L., Williamson, E.J. *et al.* (2011). Annual high-dose vitamin D3 and mental well-being: randomised controlled trial. *British Journal of Psychiatry*, 198, 357–364.

Sarris, J., Lake, J., and Hoenders, R. (2011a). Bipolar disorder and complementary medicine: Current evidence, safety issues, and clinical considerations. *Journal of Alternative and Complementary Medicine*, 17, 881–890.

Sarris, J., Panossian, A., Schweitzer, I., Stough, C., and Scholey, A. (2011b). Herbal medicine for depression, anxiety and insomnia: A review of psychopharmacology and clinical evidence. *European Neuropsychopharmacology*, 21, 841–860.

Schmidt, P.J., Daly, R.C., Bloch, M. *et al.* (2005). Dehydroepiandrosterone monotherapy in midlife-onset major and minor depression. *Archives of General Psychiatry*, 62, 154–162.

Schulz, V. (2006). Safety of St. John's Wort extract compared to synthetic antidepressants. *Phytomedicine*, 13, 199–204.

Shelton, R.C., Keller, M.B., Gelenberg, A. *et al.* (2001). Effectiveness of St John's wort in major depression: A randomized controlled trial. *Journal of the American Medical Association*, 285, 1978–1986.

Silber, B.Y. and Schmitt, J.A. (2010). Effects of tryptophan loading on human cognition, mood, and sleep. *Neuroscience and Biobehavioral Reviews*, 34, 387–407.

Simeon, J., Nixon, M.K., Milin, R., Jovanovic, R., and Walker, S. (2005). Open-label pilot study of St. John's wort in adolescent depression. *Journal of Child and Adolescent Psychopharmacology*, 15, 293–301.

Simopoulos, A.P. (2006). Evolutionary aspects of diet, the omega-6/omega-3 ratio and genetic variation: nutritional implications for chronic diseases. *Biomedicine and Pharmacotherapy*, 60, 502–507.

Smith, C.A., Hay, P.P., and MacPherson, H. (2010). Acupuncture for depression. *Cochrane Database of Systematic Reviews*, 1, CD004046.

Stoll, A.L., Severus, W.E., Freeman, M.P. *et al.* (1999). Omega 3 fatty acids in bipolar disorder: A preliminary double-blind, placebo-controlled trial. *Archives of General Psychiatry*, 56, 407–412.

Streeter, C.C., Whitfield, T.H., Owen, L. *et al.* (2010). Effects of yoga versus walking on mood, anxiety, and brain GABA levels: A randomized controlled MRS study. *Journal of Alternative and Complementary Medicine*, 16, 1145–1152.

Su, K., Huang, S., Chiu, C., and Shen, W. (2003). Omega-3 fatty acids in major depressive disorder: A preliminary double-blind, placebo-controlled trial. *European Neuropsychopharmacology*, 13, 267–271.

Sublette, M.E., Ellis, S.P., Geant, A.L., and Mann, J.J. (2011). Meta-analysis: Effects of eicosapentaenoic acid in clinical trials in depression. *Journal of Clinical Psychiatry*, 72, 1577–1584.

Sublette, M.E., Hibbeln, J.R., Galfalvy, H., Oquendo, M.A., and Mann, J.J. (2006). Omega-3 polyunsaturated essential fatty acid status as a predictor of future suicide risk. *American Journal of Psychiatry*, 163, 1100–1102.

Szegedi, A., Kohnen, R., Dienel, A., and Kieser, M. (2005). Acute treatment of moderate to severe depression with hypericum extract WS 5570 (St John's wort): Randomised controlled double-blind non-inferiority trial versus paroxetine. *British Medical Journal*, 330, 503.

Tiemeier, H., Van Tuijl, H.R., Hofman, A. *et al.* (2002). Vitamin B12, folate, and homocysteine in depression: The Rotterdam Study. *American Journal of Psychiatry*, 159, 2099–2101.

Tolppanen, A.M., Sayers, A., Fraser, W.D. *et al.* (2011). The association of serum 25-hydroxyvitamin D(3) and D(2) with depressive symptoms in childhood: A prospective cohort study. *Journal of Child Psychology and Psychiatry*, 53, 757–766.

Uebelacker, L.A., Epstein-Lubow, G., Gaudiano, B.A. *et al.* (2010). Hatha yoga for depression: Critical review of the evidence for efficacy, plausible mechanisms of action, and directions for future research. *Journal of Psychiatric Practice*, 16, 22–33.

Vadiraja, H.S., Raghavendra, R.M., Nagarathna, R. *et al.* (2009). Effects of a yoga program on cortisol rhythm and mood states in early breast cancer patients undergoing adjuvant radiotherapy: A randomized controlled trial. *Integrative Cancer Therapies*, 8, 37–46.

Van Diermen, D., Marston, A., Bravo, J. *et al.* (2009). Monoamine oxidase inhibition by Rhodiola rosea L. roots. *Journal of Ethnopharmacology*, 122, 397–401.

Vidal-Alaball, J., Butler, C.C., Cannings-John, R. *et al.* (2005). Oral vitamin B12 versus intramuscular vitamin B12 for vitamin B12 deficiency. *Cochrane Database of Systematic Reviews*, 3, CD004655.

Wilkins, C.H., Sheline, Y.I., Roe, C.M., Birge, S.J., and Morris, J.C. (2006). Vitamin D deficiency is associated with low mood and worse cognitive performance in older adults. *American Journal of Geriatric Psychiatry*, 14, 1032–1040.

Wolfe, A.R., Ogbonna, E.M., Lim, S., Li, Y., and Zhang, J. (2009). Dietary linoleic and oleic fatty acids in relation to severe depressed mood: 10 years follow-up of a national cohort. *Progress in Neuropsychopharmacology and Biological Psychiatry*, 33, 972–977.

Wolkowitz, O.M., Reus, V.I., Keebler, A. *et al.* (1999). Double-blind treatment of major depression with dehydroepiandrosterone. *American Journal of Psychiatry*, 156, 646–649.

Zanarini, M. and Frankenburg, F. (2003). Omega-3 fatty acid treatment of women with borderline personality disorder: A double-blind, placebo-controlled pilot study. *American Journal of Psychiatry*, 160, 167–169.

Chapter

19

Cognitive behavior therapy

Michael E. Thase

Cognitive therapy (CT) is one of the most influential, best studied, and most widely practiced systems of psychotherapy. A member of a much larger "family" of interventions known as cognitive behavior therapy (CBT), CT was first developed by Aaron T. Beck and his students and colleagues in the late 1960s and early 1970s. The centerpiece of Beck's particular model of therapy is the theory that maladaptive information processing and faulty ways of thinking about oneself, the world around, and one's future play critical roles in the development and maintenance of various forms of psychopathology. Most intensively studied in depression, CT has been adapted for treatment of bipolar disorder, the full spectrum of anxiety disorders, personality disorders, and schizophrenia. For treatment of depression, including major depressive disorder (MDD) and dysthymic disorder, CT may be used either alone or in combination with an appropriate medication management strategy. For bipolar disorder, CT is typically used as an adjunctive therapy for patients who have not obtained adequate benefit from medication strategies. Across disorders, the overarching aims of CT are to: (1) educate patients about their conditions and to help them gain greater awareness of the functional relationships between how and what they are thinking and their emotional and behavioral difficulties, and (2) to learn and master more adaptive ways of coping with their problems. These efforts usually include behavioral activation strategies, such as graded task assignments and scheduled participation in activities intended to increase involvment in activities that are associated with feelings of fulfillment (mastery) and enjoyment (pleasure), and a number of cognitive exercises, as exemplified by the use of a Daily Record of Dysfunctional Thoughts, to develop alternative, more rational, responses to the cognitive

disturbances that are associated with negative states of emotional arousal and problematic behavior. This chapter will briefly describe the theoretical underpinnings and basic techniques of CT as used for treatment of depression. Relevant treatment outcome research and future directions also will be discussed.

The cognitive model of depression

A central tenet of CT is that psychopathological states are characterized by errors in information processing, which in turn elicit or provoke the emotional and behavioral symptoms of depression or mania/hypomania (Beck, 1976, Wright *et al.* 2006). These information processing errors include misperceptions, errors in logic, and biases in memory recall (see Table 19.1; Beck *et al.* 1979). Depressed people, for example, have selective recall of mood-congruent negative memories, are more likely to minimize or disqualify the meaning of a positive event, and tend to personalize and overgeneralize – or think more globally – about the impact of a negative life event. Should the depressed individual switch into hypomania and mania, by contrast, the change in mood state would be associated with underestimation of risks, overestimation of opportunities and/or probabilities for success, and a mood-dependent impairment in the ability to perceive the impact that one's behavior has on others. In both cases, the information processing errors serve to support or maintain the pathological mood disturbance.

In addition to errors in information processing, individuals suffering from mood disorders usually show evidence of two other types of cognitive symptoms. At the "surface" are the thoughts, ideas, and mental images associated with the mood state, which

Clinical Handbook for the Management of Mood Disorders, ed. J. John Mann, Patrick J. McGrath, and Steven P. Roose.
Published by Cambridge University Press. © Cambridge University Press 2013.

Table 19.1 Cognitive errors associated with automatic negative thoughts

All or none thinking:	Using rigid dichotomies (e.g., good vs. bad, perfect vs. defective, or success vs. failure) to describe to oneself a life event (also called "black or white thinking")
Arbitrary inference:	Reaching a negative conclusion without examining the supporting evidence (also known as jumping to a conclusion)
Catastrophization:	Predicting a terrible or catastrophic outcome of a recent or impending event without examining the likelihood of other outcomes
Fortune telling:	Imaging what another person is thinking without considering other possibilities (also called mind reading)
Magnification and minimization:	Over- or undervaluing the impact or importance of an event or interchange without considering alternate possibilities
Personalization:	Attributing the outcome of an event to a negative personal characteristic or trait without examining other causal possibilities
Selective abstraction:	Reaching an unfounded conclusion based on only a small portion of the available data

(*Source:* Beck *et al.* 1979)

are referred to as automatic negative thoughts, and at a "deeper" (in the Piagetian sense) level are dysfunctional attitudes and underlying basic beliefs, also known as schema. Automatic negative thoughts occur almost instantaneously when a person is in a situation that provokes or elicits a negative change in mood; hence they are sometimes called "hot" thoughts. Beck (1976) coined the term "the cognitive triad" to reflect the fact that most depressed people have automatic negative thoughts about themselves, their world, and their future, which in turn underpin common cognitive symptoms of depression, such as hopelessness, pessimism, helplessness, and worthlessness.

Automatic negative thoughts are usually tacitly accepted as the "truth." A common example drawn from everyday life is the thought "This ALWAYS happens to me," that accompanies the annoying reality of having picked the slowest line at the bank or grocery. Of course, no one *always* picks the wrong line; the numerous times in which one picked the fastest line are simply not recalled in the moment of affective arousal and, removed from the emotional state, it is relatively easy to restate the problem in less upsetting terms (i.e., "It is annoying that I picked the slowest line

today. I was hoping to get out of here quickly and move on to other more enjoyable activities. I need to take a deep breath, relax, and make the best of this, and not let it ruin my afternoon!"). The perceived accuracy of emotionally charged, yet objectively irrational thoughts is called emotional realism, which (to borrow from Descartes) can be succinctly summarized as "because I feel it, it must be true." From this vantage point, experiential therapies that encourage patients to "go with their feelings" may be encouraging patients to go in the wrong direction. From the CT perspective, while it is important to validate feelings, it is also essential to examine the thoughts and thought processes that accompany emotions, as reflected by Beck's assertion that "emotion is the royal road to cognition."

Most people do not need to closely examine the veracity of their automatic thoughts or subject them to rational analysis, in large part because the uncomfortable emotional states that are triggered by these thoughts typically resolve and life goes on without too many adverse consequences. Indeed, in states of well-being, automatic negative thoughts may account for only a small percentage of one's mental activities. However, the cognitive model of depression posits that people prone to depressed mood are predisposed to develop more persistent and overwhelming states of emotional distress during times of adversity because they have more rigid, enduring negative attitudes and beliefs, which in turn serve to organize perception and recall in such a way so as to perpetuate the automatic negative thoughts. Thus, getting into a slow line at the grocery might have a more persistently negative impact on mood if one truly believed that "I can't do anything right!" Indeed, in states of depression or pathological elation, the frequency of "hot thoughts" can dominate one's state of mind to the extent that more than 80% of the thoughts were negatively valenced. For such individuals, one's mood may still fluctuate from "not so bad" to "much, much worse," and the simple exercise of thought recording can rapidly lead to identifying the link between automatic negative thoughts and worsening of mood.

Some "less than introspective" individuals report that, at the outset of therapy, they do not experience automatic negative thoughts. Although it is perhaps plausible that some people actually do not have automatic negative thoughts, it is more likely that awareness of one's mental life may be thought of as a dimensional concept and that some people are simply less able to identify their thoughts than others. For such

Table 19.2 Functional and dysfunctional attitudes and beliefs

Functional	If I have a fair chance, I can succeed
	No matter what happens, I'll survive
	People can trust me
	I'm lovable
	People respect me
	I like to be challenged
	People can count on me
Dysfunctional	I must be perfect at all times
	I must succeed in order to be liked
	I'm a phony
	Without romantic love, I'm nothing
	I don't have what it takes to succeed
	The world is a harsh and unfair place

(*Source:* Beck et al. 1979)

individuals, the use of the therapeutic tactics of guided discovery and the "downward arrow" technique may be helpful to identify the close relationship between thinking and feeling (Beck *et al.* 1979, Wright *et al.* 2006).

As noted above, attitudes and schema are posited to be "deeper" organizing structures in the cognitive model of psychopathology. Although one can usually infer dysfunctional attitudes by grouping together thematically linked automatic thoughts, which in turn usually can be organized into attitudes and beliefs about one's worth being tied to success in intimate affective relationships or performance in personally relevant achievement domains. In this regard, the cognitive model owes some heritage to Freud's observations about the importance of love and work to well-being. Self-report tools such as the Dysfunctional Attitude Scale also can be used to identify problem areas and to monitor for adaptive changes during the course of therapy. The term schema is used to describe an even deeper level of cognitive structure that is posited to be responsible for implementing screening, filtering, organizing, and coding information to conform to one's basic rules of life (Beck *et al.* 1979). Examples of maladaptive schema are provided in Table 19.2.

The early writings of Beck can rightfully be considered to reflect "cognitive primacy" (i.e., that dysfunctional attitudes and pathological schema predispose to cognitive errors), which in turn provoke/elicit emotional or behavioral symptoms within the context of real or imagined adversity (Beck, 1976). In particular, the emphasis of CT on obtaining change in dysfunctional attitudes and schema to ensure that therapy has a more enduring or durable effect represents the largest paradigmatic difference for this model

of intervention as compared to other, more behaviorally focused therapies. It is true that "pathological schema" cannot be directly observed and are unlikely to be localized in one particular area of the brain and, as such, are by definition a kind of hypothetical construct. Nevertheless, anyone who has learned how to tie shoelaces or a bow tie, or ride a bike, or has mastered the concept of conservation of volume has collected evidence that schema do exist in everyday life. It is likewise true that the interactive and dynamic relationships between a life event, a particular thought or memory, the accompanying change in emotional tone, and any corresponding behavior change illustrate that there are multiple targets for intervention. Most contemporary theoreticians accept that depression and bipolar disorder have complex etiologies that involve genetic, other biological, social, and interpersonal influences – in addition to cognitive processes – and that change in dysfunctional cognitive processes also can be achieved through biological processes mediated by effective psychopharmacological interventions (see, for example, Wright and Thase, 1992).

Therapeutic strategies

CT was first developed as a time-limited treatment of depression. Although longer courses of CT are sometimes used to treat individuals with more chronic or complex conditions, CT typically consists of 6 to 20 sessions conducted over 6 to 16 weeks. Twice weekly sessions are recommended for more severely depressed individuals. As a successful course of therapy approaches completion, therapists often use every other week or monthly sessions to ensure that the patient is able to maintain gains with progressively less therapeutic support.

CT is typically conducted as an individual therapy, though it is readily delivered in groups and some might even argue that the potential of group therapy to make this treatment more available for far greater numbers of patients has been woefully underutilized. Individual sessions of CT typically last 45 to 60 minutes, whereas group therapy sessions usually last 90 to 120 minutes.

When CT is properly performed, a trained observer can easily differentiate it from other forms of psychotherapy by use of a small number of reliable characteristics, as described below. A session of CT should begin with an explicit agenda of activities to be conducted, including a brief review of symptomatic status or a "progress report." After the first session, the progress report should almost always consist of a review of the self-help exercises or homework that were assigned at the previous session. Indeed, the use of homework to extend the scope of intervention outside of the conventional once or twice a week model of treatment is so essential to the process of therapy that one might conclude that if there is no homework, than it is not CT. Like other therapies that are sometimes described as directive, the therapist should have a relatively high activity level and it should be evident that the therapist is guiding and/or managing the time flow of the session to ensure that the agenda is addressed. Perhaps more unique to CT among the directive therapies is the therapist's explicit use of Socratic questioning to actively engage the patient in the process of learning about the cognitive model of psychopathology and eliciting personally relevant examples for intervention. Socratic questioning is but one way that the therapist tries to foster a process referred to as collaborative empiricism, which implicitly reflects that the dyad will work as a team, using methods that have been shown to work and applying them flexibly to meet the specific needs and talents of the individual. Another way that collaborative empiricism is fostered is by the therapist's use of summaries or check-ins at each transition point in the session to elicit and answer questions and to ensure that the patient has understood the material covered during that segment of the session. This process is similarly accomplished at the end of each session by asking the patient for his/her appraisal of the session, i.e., "What are your thoughts (or how do you feel) about what we've accomplished today?"

The first one or two sessions of CT are typically spent obtaining a history, teaching the patient about the cognitive model, constructing a problem list, and – whenever possible – illustrating the personal relevance of the approach. This usually can be accomplished by capitalizing upon a visible mood shift during the course of the interview or by asking the patient about his or her thoughts or concerns about starting therapy. Though ultimately focused on helping patients to improve in the "here and now," it is of course also important for the therapist to have basic information about the patient's life story, including family background, developmental and social histories, medical history, and past experiences with psychotherapy.

An important aspect of socialization is communicating the essential nature of homework and, if possible, obtaining a shared "vision" that completing homework assignments will increase the likelihood that therapy will be helpful. For this reason, the first session of therapy should always include a relatively simple homework assignment, such as reading the pamphlet *Coping with Depression* and writing comments on the margin or denoting passages that are either particularly relevant or don't make sense. One other early homework assignment is to begin to complete a daily "hour-by-hour" charting of activities and moods, which of course will provide the source data for the initial in-session work on the relationships between emotions, behaviors, and thoughts.

A meta-message of the socialization process that should be clear to new patients is that CT will be more than simply talking about problems and that the therapist's job is to do much more than simply listen and facilitate ventilation. Rather, the purpose of therapy is to operationalize specific problems and issues that are contributing to their difficulties, and to learn, practice, and ultimately master strategies that will improve one's ability to cope with mood symptoms, and to feel and function better. Thus, after the first session, it is common for a therapy session to be devoted to only two or three segments of work focused on specific goals or problems.

People who have extensive histories of more conventional therapy sometimes chafe at the structure of CT or even find the idea of focusing on specific problems to be somewhat derivative or oppressive. An accomplished therapist will recognize such reactions and will address them within the session. For example, "I noticed that you crossed your arms and changed your posture a moment ago, which I worry might suggest that somehow I have missed the mark or said something that didn't 'sit well' with you. Do you mind if we spend a few moments talking about what's happening right now, between you and I?" Such an intervention can have manifold benefits by preventing an alliance rupture and improving the therapeutic alliance. For example, eliciting the patient's automatic negative thoughts about the sense of being "cut off" by the therapist might help to clarify the patient's skepticism about the therapy or belief that it is important to ventilate and that a therapy that doesn't facilitate this is unlikely to work. Although it is true that CT is not specifically about fostering the therapeutic relationship, it is also true that a strong alliance is an important element of a productive course of therapy.

Behavioral interventions

There is a wide range of latitude in how much or how little behavioral strategies are used in CT. Many therapists emphasize behavioral strategies, starting with behavior and mood recording, early in the course of therapy as a practical means to help people get moving and as a platform upon which to identify the relationship between dysfunctional patterns of thinking and depressive symptoms. Three of the most commonly used techniques, which can be called behavioral activation strategies, are described below (also, see Wright *et al.* 2006).

Typically introduced in the second or third session, activity scheduling is used to help patients first recognize and then remedy problems of inertia (i.e., volitional inhibition), decreased operant responding (i.e., reduced interest and anhedonia, as revealed by a low rate of involvement in pleasurable acitivities), and various behavioral deficits and excesses (e.g., sitting alone or pacing about) (Beck *et al.* 1979, Wright *et al.* 2006). The patient is asked to use the activity log to record on an hourly basis what he or she is doing and, using a simple ordinal scale (i.e., 0–10) to rate each segment for mastery (M) and pleasure (P).

Almost all clinically depressed individuals will have periods of each day when they are alone and not actively engaged in some activity; characteristically, these times will have low M and P scores. Some formerly pleasurable activities, such as listening to music, reading, or watching television may likewise garner low M or P scores because of mood-dependent changes in preference (i.e., depressed people tend to gravitate toward sad music) or the activity reveals frustrating difficulties with concentration or memory. After noting the apparently functional relationship between how one is spending his or her time and mood, the therapist suggests that many people are helped by planning and following through with specific activities that have been shown to either improve mood or provide some increase in M and P ratings. The patient is then helped to identify particular activities that they might have enjoyed or felt good about doing during similar times when they were well or at least feeling better. The activities are sorted for practicability (i.e., access, cost, and ease of implementation) and a plan is implemented to engage in one or two such activities during each day during a habitually "down" time. The net result of such behavioral assignments is that most people will report feeling better and/or accomplishing

more and, even when not highly successful, the automatic negative thoughts that characteristically accompany attempts to implement behavioral assignments can become grist for the therapeutic mill.

The second widely used behavioral technique, the graded task assignment, is used to help patients address more complex, multi-step situations that are perceived as too hard or overwhelming. Depression is a state of low energy, pessimism, and impaired concentration, and procrastination is one coping tactic that is both highly practicable and, within the moment, reliably effective. The prototypic example of a graded task assignment is the example of moving a 300 lb boulder by breaking it down into 5 or 10 smaller chunks. Although our patients seldom have to move giant boulders, they are often behind on completing tax forms, paying bills, home repairs, and other tasks that are ultimately necessary to ensure sustained well-being. Thus, the complex task is identified and "de-chunked" into discrete units of activity that can be accomplished within a 30–60 minute time frame, and these component activities are built into the activity schedule. Whereas many of the activities chosen for behavioral assignments are aimed to increase feelings of pleasure, graded task assignments are largely intended to improve feelings of mastery and self-efficacy, which in turn help to reduce feelings of hopelessness and helplessness.

A third behavioral strategy, the coping card, is used to facilitate the transition from a more behavioral focus of therapy to cognitive interventions. A coping card is, quite simply, a brief scripted response to help initiate an action or to rebut a commonly experienced automatic thought. Often written or typed on a 3 × 5 index card, which can easily fit in a shirt pocket or a purse, the coping card can be retrieved on a moment's notice to help marshal a response to thoughts such as "you're not good enough," "you're a hopeless case – don't even try," or "nothing you do ever works."

Cognitive interventions

Many cognitive therapists believe that the "real" work of CT occurs after the patient has begun to make progress using behavioral strategies and is beginning to recognize and modify automatic thoughts. For this reason, some therapists use these strategies from the outset of therapy, coincident with self-monitoring and activity scheduling. Whether formal cognitive assignments are introduced earlier or later, it is extremely useful to use mood or behavioral shifts within therapy sessions as a means to illustrate the impact of automatic negative thoughts and to begin to teach about the ways in which these thoughts can be distorted or illogical, and ultimately counterproductive.

Perhaps the most frequent procedure used within sessions of CT to begin to elicit and challenge automatic negative thoughts is Socratic questioning, specifically as applied using guided discovery and the downward arrow techniques. As illustrated in the example below, this process uses a series of inductive questions that are intended to reveal dysfunctional thought patterns.

Therapist: "What things seem to make your mood lower or more depressed?"

Mr. J: "Lots of things. Actually, I'm depressed most of the time."

Therapist: "That's certainly possible, but do you mind if we take a moment and try to check out if there are at least some factors that can make your mood worse?"

Mr. J: "Okay."

Therapist: "Great – I'm glad that you're at least willing to give this a try. Can you think of a circumstance in which your level of depression is relatively low and another situation where your depression is much higher?"

Mr. J: "Sure. The last time that I did not feel too depressed was over the weekend when my son was visiting and we were watching the baseball game together. This morning my depression was at it highest level when I was getting ready to go to work and was thinking about having to tell my boss that I had not been able to finish my work on a very important account."

Therapist: "So, it does sound like there's quite a bit of fluctuation in how you are feeling at different times."

Mr. J: "Okay – I see your point – but the low times really dominate my life."

Therapist: "I understand your point. Do you mind if we spend a little more time examining the differences between these times?"

Mr. J: "Sure, but in this case the answer's pretty simple. I love my son and I love baseball. I hate being behind in my work and I really hate having to tell my boss that I'm not able to get my work done. Case closed, right?"

Therapist: "I think you've 'nailed' the largest differences, but I wonder if there might be some other relevant factors, which might help us devise a plan to to help you work out of this depression."

Mr. J: "Okay. What do you have in mind?"

Therapist: "Well, for instance, why don't we take a look at the different thoughts that you have about these situations. When you think about talking to your boss, what thoughts are on your mind?"

Mr. J: "He'll be disappointed in me and probably mad. He'll realize that I can't be counted on to deliver and maybe even shouldn't be trusted with new projects. Maybe he'll even fire me or – at best – insist that I take a leave of absence. That frankly would be the last straw for me – I'd be a complete failure."

Although this example illustrates how Socratic questioning can be used to elicit automatic negative thoughts in the early sessions of CT, it should be clear that additional discussion would be needed to help the patient recognize the extent to which these "hot thoughts" are influenced by cognitive biases and thus represent distortions rather than facts.

Outside sessions, thought recording is the most frequently used method for identifying automatic thoughts (Beck, 1995, Wright *et al.* 2006). The most common techniques to begin thought recording are the two- and three-column methods. In the two-column method the patient is asked to look for periods of increased depressive feelings and to write down the accompanying thoughts. In the three-column technique, patients are asked to identify distressing situations and to record their mood and thoughts. Like mood charting, these methods help patients to begin to recognize the inter-relationships of situations, feelings and thoughts.

As automatic negative thoughts are identified, some therapists encourage patients to learn to label the particular type of cognitive distortion reflected by the negative thought (e.g., is this an example of overgeneralization or catastrophizing?). There are likewise some patients who find the process of labeling different types of negative thinking to be a valuable activity, whereas others find this task to be of only passing interest and are able to move on to trying to change the thoughts.

Modifying automatic thoughts

The most commonly used techniques for modifying automatic negative thoughts include examining the evidence (i.e., developing a pros and cons list) and generating alternatives (i.e., more rational responses). When these techniques are used during sessions, the process is facilitated by Socratic questioning. Similarly, when the thought recording has occurred as part of a homework session, the therapist and patient work collaboratively to review, critique, and improve the impact of the strategy.

As the cognitive model dictates that automatic negative thoughts are the product of distorted information processing, examining the evidence that justifies or "proves" the validity of the thought is a major component of collaborative empiricism. Thus, it is suggested that the thought should be looked at as a hypothesis, which in turn can be tested by collecting the relevant evidence for and against the hypothesis. A five-column sheet, sometimes called the Daily Record of Dysfunctional Thoughts (DRDT)(Beck *et al.* 1979), is the standard form used for this portion of the therapy. The five columns identify the situation (in which an upsetting event occurred), the mood, the accompanying automatic negative thoughts, the rational alternatives or evidence for and against, and the outcome (i.e., change in mood). Regular use of the DRDT will usually result in the development of a strategy to manage low or dysphoric moods "in the moment" and can also lead to adaptations to address the deeper schematic beliefs.

Adapting CT for bipolar disorder

As described by Basco and Rush (2005), specific CT methods for bipolar disorder focus on psychoeducation, self-monitoring to improve recognition of early warning signs, and increasing medication adherence. In fact, an early study by Cochran (1986) demonstrated that CT could significantly improve outcomes simply by increasing medication adherence. Dysfunctional cognitions about medication can be modified with CT, and behavioral interventions, such as reminder systems and behavioral plans to overcome obstacles to adherence, can be used. There are no specific CT methods used for treatment of mania, although some hypomanic individuals can use DRDTs and rational rebuttal strategies. No modifications of the methods used to treat depressive episodes are usually needed.

What is the best way to learn CT?

Given the broad impact of CT, most mental health practitioners trained in the past several decades have completed some coursework and received some supervised introduction to this form of therapy. For example, competency in CT – as evidenced by faithful completion of one or two supervised training cases – is now one of the core competence areas for psychiatric residents. Learning about CT during training is only a starting point, however, and some form of advanced training and ongoing supervision is usually necessary before one can truly master and sustain compe-

tence in this model of therapy. It is simply too easy for therapists who have had more training in more conventional therapies to fall back on less directive and less systematized approaches, incorporating some cognitive interventions within a more eclectic therapy. One excellent source for advanced training is the extramural fellowship program of The Beck Institute (www.beckinstitute.org). A second useful resource is the website for The Academy of Cognitive Therapy (www.academyofct.org). A list of other training programs is provided in the book *Learning Cognitive Therapy* (Wright *et al.* 2006).

Efficacy of treatment

The efficacy of CT has been subjected to hundreds of controlled investigations across a wide range of disorders. As noted earlier, CT is the most exhaustively studied psychosocial intervention for depressive disorders (Butler *et al.* 2006). In the following sections, the empirical support for CT will be briefly reviewed.

Acute phase treatment efficacy

Literally dozens of controlled trials of CT have been conducted, and meta-analyses of early studies concluded that CT is an efficacious treatment of depression, at least as compared to wait-list or nonspecific contact control conditions, and that CT is at least as effective across 3–4 months as other proven treatments (Dobson, 1989, Robinson *et al.* 1990). Early findings suggesting superior efficacy are tempered to some extent by evidence of an allegiance bias, i.e., the most positive findings are evident in studies in which it was clear that CT was the "special" treatment (Gaffan *et al.* 1995).

Perhaps the most contentious evidence of possible superiority came from meta-analyses of early studies comparing CT and antidepressants, as reviewed by Thase (2001). Among the first generation of studies, the study conducted by Beck's group at the Center for Cognitive Therapy in Philadelphia found the strongest advantage for CT (Rush *et al.* 1977). However, interpretations of this study must not only take into account a strong allegiance bias, but also the fact that the antidepressant (imipramine) was tapered and discontinued before the final outcome was measured. Two other early studies conducted in the United Kingdom also suggested an advantage for CT over pharmacotherapy (Blackburn *et al.* 1981,

Teasdale *et al.* 1984), although in both cases it is clear in retrospect that the source of the advantage was the poor performance of pharmacotherapy as provided by primary care physicians (Blackburn *et al.* 1981, Teasdale *et al.* 1984).

The primary analyses of six subsequent studies, all making greater efforts to ensure that pharmacotherapy was adequately administered, found CT and pharmacotherapy to be comparably effective across 12–16 weeks (Murphy *et al.* 1984, Elkin *et al.* 1989, Hollon *et al.* 1992, Jarrett *et al.* 1999, DeRubeis *et al.* 2005, Dimidjian *et al.* 2006). It is noteworthy that the two most recent studies (DeRubeis *et al.* 2005, Dimidjian *et al.* 2006) used selective serotonin reuptake inhibitors (rather than older-generation medications) and, hence, have greater generalizability to contemporary practice.

Among these studies, some secondary analyses of the National Institute of Mental Health (NIMH) Treatment of Depression Collaborative Research Program (TDCRP) suggested that antidepressants actually may be superior to cognitive therapy for patients with more severe depressive symptoms (Elkin *et al.* 1995). This controversial finding was not replicated in a meta-analysis of individual patient data drawn from Elkin *et al.* and three other trials (DeRubeis *et al.* 1999), nor by the results of planned analyses in the two more recent studies (DeRubeis *et al.* 2005, Dimidjian *et al.* 2006). It therefore seems unlikely that symptom severity, by itself, is a robust indicator for preferential response to pharmacotherapy vs. CT. Rather, the most parsimonious conclusion is that CT is an effective treatment for depressed outpatients and it has symptomatic benefits comparable to antidepressants across 10–12 weeks of treatment.

A seventh study (Thase *et al.* 2007) was conducted as part of the multi-center, multi-stage study known as STAR*D. In this complex trial, which also was conducted in collaboration with colleagues from the National Institute of Mental Health, patients who had not responded to a 12-week course of citalopram therapy were randomly allocated to 12 weeks of additional treatment with either CT or an alternate form of pharmacotherapy, either as an adjunct to ongoing citalopram therapy or after withdrawal of citalopram (i.e., augment or switch). Although the study was designed to have adequate power to detect moderate between-group differences, an unanticipated problem with the use of equipoise-stratified, randomization strategy resulted in obtaining only about 30% of the projected sample size. With this limitation in mind, it was nevertheless true that the outcomes were almost identical for the groups switched from citalopram to either CT or a second course of antidepressant therapy, both with respect to symptom reduction and the probability of remission. As might be expected, the CT arm was associated with fewer medication side effects than the pharmacotherapy arm. There were also no significant differences in the final outcomes of the groups receiving either CT or medications as adjuncts to ongoing citalopram therapy, although the speed of improvement was slower in the CT group than the group receiving pharmacological adjuncts.

Several controlled trials have evaluated CT as a treatment for bipolar depressive episodes. In the first, which used a mirror-image design to evaluate the outcomes of 42 patients, Scott *et al.* (2001) found that CT reduced the rate of relapse by 60% and significantly lowered depressive symptom ratings. A subsequent full-scale study in which 253 patients were randomized did not confirm the benefit of CT as compared with treatment as usual (Scott *et al.* 2006). However, in that study, response to CT was found to interact with history of prior episodes. Specifically, adjunctive CT was beneficial for patients who had suffered relatively few episodes and was actually counterproductive for patients who had experienced numerous prior bipolar episodes. In a third study, Lam *et al.* (2003) found a very strong effect of CT in lowering the relapse rate for bipolar disorder patients during the first year of follow-up. However, a subsequent 30-month follow-up suggested that the benefit of treatment began to fade after the first year post-treatment (Lam *et al.* 2005). A fourth study (Ball *et al.* 2006) found that 6 months of CT improved depressive symptoms and reduced global ratings of symptom severity. Similar benefits were observed in the psychotherapy arms of the large study of bipolar depression conducted as part of the STEP-BD study (Miklowitz *et al.* 2007). In that trial, CT was evaluated along with family-focused therapy and interpersonal social rhythms therapy in comparison to a brief psychosocial intervention known as collaborative care. Although this study was not designed to test the individual merits of the three particular forms of therapy, there was not evidence that CT was more or less effective than the other active psychosocial modalities. It therefore seems likely that CT is a useful treatment of depressive episodes at least early in the course of bipolar disorder, although further research is certainly needed.

Long-term outcome studies

Perhaps the strongest evidence favoring the use of CT instead of antidepressant pharmacotherapy comes from follow-up studies conducted after completion of acute phase trials. As reviewed by Vittengl and colleagues (2007), patients who have responded to acute phase therapy with CT are significantly less likely to relapse across 1 year of follow-up than patients who have responded to acute phase antidepressant therapy but who are then withdrawn from medication. With one exception, results of these studies have supported the hypothesis that short-term CT is associated with a relatively low risk of subsequent relapse. In fact, across 6 to 12 months after completion of acute phase CT, patients are about as likely to remain well as those who receive ongoing continuation phase pharmacotherapy (i.e., the guideline-specified strategy for people who respond to antidepressant medications (Evans et al. 1992, Hollon et al. 2005). Thus, for many patients, acute phase CT has a durable therapeutic effect.

Thase et al. (1992) proposed that the likelihood of sustained benefit following a time-limited course of CT could be reliably estimated by examining the rapidity and course of symptom reduction. Specifically, Thase and colleagues found that depressed people who responded rapidly and completely during the first 12 weeks of acute phase therapy had only a 10% relapse rate for the subsequent year, whereas patients with slower, less complete, or more labile courses of improvement had a 50+% relapse rate across 1 year of untreated follow-up. Jarrett et al. (2001) replicated this finding prospectively and demonstrated that, for those at greater risk, ongoing continuation phase CT sessions significantly reduced the risk of relapse.

Three other longer-term studies tested whether CT could be used in sequence with antidepressant pharmacotherapy (Fava et al. 1996, 1998; Paykel et al. 1999). Two studies targeted residual or persistent subsyndromal depressive symptoms in patients receiving antidepressant medications (Fava et al. 1996, Paykel et al. 1999). In the 6-year follow-up of the first study, the relapse rate among the patients who received CT was 40%, as compared to 90% for the group that did not receive CT (Fava et al. 2004). In the second study, Paykel et al. (1999) likewise demonstrated that sequential CT significantly reduced the risk of relapse, from 47 to 29% across 68 weeks of follow-up, although the effects were not as persistent during the second and third years of follow-up. Taken together, results of these investigations of the long-term effects of CT support the use of this modality to help reduce relapse and recurrence.

In the third study, Fava et al. (1998) evaluated whether CT could be used to reduce the risk of recurrent depression among remitted patients taking antidepressant medications. They found that a course of 10 sessions of CT, conducted every other week, significantly reduced the risk of recurrent depressive episodes after discontinuation of antidepressant therapy, from 80% in the control group to 25% in the CT-treated group.

Future directions

Whereas research conducted over the past 40+ years has established CT as one of a handful of evidence-based psychosocial treatments for depression, the next generation of research may help to clarify the best indications for selecting CT for particular patients and for improving the availability of this effective form of therapy.

At present, CT is indicated as a treatment of first choice for patients with nonpsychotic episodes of MDD of a wide range of severity. There has been long-standing interest in testing the hypothesis that there may be an upper limit of illness severity, as reflected by disturbances in various neurobiological processes, beyond which psychological therapies are relatively ineffective. Consistent with this hypothesis, investigations of biological "markers" of neurobiological dysfunction, such as hypercortisolemia or disturbances of sleep electroencephalographic profiles, are associated with a poorer response to CT (Thase et al. 1996a, b). Although these findings are of heuristic interest, neither type of abnormality is particularly common in depressed outpatients, which limits the potential for application in real-world settings. More recently, Siegle and colleagues (2006) found a specific pattern of cortical activation (as measured by functional magnetic resonance imaging scanning) was correlated with a favorable response to CT. Whether this finding, if replicated, can lead to a relatively inexpensive screening test is a topic of ongoing investigation.

Beyond improving the ability to match patients with specific treatments, there is a great need to increase the availability of CT, both outside major urban areas and to a broader range of patient settings. Given the strong psychoeducational nature of CT, computer-assisted forms of therapy delivery may provide a novel and relatively inexpensive way of making therapy available for a larger number of people in a manner that is entirely consistent with the way people approach learning in the twenty-first century.

In this spirit, more recently developed CT computer- and internet-based programs incorporate multimedia, virtual reality, and palm-top technologies. For example, "Good Days Ahead: The Multimedia Program for Cognitive Therapy" (Wright *et al.* 2004) incorporates video and audio clips, as well as interactive self-help exercises, and a library of tools for self-monitoring and self-help exercises. This particular program was not, however, intended for "stand-alone" use and, rather, should be viewed as a means to increase the efficiency of therapy. A small randomized trial of evaluating this program found that patients could achieve outcomes comparable to conventional CT with only half of the face-to-face time with a therapist (Wright *et al.* 2005).

The efficacy of a second, less elaborate multimedia CT program, "Beating the Blues," has been evaluated as a "stand-alone" treatment of depression in primary care patients (Proudfoot *et al.* 2004). In this trial, patients who participated in the internet-delivered CT program experienced significant improvements in depressive and anxiety symptoms.

These examples only scratch at the surface of what might be possible to improve the dissemination, efficiency, and acceptability of CT.

References

Ball, J.R., Mitchell, P.B., Corry, J.C. *et al* (2006), A randomized controlled trial of cognitive therapy for bipolar disorder: Focus on long-term change. *Journal of Clinical Psychiatry* 67, 277–286.

Basco, M.R. and Rush A.J. (2005). *Cognitive-Behavioral Therapy for Bipolar Disorder*. New York: Guilford.

Beck, A.T. (1976). *Cognitive Therapy and the Emotional Disorders*. New York: International Universities Press.

Beck, A.T. (1993). Cognitive therapy: Past, present, and future. *Journal of Consulting and Clinical Psychology*, 61, 194–198.

Beck, J. (1995). *Cognitive Therapy: Basics and Beyond*. New York: Guilford.

Beck, A.T., Greenberg, R.L., Beck, J. (1995). *Coping with Depression* (a booklet). Bala Cynwyd, PA: The Beck Institute.

Beck, A.T., Rush, A.J., Shaw, B.F. *et al.* (1979). *Cognitive Therapy of Depression*. New York: Guilford.

Blackburn, I.M., Bishop, S., Glen, A.I.M. *et al.* (1981). The efficacy of cognitive therapy in depression: A treatment trial using cognitive therapy and pharmacotherapy, each alone and in combination. *British Journal of Psychiatry*, 139, 181–189.

Butler, A.C., Chapman, J.E., Forman, E.M. *et al.* (2006). The empirical status of cognitive-behavioral therapy: A review of meta-analyses. *Clinical Psychology Reviews*, 26, 17–31.

Cochran, S.D. (1986). Compliance with lithium regimens in the outpatient treatment of bipolar affective disorders. *Journal of Compliance in Health Care*, 1, 151–169.

Covi, L. and Primakoff, L. (1988). Cognitive group therapy. In Frances, A.J. and Hales, R.E., eds., *The American Psychiatric Press Review of Psychiatry*. Washington, DC: American Psychiatric Press, 608–616.

DeRubeis, R.J., Gelfand, L.A., Tang, T.Z. *et al.* (1999). Medication versus cognitive behavior therapy for severely depressed outpatients: Mega-analysis of four randomized comparisons. *American Journal of Psychiatry*, 156, 1007–1013.

DeRubeis, R.J., Hollon, S.D., Amsterdam, J.D. *et al.* (2005). Cognitive therapy vs medications in the treatment of moderate to severe depression. *Archives of General Psychiatry*, 62, 409–416.

Dimidjian, S., Hollon, S.D., Dobson, K.S. *et al.* (2006). Randomized trial of behavioral activation, cognitive therapy, and antidepressant medication in the acute treatment of adults with major depression. *Journal of Consulting and Clinical Psychology*, 74, 658–670.

Dobson, K.S. (1989). A meta-analysis of the efficacy of cognitive therapy for depression. *Journal of Consulting and Clinical Psychology*, 57, 414–419.

Elkin, I., Shea, M.T., Watkins, J.T. *et al.* (1989). NIMH Treatment of Depression Collaborative Research Program, I: general effectiveness of treatments. *Archives of General Psychiatry*, 46, 971–982.

Elkin, I., Gibbons, R.D., Shea, M.T. *et al.* (1995). Initial severity and differential treatment outcome in the National Institute of Mental Health Treatment of Depression Collaborative Research Program. *Journal of Consulting and Clinical Psychology*, 63, 841–847.

Evans, M.D., Hollon, S.D., DeRubeis, R.J. *et al.* (1992). Differential relapse following cognitive therapy and pharmacotherapy for depression. *Archives of General Psychiatry*, 49, 802–808.

Fava, G.A., Grandi, S., Zielezny, M. *et al.* (1996). Four-year outcome for cognitive behavioral treatment of residual symptoms in major depression. *American Journal of Psychiatry*, 153, 945–947.

Fava, G.A., Rafanelli, C., Grandi, S. *et al.* (1998). Prevention of recurrent depression with cognitive behavioral therapy. *Archives of General Psychiatry*, 55, 816–820.

Fava, G.A., Ruini, C., Rafanelli, C. *et al.* (2004). Six-year outcome of cognitive behavior therapy for prevention of recurrent depression. *American Journal of Psychiatry*, 161, 1872–1876.

Gaffan, E.A., Tsaousis. I., and Kemp-Wheeler, S.M. (1995). Researcher allegiance and meta-analysis: the case of cognitive therapy for depression. *Journal of Consulting and Clinical Psychology*, 63, 966–980.

Hollon, S.D., DeRubeis, R.J., Evans, M.D. *et al.* (1992). Cognitive therapy and pharmacotherapy for depression: singly and in combination. *Archives of General Psychiatry*, 49, 774–782.

Hollon, S.D., DeRubeis, R.J., Shelton, R.C. *et al.* (2005). Prevention of relapse following cognitive therapy vs medications in moderate to severe depression. *Archives of General Psychiatry*, 62, 417–422.

Jarrett, R.B., Schaffer, M., McIntire, D. *et al.* (1999). Treatment of atypical depression with cognitive therapy or phenelzine: A double-blind, placebo-controlled trial. *Archives of General Psychiatry*, 56, 431–437.

Jarrett, R.B., Kraft, D., Doyle, J. *et al.* (2001). Preventing recurrent depression using cognitive therapy with and without a continuation phase: A randomized clinical trial. *Archives of General Psychiatry*, 58, 381–388.

Lam, D.H., Watkins, E.R., Hayward, P. *et al.* (2003). A randomized controlled study of cognitive therapy for relapse prevention for bipolar affective disorder: Outcome of the first year. *Archives of General Psychiatry*, 60, 145–152.

Lam, D.H., McCrone, P., Wright, K. *et al.* (2005). Cost-effectiveness of relapse-prevention cognitive therapy for bipolar disorder: 30-month study. *British Journal of Psychiatry*, 186, 500–506.

Miklowitz, D.J., Otto, M.W., Frank, E. *et al.* (2007). Psychosocial treatments for bipolar depression: A 1-year randomized trial from the Systematic Treatment Enhancement Program. *Archives of General Psychiatry*, 64, 419–427.

Murphy, G.E., Simons, A.D., Wetzel, R.D. *et al.* (1984). Cognitive therapy and pharmacotherapy, singly and together in the treatment of depression. *Archives of General Psychiatry*, 41, 33–41.

Paykel, E.S., Scott, J., Teasdale, J.D. *et al.* (1999). Prevention of relapse in residual depression by cognitive therapy. *Archives of General Psychiatry*, 56, 829–835.

Proudfoot, J., Ryden, C., Everitt, B. *et al.* (2004). Clinical efficacy of computerised cognitive-behavioural therapy for anxiety and depression in primary care: Randomised controlled trial. *British Journal of Psychiatry*, 185, 46–54.

Robinson, L.A., Berman, J.S., and Neimeyer, R.A. (1990). Psychotherapy for the treatment of depression: A comprehensive review of controlled outcome research. *Psychology Bulletins*, 108, 30–49.

Rush, A.J., Beck, A.T., Kovacs, M. *et al.* (1977). Comparative efficacy of cognitive therapy and pharmacotherapy in the treatment of depressed outpatients. *Cognitive Therapy Research*, 1, 17–37.

Scott, J., Garland, A., and Moorhead, S. (2001). A pilot study of cognitive therapy in bipolar disorders. *Psychological Medicine*, 31, 459–467.

Scott, J., Paykel, E., Morriss, R. *et al.* (2006). Cognitive-behavioural therapy for severe and recurrent bipolar disorders: Randomized controlled trial. *British Journal of Psychiatry*, 188, 313–320.

Siegle, G.J., Carter, C.S., and Thase, M.E. (2006). Use of fMRI to predict recovery from unipolar depression with cognitive behavior therapy. *American Journal of Psychiatry*, 163, 735–738.

Teasdale, J.D., Fennell, M.J.V., Hibbert, G.A. *et al.* (1984). Cognitive therapy for major depressive disorder in primary care. *British Journal of Psychiatry*, 144, 400–406.

Thase, M.E. (2001). Depression-focused psychotherapies. In Gabbard, G.O., ed., *Treatments of Psychiatric Disorders, Third Edition, Vol. 2*. Washington, DC: American Psychiatric Publishing, 1181–1227.

Thase, M.E., Simons, A.D., McGreary, J. *et al.* (1992). Relapse after cognitive behavior therapy of depression: potential implications for longer courses of treatment? *American Journal of Psychiatry*, 149, 1046–1052.

Thase, M.E., Dubé, S., Bowler, K. *et al.* (1996a). Hypothalamic-pituitary-adrenocortical activity and response to cognitive behavior therapy in unmedicated, hospitalized depressed patients. *American Journal of Psychiatry*, 153, 886–891.

Thase, M.E., Simons, A.D., and Reynolds, C.F., III (1996b). Abnormal electroencephalographic sleep profiles in major depression. *Archives of General Psychiatry*, 53, 99–108.

Thase, M.E., Friedman, E.S., Biggs, M.M. *et al.* (2007). Cognitive therapy versus medication in augmentation and switch strategies as second-step treatments: a STAR*D report. *American Journal of Psychiatry*, 164, 739–752.

Vittengl, J.R., Clark, L.A., Dunn, T.W., and Jarrett, R.B. (2007). Reducing relapse and recurrence in unipolar depression: A comparative meta-analysis of cognitive-behavioral therapy's effects. *Journal of Consulting and Clinical Psychology*, 75, 475–488.

Wright, J.H. and Thase, M.E. (1992). Cognitive and biological therapies: A synthesis. *Psychiatric Annals*, 22, 451–458.

Wright, J.H., Basco, M.R., and Thase, M.E. (2006). *Learning Cognitive-Behavior Therapy: An Illustrated Guide (Core Competencies in Psychotherapy Series)*, Gabbard, G.O., series ed. Arlington, VA: American Psychiatric Publishing.

Wright, J.H., Thase, M.E., Beck, A.T. *et al.* (eds.) (1993). *Cognitive Therapy with Inpatients: Developing a Cognitive Milieu*. New York: Guilford.

Wright, J.H., Wright, A.S., Albano, A.M. *et al.* (2005). Computer-assisted cognitive therapy for depression: Maintaining efficacy while reducing therapist time. *American Journal of Psychiatry*, 162, 1158–1164.

Wright, J.H., Wright, A.S., and Beck, A.T. (2004). *Good Days Ahead: The Multimedia Program for Cognitive Therapy*. Louisville, KY: MindStreet.

Interpersonal therapy

Myrna M. Weissman, Annie E. Rabinovitch, and Helen Verdeli

Introduction

Interpersonal psychotherapy (IPT) is a time-limited, evidenced-based therapy, initially developed to treat major depressive disorder (MDD) in adults (Klerman *et al*. 1984, Weissman *et al*. 2000, 2007, Markowitz and Weissman, 2012). A number of clinical trials have demonstrated the efficacy of IPT for major depression, either as a monotherapy or in combination with medication. A recent meta-analysis conducted by Cuijpers and colleagues (2011) summarizing results from 38 randomized, controlled clinical trials including 4356 patients concluded that IPT is among the most empirically validated treatments for depression. IPT has been adapted for a number of mood disorders and patient populations, e.g., depressed adolescents (Mufson *et al*. 2004), depressed elderly (Hinrichson and Clougherty, 2006), dysthymic adults (Markowitz, 1998, Markowitz *et al*. 2005), adults (Frank, 2005) and adolescents (Hlastala *et al*. 2010) with bipolar disorder, borderline personality disorder (Swartz *et al*. 2005), pregnant and post-partum mothers (O'Hara *et al*. 2000, Spinelli and Endicott, 2003). An expanding body of research focuses on integrating IPT into primary care with middle-aged adults, older adults, and adolescents (Klerman *et al*. 1987, Schulberg *et al*. 2002, Menchetti *et al*. 2010). A summary of the clinical trials can be found in Weissman *et al*. (2007) and Markowitz and Weissman (2012). Since then, there have been two additional, updated manuals: Interpersonal Psychotherapy: Evaluation Support and Triage (IPT:EST) (Weissman and Verdeli, 2012) and IPT for a group in Uganda (IPT:GU) (Clougherty *et al*. 2003). The Weissman *et al*. 2007 manual is the most clinician-friendly and has scripts to guide novice therapists. IPT manuals have been translated into Spanish, German, Dutch, French, Italian, Portuguese, Korean, and Japanese.

Fundamental to IPT is the idea that depressive episodes typically occur in the context of interpersonal events and crises. Some common events might include the dissolution of a marriage, death of a loved one, job loss, diagnosis of a medical illness, etc. Such events can cause disruptions of significant attachments and social roles, and serve as triggers of depressive episodes. Four interpersonal problem areas form the focus of IPT: grief, interpersonal disputes, role transitions, and interpersonal deficits. Obviously there are many potential contributions to depression, including genetics, personality, and early childhood experiences, however, the treatment focuses on the relationship between the onset of patients' current depression symptoms and interpersonal problems associated with the onset.

The IPT therapist conceptualizes depression in three parts (Weissman *et al*. 2007):

1. *Symptoms*. The emotional, cognitive, and physical symptoms associated with depression (e.g., depressed and anxious mood, anhedonia, disturbances in eating and sleeping, fatigue, etc.).
2. *Social and interpersonal life*. Patients' relationships with important people in their lives (e.g., family, friends, colleagues).
3. *Personality*. The enduring patterns underlying how people manage life, including how patients assert themselves, express anger and hurt feelings, and maintain self-esteem. Personality also encompasses specific traits such as shyness, aggression, inhibition, and suspiciousness. IPT does not to attempt to treat an individual's personality difficulties.

Clinical Handbook for the Management of Mood Disorders, ed. J. John Mann, Patrick J. McGrath, and Steven P. Roose.
Published by Cambridge University Press. © Cambridge University Press 2013.

IPT phases

In clinical trials, the duration of IPT for depression typically ranges from 8–16 sessions and is conducted in three distinct phases: initial, middle, and termination. Maintenance treatment for as long as 3 years has also been described (Frank *et al.* 1990). In clinical practice, treatment length varies, but is always specified in the initial phase. If needed, at the end of the prescribed acute treatment the therapist and patient may contract for a specific number of weekly sessions with a redefined aim or maintenance sessions (usually monthly) aiming to prevent relapse.

Initial phase

During the initial phase, which can be 2–4 sessions, the therapist administers a standard diagnostic assessment, as well as symptom checklists such as the Hamilton Rating Scales for Depression (Hamilton, 1960) and Anxiety (Hamilton, 1959) or the Beck Depression Inventory (Beck, 1996) to make a clinical diagnosis and to assess symptom severity and co-morbidity. A detailed history and a review of the current important relationships (interpersonal inventory) is taken. The interpersonal inventory clarifies the patient's interpersonal situation around the onset of the current episode in order to select an interpersonal focus for treatment within at least one of the four IPT problem areas, identifies strengths and weaknesses in the patient's support and resources, and determines the patient's need for medication based on symptom severity, previous experience with medication, and patient preference.

In the initial treatment phase, the therapist: (1) educates about depression and provides hope that it is a treatable condition, (2) assists in managing consequences of depression and creating conditions to heal from the current episode, and (3) jointly selects with the patient one or two interpersonal problems areas as a focus throughout the duration of the treatment.

Once a treatment formulation is developed, the therapist establishes a treatment contract and jointly considers practical and financial issues to determine the precise number of treatment sessions. The therapist may refer back to this contract later in treatment if the focus strays from the agreed-upon problem area.

Therapists are to complete the following tasks in the initial sessions. The questions to guide these tasks are outlined in the Weissman *et al.* 2007 manual:

- Review the symptoms of depression and make a diagnosis.
- Explain depression and the various treatment options available.
- Evaluate the need for adjunct medication treatment which is based on severity of symptoms, patient preference, and past experience.
- Review details of the patient's life and the onset of the episode of depression to identify the context in which the depressive episode has arisen.
- Present a treatment formulation, linking the patient's illness to an interpersonal focus (one or more of the four problem areas: grief, disputes, transitions, and deficits).
- Establish a treatment contract based on the treatment formulation linking depression onset to an interpersonal event, and educate the patient about what to expect in treatment.
- Assign the "sick role:" explain to patients that they are suffering from an episode of depression that does not allow them to function at an optimal level; inform them that they may need to temporarily lower expectations for what they are able to accomplish, but with treatment they should recover from the current depressive episode and return to normal functioning.

The following is a dialogue between a patient, Michael, and his therapist in the initial phase of treatment (session 2). Michael is a 39-year-old man who sought help for depression. It should be noted that prior to this interview, the therapist conducted a thorough clinical interview with Michael to make the diagnosis, evaluate suicide risk, and assess the need for medication. In this case, the patient preferred not to take medication. He had a moderately severe first episode of major depression, mild anxiety symptoms, and no substance-abuse history.

Therapist: You've shared a lot with me today about the problems you've been experiencing over the past 2 months. You reported difficulty staying asleep at night … you've lost your appetite and told me that you've shed 9 pounds in the last 5 weeks … you mentioned having difficulty concentrating, feeling far more tired than you used to … even walking a few blocks to the Starbucks near your home to get a cup of coffee has felt like an effort … you also reported feeling really down on yourself and irritable. Michael, these are symptoms of depression. Depression is …

Michael: I just feel…I feel exhausted. My life is a complete mess…"depression," you call it? (sarcastic)…I'm a lost cause.

Therapist: It's not your fault that you have depression. And it isn't a failing. Depression is common, and fortunately we have plenty of good, proven treatments for it. Your main job for now needs to be taking care of yourself, cutting back on the stresses in your life as much as possible, and making sure that the circumstances around you allow you to get better.

Michael: I don't have time to take care of myself! Between the money my wife is bringing in and my unemployment check we barely have enough to pay the monthly mortgage on our home…(loud and panicked)

Therapist: What if you had another illness? Say a bad case of the flu or pneumonia. Have you ever had pneumonia?

Michael: Sure I have. Back a few winters ago. But that's different. I had a fever something terrible…thought I was going to have to go to the ER. The thing lasted about 2 months.

Therapist: (nodding head thoughtfully)…Did you have the same expectations for yourself during that time? Did you think you should get the same amount done, even though you were ill?

Michael: Aw c'mon. You're equating *pneumonia* with depression?

Therapist: I am. Depression is a real illness, too. It has symptoms, among them the ones you mentioned before: irritability, sleep and appetite problems, low energy and motivation. This is typical depression. The good news is that we have some very effective ways to treat it. But for now, until you're feeling a little better, you may need a little extra help from family and friends to do all of the things that you need and want to do. As we make progress in treatment, you'll start improving, but it's going to take a little time.

Michael: I sure hope so…(more relaxed now) I don't know how much longer I can take this…always feeling like a failure and not being able to do anything.

Having given Michael's symptoms a name, provided hope, and assigned him the "sick role," the therapist proceeds to explore the interpersonal context of Michael's depression. The following is an excerpt from his third session:

Therapist: Michael, you began noticing your symptoms of depression about 2 months ago, in the fall. What was going on for you at that time? Can you recall?

Michael: Yup. At the beginning of September I get pulled into my boss's office. He tells me that the company has taken an unexpected turn and my position is being terminated.…can you believe it? Almost 17 goddamn years on the job and they "snip" fire me just like that (gesturing with his hand as if cutting with scissors)…ungrateful is what they are…I busted my butt for them…

Therapist: I see. And how has your life changed since losing your job?

Michael: Well, for one thing, my wife had to go out and get a part-time job because my unemployment check couldn't cover the mortgage on our home…for all these years, I've prided myself on being able to support my family…now I can't even hold down a job. She's the breadwinner…she's the one trying to put dinner on the table…

Therapist: That sounds like a very large adjustment to make.

Michael: You bet it is…and what's worse, I can't find the energy to get up and look for a new job. My son Justin leaves for school in the morning, my wife takes off for work, and I'm just home…on the couch…kind of feels like I'm paralyzed…stuck.

Therapist: When you lost your job, what happened?

Michael: Well, my wife freaked out…and I can understand that, it's not easy for us to make ends meet. A friend of hers knew of an opening at a bookstore 'round the corner from our house. She got hired there. You know, she was supportive at first. But even then, I could see in her eyes the disappointment. Like I let her down…her and Justin…and maybe she's right…recently we've been fighting…over little things like whose gonna' pick up Justin from soccer practice, or what to order from the Chinese restaurant.…I mean screaming matches…it's never been like that between us.

Therapist: I can hear in your voice how upsetting those fights with your wife are for you. How have things been with your son, Justin?

Michael: He's just a kid, you know…but he can tell something's up. We used to watch the ball game on T.V. at night…he'd tell me about school…and now he just goes straight to his room. Maybe it's the age he is, but sometimes it feels like he can't even stand to be in the same room as his old man anymore.

Upon exploring the interpersonal circumstances that surrounded the onset of Michael's depression symptoms, the therapist links the loss of Michael's job and the role transition from being employed to unemployed to the current depression episode. The therapist also hypothesizes that, while the loss of Michael's job triggered the episode, the subsequent dispute between Michael and his wife (secondary to Michael's role transition) has perhaps exacerbated his depression.

At this point the therapist shares her understanding of Michael's problems, explains the treatment course, and makes a treatment contract, also known as the interpersonal formulation:

Therapist: Michael, from the information we have gathered over the past few sessions, it seems that your depression symptoms arose right around the time that you lost your job at the beginning of September. It's been a really hard adjustment for you. You told me how demoralized you felt, and like you'd "let your family down." That's when the depression symptoms began to kick in: your trouble sleeping, your lack of appetite, your fatigue and irritability. And the pressure you're feeling to get another job just gets you down more, which makes it harder to look for new work, and so on in a vicious cycle. On top of that, you've been arguing with your wife more, which also impacts your mood.

Michael: Yep...sounds about right.

Therapist: We'll be talking about these important changes that triggered your depression, and we'll try to find ways to help you feel confident in negotiating these problems...searching for a new job, and how to manage your interactions with your wife. I want to remind you that we will be meeting every week for the next 13 weeks, as we discussed. To make the best use of treatment, it's important that you come on time and that you reschedule if you need to miss an appointment.

Middle phase

The majority of the therapeutic work takes place in this phase of treatment. The therapist helps the patient clarify how he is affected by and affects his interpersonal environment, and builds relational skills to counteract symptoms of depression and manage interpersonal difficulties more effectively. Although the interpersonal problems identified may have a long history, the therapist focuses on how these problems relate to the development of the patient's depression symptoms and how they manifest themselves in the here-and-now of the patient's relationships.

At the start of each session, the therapist assesses the patient's depression symptoms, noting any changes that occurred over the course of the week and linking symptom changes to interpersonal interactions and events. The therapist might ask, "How have things been since we last met?" If the patient responds by addressing mood (e.g., "I've been feeling just terrible"), the therapist inquires about the interpersonal context and attempts to link the depressed mood with interpersonal circumstances. Alternatively, if the patient answers the initial question by reporting an event e.g., "Well, I had a big fight with my husband," the therapist links the event to mood. The therapist might respond, "I'm sorry to hear that. How did it make you feel? What were your symptoms?" Subsequently, the therapist should further explore the event, the patient's associated feelings (e.g., What happened? How did

the patient feel about what happened? What did the patient wish or expect to happen? What were the specifics of the event? And did symptoms emerge?).

The sample questions used in the initial phase to determine the problem area, and the goals and strategies for the problem area, which is the work of the middle phase, are described in Table 20.1.

In the middle phase of IPT, the therapist utilizes a number of standard techniques, including social activation to help the patient re-engage in pleasurable activities; communication analysis to examine and identify problems in communication that may be perpetuating interpersonal disputes; clarification to shed light on a statement or make the patient more aware of what is being communicated; and direct elicitation of information to obtain specific information that might be needed to demonstrate a point (e.g., identifying a patient's role in an interpersonal dispute).

The following is an excerpt from session 6, in the middle phase of Michael's therapy. Role transitions were the primary problem area...

Therapist: Michael, how are you doing today?

Michael: I'm alright.

Therapist: How are your sleeping and eating?

Michael: I've been sleeping a little better, and trying to eat three square meals a day, but I'm still having a hard time concentrating, and I'm having difficulty mustering the energy to get off the damn couch and look for work...things with my wife are still strained, too.

Therapist: I'm glad to hear that your eating and sleeping have improved. Today I was hoping that we could talk a bit about your job...what it meant to you...

Michael: Losing my job, it feels like I lost some of the best years of my life. I mean, being a computer technician seems kind of boring to the average guy, but to me it's like a science...you are presented with a problem and you're like a detective searching for clues that might point you in the direction of a solution. It takes a level of creativity too, you know.

Therapist: It's clear from what you've said here that your job was important to you. It helped support your family financially, but it also was deeply fulfilling to you on a personal level. It sounds like it gave you a real sense of purpose.

Michael: It did. It really did. I used to get up early in the morning...around 5 a.m. or so...make breakfast...go for a jog...get to work around 7:30 a.m. I had so much energy. I was part of a team at work...they called us the "techies..." (chuckling lightly). I worked there for almost 20 years...I told you that. Then they just get rid of me...the company...for all the work I put in...And now...you know I try to spend

Table 20.1 Goals, strategies, and sample questions for the problem areas

Goals	Strategies	Sample questions
Grief – death of people important to the patient		
• Facilitate mourning of the deceased loved one • Re-engage with the world by breaking social isolation and refocusing on relationships and interests	• Start with the sequence of events before, during, and after the death • Help the patient to reconstruct the relationship with the deceased and to view it in a balanced way • Assist the patient in facing the future without the loved one, in developing new skills, and in deepening social support	*"Did someone you care about die?"* *"Was it the anniversary of someone's death?"* *"Were you thinking about someone who died?"*
Interpersonal disputes – overt or covert disagreements with a significant other		
• Identify the stage of the dispute[a] • Identify and modify mismatched expectations and/or maladaptive communication between the two parties • Assist the patient in actively resolving the dispute	• Explore interactions between the parties to identify discordant expectations that led to the dispute • Explore patient's wishes about the relationship • Modify maladaptive communication patterns • Support the patient in trying out new communication skills to resolve the dispute (and as a result either improve a relationship or end a destructive one)	*"Were you having problems with your spouse or partner?"* *"Were you having problems with your children?"* *"Were you having problems at work?"*

[a]**Identify stages of disputes**

Renegotiation:	The two parties are still communicating, and both want to resolve dispute, but have been unsuccessful so far.
Impasse:	The parties have failed in resolving the dispute and have stopped trying. They still want to be together but are "stuck." The therapist helps to move the impasse into either a renegotiation or a dissolution.
Dissolution:	One or both parties want to end the relationship. The therapist explores whether the person wants to try one more time. If this fails, the therapist helps the patient in moving away from the relationship.

Goals	Strategies	Sample questions
Role transitions – positive or negative life changes		
• Mourn the loss of the old role • Develop new skills and social support to handle the new role	• Elicit feelings about loss of the old role • Identify positive and negative aspects of the old role • Identify positive and negative aspects of the new role • Assist patient in reducing social isolation and in finding resources and skills to handle the new role better	*"Did your children leave home?"* *"Did you start a new job?"* *"Did you retire?"*
Interpersonal deficits – difficulty initiating and/or sustaining relationships or a paucity of relationships		
• Reduce social isolation by improving social skills	• Review past and current relationships to identify recurrent patterns • Rehearse new social skills for the formation of new relationships and the deepening of existing relationships	*"Were you put in a situation where you had to meet new people?"* *"Were you lonely?"* *"Were you bored?"*

[a] adapted from Weissman *et al.* (2007)

a couple hours in the morning searching for jobs on the internet…there's not much out there…and I'm tired of camping out at Starbucks all morning…mindlessly staring at my computer screen…now *that's* depressing.

Therapist: (nodding)…so by losing your job you also lost structure around which to plan your day. It also sounds like you lost a part of your identity as a "techie" and a part of your team at work.

Michael: Mmm…(murmurs in agreement)

Having identified this role transition as an interpersonal trigger of depression, the therapist attempts to reduce Michael's sense of isolation, and help him re-engage in pleasurable pastime activities despite his lack of motivation and depression symptoms:

Therapist: What if you could set up a schedule for yourself? Write it out even. What would this look like?

Michael: I don't know. Maybe I would wake up at 6 a.m. and go for a jog...by 8:30 a.m. begin my job search. Uh, I guess I could make goals for myself as to what I'd like to accomplish for the day.

Therapist: What sort of goals are you thinking of?

Michael: Well, maybe I'll try to submit two applications each day. I could also relocate to the public library...give myself a break from the coffee shop.

Therapist: So maybe you could turn your job search into a job in and of itself. What are your thoughts on that?

Michael: Yeah. That's actually a pretty good idea. If I can just break the cycle...get up and take the steps that need to be taken to find a job and get my life back on track. Stop wasting hours sitting on the couch and bemoaning what's happened...

Therapist: Sometimes when people become depressed they isolate themselves from other people...loved ones and friends. I think it is important that you provide yourself with daily structure, and also reach out to friends...take advantage of your support network.

Michael: It has been a long time since I've seen my buddies. We used to get together every Sunday and play softball...then head to the tavern for a beer.

Therapist: Could you give your friends a call this week and set up a softball game for this upcoming weekend?

Michael: Sure...yeah...I could do that.

The therapist also addresses the secondary interpersonal problem area sustaining Michael's current episode, his disputes with his wife:

Therapist: Great. I also want to address some of the issues that you are having with your wife. You've mentioned that the two of you have begun arguing more than you ever did in the past. You also expressed that you didn't think she respected you as she once did.

Michael: My wife thinks I've let down the family...I know it...and the fighting...it's relentless...it's like she's waiting to jump down my throat at the slightest provocation. My wife used to look at me with such adoration, tussle my hair...now she won't so much as look in my direction...unless we're fighting.

Therapist: That makes the situation even more difficult for you What are some things that you would like to change about your relationship with your wife?

Michael: I guess I just want my wife to get off my back a little...cut me a little slack. I already feel bad enough about losing my job and forcing her to go out and work.

The therapist implements communication analysis technique to examine and identify problems in communication between Michael and his wife. The therapist elicits a concrete example of when communication broke down, how the conversation became derailed, and what Michael perhaps intended to say, but did not (direct elicitation technique):

Therapist: Michael, did you experience a specific altercation with your wife this past week that was especially upsetting to you?

Michael: Hmmm (thinking)...Yeah. On Tuesday morning my wife had asked me to pick up a list of groceries from the supermarket. I spent most of the day working on my resume and looking for job openings online. The groceries just slipped my mind. Anyhow, my wife comes home from work that evening, sees that I haven't been to the supermarket...she's missing a couple of ingredients she needs to make dinner and she just flies off the handlebars.

Therapist: When you say she "flew off the handlebars" what do you mean exactly? (clarification technique) She became very angry?

Michael: Yeah. She starts laying into me. She told me that if I wasn't going to work, or taking care of the cleaning, cooking and laundry, the least I could do is pick up a small list of groceries.

Therapist: How did that make you feel?

Michael: Oh, so crappy. Worthless. I wondered if she was right.

Therapist: (nodding empathetically) How did you respond to your wife?

Michael: I didn't know what to say. I just said I was sorry. She interrupted me...began accusing me of loading all of the household responsibilities on her. Meanwhile, she said I was just wallowing in my own sadness.

Therapist: Are there things that you wanted to communicate to your wife, but felt you couldn't?

Michael: Yeah. I was gonna explain to her that I was looking for work all day and simply forgot to get the groceries. I wanted to tell her that I'm doing the best I can...I'm seeking treatment to handle my depression and taking steps to find employment...Maybe remind her that this is a time when the two of us need to stick together and support one another.

Therapist: I see. Is there a time either today or tomorrow when you could speak to her about how the conversation on Tuesday made you feel? Maybe tell her some of things that you just told me, that you are doing the best you can, you are in treatment for depression, looking for employment, and really need her support right now?

Michael: I could do that. Justin goes to bed around 10 p.m. usually. I could bring it up with her when we are watching T.V. in our room, you know, unwinding. And she's usually real receptive about stuff. Anytime I've needed to talk to her, I mean *really* talk...

Therapist: Michael, that sounds like a great plan.

Termination phase

In the initial phase of treatment, the therapist and patient make an explicit contract about the frequency and length of treatment. Termination is periodically mentioned throughout treatment, and several sessions prior to the agreed-upon end, the upcoming termination becomes more of a focus. What has been accomplished, and what work remains to be done is discussed. The patient is encouraged to explore and express feelings surrounding treatment termination.

The goals of the termination phase are to: (1) help the patient recognize that separations (i.e., dissolution of therapist–patient relationship) are role transitions and thus may bring about normal sadness that is not the same as depression, (2) support the patient's sense of independence and competence if treatment is to end, (3) relieve any sense of guilt or self-blame in the event that treatment has not been successful, and explore alternative treatment options available, and (4) discuss continuation or maintenance treatment if IPT treatment has been acutely successful, but the patient is still at risk for relapse or recurrence.

The following is an excerpt from Michael's penultimate session:

Therapist: Michael, you have made some significant gains in the last 4 months. First of all, your depression symptoms have improved: you describe sleeping better and eating better, you're feeling more motivated and energetic, and not so irritable. All these improvements have helped you to secure two upcoming job interviews.

Michael: (smiling and shaking his head)...Yep, you know, in the beginning I was doubtful that I'd get my life back on track...what with being laid off and those fights with my wife...she's beginning to come around...she even gave me a backrub before bed on Wednesday night...I'm still fighting back feelings of failure and disappointment...I mean what if these two interviews fall through?

Therapist: That's one of the things that remain for you to keep working on going forward from here. But what you've done during the last few months has been enough to improve your mood. The work you'll do in the future should help keep you from getting depressed again. We're almost finished for today.

Next week is our last session, and I'd like to hear about your feelings about termination, to look at what situations might arise in your future that you think might trigger another depression, and to look at what skills you've developed during our work that you might use to manage those situations.

Maintenance treatment

At the end of acute treatment, many patients are still symptomatic. Even those with full remission have a moderately high rate of recurrence or relapse. Patients who have experienced multiple depressive episodes have a particularly high (over 80%) probability of recurrence (Judd *et al.* 1998, 2000). Thus, in the termination phase of IPT, a discussion of the risk of relapse or recurrence is included. Patients should be advised to seek further help as needed and a review of the events which trigger episodes is completed. Maintenance IPT (IPT-M) with or without medication is an option. There is considerable evidence for the efficacy of IPT weekly as a continuation therapy for 6 months (Klerman *et al.* 1984), or monthly for 3 years as maintenance therapy (Frank *et al.* 1990).

The objective of maintenance treatment is to prevent recurrences of depression, to keep the patient asymptomatic, and to manage triggers of future episodes. IPT-M focuses on interpersonal functioning and mood in relation to life events. In terms of time limit and frequency, a time-specified contract is arranged between therapist and patient. At the end of the agreed-upon time frame, the therapist and patient again discuss and renegotiate termination.

In IPT-M, the therapist and patient work collaboratively, watching for signs that depression symptoms have returned which may have preceded the onset of prior episodes of depression. Additionally, both parties are mindful of interpersonal disturbances that might set off a depressive episode (Frank *et al.* 1991). The interpersonal problem areas can shift in response to changing life circumstances if treatment continues over an extended time.

Adaptations and training

IPT has had numerous adaptations for different age groups, disorders, cultures, and formats. Some of these adaptations have specific manuals. A 2012 book summarizes many of these adaptations (Markowitz and Weissman, 2012), including depressed adolescents, older individuals, post-partum depression, depressed medically ill or hospitalized patients, low-income patients, cultural variations for use in developing countries, for use in groups, by telephone, and for patients with eating disorders, post-traumatic stress disorder, social anxiety disorder, borderline personality disorder, or bipolar disorder. A new three-session adaptation, Interpersonal Psychotherapy: Evaluation, Support, and Triage (IPT:EST) has been developed to help primary care and other health workers evaluate, offer support, and determine appropriate triage for patients who screen positive for depression (Weissman and Verdeli, 2012). There are other adaptations of IPT (individual and group) in low- and middle-income countries (Verdeli *et al.* 2003).

IPT is included in some training programs in psychiatric residency, psychology, and social work. Other opportunities for learning IPT include the Continuing Medical Education (CME) programs at the American Psychological Association and the American Psychiatric Association annual meeting. Individual practicum workshops are also offered by experienced IPT therapists. There is an International Society of IPT and a website (http://interpersonalpsychotherapy.org/) which lists available trainers, workshops, and new manuals.

Future

The future of IPT and of psychotherapy in general is somewhat guarded in the United States, but not elsewhere. Psychotherapy in the USA has had a diminishing role in outpatient mental health treatment. A larger and increasing proportion of patients receive psychotropic medication alone, and visits to office-based psychiatrists, that include psychotherapy, have declined by nearly one-third (Olfson and Marcus, 2010). The number of psychotherapy sessions per patient has also decreased. At the same time, training in evidence-based psychotherapy occupies only a small portion of psychotherapy training in psychiatric residency, psychology, or social work programs (Weissman *et al.* 2006). Psychotherapy has been under pressure from managed care and the forces of health care cost. Psychiatry is increasing its training to include genetics, neuroscience, and brain imaging. These same trends are not found in Canada and Western countries where IPT institutes have been formed, and primary care doctors receive training in IPT or in mental health programs in developing countries (Verdeli *et al.* 2003). Of note are the numerous translations of IPT and its adaptation and training in Uganda,

Goa, Ethiopia, Haiti, and Nigeria. As it has become clearer that depression may hinder HIV and maternal and child health care as well as recovery from disasters, demands for IPT have increased in developing countries for health workers. The IPT model which deals with grief, disputes, and transitions is readily useful for countries dealing with the aftermath of earthquakes, civil war, and loss of lives from HIV. The social and economic benefits of parity may be better recognized outside of the USA.

So what will the future hold? Clearly the trend for research in personalized psychiatry, determining biomarkers for specific treatments in specific patients, will have some results in the next decade. Thus far, the few studies in depression focus on medication, but psychotherapy will undoubtedly be included if there is any success with medication biomarkers. For now, common sense will need to prevail so that patients with clear interpersonal problems in association with depression onset may receive IPT and those who do not like to talk about relationships or do not have many relationships may be referred to cognitive behavior therapy (CBT). Of course, scientific study should overrule common sense.

There is a clear need to reduce health care cost, which can be done by reducing time and frequency, and task shifting to nondoctoral-level therapists. IPT has already passed this test by specifying time limits and in success in training health workers; the success for the latter has been tested in controlled clinical trials (Verdeli *et al.* 2003). More needs to be done in delivering psychotherapy with computer applications and web-based interactive training. CBT is further ahead of IPT in this regard.

There is increasing evidence that for depression both medication and psychotherapy have effects on the brain and that the relationship between the brain and environment is bidirectional. This means that understanding better how psychotherapy and medication can be best applied to the individual patient is the critical task. The struggle over which treatment is "better" and treatment recommendations made simply on the basis of what is available or cheapest hopefully will vanish. The future of IPT and of psychotherapy has many challenges.

References

Beck, A., Rush, A., Sha, B., and Emergy, G. (1979). *Cognitive Therapy of Depression*. New York: Guilford.

Beck, A.T., Steer, R.A., and Brown, G.K. (1996). *Manual for Beck Depression Inventory II (BDI-II)*. San Antonio, TX: Psychology Corporation.

Beck, J. (1995). *Cognitive Therapy: Basics and Beyond*. New York: Guilford.

Clougherty, K.F., Verdeli, H., and Weissman, M.M. (2003). Interpersonal psychotherapy for a group in Uganda (IPT:GU). Copyrighted unpublished manual.

Cuijpers, P., Geraedts, A.S., van Oppen, P. *et al.* (2011). Interpersonal psychotherapy for depression: A meta-analysis. *American Journal of Psychiatry*, 168, 581–592.

Frank, E. (2005). *Treating Bipolar Disorder: A Clinician's Guide to Interpersonal and Social Rhythm Therapy*. New York: Guilford.

Frank, E., Kupfer, D.J., Wagner, E.F., McEachran, A.B., and Cornes, C. (1991). Efficacy of interpersonal psychotherapy as a maintenance treatment for recurrent depression: Contributing factors. *Archives of General Psychiatry*, 48, 1053–1059.

Frank, E., Kupfer, D.J., Perel, J.M. *et al.* (1990). Three-year outcomes for maintenance therapies in recurrent depression. *Archives of General Psychiatry*, 47, 1093–1099.

Hamilton, M. (1959). The assessment of anxiety states by rating. *British Journal of Medical Psychology*, 32, 50–55.

Hamilton, M. (1960). A rating scale for depression. *Journal of Neurology, Neurosurgery and Psychiatry*, 23, 56–62.

Hinrichsen, G.A. and Clougherty, K.F. (2006). *Interpersonal Psychotherapy for Depressed Older Adults*. Washington, DC: American Psychological Association.

Hlastala, S.A., Kotler, J.S., McClellan, J.M., and McCauley, E.A. (2010). Interpersonal and social rhythm therapy for adolescents with bipolar disorder: Treatment development and results from an open trial. *Depression and Anxiety*, 27, 457–464.

Judd, L.L., Akiskal, H.S., Maser, J.D. *et al.* (1998). Major depressive disorder: A prospective study of residual subthreshold depressive symptoms as predictor of rapid relapse. *Journal of Affective Disorders*, 50, 97–108.

Judd, L.L., Akiskal, H., Zeller, P.J. *et al.* (2000). Psychosocial disability during the long-term course of unipolar major depressive disorder. *Archives of General Psychiatry*, 57, 375–380.

Klerman, G.L., Weissman, M.M., Rounsaville, B., and Chevron, E.S. (1984). *Interpersonal Psychotherapy of Depression*. New York: Basic Books.

Klerman, G.L., Budman, S., Berwick, D. *et al.* (1987). Efficacy of a brief psychosocial intervention for symptoms of stress and distress among patients in primary care. *Medical Care*, 25, 1078–1088.

Markowitz, J.C. (1998). *Interpersonal Psychotherapy for Dysthymic Disorder*. Washington, DC: American Psychiatric Press.

Markowitz, J.C. and Weissman, M.M. (2012). *Casebook of Interpersonal Psychotherapy*. New York: Oxford University Press.

Markowitz, J.C., Kocsis, J.H., Bleiberg, K.L., Christos, P.J., and Sacks, M. (2005). A comparative trial of psychotherapy and pharmacotherapy for "pure" dysthymic patients. *Journal of Affective Disorders*, 89, 167–175.

Menchetti, M., Bortolotti, B., Rucci, P. *et al.* (2010). Depression in primary care: Interpersonal counseling vs selective serotonin reuptake inhibitors. The DEPICS Study. A multicenter randomized controlled trial. Rationale and design. *BMC Psychiatry*, 10, 97.

Mufson, L., Pollack, D.K., Moreau, D., and Weissman, M.M. (2004). *Interpersonal Psychotherapy for Depressed Adolescents, Second Edition*. New York: Guilford.

O'Hara, M.W., Stuart, S., Gorman, L.L., and Wenzel, A. (2000). Efficacy of interpersonal psychotherapy for postpartum depression. *Archives of General Psychiatry*, 57, 1039–1045.

Olfson, M. and Marcus, S.C. (2010). National trends in outpatient psychotherapy. *American Journal of Psychiatry*, 167, 1456–1463.

Schulberg, H.C., Raue, P.J., and Rollman, B.L. (2002). The effectiveness of psychotherapy in treating depressive disorders in primary care practice: Clinical and cost perspectives. *General Hospital Psychiatry*, 24, 203–212.

Spinelli, M.G. and Endicott, J. (2003). Controlled clinical trial of interpersonal psychotherapy versus parenting education program for depressed pregnant women. *American Journal of Psychiatry*, 160, 555–562.

Swartz, H.A., Pilkonis, P.A., Frank, E., Proietti, J.M., and Scott, J. (2005). Acute treatment outcomes in patients with bipolar I disorder and co-morbid borderline personality disorder receiving medication and psychotherapy. *Bipolar Disorders*, 7, 192–197.

Verdeli, H. and Weissman, M.M. (2011). Interpersonal Psychotherapy. In Corsini, R.J. and Wedding, D., eds., *Current Psychotherapies, Ninth Edition*. Pacific Grove, CA: Brooks/Cole, 383–414.

Verdeli, H., Clougherty, K., Bolton, P. *et al.* (2003). Adapting group interpersonal psychotherapy for a developing country: Experience in rural Uganda. *World Psychiatry*, 2, 114–120.

Weissman, M.M. and Verdeli, H. (2012). Interpersonal psychotherapy: Evaluation, support and triage. For special issue of *Clinical Psychology and Psychotherapy*. Published online in Wiley Online Library, doi: 10.1002/cpp.1775.

Weissman, M.M., Markowitz, J.C., and Klerman, G.L. (2000). *Comprehensive Guide to Interpersonal Psychotherapy*. New York: Basic Books.

Weissman, M.M., Markowitz, J.C., and Klerman, G.L. (2007). *A Clinician's Quick Guide to Interpersonal Psychotherapy*. New York: Oxford University Press.

Weissman, M.M., Verdeli, H., Gameroff, M.J. *et al.* (2006). National survey of psychotherapy training in psychiatry, psychology, and social work. *Archives of General Psychiatry*, 63, 925–934.

Chapter

21

Dialectical behavior therapy for mood disorders

Megan S. Chesin and Barbara H. Stanley

Overview

This chapter will provide an overview of dialectical behavior therapy (DBT), a form of cognitive behavior therapy (CBT) and a newer generation psychotherapy or "third-wave" treatment, combining behaviorally oriented change techniques with acceptance-based strategies. DBT was originally designed as a treatment for chronically suicidal and self-injuring individuals (Linehan, 1987). It has been manualized as a treatment for individuals with borderline personality disorder (BPD) (Linehan 1993a, b) and adapted for individuals with depression, eating disorders, substance abuse and geriatric populations. Furthermore, with its focus on emotion regulation, it can be used for individuals with bipolar disorder (BD). We will provide a description of DBT, including the stages of treatment, how it differs from other forms of CBT, the empirical support for this treatment approach, and clinical vignettes demonstrating its application to mood disorders.

Description of DBT

DBT is a principles-driven, as opposed to a protocol-driven, treatment and, thus, "organizes strategies into protocols and structures therapy and clinical decision making" (Koerner and Dimeff, 2007, p. 2). The content of individual treatment sessions is not proscribed as it can be in other protocol-driven CBT approaches, i.e., This allows the therapist to "respond quickly to an ever-changing clinical picture" (Koerner and Dimeff, 2007, p. 2).

DBT (Linehan, 1993a) includes five domains or targets of comprehensive psychosocial treatment: enhancing patient capabilities, improving motivation for change and treatment, enhancing generalization of skillful responses to the environment, enhancing therapist capabilities and motivation, and structuring the environment to improve patient amenability to treatment. In DBT, these domains or targets are addressed through four modes of treatment: individual psychotherapy, group skills training, individual coaching between sessions (usually on the phone), and the therapist consultation meetings.

Individual psychotherapy in DBT treatment is organized into stages and then targets within stages. In the initial phase, life-threatening behaviors, i.e., suicide-related actions and urges, therapy-interfering behavior that can lead to early treatment dropout (e.g., lateness, nonattendance) and behaviors that seriously impact the quality of life (e.g., severe problems with relationships, substance abuse) are targeted. These problems are addressed in a hierarchical manner with life-threatening behaviors always addressed as a first priority. This focus reflects the origins of DBT as a treatment for chronically suicidal individuals with BPD, but also makes DBT particularly relevant to mood disorders, with their high incidence of suicidal behavior. Symptoms and problem behaviors are tracked on diary cards (Linehan, 1993b), a tool on which patients record their daily emotional experiences and behaviors. Thus, agenda-setting for individual DBT therapy sessions proceeds directly from the therapist's and patient's review of the diary card at the beginning of a session.

DBT incorporates several assumptions about patients and the treatment. For example, the treatment approach explicitly acknowledges that, while patients are struggling and their coping strategies are inadequate, they are, in fact, doing the best that they can. At the same time, there is a strong emphasis on change, as things cannot remain in the status quo (Linehan, 1993a). The agreements made by DBT patients and their clinicians are another foundational

Clinical Handbook for the Management of Mood Disorders, ed. J. John Mann, Patrick J. McGrath, and Steven P. Roose. Published by Cambridge University Press. © Cambridge University Press 2013.

element of DBT. At the outset of treatment, the requirements for both the clinician and patient are outlined. One important condition is that patients must agree to work on suicidal behaviors and problems that interfere with therapy as they arise. This focus again reflects the origins of DBT as a treatment for chronically suicidal individuals and individuals with BPD. Commitment to working on suicidal behaviors and problems that interfere with therapy may be more applicable to mood-disordered patients with co-morbid personality disorder than mood-disordered patients without personality pathology. However, for patients with depression or BD who become suicidal, they can often experience fluctuating motivation to discuss suicidal feelings and plans. This commitment to maintain this focus can be very useful.

There are three categories of core strategies employed in DBT: change strategies, acceptance and validation strategies, and dialectical strategies. *Change strategies* in DBT, for the most part, are based on learning principles. Behaviors are understood as maintained through either operant or classical conditioning. If a maladaptive behavior is maintained through operant conditioning, removal of reinforcers is likely to be helpful along with positive reinforcement of adaptive behaviors. If a maladaptive behavior is maintained through respondent (classical) conditioning, loosening the connection between the conditioned and unconditioned stimuli is attempted. Many of the change procedures and strategies used to alter the problem behaviors and symptoms are consistent with those used in CBT. They include behavioral analysis and skills training, as well as didactic instruction.

Aspects of Eastern philosophy are an important component of DBT (Robbins, 2002). In particular, there is a strong focus on *acceptance and validation strategies*. Linehan (1987) noted that an exclusive focus on change in therapy can be viewed as not understanding the patient's pain and as invalidating the credibility of the therapist or therapy. This DBT strategy involves acceptance of whatever is valid about the patient's reactions and an effort to decrease suffering. However, not attending to the need for change is just as invalidating because it does not help to move the patient forward. Therefore, acceptance and validation are combined with change strategies.

Dialectical strategies, in which polar opposite positions are synthesized to make a cohesive whole, are the third set of core strategies. A dialectical world view is the overarching perspective in DBT and is manifest in the strategies and assumptions of the treatment. Therapists create a balance between accepting patients' dysfunctions and helping patients modify their thinking and behavior (Stanley and Brodsky, 2009). One dialectic strategy is called the "devil's advocate technique." An example of this technique is challenging patients to express why they would want to give up cutting themselves given that it "works" for them, i.e., provides relief from emotional distress. Patients are, thus, compelled to argue against the behavior and justify stopping it. Similarly, when the patient and therapist are "stuck" in-session and find themselves having difficulty agreeing on common goals, dialectical strategies are helpful for initiating progress (Linehan, 1993a). At the same time, problem behaviors are addressed in individual therapy, deficits in emotion regulation, cognitive and behavior control, and interpersonal skills are remedied in separate skills training sessions (Linehan, 1993a).

Clinical vignette

Ms. T is a 26-year-old depressed female with a history of chronic suicide ideation as well as multiple suicide attempts and psychiatric hospitalizations. Ms. T often uses prescribed antianxiety or sleeping medications, sometimes in higher doses than prescribed, to dampen the intensity of her emotional experience, to "zone out," and to reduce the likelihood she will "act-out." During the eighth session of treatment, Ms. T reported that she had been minimizing the extent of her suicidal urges and that during the last session, she under-reported her suicidal ideation, which included a plan. She also reported she had taken some steps to procure her intended means. She said she had not reported her suicidal thoughts during the previous session because she was afraid of being hospitalized and of overwhelming the therapist. The patient's fears were validated. In the past, reporting suicidal ideation with a plan had led to hospitalization against her wishes. An assessment of current suicidal ideation as well as access to means was then conducted. The patient reported she was no longer suicidal due to the removal of the primary trigger from her life. A behavioral chain analysis of the most recent experience of high suicidal urges was conducted. Feelings of sadness, hopelessness, and boredom figured prominently on the chain of events preceding the high suicidal urges. Ms. T and the therapist discussed using emotion-regulation skills and distress-tolerance skills to manage future intense emotional experiences. Ms. T and the therapist also discussed using phone coaching. The patient expressed that she did not want to overwhelm or burn out the therapist. The therapist assured the patient that she would let the patient know when she was in danger of overwhelming the therapist. The therapist and patient developed a safety plan (Stanley and Brown, 2012), which included identifying early warning signs of impending suicidal crisis (e.g., staring into space for extended periods of time in her bedroom) and committing to contacting the therapist for phone coaching when these warning signs occurred if strategies employed on her own did not work. The therapist also used the opportunity to openly discuss the patient's minimization of suicidal thoughts during the last session and how such minimization had an impact on the therapeutic relationship. The therapist and patient decided to target concealing important thoughts and feelings in treatment.

This case illustrates a DBT approach to managing multiple problem behaviors in one session, prioritizing suicidal behaviors over therapy-interfering behaviors. It also exemplifies how validation is balanced with change to keep the patient and therapist working together on priority targets.

Underpinnings of DBT

In DBT, emotion dysregulation, defined as difficulty modulating experience and reactions, reorienting attention, and organizing behavior towards goal-directed activities during an emotional experience (Gross and Thompson, 2007), is conceptualized as a core difficulty (Linehan, 1993a). For individuals who have co-morbid depression, emotion dysregulation can be manifest in one of two ways: mood reactivity and constricted affect expression. Thus, in this model, dysfunction in other areas, including behavioral, interpersonal, intrapersonal, and cognitive dysfunction, are viewed as emanating from emotion dysregulation or maladaptive attempts to manage emotions. Emotion dysregulation, in turn, is posited to develop, in part, from the transaction of an invalidating environment (e.g., an individual's private experiences are trivialized or denied, or the individual has been victimized) and biological dysfunction in regulating emotions which may include heightened emotional sensitivity to stimuli, intense magnitude of emotional experience, and prolonged emotional arousal (Linehan, 1993a).

Distinguishing DBT and CBT

DBT is a comprehensive treatment which draws upon and combines aspects of a variety of therapies and philosophical approaches. DBT was among the first treatments to formally combine Eastern ideas, e.g., acceptance, with CBT (Hayes, 2004). Incorporation of a dialectical world view remains a unique feature of DBT (Koerner and Dimeff, 2007). In 2003, Verheul et al. identified intersession coaching, attendance to therapist burnout, and consistent monitoring of suicidal behavior and nonsuicidal self injury as distinguishing features of DBT. Although learning principles are prominent in all forms of CBT, some forms of CBT emphasize the importance of, and therefore focus on, the role of cognitions. Other forms of CBT place an emphasis on behavior (Stanley and Brodsky, 2009). For example, the CBT developed by Beck emphasizes the importance of distorted cognitions (Beck et al. 2003). DBT places a greater emphasis on emotion dysregulation. This focus does not imply that DBT never examines distorted cognitions nor that Beck's CBT ever examines behavioral reinforcers.

Cognitive behavior therapy (CBT) has established efficacy in the treatment of depression and anxiety disorders. However, patients with co-morbid depression and BPD have difficulty tolerating standard CBT (Dimeff and Linehan, 2001). CBT emphasizes change strategies that are very difficult for individuals with co-morbid BPD to accept and utilize. They can experience the strong focus on change as being criticized, told that what they are doing is "wrong," and a sense that the clinician does not understand and appreciate their emotional suffering and how difficult it is for them to change. Consequently, this can exacerbate their severe self-criticism and may result in early treatment dropout. To counteract this tendency, DBT emphasizes the importance of balancing the use of change strategies with acceptance and validation techniques. This balance is crucial because both acceptance and change have been identified as important aspects of successful psychotherapy. There are some problems that trouble patients that cannot be changed and, therefore, ways to accept them must be found. For example, patients who were abandoned or neglected in their childhood may feel that it was unfair and that they deserve reparations and/or apologies. Most of the time neither of these are forthcoming. Patients can get entrenched in not accepting their past and, consequently, are unable to move beyond a stance that it should not have happened to them. Acceptance of that past is the only way to move beyond it. Furthermore, acceptance and change have a dynamic interplay which results in a "dialectic." Increasing acceptance enables greater change. At the same time, greater change allows for increased tolerance and acceptance of what cannot be changed.

Clinical vignette

Ms. U is a 26-year-old white female with a history of nonsuicidal self-injury (mostly head banging) and passive suicidal ideation. She has no history of suicide attempt or psychiatric hospitalization.

Ms. U began DBT with reluctance. She was concerned by the time and effort required. She was considering medication as an alternative to DBT. However, she pursued DBT at the suggestion of her CBT therapist. Both Ms. U and her prior therapist agreed CBT was not helping Ms. U. Upon entering treatment, Ms. U was most concerned with her lack of self-worth, her chronic feelings of emptiness and sadness, as well as her difficulties maintaining her independence in intimate relationships. In the first session, Ms. U and the therapist discussed emotion dysregulation as the core difficulty in BPD and how other problem behaviors (e.g., behavioral and cognitive dysregulation) stem from chronic emotional dysregulation. Ms. U said these difficulties and the biosocial theory used to explain the development of such difficulties reflected her experiences quite well. She remarked she felt very well understood and agreed to come back the next week. After the second week, Ms. U agreed to 6 months of treatment. Over the course of treatment, the therapist focused on validating the client, especially her emotional experiences. The therapist also modeled a nonjudgmental stance towards the client's behavior and searched with the client to understand why she was doing what she later regretted. By the end of treatment, the patient was better able to notice her self-judgment and sometimes even let go of it, as well as validate herself. In the context of increased self-acceptance, she was freer to understand why she was doing what she was doing and thus how she might do things differently in the future. By the end of treatment, secondary to managing

better and being less judgmental, her depression was remitted and she was content with her life.

This clinical vignette shows how DBT focuses on acceptance and balancing change and acceptance throughout treatment. It also demonstrates how patients familiar with CBT treatment might experience, and benefit from, an approach with such balance.

Empirical support for DBT

As mentioned earlier, DBT was originally designed as a treatment for chronically suicidal patients and/or patients with chronic nonsuicidal self-injury, defined as the intentional, direct destruction of one's own body tissue without any conscious intent to die (Linehan, 1987, Favazza, 1998). Because chronic nonsuicidal self-injury and repetitive suicidal behavior occur frequently in BPD (American Psychiatric Association, 2000, Jacobson and Gould, 2007), DBT was quickly considered to be, and tested as, a treatment for BPD. Most randomized controlled trials (RCTs) of DBT have tested the treatment in individuals with BPD, with the majority, but not all (Koons et al. 2001, Verhuel et al. 2003, Clarkin et al. 2007), requiring that sample members also have a history of deliberate self-harm, i.e., self-inflicted injury with and without suicidal intent.

Primary outcomes assessed in trials of DBT align with the treatment targets of the initial phase of DBT and, thus, include suicidal behaviour and self–injury, as well as psychiatric hospitalization and treatment retention. Findings from seven RCTs conducted by six different groups (Linehan et al. 1991, 1999, Koons et al. 2001, Verhuel et al. 2003, Linehan et al. 2006, Clarkin et al. 2007, McMain et al. 2009, Carter et al. 2010) show DBT is an effective and efficacious treatment for self-injury and suicidal behavior among individuals with BPD. Findings from the three RCTs comparing DBT to active treatments are particularly noteworthy. Linehan et al. (2006) found participants receiving DBT, as compared to individuals receiving treatment by experts, were significantly less likely to make a suicide attempt during treatment and for 1 year post-treatment. Clarkin et al. (2007) found greater reductions in suicidality among participants receiving DBT and transference-focused psychotherapy (Clarkin et al. 1999) than among patients receiving supportive psychotherapy. McMain et al. (2009) found patients receiving DBT and those receiving general psychiatric management plus psychodynamic psychotherapy realized reductions in the frequency of suicide episodes. Of the three other RCTs assessing suicidality (Linehan *et al.* 1991, Koons *et al.* 2001, Verhuel *et al.* 2003), one (Koons *et al.* 2001) found reductions in suicidality among BPD patients such that DBT participants realized greater reductions in suicidal ideation than those receiving treatment-as-usual.

Findings demonstrating the efficacy of DBT for nonsuicidal self-injury or deliberate self-harm are more robust. Among six RCTs assessing nonsuicidal self-injury or deliberate self-harm (Linehan *et al.* 1991, 2006, Koons *et al.* 2001, Verhuel *et al.* 2003, McMain *et al.* 2009, Carter *et al.* 2010), all but one (Carter *et al.* 2010) found DBT participants showed decreases in self-injury over treatment, with Linehan *et al.* (1991) and Verhuel *et al.* (2003) finding greater reductions in self-injury among DBT patients than treatment-as-usual patients.

Rates of attrition and hospitalization among BPD individuals receiving DBT are relatively low. Linehan *et al.* (1991, 2006) found BPD patients were less likely to present at the emergency room and be admitted than both treatment-as-usual patients and patients receiving treatment by experts. McMain *et al.* (2009) found similar and significant reductions in emergency room visits and days of hospitalization among BPD patients receiving DBT and general psychiatric management plus psychodynamic psychotherapy. Rates of attrition ranged from 61% (McMain *et al.* 2009) to 83% (Linehan *et al.* 1991). With one exception (McMain *et al.* 2009), these rates were significantly better than retention rates among BPD participants receiving other psychological treatment.

Additional evidence for the efficacy and effectiveness of DBT comes from numerous less well-controlled studies which have been conducted (see Dimeff and Linehan, 2006, for a review). Unlike any other therapy for BPD, DBT has been designated an empirically validated treatment for BPD (Chambless *et al.* 1998). In 2001, the American Psychiatric Association recommended using DBT or psychodynamic psychotherapy and adjunctive psychopharmacotherapy to treat BPD (American Psychiatric Association, 2001).

DBT for mood disorders

One rationale for using DBT to treat mood disorders is the significant co-morbidity between BPD and mood disorders. Findings from a large-scale epidemiological study conducted in the US general population (National Epidemiologic Survey on Alcohol and Related Conditions) show at least 75% of BPD individuals have a lifetime mood disorder (Grant *et al.* 2008). Major depressive disorder, in particular, is highly co-morbid with BPD. The lifetime prevalence of major depressive disorder among community members with BPD is 32% (Grant, 2008). In clinical studies, rates are much higher, with 85% of BPD patients having major depressive disorder at some point in their lifetime (e.g., Zanarini *et al.* 1998). BD also co-occurs with BPD, albeit at lower rates. Methodologically rigorous clinical studies (i.e., McLean Study of Adult Development, Collaborative Longitudinal Personality Disorders Study) show 8–10% of BPD patients have co-morbid BD-II and 12% of BPD patients have co-morbid BD-I (Gunderson *et al.* 2006). Epidemiological data on rates of co-morbidity between BD-II and BPD mirror findings from clinical studies. Rates of BD-I among BPD community members are, however, higher. Thirty-two percent of community members with BPD also had BD-I (Grant *et al.* 2008). It is surprising that epidemiological data show higher rates of co-morbidity than clinical data (Gunderson *et al.* 2006). Less rigorous assessment methods coupled with significant overlap in the clinical characteristics of BD and BPD, e.g., affective liability and impulsivity, may explain the surprisingly high rates observed in the epidemiological study (Gunderson *et al.* 2006). Nonetheless, the association between mood disorders, excepting dysthymia, and BPD seems robust. When sociodemographic variables and all other psychiatric disorders are controlled, individuals with BPD are at six times greater risk for BD and three times greater risk for major depression than those without BPD. Further, Gunderson *et al.* (2006) found rates of BD among BPD patients were higher than rates among patients with other personality disorders. Grant *et al.* (2008) concluded the association between BPD and mood disorder is neither accounted for by other disorders nor by factors common to psychopathology. Instead, there are unique factors which explain the co-morbidity of mood disorder and BPD.

Another rationale for the use of DBT in mood disorders stems from the overlap in skills taught in DBT with behavioral activation, an effective component of cognitive therapy for reducing depression (Jacobson *et al.* 1996). In DBT, emotion-regulation skills and interpersonal effectiveness skills teach patients to "get active, approach and do things that make one feel competent and confident," to schedule pleasurable activities and activities which give a sense of mastery into daily routines, and to communicate effectively (Linehan, 1993b). In other words, skills taught and employed in DBT parallel behavioral activation in cognitive therapy.

The third, and perhaps most compelling reason to use DBT for mood disorders derives from DBT trials suggesting DBT is a feasible and effective treatment for individuals with mood disorder. Lynch *et al.* (2003, 2007) tested the feasibility, acceptability, and preliminary effectiveness of DBT for depressed older adults (aged 55 and older) in two RCTs. Lynch *et al.* (2003) compared medication to medication plus group DBT skills training plus weekly telephone coaching. They found individuals receiving DBT skills plus medication were more likely to remit, as indicated by scores on clinician-administered and self-reported depression measures, than patients receiving medication only. Significant decreases in self-reported depression and hopelessness were observed among DBT skills participants pre- to post-treatment, though gains among DBT skills participants were not significantly greater than those among patients receiving medication only. DBT skills training and telephone coaching as an adjunctive to medication management also proved acceptable and feasible, as indicated by low dropout rates and participant feedback. In a second trial, Lynch *et al.* (2007) compared 6 months of standard DBT plus medication to medication only among depressed older adults who had not remitted after 8 weeks of psychopharmacotherapy. A similar, small to moderate effect (Cohen's $d = 0.3–0.49$) of treatment on depression was observed for both treatments. Lynch *et al.* (2007) concluded DBT for depression among older individuals was a treatment with clinical promise.

In all five RCTS of DBT that have evaluated depressive symptoms as a secondary outcome, patients receiving DBT had significant reductions in depressive symptoms (Linehan *et al.* 1991, 2006, Koons *et al.* 2001, Clarkin *et al.* 2007, McMain *et al.* 2009). Notably, in 2012, Bedics *et al.* found significant reductions in depressive symptoms were maintained 1 year post-treatment, and Koons *et al.* (2001) found self-reported reductions in depressive symptoms were greater in DBT compared with treatment-as-usual participants. Superiority of DBT vs. treatment-as-usual in reducing depressive symptoms was also observed in a controlled trial conducted in a routine public mental health setting (Pasieczny

and Connor, 2011). Specifically, Pasieczny and Connor found large reductions (Cohen's $d = 1.23$) in self-reported depression among BPD patients receiving DBT, the large majority of whom had co-morbid major depression or BD. Additional support for the potential effectiveness of DBT for treating mood disorder include studies showing improvements in symptoms associated with mood disorder. Bedics *et al.* (2012) found DBT patients compared to BPD patients receiving treatment by experts (non-DBT) realized significantly greater increases in self-love, protection, and affirmation, and were conversely, less attacking towards themselves, over the course of treatment. These relative gains in self-reported self-affiliation were maintained for 1 year post-treatment. Carter *et al.* (2010) found BPD individuals receiving DBT, compared to BPD individuals maintained in treatment-as-usual while awaiting DBT, reported greater reductions in the number of days spent in bed during treatment.

High retention rates in the DBT arm of two RCTs of DBT for BPD in which sample members had significant rates of co-morbid major depression further shows DBT is an acceptable and feasible treatment for individuals with major depression (Linehan *et al.* 2006, McMain *et al.* 2009). Linehan *et al.* (2006), in a sample in which 70% of BPD patients had a co-morbid condition, found 80% of those randomized to DBT maintained in treatment. This retention rate was significantly higher than the rate observed among patients treated by experts.

On the other hand, using DBT to treat patients without multiple difficulties and extreme behavioral dysregulation, e.g., depressed patients, perhaps, may be akin to "killing a fly with a sledge-hammer," or an unnecessary or even ineffective use of resources (Koerner *et al.* 2007). Koerner *et al.* (2007) in fact warn against using DBT when etiological theories or theories of change for the disorder do not match well to those of DBT. In alignment with this contention, some data show treatment gains among more severe DBT patients are greater than those among less severe patients. Verhuel *et al.* (2003) in comparing DBT to treatment-as-usual for women with BPD, found those women with a history of repeated self-harm behavior receiving DBT self-harmed less than those receiving treatment-as-usual. Further, among patients with fewer lifetime episodes of self-harm, reductions in self-harm over the course of treatment appeared similar (and similarly minimal) in both the treatment-as-usual and DBT conditions. Only one

(Koons *et al.* 2001) of five of the RCTs which evaluated depression outcomes among BPD patients found gains were specific to DBT. Linehan *et al.* (2006) reconciled differing views and explained limited empirical support for DBT for depression by stating, "findings fit the 2-stage model of DBT that targets out-of-control behaviors first (stage 1 target) among more severe patients (stage 1 DBT target) and targets 'quiet desperation' such as depression (stage 2 DBT target) among less severe patients who demonstrate behavioral control" (p. 765).

While there is some evidence supporting DBT for major depression, all RCTs of standard DBT, including those testing DBT in elderly depressed patients (Lynch *et al.* 2007), excluded individuals with BD. A few less well-controlled studies of DBT for BPD have included small numbers of BD patients (e.g., Pasieczny and Connor, 2011). Thus, using DBT for BD is not supported by secondary data. Koerner *et al.* (2007), in fact, warn against using DBT for BD, stating, "DBT is not a panacea and should not be used as a first-line treatment if there is already another evidence-based practice for the problem or population. For example, it would be a mistake to offer DBT to patients with BD who had apparently failed at conventional treatment before being certain that *in fact* evidence-based treatments for these disorders had been provided with good fidelity to those protocols" (pp. 25–26).

Adaptations of DBT

Adapting DBT is different from adopting DBT. In the latter, DBT, e.g., the modes of treatment delivery, may be changed to meet the needs of the setting or target population. The original DBT model, including the principles, assumptions, theories, and functions, is, however, maintained. Programs which adopt comprehensive DBT benefit from the existing evidence base. Alternatively, a program may forgo delivering comprehensive DBT and instead offer DBT-informed services or portions of the model (e.g., skills training). A third option is adapting DBT. When DBT is adapted, systematic innovations to biosocial theory and the treatment model are made. Such changes are based on empirical and theoretical understanding of what works for the targeted population or in the targeted setting. Outcomes are then evaluated, and systematic refinements and re-evaluations are conducted. Adapting DBT is, in other words, like developing a new treatment (Rounsaville *et al.* 2001).

Upon considering the costs and benefits associated with each option, Koerner *et al.* (2007) conclude, "the evidence to date supports adopting the standard model (unless one is adopting an adaptation that has itself become evidence-based)" (p. 34).

Nonetheless, a number of adaptations of DBT have been made, with promising results (Linehan *et al.* 1999, 2002, Stanley *et al.* 2007). These include adaptations for higher levels of care, forensic, adolescent, substance use disorder, and eating disordered populations (Dimeff and Koerner, 2007). Stanley *et al.* (2007) shortened the treatment from 1 year to 6 months. Two adaptations for mood disorder have been developed, one for adolescents with BD (Goldstein *et al.* 2007) and one for treatment-resistant depressed elders (Lynch *et al.* 2007).

Lynch (2000, Lynch *et al.* 2007) adapted DBT for depressed elderly individuals (aged 55 or older) who were treatment-resistant or who had a co-morbid personality disorder. Primary adaptations included addition of two targets, reducing behaviors functionally related to depression and increasing openness to experience, as the highest third-level primary targets (Lynch, 2000, Lynch and Cheavens, 2007). Reconciling unresolved grievances and decreasing behaviors functionally related to depressive relapse are additional targets (Lynch, 2000, Lynch and Cheavens, 2007). Additional changes to the structure and content of treatment (e.g., secondary targets, skills, length and frequency of treatment) reflect knowledge of difficulties and patterns in depression (Lynch, 2000, Lynch and Cheavens, 2007). The biosocial theory was also accordingly adapted. Rigid, maladaptive coping is conceptualized as the core difficulty. It is posited to result from the interaction of a biological predisposition towards negative affect and environmental experiences which reinforce maladaptive rigid coping. Additionally, avoidance of experiences which may reinforce more adaptive ways of coping with negative affect is posited to contribute to pathology (Lynch and Cheavens, 2007). DBT adapted for depressed, elderly individuals with co-morbid personality disorder has not yet been tested (Lynch *et al.* 2007).

Goldstein *et al.* (2007) adapted the adolescent version of DBT (Miller *et al.* 2007) for BD adolescents. Adaptations included changes to the length and timing of treatment and the content of skills training for family members and adolescents. These changes were made to increase the likelihood that skills would be applicable, useful, and utilized during different mood episodes. The biosocial theory was also expanded to reflect limited understanding of specific environmental risk factors for BD (Goldstein *et al.* 2007). In a small, open pilot trial, Goldstein *et al.* (2007) found BD adolescents realized significant reductions in suicidal ideation and depressive symptoms pre- to post-DBT treatment. It was also found to be acceptable to patients and their family members, as indicated by high treatment attendance rates and satisfaction ratings (Goldstein *et al.* 2007).

Future directions

DBT is an efficacious treatment proven to reduce suicidal behavior and nonsuicidal self-injury. DBT has been adapted for both bipolar adolescents and geriatric patients with treatment-resistant depression or depression co-morbid with BPD. Only small pilot and feasibility studies, however, have tested the acceptability and preliminary effectiveness of DBT for mood disorders. Large-scale randomized trials are thus needed to evaluate the efficacy of DBT adapted for mood disorders.

References

American Psychiatric Association (2000). *Diagnostic and Statistical Manual of Mental Disorder, Fourth Edition, Text Revision*. Washington, DC: American Psychiatric Association.

American Psychiatric Association (2001). *Practice Guideline for the Treatment of Patients with Borderline Personality Disorder*. Arlington, VA: American Psychiatric Publishing.

Beck, A.T., Freeman, A., and Davis, D.D. (2003). *Cognitive Therapy of Personality Disorders, Second Edition*. New York: Guilford.

Bedics, J.D., Atkins, D.C., Comtois, K.A., and Linehan, M.M. (2012). Treatment differences in the therapeutic relationship and introject during a 2-year randomized controlled trial of dialectical behavior therapy versus nonbehavioral psychotherapy experts for borderline personality disorder. *Journal of Consulting and Clinical Psychology*, 80, 66–77.

Carter, G.L., Willcox, C.H., Lewin, T.J., Conrad, A.M., and Bendit, N. (2010). Hunter DBT project: Randomized controlled trial of dialectical behaviour therapy in women with borderline personality disorder. *Australian and New Zealand Journal of Psychiatry*, 44, 162–173.

Chambless, D.L., Baker, M.J., Baucom, D.H. *et al.* (1998). Update on empirically validated therapies, II. *The Clinical Psychologist*, 51, 3–16.

Clarkin, J.F., Yeomans, F., and Kernberg, O.F. (1999). *Psychotherapy of Borderline Personality*. New York: John Wiley and Sons.

Clarkin, J.F., Levy, K.N., Lenzenweger, M.F., and Kernberg, O.F. (2007). Evaluating three treatments for borderline personality disorder: A multiwave study. *American Journal of Psychiatry*, 164, 922–928.

Dimeff, L. and Linehan, M.M. (2001). Dialectical behavior therapy in a nutshell. *The California Psychologist*, 34, 10–13.

Dimeff, L.A. and Linehan, M.M. (2006). *Summary of Research on DBT* [online]. Available: http://behavioraltech.org/downloads/dbtSummaryOfData.pdf (accessed October 2012).

Dimeff, L.A. and Koerner, K. (eds.) (2007). *Dialectical Behavior Therapy in Clinical Practice: Applications Across Disorders and Settings*. New York: Guilford.

Favazza, A.R. (1998). The coming of age of self-mutilation. *Journal of Nervous and Mental Disease*, 186, 259–268.

Goldstein, T.R., Axelson, D.A., Birmaher, B., and Brent, D.A. (2007). Dialectical behavior therapy for adolescents with BD: A 1-year open trial. *Journal of the American Academy of Child and Adolescent Psychiatry*, 46, 820–830.

Grant, B.F. Chou P., Goldstein R.B. *et al.* (2008). Prevalence, correlates, disability, and comorbidity of DSM-IV borderline personality disorder: Results from the Wave 2 National Epidemiologic Survey on Alcohol and Related Conditions. *The Journal of Clinical Psychiatry*, 69, 533.

Gross, J.J. and Thompson, R.A. (2007). Emotion regulation: Conceptual foundations. In Gross, J.J., ed., *Handbook of Emotion Regulation*. New York: Guilford, 3–24.

Gunderson, J.G., Weinberg, I., Daversa, M.T., and Kueppenbender, K.D. (2006). Descriptive and longitudinal observations on the relationship of borderline personality disorder and bipolar disorder. *The American Journal of Psychiatry*, 163, 1173–1178.

Hayes, S.C. (2004). Acceptance and commitment therapy, relational frame theory, and the third wave of behavioral and cognitive therapies. *Behavior Therapy*, 35, 639–665.

Jacobson, C.M. and Gould, M. (2007). The epidemiology and phenomenology of non-suicidal self-injurious behavior among adolescents: A critical review of the literature. *Archives of Suicide Research*, 11, 129–147.

Jacobson, N.S., Dobson, K.S., Truax, P.A. *et al.* (1996). A component analysis of cognitive-behavioral treatment for depression. *Journal of Consulting and Clinical Psychology*, 64, 295–304.

Koerner, K. and Dimeff, L.A. (2007). Overview of dialectical behavior therapy. In Dimeff, L.A. and Koerner, K., eds., *Dialectical Behavior Therapy in*

Clinical Practice: Applications Across Disorders and Settings. New York: Guilford, 1–18.

Koerner, K., Dimeff, L.A., and Swenson, C.R. (2007). Adopt or adapt? Fidelity matters. In Dimeff, L.A. and Koerner, K., eds., *Dialectical Behavior Therapy in Clinical Practice: Applications Across Disorders and Settings.* New York: Guilford, 19–36.

Koons, C.R., Robins, C.J., Lindsey Tweed, J. *et al.* (2001). Efficacy of dialectical behavior therapy in women veterans with borderline personality disorder. *Behavior Therapy*, 32, 371–390.

Linehan, M.M. (1987). Dialectical behavioral therapy: A cognitive behavioral approach to parasuicide. *Journal of Personality Disorders*, 1, 328–333.

Linehan, M.M. (1993a). *Cognitive-Behavioral Treatment of Borderline Personality Disorder.* New York: Guilford.

Linehan, M.M. (1993b). *Skills Training Manual for Treating Borderline Personality Disorder.* New York: Guilford.

Linehan, M.M., Armstrong, H.E., Suarez, A., Allmon, D., and Heard, H.L. (1991). Cognitive-behavioral treatment of chronically parasuicidal borderline patients. *Archives of General Psychiatry*, 48, 1060–1064.

Linehan, M.M., Schmidt, H., Dimeff, L.A. *et al.* (1999). Dialectical behavior therapy for patients with borderline personality disorder and drug-dependence. *The American Journal on Addictions*, 8, 279–292.

Linehan M.M., Dimeff L.A., Reynolds S.K. *et al.* (2002). Dialectical behavior therapy versus comprehensive validation plus 12-step for the treatment of opioid dependent women meeting criteria for borderline personality disorder. *Drug and Alcohol Dependence*, 67, 13–26.

Linehan, M.M., Comtois, K.A., Murray, A.M. *et al.* (2006). Two-year randomized controlled trial and follow-up of dialectical behavior therapy vs. therapy by experts for suicidal behaviors and borderline personality disorder. *Archives of General Psychiatry*, 63, 757–766.

Lynch, T.R. (2000). Treatment of elderly depression with personality disorder comorbidity using dialectical behavior therapy. *Cognitive and Behavioral Practice*, 7, 468–477.

Lynch, T.R. and Cheavens, J.S. (2007). Dialectical behavior therapy for depression with comorbid personality disorder: An extension of standard dialectical behavior therapy with a special emphasis on the treatment of older adults. In Dimeff, L.A. and Koerner, K., eds., *Dialectical Behavior Therapy in Clinical Practice: Applications Across Disorders and Settings.* New York: Guilford.

Lynch T.R., Morse J.Q., Mendelson T., and Robins C.J. (2003). Dialectical behavior therapy for depressed older adults: a randomized pilot study. *American Journal of Geriatric Psychiatry* 11, 1–13.

Lynch, T.R., Cheavens, J.S., Cukrowicz, K.C. *et al.* (2007). Treatment of older adults with co-morbid personality disorder and depression: A dialectical behavior therapy approach. *International Journal of Geriatric Psychiatry*, 22, 131–143.

McMain, S.F., Links, P.S., Gnam, W.H. *et al.* (2009). A randomized trial of dialectical behavior therapy versus general psychiatric management for borderline personality disorder. *American Journal of Psychiatry*, 166, 1365–1374.

Miller, A., Rathus, J.H., and Linehan, M.M. (2007). *Dialectical Behavior Therapy with Suicidal Adolescents.* New York: Guilford.

Pasieczny, N. and Connor, J. (2011). The effectiveness of dialectical behaviour therapy in routine public mental health settings: An Australian controlled trial. *Behaviour Research and Therapy*, 49, 4–10.

Robbins, C.J. (2002). Zen principles and mindfulness practice in dialectical behavior therapy. *Cognitive Behavioral Practice*, 9, 50–57.

Rounsaville, B.J., Carroll, K.M., and Onken, L.S. (2001). A stage model of behavioral therapies research: Getting started and moving on from stage I. *Clinical Psychology: Science and Practice*, 8, 133–142.

Stanley B. and Brodsky B. (2009). Dialectical behavior therapy. In Oldham, J.M., Skodol, A.E., and Bender, D.S., eds., *Essentials of Personality Disorders, First Edition.* Washington, DC: American Psychiatric Publishing, 235–251.

Stanley, B. and Brown, G.K. (2012). Safety planning intervention: A brief intervention to mitigate suicide risk. *Cognitive and Behavioral Practice*, 19, 256–264.

Stanley, B., Brodsky, B., Nelson, J.D., and Dulit, R. (2007). Brief dialectical behavior therapy (DBT-B) for suicidal behavior and non-suicidal self injury. *Archives of Suicide Research*, 11, 337–341.

Verheul, R., Van Den Bosch, L.M., Koeter, M.W., De Ridder, M.A., Stijnen, T., and Van Den Brink, W. (2003). Dialectical behaviour therapy for women with borderline personality disorder. *The British Journal of Psychiatry*, 182, 135–140.

Zanarini, M.C., Frankenburg, F.R., Dubo, E.D. *et al.* (1998). Axis I comorbidity of borderline personality disorder. *American Journal of Psychiatry*, 155, 1733–1739.

Chapter

22

The psychodynamic treatment of mood disorders

Deborah L. Cabaniss, Diana E. Moga, and Aerin M. Hyun

Introduction

Psychodynamic psychotherapy is a treatment based on the premise that conscious thoughts, feelings, and behavior are affected by unconscious mental activity. It is called by many different names, including expressive psychotherapy, exploratory psychotherapy, or insight-oriented psychotherapy. Its basic theory of therapeutic action is that, in the context of the relationship with the therapist, patients can benefit from learning about their unconscious thoughts and feelings. This can help them to become more aware of maladaptive coping mechanisms and fantasies that are leading to symptoms and problematic character patterns, and it can help the therapist to support their weakened ego functions (Cabaniss *et al.* 2011).

Prior to the advent of antidepressant medication and manualized psychotherapies in the second half of the twentieth century, virtually all mood disorders were treated with psychodynamic psychotherapy or psychoanalysis. Today psychodynamic psychotherapy for mood disorders spans a wide range of short-term (generally 12–24 sessions) and long-term psychotherapies (typically lasting over 6 months or a year) based on different psychodynamic theories and a multitude of books and treatment manuals. The common denominator making these treatments "psychodynamic" is their focus on underlying psychological conflicts and deficits that increase a person's vulnerability to depression. Thus, these treatments have goals that, in addition to symptom relief, explore the person's development, self-experience, relationships with others, and characteristic coping mechanisms. They often use the patient's previous experience of the therapist to illuminate ways in which the person thinks about him/herself and interacts with others (e.g., transference).

This chapter will review:

- The evidence base for the use of psychodynamic psychotherapy in mood disorders.
- Three models of psychodynamic psychotherapy that have been used in mood disorders.
- Basic techniques for conducting psychodynamic psychotherapy in mood disorders.

The evidence base for psychodynamic psychotherapy in mood disorders

Depression

As the number of effective treatments for depression increases, and newer antidepressants with more tolerable side-effect profiles are developed, there is increasing pressure to provide research evidence for the efficacy of psychodynamic psychotherapy for depression. While research supporting the efficacy of psychodynamic psychotherapy has been slower to emerge compared to that for cognitive behavior therapy (CBT) or interpersonal psychotherapy (IPT), this body of literature has steadily increased. Psychodynamic psychotherapy is now included as an evidence-based psychotherapy for depression in the most recent APA practice guidelines for the treatment of major depressive disorder (2002).

Short-term psychodynamic psychotherapy (STPP)

Because short-term psychodynamic psychotherapy (STPP) was initially used in research as a comparator arm for newly emerging therapies such as CBT, it was often delivered in an unstructured way (using inexperienced or untrained therapists, no treatment manuals, no adherence measures, undefined length of time) or by therapists who lacked allegiance to the

---

treatment. Under such conditions STPP was found to be inferior to CBT (Churchill *et al.* 2001). However, Leichsenring's (2001) meta-analysis of STPP vs. CBT, which included only large, systematically conducted studies (defined as: using clearly defined depressive populations, manualized treatments, and trained therapists; lasting at least 13 sessions; and measuring their adherence to the treatment and competence – these studies are marked in Table 22.1 by asterisks), found that STPP and CBT were equally effective for depressive symptoms and that they did not differ significantly in response or remission rates.

Since this meta-analysis, newer randomized controlled trials have compared STPP to more purely supportive therapies (Table 22.1) or to medications for major and minor depressions. Burnard *et al.* (2002) randomized 95 patients with major depression of at least moderate severity (a Hamilton Depression Rating Scale, or HDRS, of at least 20) to either clomipramine alone (control arm) or combined treatment with clomipramine and STPP (treatment arm, consisting of the clomipramine protocol plus 10 weeks of STPP using manual-trained therapists supervised by a psychoanalyst and monitored for adherence). A particular strength of this study is that the authors matched the amount of time spent with the therapist in the treatment arm with the amount of supportive care provided by the psychiatrist in the control group (consisting of empathic listening, guidance, support, and facilitation of an alliance), allowing the treatment effects to be specifically attributed to psychodynamic treatment rather than other common therapeutic factors. No difference was found between the control and treatment arms in the HDRS scores; however, patients in the active treatment arms were less likely to experience treatment failure (defined as a major depressive episode still present at the end of 10 weeks), had better ratings of function and fewer days of hospitalization, and also lost fewer days of work during treatment. In addition, the cost analysis indicated mean savings of $2311 per patient when the indirect costs of sick leave were added to the costs incurred by hospitalization.

In a small study of 30 patients with dysthymia or minor depression randomized to brief dynamic therapy (BDT, a manualized form of STPP that focuses on a focal problem or life event precipitating depression), brief supportive psychotherapy, or wait list controls, Maina *et al.* (2005) found that both the BDT and the supportive psychotherapy arms showed improvements in the HRDS compared to wait is list controls by the end of 6 months. However, patients treated with BDT showed a statistically significant further improvement in their depressive symptoms at 6-month follow-up compared to those treated with supportive psychotherapy. A similar effect at the 6-month follow-up was observed when BDT and brief supportive therapy were added to medication treatment in a sicker population of patients with major depressive disorder (Maina *et al.* 2007). Both treatment arms showed an average decrease of 10 points in the mean HDRS from baseline at the end of treatment; however, at the 6-month follow-up point the BDT arm continued to show improvement, while maintained on antidepressants (a further decrease of 4 points from end of treatment), whereas the supportive arm showed a worsening of HDRS mean scores (an increase of 3 points). Both Burnard and Maina's studies indicate a specific effect of short-term psychodynamic treatment in improving depressive symptoms when added to antidepressant medications, as compared to supportive psychotherapy. In addition Maina's studies suggest that brief psychodynamic treatment continues to affect patients over time while they are maintained on antidepressant medication. This cannot be explained by the passage of time alone, as supportive therapy does not show the same benefit in two separate trials.

Two studies that compared the efficacy of STPP to antidepressant medication found them to work equally well in depressed patients. Salminen *et al.* (2008) randomized 51 patients with mild or moderate major depression (HDRS of 15 or greater) to either 16 weekly sessions of psychodynamic psychotherapy, or 16 weeks of treatment with fluoxetine up to 40 mg, administered by a general practitioner. The authors found no difference in HDRS, Beck Depression Inventory (BDI), or an assessment of functional capacity at the end of the 4-month study between the psychodynamic psychotherapy and the fluoxetine group, and remission rates (HDRS less than 7) corresponded to 46% and 48%, respectively. Limitations of this study include that the study did not control for time spent with a clinician (making it difficult to exclude the effects of common therapeutic factors), and that fluoxetine was only titrated to a moderate dose (raising the possibility that more patients would have responded to a higher dose). De Maat's (2008) meta-analysis pooled data from three separate randomized control trials (Jonghe *et al.* 2001, 2004, Dekker *et al.* 2005) of patients with major

Table 22.1 Randomized controlled trials of short-term psychodynamic psychotherapy (STPP) compared to other therapies in the treatment of depression (with or without combined pharmacotherapy)

Study	Diagnosis	Population	Patients in STPP arm	Comparison groups	Manuals used	Treatment duration	Outcome
Hersen et al. 1984	Unipolar depression Feighner Raskin Scale >7	Women outpatients	22	STPP+placebo, social skills+ placebo, amitriptyline alone, social skills+amitriptyline	No information	12 sessions + 6–8 maintenance sessions	No difference in outcomes between STPP and social skills training at treatment end and at 6-months follow-up
Thompson et al. 1987; Gallagher-Thompson et al. 1990	MDD as defined by RDC, BDI>17, HDRS>14	Outpatients > 60 years old without cognitive impairment. Not on anti-depressant medications	24	Behavioral therapy, CBT, STPP, delayed treatment control	Horowitz and Kaltreider, 1979	16–20	No difference between behavioral therapy, CBT, and STPP, all showed improvement over delayed treatment control. No significant difference at 1- and 2-year follow-up
Gallagher-Thompson and Steffen, 1994	Major, minor or intermittent depressive disorder by RDC, BDI>10	Primary care-givers, mean age of 62. Not on antidepressant medications	30	CBT vs. STPP	Mann 1973, Rose and Del-Maestro, 1990	16–20	No significant difference between the two therapies at treatment ending and 3-month follow-up
The Sheffield Psychotherapy Project: Shapiro et al. 1994; 1-year follow-up: Shapiro et al. 1995	DSM-III MDD BDI>16	White-collar workers in England. On stable medications without major co-morbidities	58	8 vs. 16 sessions of CBT or STPP	Shapiro and Firth, 1985	8 vs. 16	Advantage to CBT over STPP in BDI at end of treatment. No difference on six other measurements. No difference at 3-month follow-up. At 1-year follow-up, 8 session STPP less effective than other conditions. No difference between 16 sessions of STPP and CBT
Barkham et al. 1996: Replicating the second Sheffield Psychotherapy Project	Same as above	Outpatients from three national health sites in England. Medications allowed	18	8 vs. 16 sessions of CBT or STPP	Shapiro and Firth, 1985	8 vs. 16	Advantage of CBT compared to STPP only on IIP scale and only at end of treatment, not 3-month or 1-year follow-up
Maina et al. 2005	DSM-IV dysthymic disorder, adjustment disorder with depressed mood, or depressive disorder NOS. HDRS 8–15	Outpatients with recent precipitant life event in Italy. Major co-morbidities and antidepressant medication use excluded	10	Wait list, brief supportive therapy, and BDT	Malan, 1976	15–30 sessions	BDT more effective than brief supportive therapy at follow up evaluation. Both treatment conditions improved compared to wait-list control
Burnard et al. 2002	MDD by DSM-IV and HDRS>20	Outpatients 20–65 in Switzerland. Major co-morbidities excluded	35	Clomipramine+ STPP vs. clomipramine + supportive care	Authors own dynamic model	10 weeks (number of sessions not specified)	No difference between groups in HDRS scores. However, patients receiving STPP less likely to experience treatment failure (MDD still present at 10 weeks) and with lower rates of hospitalization-> STPP found to be cost-effective

Table 22.1 (cont.)

Study	Diagnosis	Population	Patients in STPP arm	Comparison groups	Manuals used	Treatment duration	Outcome
Maina et al. 2007	MDD in DSM-IV-R and HDRS>15	Outpatients with a precipitant life event or focal stressor 18–65 in Italy without major co-morbidities	18	BDT+ celexa or paxil vs. brief supportive therapy + celexa or paxil	Malan, 1963	6 months of 15–30 weekly sessions	No difference at 6 months, but patients in BDT continued to improve and had significantly lower HDRS and HAM-A scores and better assessment of function scores at 1 year compared to patients in brief supportive therapy

depression. In the first trial, patients were randomized to either medication alone (a pharmacological algorithm involving three steps as clinically indicated: an SSRI, a TCA, and an MAOI) or to combined treatment with medication and short-term psychodynamic supportive psychotherapy (SPSP). SPSP is a manualized short-term treatment that leans towards the supportive end of the supportive–expressive spectrum, while maintaining a relational emphasis in which the transference is used to understand the patient and effect psychotherapeutic change. Remission rates (HDRS less than 7) were significantly higher at the end of the study for the patients in combined treatment compared to medication alone. Furthermore, the pharmacotherapy dropout rate was lower in the combined treatment arm than in the pharmacotherapy arm (22% vs. 40%, respectively). Although once again time spent with a clinician was not controlled for, this study does indicate that the addition of psychodynamic psychotherapy to medication treatment can help improve response and medication adherence in depressed patients.

De Jonghe et al.'s 2004 study compared patients in SPSP to patients in SPSP with medication (a four-step algorithm using an SNRI, an SSRI, a TCA, and a TCA plus lithium). No significant difference was found in remission rates between the groups. In a third study, Dekker et al. (2005) compared two different lengths of combined treatment (8 or 16 sessions) and found no significant difference between the two treatment intensities.

Finally, de Maat et al. (2008) pooled the patients in these studies in a mega-analysis to indirectly compare the effects of SPSP, pharmacotherapy, and their combination. No significant differences were found in the remission and response rates by HDRS in the pharmacotherapy vs. psychotherapy arms (24.4 vs. 30.9%, respective remission rates; 35.6 and 40.2%, respective

response rates); however, combined treatment had a significantly higher remission rate when compared to pharmacotherapy alone (24.4% vs. 40.4%). There was no significant difference between SPSP alone and combined treatment.

Overall, these studies indicate that in the minor depressive disorders as well as mild and moderate major depression, STPP is an effective treatment option. Its efficacy is comparable to CBT and to medication treatment. In addition, STPP has demonstrated added efficacy when combined with pharmacotherapy in improving depressive symptoms, decreasing functional impairment and the need for hospitalization, and improving compliance with pharmacotherapy.

Long-term psychodynamic psychotherapy (LTPP)

There are currently no published randomized controlled trials of LTPP in a homogeneous depressed population. Long-term psychotherapy is harder to study due to cost and higher likelihood of attrition, and often lends itself more favorably to naturalistic or observational studies. For example, Bond and Perry (2004) conducted a 3-year, naturalistic study of LTPP in outpatients with both Axis 1 and Axis II disorders (73% of whom had depressive disorders) with or without concomitant medications. They found that those patients with depressive symptoms at intake improved significantly, both in terms of their depressive symptomatology and in their overall defensive functioning. Leichsenring and Rabung's (2008) meta-analysis of LTPP (defined here as over 1 year) for patients with complex mental disorders (i.e., personality disorders, chronic or multiple mental disorders) included 11 randomized controlled trials and 12 observational studies of patients with anxiety, depressive, eating, and personality disorders. The authors found that patients treated with LTPP fared better in terms of target symptoms and personality functioning compared to shorter forms of psychotherapy. In the Helsinki psychotherapy study (Knekt *et al.* 2008), 326 outpatients with mood (84.7%) or anxiety disorders were randomly assigned to three treatment groups (LTPP, STPP, or solution-focused psychotherapy) and were followed up for 3 years using the HDRS and the Beck Depression Inventory (BDI) to monitor depressive symptoms. Although at 1-year follow-up STPP was found to be more effective than LTPP in terms of depressive symptomatology, after 3 years LTPP was found to be more effective than both for reducing depressive symptoms (Knekt *et al.* 2011).

Thus, despite the lack of conclusive evidence for the efficacy of LTPP for depressive disorders, these naturalistic studies suggest that depressed patients may continue to improve with longer-term psychodynamic psychotherapy and that their improvement may be related to the development of more adaptive coping mechanisms.

Post-partum depression

In the one published study of psychodynamic psychotherapy for post-partum depression (PPD) (Cooper *et al.* 2003) subjects were randomly assigned to receive routine primary care, nondirective counseling, CBT, or psychodynamic therapy and were assessed at 4.5, 9, 18 and 60 months post-partum. Participants were assessed using the Edinburgh Postnatal Depression Scale (EPDS; as a self-report measure) and the depression section of the Structured Clinical Interview for the DSM-III-TR (SCID). Additionally, provider adherence was examined (using Therapist Rating Scale), as well as the children's cognitive and emotional development and the quality of the mother–infant interactions. While maternal mood improved with all three treatments at 4.5 months, only psychodynamic therapy produced a reduction in depression that was significantly superior to control. However, this benefit was no longer apparent by 9 months post-partum, and treatment did not reduce subsequent episodes of PPD. Limitations of the study were its small size and the brief period of treatment. It should be borne in mind that episodes of major depression, including post-partum depression, last about 6 months, and therefore measuring treatment outcome beyond 6 months begins to detect an increasing number of patients whose depression has remitted spontaneously, making the detection of a treatment effect more difficult. Further studies are needed to understand the underlying psychodynamics

of post-partum depression, as well as the efficacy and effectiveness of psychodynamic psychotherapy in PPD.

Bipolar disorder

Gonzalez and Prohoda (2007) found that psychodynamic group therapy for bipolar patients led to improvement in depressive, but not manic symptoms, and recommended that this form of treatment should be considered as adjunctive to psychopharmacologic management of acute bipolar illness. The current APA practice guidelines recommend the use of psychotherapy of any kind for bipolar illness only during the maintenance period of illness. The guidelines do note the role that group therapy may play in treating individuals with bipolar illness, as well as the fact that evidence suggests that prognosis is more favorable for those receiving monthly supportive psychotherapy addressing illness management, interpersonal difficulties, and co-morbidities.

Models of psychodynamic psychotherapy used in depression

To illustrate the types of psychodynamic psychotherapy that are used to treat mood disorders, we will outline three models that have a substantial research basis and are used in teaching psychodynamic psychotherapy for depression. They are:

1. Brief dynamic therapy (BDT).
2. Psychodynamic treatment of depression model of Busch *et al.* (2004).
3. Supportive expressive psychotherapy (SE).

All three models focus on long-standing difficulties in relationships as a source of painful feelings of disappointment, anger, and blame, which, when internalized, lead to a sense of helplessness and worthlessness, and a wish to isolate oneself from others. They use the therapeutic relationship to collaboratively examine the emergence of this pattern with the therapist, allowing the patient to then learn experientially about him/herself in relationships. This experience then provides the impetus for growth and change.

BDT is a short-term, focused form of psychodynamic psychotherapy that is usually conducted in 16–20 sessions. During an extended evaluation period (two to five, 45-minute sessions), the therapist discerns problematic patterns in the patient's interpersonal relationships with family members and other individuals, and in the emerging transference with the therapist. These core relational patterns generally contribute to the depressive symptoms that led the individual to seek treatment in the first place. They are brought to the patient's attention during the course of the initial evaluation period and then are used to establish a focus for the treatment. The goal of the treatment is for patients to change something about these problematic patterns within the time-limited period of the treatment. The treatment is broken down into opening, middle, and termination phases. In the opening phase (two to five sessions), a focus is established and offered to the patient. The middle phase (10–12 sessions) is spent deepening the focus, particularly in the context of the developing transference. Termination is spent reflecting on what the patient has learned about his/her interpersonal patterns, as well as about the ending of the treatment and what it means to the patient. Termination may also involve examining and confronting how the patient deals with endings in general. The optimism of the beginning and middle sessions gives way to the sadness of terminating, and these are also closely examined within the treatment (Mann, 1973).

Psychodynamic Treatment of Depression (Busch *et al.* 2004) outlines a core dynamic formulation for depression in which "narcissistic vulnerability is seen as fundamental to the susceptibility to depression." They suggest that people who have this vulnerability more easily experience disappointment and rejection, which they translate into rage. The introjection of that rage results in feelings of depression, guilt, and worthlessness. Using this basic model, they offer a manual for the treatment of depression that focuses on helping to mitigate the vulnerability to depression. Their model involves three phases:

- Phase 1 – Beginning of treatment. In this phase, patient and therapist explore stressors, perceptions, and feelings related to the onset of the depression and link them to core dynamics, including narcissistic vulnerability, conflicted anger, guilt, and shame, and various defenses.
- Phase 2 – Treating vulnerability to depression. Using exploration of feelings, fantasies, and their transference, patients gain increased understanding of the way in which they turn disappointing experiences into depression.

- Phase 3 – Termination. This phase deals with narcissistic vulnerabilities that arise in the context of leaving treatment, and consolidates gains.

As exemplified by the outline provided above, brief dynamic psychotherapy offers a focused approach based on psychodynamic principles, with a nicely outlined, accessible manual for practitioners.

SE therapy aims at symptom relief and limited changes in personality structure by means of developing patients' insight into their conflictual relationship patterns, or core conflictual relationship themes (CCRT) in the context of a supportive relationship with the therapist (Luborsky, 1984). SE therapy manuals have been developed for a variety of Axis I and II disorders, including depression (Luborsky *et al.* 1995). SE therapy can be carried out as either a short-term and highly focused treatment or as a long-term treatment for up to several years. After an initial period in which the therapist works actively to foster a strong therapeutic alliance using specific supportive techniques outlined in the manual, patient and therapist formulate the patient's main relationship problems as modeled by the CCRT. A CCRT has three components:

1. The patient's wishes, needs, and interpersonal intentions, e.g., " I wish that X would notice me."
2. An anticipated response from the other, e.g, "but X will probably ignore me," or a subjective perception of how the other has responded, "he smiled but only to be polite."
3. A response from the self or reaction (feelings, behavior) to the anticipated or perceived response from the other, e.g., "I can never get anyone to notice me."

A typical CCRT that occurs in depression (Vanheule *et al.* 2006) involves the patient's wish to be happy and understood by others, along with the perception of others' dislike that stands in conflict with these wishes. The patient then reacts by disliking others, and also feeling helpless to fulfill their wishes, leading to chronic hopelessness about ever being happy. Thus, helplessness and disliking others are defensive ways of responding to what is perceived as a rejecting or hostile environment to the patient's narcissistic needs and wishes. When treating depression, the therapist helps the patient link the CCRT to his current relationship difficulties and past significant relationships.

Guidelines for conducting psychodynamic psychotherapy in patients with mood disorders

Many psychodynamic techniques and interventions can be potentially helpful in the treatment of patients with mood disorders. These can be used alone or in combination with medication; note that it is important to remember that the presence of moderate to severe neurovegetative symptoms strongly suggest the need for medication in addition to psychotherapy.

Below, we will outline some of the basic techniques of psychodynamic psychotherapy to use with patients with mood disorders.

Beginning the treatment: Assessment, alliance and goal setting

Assessment

The evaluation of every patient needs to begin with a comprehensive assessment of symptoms, ego functions, coping strategies, super-ego function, and strengths and weaknesses. Discovering whether difficulties with mood regulation and weakened ego function are chronic or acute is key to forming reasonable goals for the treatment. As above, significant neurovegetative symptoms strongly suggest the need for combined treatment, while the presence of ego weakness suggests the need for ego support.

Alliance

A strong alliance is key for any treatment (DeFife and Hilsenroth, 2011) but it is particularly important for patients with mood disorders. Hopeless and helpless, patients with depression need to feel that the therapist is working with them and for them. Therapists can build alliance with this population by actively demonstrating interest, empathy, and understanding (Cabaniss *et al.* 2011), as in the following example:

> Patient: I just feel so terrible. I don't think that anyone could help me. And who would want to?
>
> Therapist: You have really been suffering – I can hear that in your voice and and in your story. I'm really glad that you came in when you did: I think that with medication and therapy we can work together to help you feel better.

This therapist is collaborative, empathic, and builds hope, which has been shown to be central to good therapeutic outcome. In mania, denial, omnipotence, and irritability pose a challenge to forming alliance; here again building trust by trying to understand the patient's experience is key. The therapist with a good alliance can help the patient with compliance, both with medication and psychotherapy (Gutheil, 1978), which can be an important part of psychodynamic psychotherapy with this population.

Goals

Working collaboratively to help patients with mood disorders to set realistic goals can be extremely therapeutic. This fosters alliance and helps to allow them to experience success as they recover, as in the following exchange:

> Patient: I have to get better in 2 weeks so that I can go back to school. If I don't it will be a disaster.
>
> Therapist: You have been very depressed – that's something that schools understand. Let's think together about what might be reasonable to expect in a few weeks. I think, for example, that you might start sleeping better, which would be a great start.

Once acute symptoms have diminished, the therapist and patient can work together to set new longer-term goals, including shifts in patterns relating to sense of self, relationships with others, and coping mechanisms.

Conducting the treatment

Both supporting and uncovering psychodynamic interventions can be helpful with the depressed patient.

Supporting weakened ego function

Mood disorders can lead to both acute and chronic weakness of many ego functions. Impairment of self-esteem management is a common problem in depression, often requiring encouragement and motivation during the acute phases, as well as support of strengths that the patient might not be able to utilize for buoying self-regard. Judgment and impulse control are often problematic in both depression and mania, putting patients at risk of self-harm during the acute phases of the illness. Interventions designed to ensure safety, such as jointly thinking through consequences, thinking of alternatives, and, when necessary, containing interventions such as hospitalization are often indicated. Patients with mood disorders often lack self-awareness, diminishing their ability to separate themselves from their current symptoms, thus modeling reflective function and psychoeducation can be very helpful at this time. Because these patients also frequently use less adaptive defenses, supportive interventions such as reinforcing adaptive defense mechanisms and discouraging less adaptive defenses are key therapeutic tools. Here is an example of an exchange with an acutely depressed patient using predominantly supporting interventions:

> Patient: I'm just a terrible mother – here I am, unable to even do things for myself and it's a time that my daughter really needs me.
>
> Therapist: I know that you feel that way, but many people feel that way when they're depressed (psychoeducation). Let's think together for a minute about your relationship with your daughter (modeling self-reflection). Didn't you tell me that she's applying to your alma mater? That sounds like she sees you as someone she'd like to emulate (reminding patient of strengths).
>
> Patient: You're right – it's hard to remember that when I feel so bad.

Uncovering unconscious thoughts and feelings

Although no one knows whether unconscious conflicts cause depressions, clinical experience tells us that many depressed people have similar unconscious thoughts, feelings, and fantasies. Interpreting these unconscious elements means helping patients to become consciously aware of them. This can help depressed patients to gain self-awareness and can aid recovery. For example, many depressed patients have unconscious fantasies, which, if uncovered, can be more thoughtfully considered and challenged. Here is an example:

> Patient: I feel so depressed – everyone tells me that I should take a semester off from school – and part of me agrees – but I can't get myself to do it – I don't know why.
>
> Therapist: Well, I remember that you told me that your father was very critical of your decision to take a year off between high school and college, and that he called you a failure. Perhaps you feel that taking time off now would mean that, too.
>
> Patient: I hadn't thought of that but I think that you're right – and the thing is, that didn't hurt my career at all.

Note that this kind of intervention requires the patient to be able to tolerate some affect and anxiety, since thoughts and feelings are unconscious because they are difficult to consciously experience.

Common themes

Common unconscious fantasies in depressed patients involve deserving punishment, being unlovable or worthless, and being completely helpless. As in the three models of psychodynamic therapy discussed above, problematic interpersonal patterns, often involving expectations of abandonment and disappointment, are also common. People often need to mourn the loss of their "undepressed" self, as in the following example:

> Patient: I know that I feel better when I take the medication, but I just keep them in the drawer. I only remember that I have them when I'm here.
>
> Therapist: Maybe you'd like to forget that you're depressed – taking a pill daily would remind you of that.
>
> Patient: I hate that. I'd like the whole thing to disappear – like waking up from a bad dream.

Discussions like this one can help people to acknowledge these fantasies in order to accept their depression and to aid their recovery.

Women with post-partum depression are thought to struggle with conflicts regarding dependency, anger, and motherhood (Blum, 2007). Helping them to freely discuss feelings that may feel very shameful to them, including aggressive feelings towards their children and ambivalent feelings about being a mother, can help them to normalize their experience and diminish their depressive symptoms.

Bipolar patients, particularly after manic episodes, often struggle with conflicts over aggression. Allowing them to talk about these feelings can help them to integrate the loving and aggressive ways that they think about themselves and others (Gabbard, 2005). In remission, they may also disconnect from their "manic selves" and Gabbard suggests that helping them to piece together the disparate parts of their lives into a coherent narrative can be extremely therapeutic (p. 228). This may also be helpful in patients with chronic depression.

Transference

Interpretation of the transference can be a powerful way to help patients with mood disorders to improve their sense of themselves and their relationships with others. For example, depressed patients who long for closeness but fear rejection may initially idealize the therapist, but soon feel disappointed by him/her. Interpretation of this reaction to the therapist can help the patient to understand the way in which their fantasies compound their disappointment in others and contribute to their depressed mood. This understanding is powerful because it occurs on an emotional–experiential level in the room with the therapist. The ability to discuss one's feelings toward the therapist openly and have the therapist respond in a curious, nondefensive way, and to collaboratively utilize these feelings to learn something new about oneself is unique to psychodynamic psychotherapy and provides a transformative experience which can potentially lead to long-term change.

Countertransference

Staying aware of one's countertransference during the treatment is key to being able to treat a hopeless and helpless patient with a mood disorder. Particularly during the acute phase of depression, the patient's relentless despair and pessimism can easily make even the most seasoned therapist bored, fatigued, paralyzed, and even dislike the patient. Similarly, the bipolar patient's continuous disavowal of illness, both during and after manic episodes, can feel exasperating. Discussing this with a supervisor or peer can be extremely helpful during this kind of treatment.

Recommendations and conclusions

A growing body of literature now supports the role of psychodynamic psychotherapy in the treatment of depression. Used alone or in combination with medication, it can provide symptomatic relief, as well as help depressed patients to have more a more realistic sense of themselves and their relationships with others, and can improve overall functioning. Supportive interventions should predominate in the acute phase of the illness with judicious use of expressive interventions, especially to counteract negative countertransference and treatment-interfering behaviors. Supportive interventions can also be helpful as an adjunct to medication in the treatment of bipolar disorder, with the goals of integrating loving and aggressive feelings, helping patients to have a more cohesive life experience, and decreasing denial of illness. While further studies are needed, the evidence base is growing for the use of psychodynamic psychotherapy in this population.

References

American Psychiatric Association (2002). *Practice Guidelines for Bipolar Disorder* [online]. Available: http://www.psych.org/psych_pract/treatg/pg/prac_guide.cfm (accessed April 2002).

American Psychiatric Association (2010). *Practice Guidelines for the Treatment of Patients with Major Depressive Disorder, Third Edition.* Washington DC American Psychiatric Association, 1–118.

Barkham, M., Rees, A., Shapiro, D. *et al.* (1996). Outcomes of time-limited psychotherapy in applied settings: Replicating the second Sheffield psychotherapy project. *Journal of Consulting and Clinical Psychology,* 64, 1079–1085.

Blum, L.D. (2007). Psychodynamics of postpartum depression. *Psychoanalytic Psychology,* 24, 45–62.

Bond, M. and Perry, J.C. (2004). Long-term changes in defense styles with psychodynamic psychotherapy for expressive, anxiety, and personality disorders. *American Journal of Psychiatry,* 161, 1665–1671.

Burnard, Y., Anderoli, A., Kolatte, E., Venturini, A., and Rosset, N. (2002). Psychodynamic psychotherapy and clomipramine in the treatment of major depression. *Psychiatric Services,* 53, 585–590.

Busch, F.N., Rudden, M., and Shapiro, T. (2004). *Psychodynamic Treatment of Depression.* Washington, DC: American Psychiatric Press Inc.

Cabaniss, D.L., Cherry, S., Douglas, C.J., and Schwartz, A. (2011). *Psychodynamic Psychotherapy: A Clinical Manual.* Oxford: Wiley.

Churchill, R., Hunot, V., Corney, R. *et al.* (2001). A systematic review of controlled trials of the effectiveness and cost-effectiveness of brief psychological treatments for depression. *Health Technology Assessment,* 5, 1–173.

Cooper, P.J., Murray, L., Wilson, A., and Romaniuk, H. (2003). Controlled trial of the short- and long-term effect of psychological treatment of post-partum depression: I. Impact on maternal mood. *British Journal of Psychiatry,* 182, 412–419.

DeFife, J.A. and Hilsenroth, M.J. (2011). Starting off on the right foot: Common factor elements in early psychotherapy process. *Journal of Psychotherapy Integration,* 21, 172–191.

de Jonghe, F., Kool, S., Aalst, G., Dekker, J., and Peen, J. (2001). Combining psychotherapy and antidepressants in the treatment of depression. *Journal of Affective Disorders,* 64, 217–229.

de Jonghe, F., Hendriksen, M., Aalst, G. *et al.* (2004). Psychotherapy and combined therapy (pharmacotherapy plus psychotherapy) in the treatment of depression. *British Journal of Psychiatry,* 185, 37–45.

Dekker, J., Molenaar, P.J., Kool, S. *et al.* (2005). Dose-effect relations in time-limited combined psycho- pharmacological treatment for depression. *Psychological Medicine*, 35, 47–58.

de Maat, S., Dekker, J., Schoevers, R. *et al.* (2008). Short psychodynamic supportive psychotherapy, antidepressants, and their combination in the treatment of major depression: A mega-analysis based on three randomized clinical trials. *Depression and Anxiety*, 25, 565–574.

Freud, S. (1917). In Mourning and melancholia. In *The Standard Edition of the Complete Psychological Works of Sigmund Freud, Vol. 14* (trans. J. Strachey). London: Hogarth Press, 237–258.

Gabbard, G.O. (2005). *Psychodynamic Psychiatry in Clinical Practice*. Washington DC: American Psychiatric Publishing.

Gallagher-Thompson, D. and Steffen, A.M. (1994). Comparative effects of cognitive-behavioral and brief-psychodynamic psychotherapies for depressed family caregivers. *Journal of Consulting and Clinical Pyschology*, 62, 543–549.

Gallagher-Thompson, D., Hanley-Peterson, P., and Thompson, L.W. (1990). Maintenance of gains versus relapse following brief psychotherapy for depression. *Journal of Consulting and Clinical Pyschology*, 58, 371–374.

Gonzalez, J.M. and Prihoda, T.J. (2007). Case study of psychodynamic group psychotherapy for bipolar disorder. *American Journal of Psychotherapy*, 61, 405–422.

Gutheil, T.G. (1978). Drug therapy: alliance and compliance. *Psychosomatics*, 19, 219–225.

Hersen, M., Himmelhoch, J.M., and Thase, M.E. (1984). Effects of social skills training, amitriptyline and psychotherapy in unipolar depressed women. *Behavior Therapy*, 15, 21–40.

Knekt, P., Lindfors, O., Härkänen, T. *et al.* (2008). Randomized trial on the effectiveness of long- and short-term psychodynamic psychotherapy and solution-focused therapy on psychiatric symptoms during a 3-year follow-up. *Psychological Medicine*, 38, 689–703.

Knekt, P., Lindfors, O., Laaksonen, M.A. *et al.* (2011). Quasi-experimental study on the effectiveness of psychoanalysis, long-term and short-term psychotherapy on psychiatric symptoms, work ability and functional capacity during a 5-year follow-up. *Journal of Affective Disorders*, 132, 37–47.

Leichsenring, F. (2001). Comparative effects of short-term psychodynamic psychotherapy and cognitive-behavioral therapy in depression: A meta-analytic approach. *Clinical Psychology Review*, 21, 401–419.

Leichsenring, F. and Rabung, S. (2008). The effectiveness of long-term psychodynamic psychotherapy: A meta-analysis. *Journal of the American Medical Association*, 300, 1551–1564.

Luborsky, L. (1984). *Principles of Psychoanalytic Psychotherapy: A Manual for Supportive Expressive Treatments*. New York: Basic Books.

Luborsky, L., Mark, D., Hole, A.V. *et al.* (1995). Supportive-expressive dynamic psychotherapy for depression: a time-limited version. In Barber J.P. and Crits-Christoph, P. eds., *Dynamic Therapies for Psychiatric Disorders (Axis I)*. New York: Basic Books, 13–42.

Maina, G., Forner, F., and Bogetto, F. (2005). Randomized controlled trial comparing brief dynamic and supportive therapy with waiting list condition in minor depressive disorders. *Psychotherapy and Psychosomatics*, 74, 3–50.

Maina, G., Rosso, G., Crespi, C., and Bogetto, F. (2007). Combined brief dynamic therapy and pharmacotherapy in the treatment of major depressive disorder: A pilot study. *Psychotherapy and Psychosomatics*, 76, 298–305.

Malan, D. (1976). *The Frontier of Brief Psychotherapy*. New York: Plenum Medical Book Company.

Mann, J. (1973). *Time-Limited Psychotherapy*. Cambridge, MA: Harvard University Press.

Salminen, J.K., Karlsson, H., Hietala, J. *et al.* (2008). Short-term psychodynamic psychotherapy and fluoxetine in major depressive disorder: A randomized comparative study. *Psychotherapy and Psychosomatics*, 77, 351–357.

Shapiro, D.A., Barkham, M., Rees, A. *et al.* (1994). Effects of treatment duration and severity of depression on the effectiveness of cognitive-behavioral and psychodynamic-interpersonal psychotherapy. *Journal of Consulting and Clinical Pyschology*, 62, 522–534.

Shapiro, D.A., Rees, A., Barkham, M. *et al.* (1995). Effects of treatment duration and severity of depression on the maintenance of gains after cognitive-behavioral and psychodynamic-interpersonal psychotherapy. *Journal of Consulting and Clinical Pyschology*, 63, 378–387.

Thompson, L.W., Gallagher, D., and Breckenridge, J.S. (1987). Comparative effectiveness of psychotherapies for depressed elders. *Journal of Consulting and Clinical Psychology*, 55, 385–390.

Vanheule, S., Desmet, M., Rosseel, Y., and Meganck, R. (2006). Core transference themes in depression. *Journal of Affective Disorders*, 91, 71–75.

Chapter

23

Combining medication and psychotherapy in the treatment of depression

Bret R. Rutherford and Steven P. Roose

Introduction

When the psychoanalytic model of the mind was the major theoretical influence in psychiatry, most American clinicians believed that the use of medication "reduces the motivation of the patient to pursue the psychotherapeutic work and deeper personality changes that are sought for in the psychoanalytic process" (Marmor, 1981). As evidence for the effectiveness of medications to treat mood disorders accumulated, other psychiatrists rejected the combination of medication and psychotherapy for the opposite reason. Biologically oriented psychiatrists saw little reason to consider nonpharmacologic treatments, whose likely mechanisms were considered by them to be persuasion and contact with a caring doctor rather than a specific treatment.

The field of psychiatry's view on combined treatment has shifted dramatically over the past 20 years. Today, many experts in mood disorders have concluded that treatment with medication and psychotherapy may be advantageous in a number of respects. One reason cited in favor of combination treatment is that it may increase the magnitude of response relative to monotherapy, resulting in fewer residual symptoms. Secondly, it is now generally accepted that combining treatments may enhance the acceptability and effectiveness of each individual treatment: psychotherapy may increase compliance with antidepressant medication and help patients tolerate side effects, while adding medication may make the problems of psychotherapy patients more tractable (Hollon *et al.* 2005). These benefits of combined therapy were initially studied with respect to cognitive behavior therapy (CBT) and interpersonal therapy (IPT), but more recent studies have investigated modalities such as psychodynamic psychotherapy

(Burnard, *et al.* 2002) and dialectical behavior therapy (DBT) (Harley *et al.* 2008).

While these arguments for combined treatment have some support from empirical studies, the pendulum may have swung too far in the direction of uncritical recommendation of combined treatment. The evidence in favor of combined treatment over monotherapy with psychotherapy or medication remains sparse. Most studies reporting superiority of combined treatment have enrolled special patient populations or have a study design that is biased against the medication comparator cell. In addition, the complexity of combining different treatment approaches has become increasingly appreciated. Rather than assuming the effects of medication and psychotherapy are simply additive, it is being asked whether the combination of these treatments may reduce their individual effectiveness. The purpose of this chapter is to review the evidence base for combined medication and psychotherapy treatment of depression, and discuss techniques and strategies for implementing combined treatment in the most effective way.

Empirical research on combined treatment

There are three primary types of randomized controlled trials comparing antidepressant medication, psychotherapy, and combined treatment, which fall into roughly chronological phases of research: (1) comparing monotherapy with medication or psychotherapy to determine which is superior, (2) comparing combined medication and psychotherapy treatment to either monotherapy, and (3) augmentation studies when patients have not fully responded to either psychotherapy or medication. Below, a

---

Clinical Handbook for the Management of Mood Disorders, ed. J. John Mann, Patrick J. McGrath, and Steven P. Roose.
Published by Cambridge University Press. © Cambridge University Press 2013.

paradigmatic example of each study type is reviewed with their merits, limitations, and implications for clinical practice.

Monotherapy studies

During the 1970s and 1980s, more pharmacologic treatment options became available, and researchers systematically began to investigate the efficacy of these treatments in clinical trials. Likewise, psychotherapy researchers began to develop treatment manuals and therapist training programs so that psychotherapies could be standardized and studied systematically. These developments eventually led to the direct comparison of treatment with medications vs. psychotherapy to determine their relative efficacy for depression, anxiety disorders, and other conditions (see Table 23.1). The first generation of trials involving medications and psychotherapy compared the two treatment modalities to determine if one was superior, but they did not usually have a combined treatment cell. A problem facing these types of trials was the difficulty of demonstrating significant differences between two active treatments, as most studies were not adequately powered to detect small but nonetheless clinically significant differences in response.

One of the more influential trials comparing psychotherapy and medication was the National Institute of Mental Health's (NIMH) Treatment of Depression Collaborative Research Program (TDCRP) (Elkin et al. 1985), whose results began to be published in 1989. The TDCRP was a multi-center clinical trial that randomized 250 outpatients with current major depressive disorder to 16 weeks of treatment with cognitive behavior therapy (CBT), interpersonal therapy (IPT), imipramine plus clinical management, or pill placebo plus clinical management. Of note, the methods have been criticized for using possibly inadequate duration of psychotherapy treatment as well as a dose of imipramine (150 mg) that results in sub-therapeutic blood levels for many patients. The study goal was to determine the relative efficacy of two psychotherapies for depression, as well as their efficacy compared to imipramine, which served as the standard reference treatment. The primary observer-rated outcome measures were the 17-item Hamilton Rating Scale for Depression (HRSD) (Hamilton, 1960) and the Global Assessment of Functioning Scale (GAS)

(Endicott et al. 1976), while the primary self-report outcome measures were the Beck Depression Inventory (BDI) (Beck et al. 1961) and the Symptom Checklist – 90 (SCL – 90) (Derogatis, 1992).

Patients enrolling in the study were 70% female, aged 35 ± 8 years, and most had recurrent depression (Elkin et al. 1989). The dropout rate was 32% in the CBT group, 23% in the IPT group, 33% in the imipramine group, and 40% in the placebo group. In the intent-to-treat analyses, patients in all four treatment conditions (including placebo) showed significant reduction in depressive symptoms over the course of the study as measured by all four of the primary outcome measures. Few significant differences were found between the treatments: imipramine was superior to placebo on the GAS measure, and IPT as well as imipramine showed a trend for superiority to placebo on the HRSD. Significantly more patients experienced remission, defined as HRSD < 7, in the imipramine and IPT groups compared to placebo, but CBT was not significantly different from either of the other active treatment groups or placebo. Follow-up analyses of the TDCRP data suggested that patients with more severe depression benefited most from imipramine as compared to either of the psychotherapy conditions (Elkin et al. 1995), but subsequent prospective trials of antidepressant medication vs. CBT for patients with severe depression have not shown significant differences between these treatments (Dimidjian et al. 2006).

Results from other studies within this first phase of research involving head-to-head comparisons of psychotherapy and medication were similar in the findings described. Some trials demonstrate a significant difference in favor of psychotherapy compared to medications (Rush et al. 1977), while others report the opposite finding (Elkin et al. 1989). However, the result found by most of the studies cited is that no significant difference was observed between the two treatment modalities (Dimidjian et al. 2006). This finding reiterates the difficulty of demonstrating significant differences between two active treatments rather than between an active treatment and baseline or a control condition. Clinically, this result also led to the consensus that either medications or psychotherapy with CBT or IPT can be a reasonable first choice for the treatment of many unipolar, nonpsychotic depressions (Agency for Health Care Policy and Research, 1993, American Psychiatric Association, 1993).

Table 23.1 Summary of research on combined treatment with medication and psychotherapy

Investigators	Diagnosis	Interventions	Sample size	Treatment duration	Results
Monotherapy Studies					
Rush *et al.* 1977	Adults with depressive disorders	CBT Imipramine	41	12 weeks	CBT > imipramine
Elkin *et al.* 1989	Adults with MDD	CBT IPT Imipramine Placebo	250	16 weeks	Imipramine > IPT > CBT > placebo
Jarrett *et al.* 1999	Adults with atypical MDD	CBT Phenelzine Placebo	108	10 weeks	CBT = phenelzine > placebo
DeRubeis *et al.* 2005	Adults with severe MDD	CBT ADs	240	16 weeks	CBT = ADs
Dimidjian *et al.* 2006	Adults with MDD	BAT CBT ADs Placebo	241	16 weeks	BAT = ADs > CBT > placebo
Combination Studies					
Blackburn *et al.* 1981	Outpatients with recurrent depression	CBT TCAs CBT + TCAs	64	20 weeks	CBT + TCAs = CBT > TCAs
Murphy *et al.* 1984	Unipolar depressive disorders	CBT Nortriptyline CBT + nortriptyline CBT+ active placebo	87	12 weeks	No differences between groups
Hollon *et al.* 1992	Outpatients with MDD	CBT ADs CBT + ADs	107	12 weeks	No differences between groups
Reynolds *et al.* 1999	Elderly with bereavement-related MDD	IPT + placebo IPT + nortriptyline Nortriptyline Placebo	84	16 weeks	IPT + nortriptyline = nortriptyline > IPT + placebo = placebo
Ravindran *et al.* 1999	Adults with DD	GCBT + placebo GCBT + sertraline Sertraline Placebo	97	12 weeks	GCBT + sertraline = sertraline > GCBT + placebo = placebo
Keller *et al.* 2000	Adults with chronic MDD	CBASP Nefazodone CBASP + Nefazodone	681	12 weeks	CBASP + nefazodone > CBASP = nefazodone
Thompson *et al.* 2001	Elderly with MDD	CBT CBT + desipramine Desipramine	102	16–20 weeks	No differences between groups
Burnard, *et al.* 2002	Adults with MDD	Psychodynamic PT + clomipramine Clomipramine	74	10 weeks	No differences between groups
Browne *et al.* 2002	Adults with DD	Brief IPT Brief IPT +sertraline Sertraline	707	24 weeks	Brief IPT + sertraline=sertraline > brief IPT
TADS Team, 2004	Children and adolescents with MDD	CBT CBT + fluoxetine Fluoxetine Placebo	439	12 weeks	CBT + fluoxetine = fluoxetine > CBT > placebo (on CGI outcome measure)

Table 23.1 (cont.)

Investigators	Diagnosis	Interventions	Sample size	Treatment duration	Results
		Combination Studies			
Paykel et al. 1995	Adults with recurrent MDD	CBT + ADs ADs	158	48-week continuation study	CBT + ADs > ADs
Frank et al. 1991	Adults with recurrent depression	IPT IPT + placebo Imipramine + IPT Imipramine Placebo	127	3-year continuation study	Imipramine = imipramine + IPT > IPT = IPT + placebo = placebo

'>' denotes statistically significant difference favoring one treatment; '=' denotes no statistically significant difference between treatments; MDD = major depressive disorder; CBT = cognitive behavior therapy; BAT = behavioral activation therapy; CBASP = cognitive behavioral analysis system of psychotherapy; GCBT = group cognitive behavior therapy; ADs = antidepressants.

Combined treatment studies

The next generation of research studies included a combined therapy treatment cell, which was compared to monotherapy with either medication or psychotherapy (see Table 23.1). Many of the initial studies having this design found little evidence supporting the superiority of combined treatment over monotherapy (Murphy et al. 1984, Hollon et al. 1992). Some researchers argued that the lack of evidence for superiority of combined treatment with medications and psychotherapy resulted from studies that were inadequately powered to detect more modest effect sizes. A more recent, larger study of combination treatment with psychotherapy and medications found combined treatment superior to monotherapy with either treatment (Keller et al. 2000).

Keller and colleagues (2000) randomized nearly 700 adults with chronic major depressive disorder to 12 weeks of nefazodone, 16–20 sessions of the Cognitive Behavioral-Analysis System of Psychotherapy (CBASP), or both. Combined treatment had a 73% response rate, which was significantly better than treatment with psychotherapy (48%) or medication (48%) alone. Rates of discontinuation were low (21–26%) and not significantly different between the treatment cells in the acute phase of the study. This study is commendable for its solid methodology and large sample size, but the special patient population enrolled (chronic depression) and the use of a psychotherapy designed specifically to treat the chronic population must be kept in mind when applying its results to clinical practice.

As another solution to the lack of statistical power characterizing many studies of combined treatment, several groups have undertaken meta-analyses of smaller individual studies to more accurately estimate the effect sizes of the differences between combined treatment and monotherapy. Thase et al. (1997) analyzed six studies comprising nearly 600 patients in which 16 weeks of treatment was provided with CBT, IPT, or combined IPT and antidepressant treatment. The primary outcome measure examined was remission of depression, as determined by HRSD < 7 at study endpoint. They found a remission rate of 37% for psychotherapy alone compared to 48% with combined therapy, which was not a significant difference. Pampalloma et al. (2004) reviewed the literature to find RCTs comparing antidepressant treatment alone to the combinations of antidepressants and psychotherapy for the treatment of depressive disorders. The authors found that combined treatment with psychotherapy and medication had a significant advantage over treatment with antidepressants alone. Patients receiving combined treatment were nearly twice as likely to experience depression response (as defined in each study) compared to antidepressants alone (odds ratio 1.86, 95% CI, 1.38–2.52).

In summary, the limited nature of the data supporting the superiority of combined treatment over monotherapy should make the clinician pause before reflexively initiating combined treatment. The significant resources required by combined treatment must be measured against this questionable benefit over monotherapy. Clinicians should consider whether sequencing treatments is a more cogent strategy, reserving combined treatment for patients who have not responded to an initial treatment.

Augmentation studies

The most recent research studies on combined treatment have attempted to answer the question of whether adding a second treatment to ongoing treatment with antidepressant medication or psychotherapy is beneficial. A unique perspective on the use of medications and psychotherapy to treat depression has been provided by the NIMH-sponsored Sequenced Treatment Alternatives to Relieve Depression (STAR*D) study, which is the largest prospective trial for depression ever conducted. A broadly representative sample of nearly 3700 patients with depression underwent successive acute treatments steps with either antidepressant medication, cognitive behavior therapy, or in some cases both (Rush *et al.* 2006). Patients whose depressions did not remit at one treatment step were encouraged to proceed with additional trials until remission was achieved. These additional trials involved either switching or augmenting treatments, and patients were allowed to express a preference for switching vs. augmenting and for medication vs. psychotherapy options. After initial treatment with citalopram, 37% of depressed patients were in remission (Trivedi *et al.* 2006). Interestingly, only 26% of participants agreed to permit randomization to the augmentation or switch options that included a CBT cell (Thase *et al.* 2007), so only 147 patients were assigned to CBT in the study. This result contrasts with survey data indicating most patients in the general population prefer psychotherapy as an initial treatment approach (Dwight-Johnson *et al.* 2000). Augmentation of citalopram with CBT resulted in a depression remission rate of 23.1%, which was not significantly different from the rate observed with augmentation with bupropion or buspirone (33.3%). Switching to CBT after unsuccessful treatment with citalopram resulted in a 25.0% remission rate, compared to 27.9% after switching to sertraline, buproprion, or venlafaxine (no significant difference). However, the authors did note that pharmacologic augmentation resulted in faster speed of depression response, and patients appeared to tolerate treatment with medication or CBT equally well.

Another important augmentation study was the REVAMP Study, conducted by Kocsis and colleagues (2009). This study of chronically depressed outpatients comprised a 12-week open-label phase, in which 808 patients received treatment with an antidepressant medication. In a second 12-week phase, the 491 patients not responding to the open-label treatment received a next-step medication option, either alone or in combination with brief supportive psychotherapy or cognitive behavioral analysis system of psychotherapy, the psychotherapy that was used in the Keller *et al.* ( ) study of chronic depression previously described. The authors found no significant differences between the three second-phase treatment options, either in the proportion of patients responding to treatment or in the change in HRSD score. Thus, combining medication treatment with psychotherapy did not appear to confer an advantage over switching to a different medication treatment.

Taken together, these studies suggest that adding psychotherapy to a medication nonresponder is no more effective than switching to a second medication, thus further questioning the belief that a combined treatment is superior to monotherapy. Of note, there are no RCTs currently available investigating different treatment options among patients who have not responded to an initial course of psychotherapy (i.e., add medication to ongoing psychotherapy, switch to medication alone, or switch to a different psychotherapy).

Methodological issues in combined treatment studies

In interpreting the above results, it is important to keep in mind several methodological difficulties that are unique to trials randomizing patients to medication and psychotherapy within a single study. In pharmacotherapy trials, randomization, a pill placebo comparison group, and double-blinding ensure that potential confounders and nonspecific factors (such as health care provider attention, patient expectations, and spontaneous remission) associated with every experimental treatment are equivalent between groups. A major difficulty in comparing psychotherapy, medication, and combined treatment is introduced by the absence of a psychotherapy placebo condition. Since no adequate psychotherapy placebo condition has been established, investigators have resorted to comparing placebo-controlled medication treatment to the open administration of psychotherapy.

To illustrate the problem with this approach, consider the Treatment for Adolescents with Depression Study (TADS), in which adolescents with major depression were randomized to CBT alone, fluoxetine alone, combined CBT and fluoxetine, and pill placebo (TADS Team, 2004). The benefit of this design is that the study can be "internally calibrated," meaning differences between the psychotherapy and medication conditions can be more easily interpreted when it is known whether or not the medication treatment condition was effective compared to placebo. However, the study compares blinded treatments (fluoxetine or pill placebo) to unblinded treatments (CBT, and combined CBT and fluoxetine). In other words, patients in the CBT alone condition knew they were receiving psychotherapy (active treatment), while patients taking pills did not know whether they were fluoxetine (active) or placebo (inactive). Similarly, patients in the combined cell knew they were receiving two active treatments rather than one (CBT alone) or possibly none (fluoxetine and pill placebo).

Comparisons between unblinded and blinded treatments are biased against the blinded treatment. Rutherford *et al.* (2009) analyzed 48 placebo-controlled and 42 comparator trials of antidepressants for major depression in adults aged 18–65. The odds of being classified as a responder to medication in comparator trials were 1.8 times the odds of being classified as a responder in placebo-controlled trials (95% CI = 1.45–2.17, $p < 0.001$), and the odds of being classified as a remitter to medication in comparator trials were 1.5 times the odds of being classified a remitter in placebo-controlled trials (95% CI = 1.11–2.11, $p < 0.001$). These results demonstrate that antidepressant response and remission rates are lower when patients and raters do not know they are receiving active treatment (i.e., placebo-controlled trials) vs. when they know they are receiving medication without knowing the exact agent (i.e., comparator trials). This situation is relevant to the open and blinded administration of treatments given to patients in many combined medication and psychotherapy studies. It appears that clinical trials comparing open to blinded treatments are significantly biased against the blinded treatment (i.e., placebo-controlled medication). Since most studies comparing medication and psychotherapy have included a placebo treatment condition (e.g., the TADS study), there is a strong possibility that the current literature under-reports

the effect of medication compared to psychotherapy and combined treatment. Future studies comparing the effect of medication to psychotherapy alone or in combination with psychotherapy must have an open medication cell to allow for unbiased comparisons.

Clinical technique in the use of combined treatment with medication and psychotherapy

Some clinicians hold that combined treatment is the optimal approach for patients with depression because medication and psychotherapy affect different dimensions of depression. However, there is little empirical evidence to support this belief, and there are some data to suggest it may be false. A very intriguing study by Tang *et al.* (2010) randomized 240 patients with moderate to severe MDD to receive antidepressant medication (an SSRI), placebo, or CBT. Patients who received antidepressant medication reported greater decreases in neuroticism and increases in extraversion, as measured by the Neuroticism-Extraversion-Openness Five Factor Inventory (NEO-FFI) than patients receiving placebo or CBT, even after controlling for depression improvement. Thus, SSRI treatment may have a salutary effect on personality distinct from its effect on depression.

Nonetheless, some clinicians, whether based on their evaluation of the evidence or because of their experience, may recommend combination treatment. As a starting treatment for a patient who is not currently receiving treatment for depression, combined treatment may be best used for patients with chronic depressive episodes complicated by co-morbid personality disorder, noncompliance, or psychosocial problems (Keller *et al.* 2000). A patient may also begin a combined treatment when medication is prescribed for the onset of a significant depressive episode in the context of an ongoing psychotherapy. Alternatively, a patient who has not fully responded to one or more medication trials may begin psychotherapy, thereby beginning a combined treatment by a different route. Irrespective of the path by which the patient is prescribed combined treatment, the prescribing clinician must recognize that the execution of this treatment plan presents unique and complex challenges, which are discussed below.

Structuring the treatment

The first question that arises is how to structure a combined treatment with medication and psychotherapy. In some cases, one psychiatrist administers both medication and psychotherapy to the patient. In other circumstances, two practitioners treat the patient – one administers psychotherapy and one prescribes medication. In a blend of these approaches, one psychiatrist is the primary practitioner, administering both psychotherapy and medication, but a consultant is involved to add expert advice and to potentially see the patient on an as-needed basis. Each of these models may be more or less appropriate for different clinical situations, and each has a unique profile of benefits and drawbacks.

In choosing the appropriate treatment model for combined treatment with medication and psychotherapy, the clinician must first assess his or her clinical strengths. Some psychiatrists feel that they are well trained in psychopharmacology but not in psychotherapy, while others may be more confident of their psychotherapy skills. Even if the clinician feels capable of delivering each type of treatment that is appropriate in a given clinical situation, the clinician may not feel able to administer them concomitantly to the same patient. For example, a clinician may decide that techniques that are important for good pharmacologic management would interfere with his or her ability to maintain an appropriate therapeutic stance in a psychodynamic treatment. In some circumstances, the practitioner may feel that a split treatment would jeopardize the quality of the treatment. For example, patients who tend to idealize and devalue different members of the treatment team (e.g., some patients with borderline personality disorder) might be better served by having one clinician administer both the psychotherapy and the medication in order to minimize the potential for manipulation and to keep all of the information in one treatment setting.

Although choosing a treatment model for administering combined treatment should be based primarily on clinical considerations, there are often logistical and financial considerations that need to be taken into account. For example, the clinician may be the only practitioner who is geographically near the patient. Other clinicians may be working in a managed care situation where the treatment options are constrained, or the patient may not be able to afford to see more than one clinician at a time. It is more common that a patient may be more able to afford psychotherapy with a non-MD practitioner, in which case it must be ensured that the pharmacologic treatment must be affordable enough for the clinician to be able to see the patient as often as necessary. In these situations, the clinician and patient need to choose options for the clinical situation that optimize the treatment plan within the context of the logistical and/or financial constraints.

Evaluation

Questions of technique begin from one's first contact with a new patient. In many cases this contact may occur in the form of a telephone call from a patient seeking a new appointment. Generally, psychotherapists will contact the psychopharmacologist before the patient to ascertain whether he or she is taking new patients and to provide clinical background. Of course, referrals also come about from the opposite direction. If preliminary communication does not occur, one should explore whether this might be an early indication the therapist is not fully in agreement with the need for medication. Psychopharmacologists treating patients who are also in therapy with a different clinician must keep in mind that their primary obligation is to the patient rather than the therapist, and in the evaluation they must not only assess the patient, but the entire treatment. In general, the MD maintains medicolegal responsibility for the patient, regardless of who else he or she might be seeing. For this reason and others, it is very helpful to speak with a patient's therapist prior to performing a psychopharmacologic evaluation to facilitate the establishment of a good working relationship, ensure the psychotherapeutic modality is compatible with medication treatment, determine whether the therapist has an appropriate degree of experience, and ensure the therapist is not philosophically opposed to medication.

When speaking with a patient to set up a consultation, it is possible to perform a brief triage over the phone. The purpose of this triage is to obtain a brief history of the presenting illness, get an initial sense of the patient's goals for the consultation, and assess the level of acuity of the patient's problems. This information allows clinicians to confirm that they have the appropriate expertise to see the patient and time in their schedule, and it allows time for logistical and financial information to be discussed so that it can be determined whether the treatment will be affordable for the patient and potentially sustainable. Speaking with patients ahead of time also prepares both clinician and patient so that the evaluation can be made as productive as possible. The patient can be instructed to prepare for the evaluation by gathering medical and psychiatric records, details of their psychopharmacologic and psychotherapeutic histories, laboratory results, neuropsychological testing, brain imaging, and other doctor's records.

In terms of the actual evaluation appointment, it is advisable to schedule the initial evaluation for a double session to allow adequate time. Though this type of evaluation may be a significant departure from standard technique for many psychotherapies, the goals of an evaluation for combined treatment are the same as for any psychiatric evaluation. For example, many psychotherapeutic assessments may focus on case formulation and an assessment of whether the patient possesses psychological mindedness or the capacity to identify automatic thoughts, which might be considered necessary to engage in a psychotherapy. Clinical diagnosis, on the other hand, is based on the phenomenological diagnostic system outlined in the DSM series. Furthermore, data on the efficacy and side effects of psychotropic medications come from studies that include patients based on phenomenologically based diagnostic systems.

By the end of a comprehensive evaluation, the psychiatrist should be in a position to make informed treatment recommendations, and if those recommendations include medication, to discuss the risks and benefits of medication. However, if the psychiatrist feels that there has not been sufficient time to finish the evaluation, or that further information must be collected from collateral history sources or prior caregivers, then recommendations should be withheld until the evaluation is complete. A clinician may at times feel pressured by the patient and/or therapist (in split treatments) to provide a prescription immediately, but that pressure must be resisted and the reasons for doing so explained. Psychiatrists prescribing medication in split treatment should determine the frequency of follow-up contact with the patient, by phone or in person, according to what they believe is optimal pharmacological management and by no other considerations. It may be necessary to see a patient weekly or more frequently when they are starting a new medication.

Informed consent

Originally, the process of informed consent was restricted to invasive procedures or participation in research. However, the concept of informed consent has been extended and is now expected to be an explicit part of the interaction between a doctor and patient whenever treatment is recommended. According to the American Medical Association, a physician has "both an ethical obligation and legal requirement" to obtain informed consent. The principles of informed consent mandate that it is the clinician's responsibility to discuss the rationale for the recommended treatment (including the evidence that supports the efficacy of the treatment). Additionally, the patient should be informed about all reasonable alternative treatments with the evidence that supports their efficacy, their possible side effects, and the risks of not using each treatment. This discussion should be documented in the patient's record.

The process of informed consent is the responsibility of the clinician regardless of professional background. To some psychotherapists, the process of a conducting a diagnostic interview to elicit phenomenology, and making treatment recommendations according to the concept of informed consent might feel intrusive and awkward. Though cognizant of the therapeutic effectiveness of psychotropic medications, a psychotherapist may still feel that the phenomenological diagnostic approach threatens the psychotherapeutic framework. Such circumstances may predispose to the incorrect clinical conclusion that psychotherapy is always the preferred treatment and medication should only be recommended for the most severe circumstances or for therapeutic stalemates. Though medication treatment is very effective for severe depression, restricting the recommendation of medication to this circumstance because of treatment allegiance to psychotherapy must be avoided.

Challenges in conducting ongoing treatment with medication and psychotherapy for depression

When combined treatments are structured as single practitioners practicing both treatments, there are potential pitfalls inherent in trying to "wear two hats" while treating the patient. Each treatment modality – psychotherapy and psychopharmacology – is challenging to administer and takes time. A psychopharmacologist is trained to carefully monitor both symptoms and side effects on a regular basis (often using structured interviews or scales), check vital signs, and suggest changes in the medication regimen when needed. If the visits are also devoted to psychotherapy, when does or should the pharmacologic management take place? Often, it is discussed "on the fly," either before or after the "real" content of the session occurs. Once a satisfactory medication regimen is established, the clinician and patient may "forget" about the medication and not discuss the pharmacologic treatment, despite the fact that the clinician is still prescribing medication for the patient. This can lead to many things being overlooked, such as changes in symptoms, side effects, and opportunities to discontinue medication after an appropriate amount of time.

Another complicating factor is that within the past decade, the cumulative evidence strongly indicates that the goal of the treatment of depression should no longer be symptom reduction, generally referred to as "response" and defined as a 50% reduction in baseline symptoms, but rather "remission" of the illness, which is generally defined as the absence of symptoms and return to premorbid baseline functioning (Paykel, 1995). The recognition that attaining remission status represents optimal treatment for depression has two significant implications for clinicians treating this illness. First, fewer than 50% of patients will achieve remission with the first antidepressant treatment prescribed; most patients require a switch in class of medication or augmentation of the initial antidepressant with a second medication (Rush *et al.* 2006). Psychopharmacologists understand that treating a depressed patient with medication often requires a series of antidepressant medications or a combination of medications given at an adequate dose for adequate duration.

Second, clinicians need a method of assessment to determine if a patient has achieved remission; they cannot simply rely exclusively on their own estimation of symptom reduction. In most studies, remission is defined as a final HRSD ≤ 7 (usual score for a depressed patient is from 15 to 30). Although rating scales may represent the gold standard for determining presence or absence of the affective disorders described in the DSM-IV, clinicians may be unschooled in their use or feel that they are awkward to use in the clinical situation. The development of easy to use self-report measures such as the Quick Inventory

for Depressive Symptoms (QIDS) (Rush *et al.* 2003) make it possible for the clinician to use the same data as used in clinical trials for making clinical decisions with respect to changing or continuing the current medication strategy.

Splitting the treatment can often free up each practitioner to concentrate solely on one treatment modality. However, many complications can arise with this type of structure. Once the split treatment is underway, the patient may feel more comfortable with one practitioner or another and is likely to discuss each treatment with the other practitioner. A patient may value the psychopharmacologist more because of the "rapid help" that comes from medication, or may value the psychotherapist more, complaining that the psychopharmacologist "never asks about my life." This type of splitting of the treatment can lead to problems. On the clinicians' side, there may exist competition over the patient stemming from conflict between differing treatment models. Confusion or overlap between roles on behalf of the clinicians can be confusing to patients, and the keeping of "secrets" between clinicians can lead to problems. In split treatment, attention to the relationship between the two clinicians is essential for a therapeutic success, and the patient should be informed of ground rules such as open communication without secrets.

The problems that may arise in split treatment are illustrated in the following vignette:

Mr. B was a 43-year-old man in an ongoing psychodynamic psychotherapy with Ms. F, a licensed social worker. Several months into the treatment, which focused largely on Mr. B's marital difficulties, he began to lose interest in his usual activities and develop insomnia, decreased appetite, and trouble concentrating at work. These symptoms worsened and began to compromise Mr. B's ability to participate in psychotherapy sessions. Though Ms. F felt these feelings might be best understood as a reaction of Mr. B's to the psychotherapy process, she reluctantly referred him to a psychopharmacologist. Dr. M diagnosed Mr. B with major depressive disorder and began to prescribe an antidepressant, but he did not call to discuss the results of his evaluation or his treatment plan with Ms. F. Two weeks after beginning the antidepressant medication, Mr. B experienced mild nausea and voiced second thoughts in a therapy session about whether taking the medication was advisable. Ms. F stated her opinion that it would be best to understand all of Mr. B's feelings in the context of their psychotherapy sessions, but that if he really was unable to tolerate the feelings developing, it was acceptable to take a medication temporarily. Mr. B decided to stop the antidepressant medication and cancel his remaining appointments with Dr. M.

In this case a lack of communication between psychopharmacologist and psychotherapist led to the patient having a negative view of treatment with medication as "second best." Had Dr. M communicated with Ms. F, the potential conflict between their treatment models might have been resolved, and Mr. B might have been encouraged to discuss his side effects and concerns with Dr. M before dropping out of treatment.

This vignette also brings up the point that it is helpful at the beginning of a split treatment for the therapist and pharmacologist to agree upon how responsibility for the patient is to be shared. Then, the patient must be educated about whom to contact in emergencies, periods of symptom worsening, or crises. In most cases the treating psychiatrist should be called during an emergency so that safety can be assessed and the need for hospitalization or other acute care considered. Communication between the clinician prescribing medication and undertaking a patient's psychotherapy is essential, especially since these clinicians may have different professional backgrounds. This communication may take place in the form of phone messages left on one another's voice mail, scheduled telephone calls, or in-person meetings. Sometimes, a session in which both practitioners are present can be helpful to ensure that all three people involved in the treatment are "on the same page." Mutual respect between the practitioners in a split treatment is essential for the development of a good working relationship in which undermining can be minimized. This type of ongoing communication can also result in mutual learning as the two practitioners share their perspectives about patients over time.

Conclusions

In light of the frequency with which combined treatment with psychotherapy and antidepressant medication appears to be prescribed, the dearth of evidence demonstrating superiority of combined treatment vs. monotherapy as an acute treatment for depression is surprising. Nonetheless, while combined treatment may not be appropriate as an initial treatment for all patients, there are some data to support its use in cases of more chronic depression, cases where depression is co-morbid with trauma or a personality disorder, or treatments in which there has been noncompliance or refractoriness to monotherapies. The decision to recommend combined treatment with psychotherapy and medications is only the first step. Executing this recommendation requires serious consideration of the preconceptions both doctor and patient bring to the treatment, logistical realities of the clinician's credentials and the patient's resources, and the nature of the illness or illnesses under treatment.

References

Agency for Health Care Policy and Research (1993). *Clinical Practice Guideline: Depression in Primary Care, Vol 2: Treatment of Major Depression.* AHCPR Publication 93–0551. Washington, DC: US Government Printing Office.

American Psychiatric Association (1993). Practice guideline for major depressive disorder in adults. *American Journal of Psychiatry*, 150.

Beck, A.T., Ward, C.H., Mendelson, M. *et al.* (1961). An inventory of measuring depression. *Archives of General Psychiatry*, 4, 53–63.

Blackburn, I.M., Bishop, S., and Glen, A.I.M. (1981). The efficacy of cognitive therapy in depression: A treatment trial using cognitive therapy and pharmacotherapy, each alone and in combination. *British Journal of Psychiatry*, 139, 181–189.

Browne, G., Steiner, M., Roberts, J. *et al.* (2002). Sertraline, and/or interpersonal therapy for patients with dysthymic disorder in primary care: 6-month comparison with longitudinal 2-year follow-up of effectiveness and costs. *Journal of Affective Disorders*, 68, 317–330.

Burnard, Y., Andreoli, A., Kolatte, E., Venturini, A., and Rosset, N. (2002). Psychodynamic psychotherapy and clomipramine in the treatment of major depression. *Psychiatric Services*, 53, 585–590.

Conte, H.R., Plutchik, R., Wild, K.V., and Karasu, T.B. (1986). Combined psychotherapy and pharmacotherapy for depression: A systematic analysis of the evidence. *Archives of General Psychiatry*, 43, 471–479.

Derogatis, L.R. (1992). *The Symptom Checklist-90-revised.* Minneapolis, MN: NCS Assessments.

DeRubeis, R.J., Hollon, S.D., Amsterdam, J.D. *et al.* (2005). Cognitive therapy vs. medications in the treatment of moderate to severe depression. *Archives of General Psychiatry*, 62, 409–416.

Dimidjian, S., Dobson, K.S., Kohlenberg, R.J. *et al.* (2006). Randomized trial of behavioral activation, cognitive therapy, and antidepressant medication in the acute treatment of adults with major depression. *Journal of Consulting and Clinical Psychology*, 74, 658–670.

Dwight-Johnson, M., Sherbourne, C.D., Liao, D., and Wells, K.B. (2000). Treatment preferences among depressed primary care patients. *Journal of General Internal Medicine*, 15, 527–534.

Elkin, I., Parloff, M.B., Hadley, S.W. *et al.* (1985). NIMH Treatment of Depression Collaborative Research Program: Background and research plan. *Archives of General Psychiatry*, 42, 305–316.

Elkin, I., Shea, M.T., Watkins, J.T. *et al.* (1989). National Institute of Mental Health Treatment of Depression Collaborative Research Program: General effectiveness of treatments. *Archives of General Psychiatry*, 46, 971–982.

Elkin, I., Gibbons, R.D., Shea, M.T. *et al.* (1995). Initial severity and differential treatment outcome in the National Institute of Mental Health Treatment of Depression Collaborative Research Program. *Journal of Consulting and Clinical Psychology*, 63, 841–847.

Endicott, J., Spitzer, R.L., Fleiss, J.L., and Cohen, J. (1976). The global assessment scale. *Archives of General Psychiatry*, 33, 766–771.

Frank, E., Prien, R.F., Jarrett, R.B. *et al.* (1991). Conceptualization and rationale for consensus definitions of terms in major depressive disorder: Remission, recovery, relapse, and recurrence. *Archives of General Psychiatry*, 48, 851–855.

Hamilton, M. (1960). A rating scale for depression. *Journal of Neurology, Neurosurgery and Psychiatry*, 23, 56–62.

Harley, R., Sprich, S., Safren, S., Jacobo, M., and Fava, M. (2008). Adaptation of dialectical behavior therapy skills training group for treatment-resistant depression. *Journal of Nervous and Mental Disease*, 196, 136–143.

Hollon, S.D., DeRubeis, R.J., and Loosen, P.T. (1992). Cognitive therapy and pharmacotherapy for depression. Singly and in combination. *Archives of General Psychiatry*, 49, 774–781.

Hollon, S.D., Jarrett, R.B., Nierenberg, A.A. *et al.* (2005). Psychotherapy and medication in the treatment of adult and geriatric depression: Which monotherapy or combined treatment? *Journal of Clinical Psychiatry*, 66, 455–468.

Jarrett, R.B., Schaffer, M., McIntire, D. *et al.* (1999). Treatment of atypical depression with cognitive therapy or phenelzine: A double-blind, placebo-controlled trial. *Archives of General Psychiatry*, 56, 431–437.

Keller, M.B., McCullough, J.P. *et al.* (2000). A comparison of nefazodone, the cognitive behavioral-analysis system of psychotherapy, and their combination for the treatment of chronic depression. *New England Journal of Medicine*, 342, 1462–1470.

Kocsis, J.H., Gelenberg, A.J., Rothbaum, B.O. *et al.* (2009). Cognitive behavioral analysis system of psychotherapy and brief supportive psychotherapy for augmentation of antidepressant nonresponse in chronic depression: The REVAMP Trial. *Archives of General Psychiatry*, 66, 1178–1188.

Marmor, J. (1981). The adjunctive use of drugs in psychotherapy. *Journal of Clinical Psychopharmacology*, 1, 312–315.

Murphy, G.E., Simons, A.D., Wetzel, R.D., and Lustman, P.J. (1984). Cognitive therapy and pharmacotherapy: Singly and together in the treatment of depression. *Archives of General Psychiatry*, 41, 33–41.

Pampalona, S., Bollini, P., Tibaldi, G. *et al.* (2004). Combined pharmacotherapy and psychological treatment for depression. *Archives of General Psychiatry*, 61, 714–719.

Paykel, E.S. (1995). Risks of not achieving remission of symptoms are well established. *Psychological Medicine*, 25, 1171–1180.

Paykel, E.S., Ramana, R., Cooper, Z. *et al.* (1995). Residual symptoms after partial remission: An important outcome in depression. *Psychological Medicine*, 25, 1171–1180.

Ravindran, A.V., Anisman, H., Merali, Z. *et al.* (1999). Treatment of primary dysthymia with group cognitive therapy and pharmacotherapy: Clinical symptoms and functional impairments. *American Journal of Psychiatry*, 156, 1608–1617.

Reynolds, C.F., Miller, M.D., Pasternak, R.E. *et al.* (1999). Treatment of bereavement-related major depressive episodes in later life: A controlled study of acute and continuation treatment with nortriptyline and interpersonal psychotherapy. *American Journal of Psychiatry*, 156, 202–208.

Rush, A.J., Beck, A.T., Kovacs, M. *et al.* (1977). Comparative efficacy of cognitive therapy and pharmacotherapy in the treatment of depressed outpatients. *Cognitive Therapy Research*, 1, 17–37.

Rush, A.J., Trivedi, M.H., Wisniewski, S.R. *et al.* (2006). Acute and longer-term outcomes in depressed outpatients requiring one or several treatment steps: A STAR*D report. *American Journal of Psychiatry*, 163, 1905–1917.

Rutherford, B.R., Sneed, J.R., and Roose, S.P. (2009). Does study design affect outcome? The effects of placebo control and treatment duration in antidepressant trials. *Psychotherapy and Psychosomatics*, 78, 172–181.

Tang, T.Z., DeRubeis, R.J., Hollon, S.D. *et al.* (2010). Personality change during depression treatment: A placebo-controlled trial. *Archives of General Psychiatry*, 66, 1322–1330.

Thase, M.E., Greenhouse, J.B., Frank, E. *et al.* (1997). Treatment of major depression with psychotherapy or psychotherapy-pharmacotherapy combinations. *Archives of General Psychiatry*, 54, 1009–1015.

Thase, M.R., Friedman, E.S., Biggs, M.M. *et al.* (2007). Cognitive therapy versus medication in augmentation and switch strategies as second-step treatments: A

STAR*D report. *American Journal of Psychiatry*, 164, 739–752.

Thompson, L.W., Coon, D.W., Gallagher-Thompson, D. *et al.* (2001). Comparison of desipramine and cognitive/behavioral therapy in the treatment of elderly outpatients with mild-to-moderate depression. *American Journal of Geriatric Psychiatry*, 9, 225–240.

Treatment for Adolescents with Depression Study (TADS) Team (2004). Fluoxetine, cognitive-behavioral therapy, and their combination for adolescents with depression: Treatment for Adolescents with Depression Study (TADS) randomized controlled trial. *Journal of the American Medical Association*, 292, 807–820.

Trivedi, M.H., Rush, A.J., Wisniewski, S.R. *et al.* (2006). Evaluation of outcomes with citalopram for depression using measurement-based care in STAR*D: Implications for clinical practice. *American Journal of Psychiatry*, 163, 28–40.

Chapter

24

Electroconvulsive therapy

Joshua Berman and Joan Prudic

Introduction

There are published reports that convulsive therapies for major psychiatric illnesses were used as early as the eighteenth century, and historical reports of its use earlier. In the 1930s, Meduna observed that the brains of epileptics had greater than average numbers of glial cells, while the brains of psychiatric patients, particularly those suffering from psychosis, had fewer glial cells. Hypothesizing that there was a biologic antagonism between convulsions and mental illness, he sought to develop a convulsive treatment for psychiatric patients, apparently unaware of the literature and lore of convulsive therapy over the past centuries. Those first reports of convulsive therapy for psychiatric illness involved camphor, which Meduna also used and obtained a 50% response, but it was soon replaced by pharmaceuticals with shorter duration, such as pentylenetetrazol. Because these agents were GABA antagonists and had noxious side effects while patients were conscious, interest in developing electricity as an alternative method of seizure induction was pursued. In 1938, Cerletti and Bini administered the first electroconvulsive treatment (ECT) and obtained a remission significant enough to allow the patient to be discharged and resume work. Electrical stimulation was more reliable and shorter acting than chemically induced convulsive therapies and replaced them by the early 1940s (Loo, 2010).

Over time, numerous improvements were made to the treatment. In 1940, curare was developed for use in preventing fractures from muscle contractions associated with the tonic phase of the seizure. In the 1950s, curare was replaced with succinylcholine and brief general anesthesia with short-acting barbiturates. There were subsequent improvements in monitoring of cardiac and respiratory status. In the following decades, efforts were also made to improve the cognitive side-effect profile of the treatment with nondominant electrode placement, development of brief and then ultrabrief square waveforms to replace sine wave induction, methods for dose calculation based on empirical seizure threshold determination, etc. The treatment also benefited from improvements in diagnostic systems and the process of informed consent. It became apparent that apart from the treatment of catatonia and related conditions, the best effects of ECT were achieved in treatment of mood disorders and that is the indication on which ECT has become more focused over time. By the 1970s, professional organizations in the USA, England, Scandanavia, Canada, etc., made recommendations for treatment delivery, education, and training (Loo, 2010).

It is estimated that 85% of patients treated in the USA have major depression, either unipolar or bipolar, as the diagnostic indication for ECT. The efficacy of ECT has been robustly established in both clinical trials and community practice (Sakeim et al. 1993, Prudic et al. 2004, Kellner et al. 2010a). Reviews indicate that response rates to ECT are 70–90%, while time to optimal response is usually shorter than antidepressants with better overall outcome than medications alone (Shelton et al. 2010).

With the widespread use of pharmacologic agents as first-line treatments, ECT is now more commonly used for those resistant to pharmaceuticals, except in the case of life-threatening illness and severe suicidal and/or psychotic symptoms. Current estimates of ECT utilization are at about 1 million treatments (100 000 patients) per year. With the recognition that depression is a chronic disease for many patients, continuation and maintenance treatments following an acute ECT course have become an increasing focus (Watts *et al.* 2011).

This chapter will review the use of ECT in the treatment of depression. We will review indications and patient selection, and relative and absolute contraindications. We will describe modes of electrode placement and current waveform, dose titration, adverse effects (including effects on cognition), course of treatment, predictors of efficacy, and management of the patient when ECT is concluded. Finally, we will discuss potential mechanisms of antidepressant action and outline areas of active research in electroconvulsive therapy.

Initial management

Indications for ECT in depression

ECT remains the most effective treatment for major depression (Sonawalla and Fava, 2001). In fact, it has been used as a standard against which other treatments, including innovative treatments such as repetitive transcranial magnetic stimulation, are compared (Thase *et al.* 2008). No treatment has ever been found to be superior to ECT in the treatment of major depression in a controlled trial.

The clinical literature demonstrating the short-term efficacy of ECT in depression includes randomized controlled trials with sham treatment or medications as alternatives, outcome data from studies involving various treatment techniques, as well as uncontrolled data and surveys of expert opinion. Historically, ECT was used as a first-line treatment in major depression, but in the modern therapeutic era, the decision to use ECT for major depression is generally governed by three considerations: severity of depression, resistance to pharmacological treatment trials, and treatment intolerance. Of these, treatment resistance is the most common. Severity can include immediate threat to life or rapid deterioration, or, alternatively, chronic illness with marked impairment of function in the setting of significant treatment resistance and/or intolerance to medications and therapy. Because ECT offers the possibility of a more rapid response than conventional antidepressants, it is especially useful when a patient is severely suicidal or has markedly decreased intake of food and liquid (Shelton *et al.* 2010).

ECT is particularly effective in treating psychotic depression and severe melancholic depression. Psychotic depression and depressions accompanied by severe agitation and anxiety can be especially responsive to ECT. Here, the severity of symptoms creates an increased level of suffering and desperation that increases the risk of suicide and calls for the possibility of a more rapid response offered by ECT. ECT can be a primary treatment for catatonia in the course of severe depression (Kellner *et al.* 2006).

ECT is also an excellent treatment for bipolar depression. While there is growing evidence for efficacy in mixed states, evidence is less clear for efficacy in rapid cycling. On occasion, treatment-emergent mania may be observed, but, in most instances, with the addition of atypical antipsychotics for mood stabilization, the antimanic and mood stabilizing properties of ECT will prevail (Medda *et al.* 2009). Of note, ECT is also a highly effective treatment for mania in its own right (Loo *et al.* 2011).

Chronic moderate depression in the patient who is medication-resistant or medication-intolerant can also be an indication for ECT; such symptoms can be more subtle, but have a catastrophic effect on overall function (Baghai and Moller, 2008).

Although ECT is not recommended for treatment of dysthymia, dysthymic patients with a major depressive episode can benefit from ECT (Dombrovski *et al.* 2005). While they may not achieve full remission, they can at least return to a dysthymic baseline from a more severe, superimposed depression (Prudic *et al.* 1993). The same can be said for some patients with co-morbid major depression and personality disorders (Feske *et al.* 2004).

Another factor affecting full remission is the presence of a co-morbid anxiety disorder. Often full remission is achieved by treating the depression first, and then switching focus to pharmacological and psychological management of the anxiety condition. The most aggressive pharmacological management of the anxiety condition is often not fully compatible with concurrent ECT because of the effects of some anxiolytic medications on seizure generation (Krystal *et al.* 1998).

Risks in the use of ECT

Absolute and relative contraindications to ECT are those conditions which will be adversely affected by the events associated with treatment – the physiological and mechanical phenomena that accompany a generalized seizure, and brief general anesthesia with induced partial paralysis and without intubation (Tess and Smetana, 2009).

Risks related to blood pressure, heart rate, and intracranial pressure

During seizure generation, there is a strong parasympathetic effect at the onset of the stimulus, and a lesser such period at the point of termination of the seizure. During the seizure itself, and for a period of hours afterward, there is higher sympathetic tone with markedly elevated heart rate and blood pressure during ictus and for several minutes postictally. The period during the seizure has been likened to a stress test, with heart rates often in the 100–150 bpm range and systolic blood pressure that may exceed 200 mm Hg (Takada et al. 2005). Clinically significant changes can be ameliorated with concurrent beta-blockade and other pharmacologic interventions. There have been questions raised about high levels of beta block reducing the efficacy of the treatment, and it is not routinely recommended (Albin et al. 2007).

Persons with uncontrolled coronary artery disease, as evidenced by EKG changes on a stress test, are at greater risk of ischemia during ECT; consequently, the treatment is generally not undertaken until corrective measures have restored functional cardiac circulation (Tess and Smetana, 2009). Patients with congestive heart failure and/or valvular heart disease can receive ECT, but consultation with a cardiologist should assess and optimize stress tolerance, risk of ischemia, risk of arrhythmia, and risks posed by periods of high afterload and high sympathetic tone from ECT. Cardiac arrythmias can be provoked by ECT, due to the changing sympathetic and parasympathetic milieu during treatment, although most arrhythmias encountered are benign. Potentially unstable arrythmias affecting hemodynamic function also require the consultation and intervention of a cardiologist prior to treatment (Rayburn, 1997).

Vascular lesions, such as unstable or nearly unstable aneurysms or recent intracerebral bleeding, would also constitute a relative contraindication. Although it is possible to optimize changes in blood pressure with intra-arterial monitoring and minute-to-minute pharmacologic intervention, blood pressure cannot be perfectly leveled. It is generally advisable to allow 2 weeks after an incident of intracerebral bleeding before undertaking ECT, and the cause of the bleeding must be fully understood and resolved. Additional pressure-sensitive conditions, such as narrow angle glaucoma, would also constitute a relative contraindication to ECT, unless relieved by surgical intervention (Takada et al. 2005).

A seizure is characterized by high cerebral demand for glucose and oxygen due to increased neuronal activity; there is accompanying increased blood flow and increased intracerebral pressure. The brain and CSF circulation can normally accommodate this increase without difficulty, but may not do so in the presence of a fixed lesion or mass. Hence, any sort of intracerebral mass or blockage of CSF flow would constitute a risk during ECT, and appropriate neurological and/or neurosurgical consultation should be obtained prior to initiating ECT (Tess and Smetana, 2009).

Pre-existing seizure disorder

Pre-existing seizure disorder is generally not a contraindication for ECT; however, in patients with seizures, it should be ascertained that the seizure is not caused by a mass lesion or vascular malformation which could constitute higher risk with ECT. In fact, ECT is anticonvulsant, so a seizure disorder would not be expected to worsen with ECT, and might ameliorate. ECT has been used to terminate status, particularly when the provoking agent has been removed. For patients who have had episodes of refractory seizures, there may be some concern about the ability to terminate the initial seizure; if such concern exists, neurological consultation should be obtained. In general, patients with seizure disorders continue their anticonvulsants during ECT on the grounds that their baseline seizure threshold is likely lower and their innate ability to terminate seizures less than patients without seizure disorder. This practice is in contrast to the termination of anticonvulsants when ECT is being used solely as a mood stabilizer (Krystal and Coffey, 1997).

Risks related to mechanical forces

While chemical paralysis, using the depolarizing agent succinylcholine, protects against muscle injury and vertebral and other fractures consequent to seizure-associated movement, there is still neck flexion associated with anesthetic technique and contraction of muscles of the face and some muscles of the neck directly stimulated by the current application in areas near the facial and trigeminal nerves. This movement is in proportion to the energy output and is not affected by the use of the paralytic agent. Patients with conditions such as cervical stenosis or vertebral compression may undergo movements that could destabilize their condition. Those who are experiencing active symptoms, e.g., paresthesias, numbness of the extremities, and impaired gait require a cautious approach. For patients with cervical stenosis, it is advisable to achieve a higher degree of paralysis with succinylcholine or similar agents. The anesthetist will also modify technique to accommodate the condition (Naguib and Koorn, 2002, Tess and Smetana, 2009).

Recent surgery, fractures, and other mechanical injuries, could, in theory, be exacerbated by movement during ECT, even with use of paralytics. In such cases, where possible, it is best to allow a period of weeks for wounds or fractures to heal, in consultation with surgical personnel. If the psychiatric status is too urgent for this waiting period, complete paralysis can reduce risk in the case of fracture (Tess and Smetana, 2009).

Risks related to anesthesia

Anesthesia for ECT is brief and, typically, does not involve intubation. The anesthetist provides pre-oxygenation and ventilates the patient using a bag mask, as well as providing monitoring of vital functions. Conditions such as chronic obstructive pulmonary disease, sleep apnea, asthma, and large habitus, which will impair the patient's ability to resume his or her own respiration effectively, can influence the risks of ECT, but, often, these can be managed. Other risks of anesthesia, e.g., pseudocholinesterase deficiency, allergy to specific anesthetic agents, aspiration, are present during ECT, but are generally held to be small. The estimated mortality associated with ECT is in the order of 1 to 4 per 100 000. The longitudinal mortality in patients who received ECT vs. other treatments is better, a regularly observed phenomenon since ECT has been used, the basis of which has not been elucidated (Watts *et al.* 2011).

Risks related to baseline cognitive status

Patients with baseline cognitive impairments can receive ECT, but are thought to be at higher risk for confusion and delirium. It is likely that these short-term impairments revert, as for other patients; since this occurs against a background of pre-existing cognitive decline, the overall clinical impression is less

than assured. Certainly, such patients have lower cognitive reserve, and caution should be exercised in their treatment. Those aspects of cognitive function most likely to be affected should be documented at baseline: orientation and memory, including recall of recent and remote events, and subjective assessment of cognitive and memory functioning (Coleman *et al.* 1996). Technique should be moderated to provide the least intensive stimulus in order to spare cognitive function.

Conducting treatment

Consent for ECT

ECT requires the consent of the patient or, in the event that the patient lacks capacity, a ruling from a legal authority regarding procedures for substituted consent if available. Objection to treatment with ECT should prompt both a sincere attempt to find alternatives, and an exploration of the basis for the objection. It is important to allay any unfounded patient fears, not only as a normal part of the doctor–patient relationship, but also because such fears may create an atmosphere of anxiety around treatment that can ultimately serve to complicate the patient's response (Ottosson, 1992). Some jurisdictions allow for treatment over objection if patients lack capacity, although this varies greatly, and clinicians are advised to be well informed about local regulation. Treatment over objection should be pursued only if the alternatives are unlikely to work, the patient is in very real danger, and prescribed legal procedures have been followed.

Consent should include a description of the treatment and a frank and accurate discussion of the risks and benefits of ECT, including risks of anesthesia, the possibility of transient cognitive impairment, and the smaller, but real, possibility of more lasting impairments, as well as the risk of relapse. The elements of the consent should be well documented, as should be the reasons for choosing ECT over other treatments (Rush *et al.* 2008).

Anesthesia for ECT

An anesthetist provides paralysis and brief general anesthesia, as well as respiratory support and hyperoxygenation, and control of heart rate and respiratory secretions. The purpose of paralysis is to prevent fractures; prior to the use of paralytic agents, the rate of fracture during a course of ECT was close to 30%, with the most serious fractures involving the vertebrae. Paralysis is achieved with succinylcholine

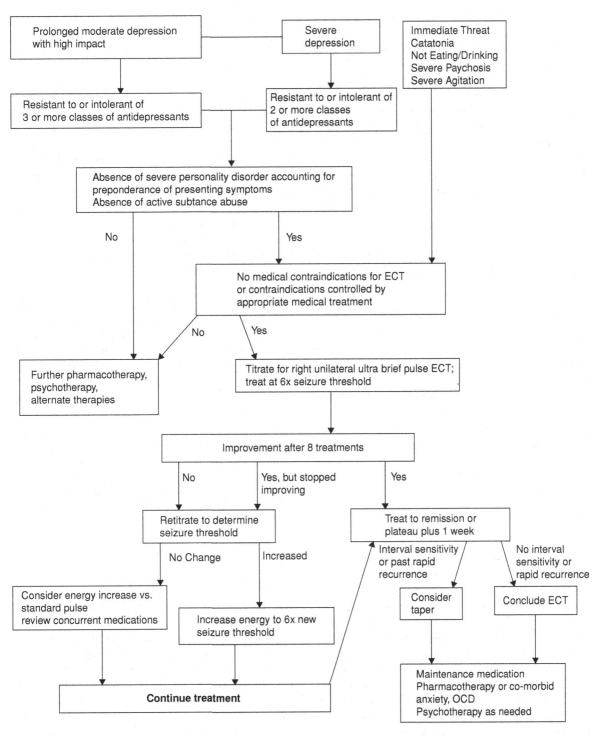

Figure 24.1 ECT algorithm

and is usually deliberately less than complete. A blood pressure cuff is applied to the right leg at the time of treatment to prevent the paralytic from affecting the foot in order to observe the full motor seizure. Besides the treatment itself, paralysis necessitates the use of an anesthetic/amnestic agent. Brevital, propofol, and etomidate are the most commonly used. Of these, propofol has the greatest impact on seizure generation and etomidate the least, but etomidate can produce myoclonus and postictal agitation, and, as such, is used less often than the others. Atropine is often given, to control airway secretions, and more importantly to prevent asystole or significant bradycardia, which can occur during the early and late portions of the seizure where there is transient parasympathetic predominance. It is especially important to use atropine in patients who are given beta-blockers and have higher risk for severe bradycardia or asystole, and those treatment sessions which may involve sub-convulsive stimulation(s) (Wagner *et al.* 2005). Hyperoxygenation beginning pre-ECT and continuing until complete recovery is the last component of modified ECT. The high neuronal activity experienced during seizure increases glucose and oxygen demand, and extra oxygenation is thought to protect the brain from these demands. Bite blocks are used to protect dentition and oral structures during electrical stimulation. Seizures longer than 3 minutes are terminated with the anesthetic agent or other suitable immediate-acting anticonvulsant medication (Weiner and Coffey, 1991, Wagner *et al.* 2005).

Electrode placement and waveform

Electrical stimulation was initially delivered as a sine wave, but modern devices use a bipolar square wave that reduces the delivery of energy to a more physiologic level and thus increases the ratio of therapeutic effect to adverse effects. Pulse width varies from ultrabrief (0.25 to 0.3 ms) through half standard (0.5 ms) up to standard (1 ms) pulses. There is no proven increase in efficacy with increased pulse width, and wider pulse width likely produces more cognitive impairment. However, in clinical practice, there seem to be some patients who respond better to standard pulse. A caveat is that these responses often occur after initiating treatment in ultrabrief pulse, and it is unclear as to whether the switch in waveform or the accumulation of more treatments is what makes the difference (Sackeim *et al.* 1993).

Electrode placements include: bitemporal (the standard bilateral placement); bifrontal; left anterior, right temporal (LART); and right unilateral. The D'Elia placement has become the most commonly used unilateral placement: one electrode is on the right temple, tangential to an imaginary line between the lateral canthus of the ear and the corner of the eye; the second electrode is just to the right and just anterior to the vertex of the skull. It is important to note when reading older ECT literature, whether other configurations were used, as results obtained with this method may not be comparable to results obtained with right unilateral ECT as it is usually performed today (Nobler *et al.* 1993, Sackeim *et al.* 1993).

There has been at least one study using left unilateral ECT; left-handers were identified as likely having speech and language function on the right by performing left- and right-sided treatments and recording the time to reorientation, then treating on the side with the shorter time. A small number of patients who oriented more quickly after left-sided treatment, continued with left unilateral ECT and efficacy was similar to that obtained with right unilateral treatment in the general population (Kellner *et al.* 2010b).

Several studies have been undertaken to compare efficacy and adverse effects between right unilateral ECT and bilateral ECT. When right unilateral ECT is dosed at five times above seizure threshold, there is no evidence that it is less effective than bilateral, and substantial evidence of fewer cognitive side effects. There is at least one study indicating that ultrabrief bifrontotemporal ECT is less effective than ultrabrief right unilateral or brief bilateral ECT; and cognitive side effects were greater than right unilateral ECT (Kellner *et al.* 2010a).

Dose titration and seizure adequacy

The most accurate way to insure that the stimulus energy is sufficient is to employ seizure titration, a method of limits technique for determining seizure threshold. Seizure threshold may be roughly estimated based on age and gender, but these estimates only account for 40% of the variance in seizure threshold. Right unilateral treatment is done at six times the seizure threshold, whether using standard pulse (1 ms) or ultrabrief pulse (0.25 to 0.3 ms). Bitemporal treatment is done at 1.5 times seizure threshold (which is generally higher than that for unilateral), and is effective with standard and half standard pulse widths. Bifrontal ECT is also performed at 1.5 times seizure threshold with efficacy comparable to other electrode placements when brief pulse waveforms are used; there is also evidence that ultrabrief bifrontal ECT is equally effective to brief pulse treatment (Abrams, 2002). The amount of brain tissue stimulated is greater for bilateral electrode placement and thought to be related to the greater adverse cognitive effects observed. There is no consistent evidence of more rapid response with any particular electrode placement (Petrides *et al.* 2009).

Seizures are assessed both by direct observation of the motor seizure and by EEG, as it is important to confirm that a seizure has terminated on EEG (Abrams, 2002). In practice, a simplified two-channel EEG is sufficient for this purpose. Seizures should be at least 15 s in duration to be considered therapeutically adequate. There is no evidence that longer seizures are more likely to be therapeutic; however, if a treatment is begun with barely adequate seizure duration, an assessment of interfering factors, such as concurrent medications or excessive anesthetic dose, should be made in order to elucidate any possibility of amelioration (Rattehalli *et al.* 2009).

Concurrent medications

Some medications are not compatible with ECT, and the procedure must be held until those medications are no longer present in circulation, or present at very low levels and their secondary effects diminished. Anticonvulsants and long-acting benzodiazepines interfere with seizure generation; besides raising seizure threshold, anticonvulsants dampen the effects of seizure, including therapeutic effects, and benzodiazepines have been associated with reduced efficacy in randomized controlled trials. It is advised to wait for 5 days to begin ECT after the last anticonvulsant dose in a nonepileptic patient, although the full effects of anticonvulsant medications take 2–3 weeks to wash out. AEDs are continued when used to treat epilepsy where reduced seizure threshold and ability to terminate neuronal firing is normalized to some extent by the medication (Naguib and Koorn, 2002).

Lithium is problematic with ECT, as patients with therapeutic lithium levels develop much more postictal confusion, bordering on delirium, and serotonin syndrome is thought to be a risk. Thus, during ECT, lithium is held for 24 hours before treatment allowing the level to drop to well below the therapeutic level (Feske *et al.* 2004). MAOIs are generally stopped

2 weeks prior to ECT, just as they are before addition of SSRIs, tricyclic, or other medications that raise monoamine levels. MAOIs are irreversible inhibitors and time is needed to produce new monamine oxidase receptors. ECT releases a surge of monoamines, so that the presence of an MAOI may increase the risk for serotonin syndrome or hypertensive crisis (Dolenc *et al.* 2004).

SSRIs are proconvulsant, as are caffeine and theophylline. Indeed these latter two are sometimes used to prolong seizures of inadequate duration. Status epilepticus has not been observed with SSRIs, but has been observed with theophylline at therapeutic levels.

There is mixed evidence of an augmenting effect of norepinephrinergic agents, e.g., nortriptyline or venlafaxine, and antipsychotics may be continued at moderate levels to manage severe agitated or psychotic depression (Sackeim *et al.* 2009).

If a patient is taking coumadin, it is advised that the dose be reduced such that the INR is equal to or less than 2.5 prior to and during treatment. Such dose adjustment should be discussed with the physician treating the condition for which the coumadin was prescribed (Mehta *et al.* 2004).

Clinical vignette

Ms. A, a 24-year-old woman with a history of seizure and 5 years of bipolar I disorder, presented for treatment of severe depression with psychotic features. A prior depressive episode had responded to six bilateral ECTs, but with some noticeable cognitive side effects that persisted several months after treatment. Her seizure disorder and mood disorder were treated with depakote 1000 qhs and trileptal 300 bid. She had been euthymic until about 2 months prior to admission, when she discontinued depakote due to concerns about weight gain and hair loss. Moderate hypomanic symptoms recurred and transitioned into a depressive episode with suicidality, delusions of guilt, and auditory hallucinations. Upon admission to the hospital, depakote was restarted along with abilify 2mg qd. Cymbalta was added as well at a dose of 30 mg qd, with no effect and the occurrence of nausea; it was discontinued. The patient was presented for consideration of a trial of ECT.

EKG, chest X-ray, and basic lab results were unremarkable with therapeutic levels of depakote and oxcarbamazepine. An MRI taken at the onset of her seizure disorder, 3 years prior, had shown no vascular lesions, hemorrhage, infarcts, or masses. Neurological examination on admission was nonfocal and it was felt that further brain imaging was not required. She was medically and neurologically cleared for ECT. Depakote and trileptal were continued for treatment of seizure disorder; abilify was maintained.

Given that right unilateral ECT is equally effective to bilateral ECT, and given her prior impairment with bilateral treatment, it was decided to treat with right unilateral, ultrabrief pulse ECT. Her seizure threshold was unremarkable. After three treatments she experienced marked improvement with near normalization of mood and cessation of delusions of guilt. After the fourth treatment she was noted to be intrusive and irritable, with pressured speech, marked insomnia, and increased energy. Auditory hallucinations increased and were accompanied by some paranoid ideation. Abilify was discontinued and risperidone was substituted at 2 mg bid. ECT was continued and by treatment #6, marked improvement was noted with reduction in all manic symptoms and near-euthymic mood. By treatment #9 the patient reported euthymic mood and no psychotic symptoms. She was continued on depakote, trileptal, and risperidone, and was reported euthymic and stable 6 months after treatment.

Course of treatment

ECT provides the possibility of responses more rapid than when patients are taking conventional antidepressants, however there is in fact a wide spectrum of rates of response. A significant number of patients show clinically useful responses after a few ECT, and many will show full recovery within 2–3 weeks (six to nine treatments), which is still sooner than one would anticipate with conventional antidepressants (Prudic et al. 2004, Dombrovski et al. 2005). It is important to note, however, that some patients may require more than 20 treatments to show significant improvement or remission; however, these patients are frequently those that have been refractory to pharmacological treatments and have significant psychiatric co-morbidity (Baghai and Moller, 2008).

Acute ECT is performed three times or two times weekly; there is no difference in efficacy, but the number of treatments needed is similar (Cameron et al. 1962, Exner and Murillo, 1973, Exner and Murillo, 1977). Hence, it will take longer to reach the required

number of treatments for response or remission with twice weekly treatment (McAllister et al. 1987, Gangadhar et al. 1993, Lerer et al. 1995, Shapira et al. 1998). ECT performed weekly is thought to have reduced efficacy except during maintenance or taper to maintenance (Janakiramaiah et al. 1998).

At present there is no evidence as to whether or when a treatment should be tapered as opposed to simply stopping some time after either remission or a response plateau is achieved. Patients who have a history of rapid recurrence after a successful course of ECT should probably be cross-tapered to the selected maintenance modalities (Kellner et al. 2006).

The total number of treatments in a course of ECT is based on clinical observation over the course of treatment. In general, we treat until we see no further improvement, either because remission has been achieved and sustained for at least a week, or because a plateau in response has been reached. A plateau in response should prompt a search for technical factors that may be preventing remission. It is useful to review medications and their effects on the patient and on the ECT course, and to perform retitration of the seizure threshold with the possibility of increasing energy if it has increased or changing pulse width if it has not. At the point of a plateau, one should also re-evaluate factors that might prevent remission which cannot be addressed by ECT. These include conditions such as psychosocial environment and life stressors, dysthymia, anxiety not related to depression, concurrent medical conditions, and characterological issues.

Adverse effects of ECT

The most common adverse effects of ECT are headache and myalgia. Some patients may develop nausea, generally in the context of headache, which is usually vascular in nature. These side effects are easily addressed: analgesics and antimigraine therapies are most frequently employed as needed. Myalgias usually resolve after a few treatments (Dinwiddie et al. 2010). Cardiopulmonary complications of illnesses which pose extra risk can usually be managed, but mortality can occur, though deaths in the setting of ECT are rare (Watts et al. 2011).

The most frequently discussed adverse effect of ECT is cognitive impairment. Disorientation, diminished processing speed, decreased anterograde and retrograde memory, and errors in visual–spatial function and word finding are greatest immediately after a treatment session, and diminish with time. Except for retrograde amnesia, other effects diminish to pre-ECT baseline for bilateral ECT, and better than baseline performance for unilateral ECT (Eschweiler *et al.* 2007). For retrograde memory deficits, use of bilateral ECT is associated with persistent effects correlated to the number of bilateral ECT received; 10–15% of patients in community practice who received bilateral ECT showed marked persistent impairment even after 6 months, as measured by the Columbia Univeristy Autobiographical Memory Interview (AMI-SF) (Sackeim *et al.* 2007).

Cognitive adverse effects can be diminished by using ultrabrief waveform, unilateral treatment, twice weekly frequency, specific dosing techniques to achieve the most efficient stimulus, minimal anesthesia dosing, and minimal concurrent use of medications (Roepke *et al.* 2011).

Clinical vignette

Mr. B, a 57-year-old man with a third episode of major depressive disorder as well as 25-year history of moderate OCD, presented for evaluation for ECT after 2 years of gradually worsening depression. Over the course, fluoxetine had been maintained for OCD treatment and other antidepressants, including bupropion and mirtazepine, were added and switched when he became symptomatic with two prior episodes of depression. In the current episode, an attempt to switch to duloxetine worsened OCD and was not tolerated due to severe headache and sweating. Addition of nortriptyline 75 mg and abilify to fluoxetine was without effect. He declined a trial of an MAOI due to concerns about adverse effects and dietary restrictions.

He had hypercholesterolemia and coronary artery disease with an LAD stent placed 2 years previously for unstable angina. His cardiogram showed no evidence of ischemia or infarct; echocardiogram and stress test were normal. His cardiologist gave clearance for ECT. Chest X-ray showed clear lungs and some calcifications in the aorta. Head CT showed mild atrophy, but no hemorrhage, mass, or infarct. Preop labs and physical examination were otherwise unremarkable.

Fluoxetine was reduced to 20 mg with some increase in OCD-like symptoms, and 1 week later he began a course of right unilateral, ultrabrief pulse ECT.

By treatments #5–6 hospital staff noted more spontaneity and some improvement in appetite and insomnia. He noted mild forgetfulness regarding events on treatment days and felt some slight worsening of balance, but was able to ambulate without assistance. He was noted to recover orientation within 20 minutes of awakening after treatment, and did not show any marked agitation or confusion. There was no further improvement through treatment #10, and the decision was made to do another dose titration. On this occasion, he was noted to have an increased seizure threshold, and stimulus intensity was raised to six times the new threshold. After five more treatments, depression remitted; some residual obsessive thoughts remained. After two more treatments, ECT was stopped; fluoxetine was raised to 40 mg; nortriptyline 75 mg and lithium 300 mg, raised to 900 mg over the course of 2 weeks, were added for maintenance treatment. By 2 months after treatment he reported feeling very well, with no discernible symptoms. He reported no lasting cognitive sequelae; MMSE was 30/30.

Maintenance treatment

While 80–90% of patients respond to ECT, and over 60% achieve remission of symptoms, the rate of recurrence of depression after ECT, in the absence of other treatment, remains high, as it would for any antidepressant regimen discontinued abruptly upon improvement (Baghai and Moller, 2008). During the first 6 months after treatment, as many as 80% of patients will experience relapse if not placed on an optimal maintenance regimen of medications and/or ECT, likely related to the fact that ECT patients are relatively resistant to standard antidepressant regimens and have severe baseline symptomatology (Sackeim *et al.* 2001).

Randomized controlled trials support two maintenance regimens that reduce the rate of relapse after ECT. One is maintenance ECT, and the other is the combination of lithium and nortriptyline or venlafaxine (Smith *et al.* 2010). When lithium, nortriptyline or venlafaxine are not tolerated, substitutions may be attempted, but the evidence for their efficacy is lacking. In general, pure SSRIs may not confer protection against recurrence in treatment-resistant patients who have had ECT, but may have value as anxiolytic agents or as treatment for co-morbid OCD. Duloxetine or venlafaxine are often substituted for nortriptyline in patients who have stopped ECT but cannot tolerate a tricyclic. Venlafaxine has been demonstrated to be equivalent in efficacy to nortriptyline in one study and is being used in a current investigation of relapse prevention. Duloxetine has not been investigated (Sackeim *et al.* 2001).

There is also evidence to suggest that lithium is the more important partner in the post-ECT combination, and it is hard to find a comparable substitute. We often use lamictal, as there is at least evidence for efficacy in preventing depression recurrence (though not specifically substantiated in the post-ECT population.) It is clear that atypical antipsychotics do not confer the protective effects of lithium, and unknown as to whether anticonvulsants are effective substitutes, but their weakness as antidepressants poses problems for their use as maintenance treatments, particularly in a unipolar population (Shelton *et al.* 2010).

A fixed schedule of ECT has been demonstrated to be equivalent to optimal pharmacologic maintenance with lithium/nortriptyline, and may be appropriate for patients who have failed or are intolerant of medication maintenance. Some patients may require both medication and a period of maintenance ECT, and such a regimen is currently under investigation (Smith *et al.* 2010). Lithium can be given during maintenance ECT, but must be stopped on the night prior to treatment to mitigate the potential for unnecessary adverse effects. Generally, anticonvulsants are avoided if ECT will be continued as maintenance (Sackeim *et al.* 2009).

Treatment alternatives for nonremission

For patients who do not respond to ECT, it should be ascertained that the course was optimized in technique and use of concurrent medications, particularly for partial responders. Intensification of stimulus, discontinuation of medications with anticonvulsant properties, including benzodiazepines, less anticonvulsant anesthesia, and change in electrode placement can be considered. Alternatives exist although they are sparse. Vagal nerve stimulation shows efficacy in a sub-set of patients with treatment-resistant depression; the response rate is low at 15–20%, but twice as high as what is a very low placebo response rate in a considerably ill and refractory group. Deep brain stimulation may be another alternative treatment and is under active investigation, having shown efficacy for some

treatment-resistant patients in several small case series (Shelton *et al.* 2010).

At this time, there is no evidence to support rTMS (repetitive transcranial magnetic stimulation) in highly treatment-resistant patients. One would expect that ECT nonresponders would fall into this group. If, however, ECT was undertaken due to treatment intolerance, there could be a case for a trial of rTMS, especially if the ECT course was aborted due to adverse effects (Loo and Mitchell, 2005).

ECT nonresponders may also be candidates for such investigational treatments as ketamine, and d-cycloserine (Heresco-Levy *et al.* 2006, Covvey *et al.* 2011).

Nonresponse or inadequate response to ECT should prompt a thorough investigation of additional clinical factors such as co-morbid anxiety, OCD, personality disorder, or substance abuse; in such instances ECT may be valuable, but unable to bring about resolution of symptoms until the other issues are addressed in a definitive manner.

Clinical pearls of therapeutic wisdom

Related to indications for treatment

Response without remission of major depression in baseline dysthymic patients may be a worthwhile therapeutic aim.

Anxiety limited to depression responds; GAD/PANIC do.

Mania and catatonia respond to unilateral treatment.

Dissociation is a risk for cognitive impairment, and exacerbation of related symptoms of PTSD.

A longer treatment with a more conservative electrode placement and pulse width can produce fewer adverse cognitive effects than a shorter, more aggressive treatment.

Related to the course of ECT

If response reaches a plateau, dosage adjustment instead of switching electrode placement is a cognitively sparing approach to enhancing response and remission of symptoms.

In treatment-emergent hypomania or mania, continued ECT with atypical antipsychotic augmentation can be a beneficial approach.

A small number of patients, usually with baseline co-morbid anxiety, can have PTSD-like symptoms related to a course of ECT, and will probably have difficulty tolerating subsequent treatments.

Related to the long-term outcome from ECT

Even remitted patients may feel best 2 months after treatment.

Treatment strategy summarized

To start treatment, determine the seizure threshold; perform right unilateral ECT at six times seizure threshold, until remission, plateau, or setback. If plateau or setback is reached with no cause external to treatment identified, recheck seizure threshold. If higher, raise energy. If no increase, consider half standard or standard pulse and retitrate in that modality. Treat to remission or plateau plus 1 week.

Future directions: improving ECT and beyond

Current clinical research on ECT aims to reduce relapse, decrease adverse effects (particularly those involving cognition), and better predict the course of treatment.

Studies on the long-term course of patients after ECT seek to identify additional medications and develop combined ECT and pharmacological protocols useful for prophylaxis of recurrence. Biomarker studies may allow better prediction both of the course of treatment and of requirements for taper, maintenance, and pharmacological prophylaxis (Christensen *et al.* 2011). Techniques such as magnetic seizure therapy (MST) and focalized electrically administered seizure therapy (FEAST) are in development with the goal of providing the efficacy of ECT, while involving more limited brain regions and, therefore, reducing adverse effects (Spellman *et al.* 2009, Hoy and Fitzgerald, 2011). Cognitive remediation is being investigated as an approach to the prevention and mitigation of the cognitive adverse effects of ECT (Choi *et al.* 2011).

As all of these research aims would be aided by a better understanding of mechanisms of action, both clinical and preclinical research seek to better identify potential therapeutic mechanisms of action. In preclinical models, electroconvulsive shock (ECS) releases the same monoamines and catecholamines that are the major targets of conventional antidepressant action – along with acetylcholine, glutamate, and multiple neuropeptides. Most of the observed effects on neurotransmitter release and production are in the same direction as those of conventional antidepressants, and the range of neurotransmitter substances involved is wider than for any single antidepressant medication. It is not yet known which of these actions are essential to therapeutic effects.

ECS in preclinical studies has been found to increase levels of such trophic factors as BDNF (brain-derived neurotrophic factor), to increase dendritic spines, and to increase the formation of neuronal precursor cells and the proliferation of glia; thus one possible set of mechanisms relates to the theory that depression involves failures of neuroplasticity and trophic function.

In one preclinical study, ECS was shown to alter histone protein deacetylation in a manner that increases transcription of BDNF message, among others. This is of particular interest because chemicals that produce the same type of histone modifications have been shown to have antidepressant-like effects in animal models over a very short time course, possibly accounting for the ability of ECT to act more rapidly than conventional antidepressants in many cases.

Another potential relationship to rapidity of action is to be found in actions of ECT on the PTEN pathway, which has been associated with the rapid effects of ketamine. ECT appears to reduce the actions of sprouty2, which exerts negative effects on glial proliferation in part via the constituents of the PTEN and Akt pathways.

In summary, ECT releases large numbers of neurotransmitters which in turn regulate a number of signal-transduction and gene-expression pathways that have been implicated in depression, as well as many whose roles in mood disorders are not yet appreciated or understood. It is likely that the greater number of ways in which ECT can access these pathways accounts in part for its higher efficacy in relation to other treatments, and also for its more varied time course with onset of action ranging from much faster than to equal to conventional antidepressants.

Understanding of these multiple effects and identification of the ones likely to convey therapeutic efficacy will not only allow for improved administration of ECT, but for the development of novel biochemical therapies as well.

References

Abrams, R. (2002). Stimulus titration and ECT dosing. *Journal of ECT*, 18, 3–9; discussion 14–5.

Albin, S.M., Stevens, S.R., and Rasmussen, K.G. (2007). Blood pressure before and after electroconvulsive therapy in hypertensive and nonhypertensive patients. *Journal of ECT*, 23, 9–10.

Baghai, T.C. and Moller, H.J. (2008). Electroconvulsive therapy and its different indications. *Dialogues in Clinical Neuroscience*, 10, 105–117.

Cameron, D.E., Lohrenz, J.G., and Handcock, K.A. (1962). The depatterning treatment of schizophrenia. *Comprehesive Psychiatry*, 3, 65–76.

Choi, J., Lisanby, S.H., Medalia, A., and Prudic, J. (2011). A conceptual introduction to cognitive remediation for memory deficits associated with right unilateral electroconvulsive therapy. *Journal of ECT*, 27, 286–291.

Christensen, T., Bisgaard, C.F., and Wiborg, O. (2011). Biomarkers of anhedonic-like behavior, antidepressant drug refraction, and stress resilience in a rat model of depression. *Neuroscience*, 196, 66–79.

Coleman, E.A., Sackeim, H.A., Prudic, J. et al. (1996). Subjective memory complaints prior to and following electroconvulsive therapy. *Biological Psychiatry*, 39, 346–356.

Covvey, J.R., Crawford, A.N., and Lowe, D.K. (2011). Intravenous ketamine for treatment-resistant major depressive disorder. *Annals of Pharmacotherapy*, 46, 117–123.

Daly, J.J., Prudic, J., Nobler, M.S. et al. (2001). ECT in bipolar and unipolar depression: Differences in speed of response. *Bipolar Disorders*, 3, 95–104.

Dinwiddie, S.H., Huo, D., and Gottlieb, O. (2010). The course of myalgia and headache after electroconvulsive therapy. *Journal of ECT*, 26, 116–120.

Dolenc, T.J., Habl, S.S., Barnes, R.D., and Rasmussen, K.G. (2004). Electroconvulsive therapy in patients taking monoamine oxidase inhibitors. *Journal of ECT*, 20, 258–261.

Dombrovski, A.Y., Mulsant, B.H., Haskett, R.F. et al. (2005). Predictors of remission after electroconvulsive therapy in unipolar major depression. *Journal of Clinical Psychiatry*, 66, 1043–1049.

Eschweiler, G.W., Vonthein, R., Bode, R. et al. (2007). Clinical efficacy and cognitive side effects of bifrontal versus right unilateral electroconvulsive therapy (ECT): A short-term randomised controlled trial in pharmaco-resistant major depression. *Journal of Affective Disorders*, 101, 149–157.

Exner, J.E., Jr. and Murillo, L.G. (1973). Effectiveness of regressive ECT with process schizophrenia. *Diseases of the Nervous System*, 34, 44–48.

Exner, J.E., Jr. and Murillo, L.G. (1977). A long-term follow-up of schizophrenics treated with regressive ECT. *Diseases of the Nervous System*, 38, 162–168.

Feske, U., Mulsant, B.H., Pilkonis, P.A. et al. (2004). Clinical outcome of ECT in patients with major depression and comorbid borderline personality disorder. *American Journal of Psychiatry*, 161, 2073–2080.

Gangadhar, B.N., Janakiramaiah, N., Subbakrishna, D.K., Praveen, J., and Reddy, A.K. (1993). Twice versus thrice weekly ECT in melancholia: A double-blind prospective comparison. *Journal of Affective Disorders*, 27, 273–278.

Heresco-Levy, U., Javitt, D.C., Gelfin, Y. et al. (2006). Controlled trial of D-cycloserine adjuvant therapy for treatment-resistant major depressive disorder. *Journal of Affective Disorders*, 93, 239–243.

Hoy, K.E. and Fitzgerald, P.B. (2011). Magnetic seizure therapy for treatment-resistant depression. *Expert Review of Medical Devices*, 8, 723–732.

Janakiramaiah, N., Motreja, S., Gangadhar, B.N., Subbakrishna, D.K., and Parameshwara, G. (1998). Once vs. three times weekly ECT in melancholia: A randomized controlled trial. *Acta Psychiatrica Scandinavica*, 98, 316–320.

Kellner, C.H., Knapp, R.G., Petrides, G. et al. (2006). Continuation electroconvulsive therapy vs pharmacotherapy for relapse prevention in major depression: A multisite study from the Consortium for Research in Electroconvulsive Therapy (CORE). *Archives of General Psychiatry*, 63, 1337–1344.

Kellner, C.H., Knapp, R., Husain, M.M. et al. (2010a) Bifrontal, bitemporal and right unilateral electrode placement in ECT: Randomised trial. *The British Journal of Psychiatry*, 196, 226–234.

Kellner, C.H., Tobias, K.G., and Wiegand, J. (2010b). Electrode placement in electroconvulsive therapy (ECT): A review of the literature. *The Journal of ECT*, 26, 175–180.

Krystal, A.D. and Coffey, C.E. (1997). Neuropsychiatric considerations in the use of electroconvulsive therapy. *Journal of Neuropsychiatry and Clinical Neuroscience*, 9, 283–292.

Krystal, A.D., Watts, B.V., Weiner, R.D. et al. (1998). The use of flumazenil in the anxious and benzodiazepine-dependent ECT patient. *Journal of ECT*, 14, 5–14.

Lerer, B., Shapira, B., Calev, A. et al. (1995). Antidepressant and cognitive effects of twice- versus three-times-weekly ECT. *American Journal of Psychiatry*, 152, 564–570.

Loo, C. (2010). ECT in the 21st century: Optimizing treatment: state of the art in the 21st century. *Journal of ECT*, 26, 157.

Loo, C., Greenberg, B., and Mitchell, P. (2011). Nonpharmacotherapeutic somatic treatments for bipolar disorder (ECT, DBS, rTMS). In Manji, H.K. and Zarate, C.A., Jr., eds., *Behavioral Neurobiology of Bipolar Disorder and its Treatment*. Berlin, Heidelberg: Springer.

Loo, C.K. and Mitchell, P.B. (2005). A review of the efficacy of transcranial magnetic stimulation (TMS) treatment for depression, and current and future strategies to optimize efficacy. *Journal of Affective Disorders*, 88, 255–267.

McAllister, D.A., Perri, M.G., Jordan, R.C., Rauscher, F.P., and Sattin, A. (1987). Effects of ECT given two vs. three times weekly. *Psychiatry Research*, 21, 63–69.

Medda, P., Perugi, G., Zanello, S., Ciuffa, M., and Cassano, G.B. (2009). Response to ECT in bipolar I, bipolar II and unipolar depression. *Journal of Affective Disorders*, 118, 55–59.

Mehta, V., Mueller, P.S., Gonzalez-Arriaza, H.L., Pankratz, V.S., and Rummans, T.A. (2004). Safety of electroconvulsive therapy in patients receiving long-term warfarin therapy. *Mayo Clinic Proceedings*, 79, 1396–1401.

Naguib, M. and Koorn, R. (2002). Interactions between psychotropics, anaesthetics and electroconvulsive therapy: Implications for drug choice and patient management. *CNS Drugs*, 16, 229–247.

Nobler, M.S., Sackeim, H.A., Solomou, M. *et al.* (1993). EEG manifestations during ECT: Effects of electrode placement and stimulus intensity. *Biological Psychiatry*, 34, 321–330.

Ottoson, J.O. (1992). Ethics of electroconvulsive therapy. *Convulsive Therapy*, 8, 233–236.

Petrides, G., Braga, R.J., Fink, M. *et al.* (2009). Seizure threshold in a large sample: Implications for stimulus dosing strategies in bilateral electroconvulsive therapy: A report from CORE. *Journal of ECT*, 25, 232–237.

Prudic, J., Sackeim, H.A., Devanand, D.P., and Kiersky, J.E. (1993). The efficacy of ECT in double depression. *Depression*, 1, 38–44.

Prudic, J., Olfson, M., Marcus, S.C., Fuller, R.B., and Sackeim, H.A. (2004). Effectiveness of electroconvulsive therapy in community settings. *Biological Psychiatry*, 55, 301–312.

Rattehalli, R.D., Thirthalli, J., Rawat, V., Gangadhar, B.N., and Adams, C.E. (2009). Measuring electroencephalographic seizure adequacy during electroconvulsive therapy: A comparison of 2 definitions. *The Journal of ECT*, 25, 243–245.

Rayburn, B.K. (1997). Electroconvulsive therapy in patients with heart failure or valvular heart disease. *Convulsive Therapy*, 13, 145–156.

Roepke, S., Luborzewski, A., Schindler, F. *et al.* (2011). Stimulus pulse-frequency-dependent efficacy and

cognitive adverse effects of ultrabrief-pulse electroconvulsive therapy in patients with major depression. *Journal of ECT*, 27, 109–113.

Rush, G., McCarron, S., and Lucey, J.V. (2008). Consent to ECT: patients' experiences in an Irish ECT clinic. *Psychiatric Bulletin*, 32, 15–17.

Sackeim, H.A., Prudic, J., Devanand, D.P. *et al.* (1993). Effects of stimulus intensity and electrode placement on the efficacy and cognitive effects of electroconvulsive therapy. *New England Journal of Medicine*, 328, 839–846.

Sackeim, H.A., Haskett, R.F., Mulsant, B.H. *et al.* (2001). Continuation pharmacotherapy in the prevention of relapse following electroconvulsive therapy: A randomized controlled trial. *Journal of the American Medical Association*, 285, 1299–1307.

Sackeim, H.A., Prudic, J., Fuller, R. *et al.* (2007). The cognitive effects of electroconvulsive therapy in community settings. *Neuropsychopharmacology*, 32, 244–254.

Sackeim, H.A., Dillingham, E.M., Prudic, J. *et al.* (2009). Effect of concomitant pharmacotherapy on electroconvulsive therapy outcomes: Short-term efficacy and adverse effects. *Archives of General Psychiatry*, 66, 729–737.

Shapira, B., Tubi, N., Drexler, H., Lidsky, D., Calev, A., and Lerer, B. (1998). Cost and benefit in the choice of ECT schedule. Twice versus three times weekly ECT. *British Journal of Psychiatry*, 172, 44–48.

Shelton, R.C., Osuntokun, O., Heinloth, A.N., and Corya, S.A. (2010). Therapeutic options for treatment-resistant depression. *CNS Drugs*, 24, 131–161.

Smith, G.E., Rasmussen, K.G., Jr., Cullum, C.M. *et al.* (2010). A randomized controlled trial comparing the memory effects of continuation electroconvulsive therapy versus continuation pharmacotherapy: Results from the Consortium for Research in ECT (CORE) study. *Journal of Clinical Psychiatry*, 71, 185–193.

Sonawalla, S.B. and Fava, M. (2001). Severe depression: is there a best approach? *CNS Drugs*, 15, 765–776.

Spellman, T., Peterchev, A.V., and Lisanby, S.H. (2009). Focal electrically administered seizure therapy: A novel form of ECT illustrates the roles of current directionality, polarity, and electrode configuration in seizure induction. *Neuropsychopharmacology*, 34, 2002–2010.

Takada, J.Y., Solimene, M.C., Da Luz, P.L. *et al.* (2005). Assessment of the cardiovascular effects of electroconvulsive therapy in individuals older than 50 years. *Brazilian Journal of Medical and Biologial Research*, 38, 1349–1357.

Tess, A.V. and Smetana, G.W. (2009). Medical evaluation of patients undergoing electroconvulsive therapy. *New England Journal of Medicine*, 360, 1437–1444.

Thase, M.E., Trivedi, M.H., Nelson, J.C. *et al.* (2008). Examining the efficacy of adjunctive aripiprazole in major depressive disorder: A pooled analysis of 2 studies. *Primary Care Companion to the Journal of Clinical Psychiatry*, 10, 440–447.

Wagner, K.J., Mollenberg, O., Rentrop, M., Werner, C., and Kochs, E.F. (2005). Guide to anaesthetic selection for electroconvulsive therapy. *CNS Drugs*, 19, 745–758.

Watts, B.V., Groft, A., Bagian, J.P., and Mills, P.D. (2011). An examination of mortality and other adverse events related to electroconvulsive therapy using a national adverse event report system. *Journal of ECT*, 27, 105–108.

Weiner, R.D. and Coffey, C.E. (1991). Practical issues in the use of electroconvulsive therapy (ECT). *Psychiatric Medicine*, 9, 133–341.

25

Transcranial magnetic stimulation and deep brain stimulation

Sarah H. Lisanby and Moacyr A. Rosa

Introduction

Transcranial magnetic stimulation (TMS) is a newer noninvasive tool for modulating brain function employing electromagnetic fields. Along with electroconvulsive therapy (ECT) and vagus nerve stimulation (VNS), TMS is one of the device-based therapies currently approved for clinical use in depression. This chapter will review the basic principles of the clinical application of TMS for the treatment of major depression.

Transcranial magnetic stimulation (TMS) refers to the administration of magnetic pulses to the brain for the purpose of altering brain function (Schlaepfer *et al.* 2010, Rosa and Lisanby, 2012). The term "repetitive transcranial magnetic stimulation" (rTMS) refers to a recurring train of TMS pulses. For simplicity, we will use the more general term TMS in this chapter. The magnetic pulses applied to the scalp induce electrical currents in the underlying superficial cortex. TMS works as an "electrodeless" electrical stimulation because it delivers an electrical current to the brain without having to use an electrode applied to the scalp. These currents are of sufficient magnitude to depolarize neurons, and when they are applied repetitively they can modulate cortical excitability, decreasing or increasing it, depending on the combination of parameters used for stimulation. The ability of TMS to noninvasively modulate brain function in a temporally and spatially targeted fashion makes it a useful tool for probing brain function in addition to its therapeutic benefit. It also presents the possibility of translating knowledge gleaned from functional imaging studies regarding circuitry underlying psychiatric and neurological disorders into a focal, circuit-guided therapeutic intervention.

Evidence for antidepressant efficacy

Between 2001 and 2003 several quantitative reviews were published on the antidepressant properties of TMS (Holtzheimer *et al.* 2001, McNamara *et al.* 2001, Burt *et al.* 2002, Martin *et al.* 2002, 2003, Couturier 2005). Most studies have shown statistically significant, though modest, antidepressant efficacy. There is meta-analytical evidence indicating that the moderate effect size presently observed is comparable to effect sizes seen in active placebo-controlled trials with pharmacological treatments (Joffe *et al.* 1996, Moncrieff *et al.* 1998, 2004). Moderate effect sizes have been observed for both tricyclic and tetracyclic agents. In sum, these findings suggest that TMS can be as effective as at least some of the commercially available antidepressant medications, though considerably less effective than electroconvulsive therapy (ECT).

Approval by the FDA was strongly influenced by an industry-sponsored multi-site study (US, Canada, and Australia) that used daily left prefrontal TMS for 4 to 6 weeks (3000 stimuli/d, intensity: 120% MT, frequency: 10 Hz, trains: 4 s; intertrain interval: 26 s). Patients had unipolar treatment-resistant depression and were medication-free during the trial. This study was sponsored by Neuronetics, Malevern, PA, and included 301 patients. Baseline depression severity on the Montgomery–Asberg Depression Rating Scale (MADRS) was 33 in the active group and 34 in the sham group, and 24-item Hamilton Rating Scale for Depression (HRSD-24) was 30 in the active and 31 in the sham group. After 4 weeks of daily treatment which was the primary endpoint, the mean drop in MADRS was 5.5 in the active and 3.6 in the sham group (just missing statistical significance with $p = 0.057$), and the mean drop in HRSD-24 was 6.5 in

---

Clinical Handbook for the Management of Mood Disorders, ed. J. John Mann, Patrick J. McGrath, and Steven P. Roose. Published by Cambridge University Press. © Cambridge University Press 2013.

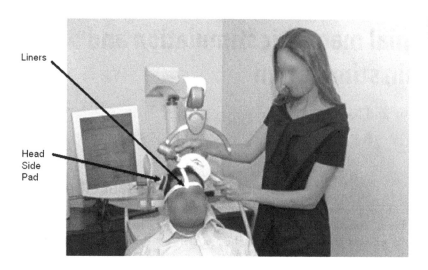

Liners

Head
Side
Pad

Figure 25.1 Front view of a typical treatment session

the active and 4 in the sham group (significant at $p = 0.012$). Mean response rate (50% drop in MADRS) at 4 weeks was 18% with active and 11% with sham ($p < 0.05$). Remission rates (MADRS < 10) did not differ between active and sham at 4 weeks (7%), but did differ at 6 weeks (14% remission with active and 5% remission with sham). Post-hoc analysis showed a strong association between treatment resistance and outcome, with the best result for patients that had failed only one medication and no difference between active and sham TMS for those who had failed two or more trials (Lisanby *et al.* 2009).

Regulatory status

In October 2008, TMS was approved by the Food and Drug Administration (FDA) in the USA for the treatment of adults with medication-resistant unipolar major depressive disorder (MDD) who have failed one adequate (but no more than one) pharmacological trial. The NeuroStar® TMS Therapy system is presently the only FDA-cleared TMS device for treatment of MDD (Figure 25.1), so the use of this device for other indications (depression refractory to more than one medication, for example), and the use of other devices are considered "off-label" use of the treatment.

The World Federation of Societies of Biological Psychiatry's guidelines (Schlaepfer *et al.* 2010), concluded that "there is sufficient class I evidence of acute efficacy for TMS in depression in medication-free unipolar depressed patients." The report goes on to recommend consideration of the use of TMS,

either monotherapy or in combination with medications, in nonpsychotic adults with major depression who have failed at least one antidepressant medication. These recommendations are somewhat broader than the FDA label, as they leave the door open for consideration of use in patients who have not failed one trial, and also those who have failed more than one trial, while the FDA labeling specifies exactly one failed trial as this was a predictor of response. The report also notes that optimal stimulation parameters are still under development, and they recommend that the dosage be determined by "a psychiatrist familiar with the relevant and recent rTMS literature."

Professional guidelines

The World Federation of Societies of Biological Psychiatry's guidelines (Schlaepfer *et al.* 2010) endorsed the International Society of Transcranial Stimulation (ISTS) guidelines concerning TMS administration (Belmaker *et al.* 2003), that stated, "Those who administer rTMS should be trained as 'first responders' in order to render appropriate care in the event of seizure. rTMS should be performed in a medical setting with appropriate emergency facilities to manage seizures and their consequences," and, "The use of rTMS should comply with regulations put forward by local regulatory bodies, medical professional organizations, and medical licensing boards. We recommend immediate responsibility and supervision by a licensed physician because of the possibility of adverse events necessitating medical intervention."

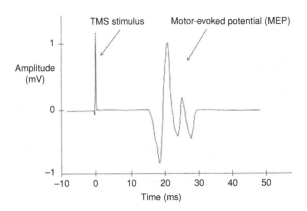

Figure 25.2 Graphic representation of motor-evoked potential

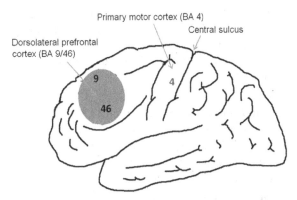

Figure 25.3 Dorsolateral prefrontal cortex (DLPFC)

Stimulation of motor cortex and determination of motor threshold

The original uses of TMS were in the study of the motor cortex and motor pathways, where there is a very simple and objective way of measuring the effects of the stimulation in the motor system. The simplest example is to hold the TMS coil over the hand area of the motor cortex. This will produce a twitch in the hand muscle represented by this part of the brain. That muscle twitch can be measured using electromyography (EMG), and is referred to as a motor-evoked potential (MEP). With TMS, it is possible to stimulate the cortical region responsible for the control of a given muscle and observe (or record with an oscilloscope) its contraction.

The size of the MEP (peak-to-peak amplitude or area under the curve) and the latency of its elicitation are some of the ways of measuring cortical excitability (Figure 25.2). The intensity needed to produce an MEP is the best available index to measure individual dosage requirement for TMS. It is used to determine what is known as motor threshold (MT). The TMS dosage is set at a percentage relative to the individual MT.

Treatment Technique

Cortical target

The cortical area that has been the main target for the treatment of depression with TMS is the dorsolateral prefrontal cortex (DLPFC). The DLPFC corresponds to the intersection between Broadmann areas 9 and 46, in the middle frontal gyrus. It is the last cerebral area

to be myelinated during development and dopamine is one of its most important neurotransmitters (Figure 25.3). This region is connected to the orbito-frontal cortex and many other regions, including the thalamus, caudate, hippocampus, and neocortical association areas (temporal, parietal, and occipital). Two main functions are linked to the DLPFC: executive function and working memory. The DLPFC is intimately linked to limbic areas implicated with mood regulation and the physiopathology of depression.

TMS parameter selection

There are a series of parameters that need to be selected when using TMS. At present it is not known what combination is considered optimal, but treatment combinations must take into account safety limits (specifically to prevent accidental seizure induction) and clinical efficacy. A specific combination of parameters was approved by the FDA for the use of TMS in the treatment of depression, and all other possible combinations would be considered "off-label" at present. The parameters that describe the TMS dosage are intensity, frequency, train duration, inter-train interval, number of trains per session, and total number of sessions.

The approval by the FDA has specific indications for combination of parameters and site of stimulation (which is the left DLPFC). On-label application of TMS treatment uses the following parameters: 120% of the patient's MT, a train duration of 4 s with frequency of 10 pulses/s (10 Hz), and a 26 s interval between trains. A treatment session lasts 37.5 minutes with a total of 3000 pulses per session. These parameters demonstrated both efficacy and safety in the largest clinical trial to date (O'Reardon *et al.* 2007, Janicak *et al.* 2008, Lisanby *et al.* 2009). Also, these parameters are within the current safety guidelines for use of TMS (Wassermann, 1998, Rossi *et al.* 2009).

Summary of treatment parameters for "on-label" use of TMS:

1. Pulses per second: 10 Hz.
2. Stimulation time (train duration): 4 s.
3. Intertrain interval: 26 s.
4. Number of pulses per session: 3000.
5. Pulse intensity: 120% of MT.
6. Coil location: left DLPFC.
7. Duration session: 37.5 min.

Initial management

TMS sessions are traditionally given daily, excluding weekends, although variations have been tried (such as three times a week, or twice daily, or with no weekend interval). Early protocols ranged between 5 to 10 days, but there is evidence for use up to 30 days, or according to clinical outcome.

A typical procedure takes approximately 40 minutes. The TMS is administered five times per week for 4 to 6 weeks. As usually happens with other psychiatric treatments, the effects of TMS may take some time to manifest. The number of sessions in an index course should be decided according to clinical response and side-effects profile.

Clinical data obtained in the randomized controlled trials (O'Reardon *et al.* 2007, Janicak *et al.* 2008, Lisanby *et al.* 2009), indicate that improvement can be seen as early as week 4, but the best response was seen at 6 weeks of daily treatment.

Physicians should evaluate the patient's clinical status at regular intervals to determine when to discontinue acute TMS. Unless tolerability or safety concerns emerge, it is recommended that a full course of 6 weeks of acute treatment be completed. Once the acute treatment course is finished, the treating psychiatrist should choose a maintenance plan for the patient. There is no controlled trial evidence available that demonstrates the efficacy of TMS beyond 6 weeks of treatment. However, in an open-label trial (Avery *et al.* 2008) some patients achieved full treatment benefit only after 12 weeks of acute treatment. As with any antidepressant treatment, symptom improvement should be evaluated at regular intervals to determine when the patient and psychiatrist decide that acute treatment is complete and further treatment is not needed. There was no evidence that the safety profile

of the TMS differed with or without concurrent medication administration.

Safety

The most serious known risk of TMS is the induction of a seizure and is the primary safety concern because it is the most severe known side effect. Several cases of accidental seizures induced by TMS have been reported, most in the early days prior to the development of the safety guidelines. Wassermann (1998) was the first to establish safety guidelines, and recently Rossi *et al.* (2009) updated this version. The safety guidelines provide the maximum duration of a train of magnetic pulses (in seconds) for each specific combination of the frequency of pulses per second and the intensity of the magnetic field (defined by percentage of motor threshold – %MT), within which TMS treatment can be administered safely with minimal risk of seizure.

The most commonly observed side effects associated with TMS are headaches, dizziness, nausea, and painful local sensation. These side effects are typically considered to be mild and respond promptly to analgesics (Wassermann, 1998, Rossi *et al.* 2009).

Maintenance treatment

At the point when the psychiatrist determines that a patient has achieved remission, or has achieved adequate symptom relief if remission cannot be reached, it is recommended that the TMS treatment be gradually tapered off as described below. Simultaneous with the TMS taper, an antidepressant continuation treatment should be chosen; or if a medication antidepressant treatment was already in progress, it should be continued. Janicak *et al.* (O'Reardon *et al.* 2007, Janicak *et al.* 2008, Lisanby *et al.* 2009) reported that clinical benefit was maintained with medication antidepressant monotherapy for up to 24 weeks of follow-up in a majority of patients. Clinical monitoring should occur on a periodic basis once TMS has been completed. Some patients may experience recurrence or relapse of illness, and the psychiatrist should re-evaluate the potential benefit of repeating the acute treatment with TMS at that time or should consider other treatment options.

Although there are still few data on continuation treatment and maintenance after response, tapering of TMS is an option. An example would be to give three treatments in the first week after the index course, two treatments in the following week and one treatment in the third week. Maintenance treatment with some antidepressant medication should always be considered.

Treatment alternatives for nonremission

Documented by controlled trials

As approved by FDA, labeled use of TMS is indicated for the treatment of major depressive disorder (MDD) in adult patients who have failed to achieve satisfactory improvement from one prior antidepressant medication (but no more than one) at or above the minimal effective dose and duration in the current episode. Off-label use of TMS in other circumstances (e.g., more refractory cases or for patients intolerant to medication) is not prohibited, and can be tried in some cases according to the clinician's judgment and experience, in accordance with state and local regulations.

Other conventional treatment alternatives

TMS seems to be an alternative for patients with mild resistance to medication, patients who cannot tolerate medication side effects, and for those that are not severe enough to justify the use of ECT or other more invasive approaches. Although with caution, it can be used as an adjunctive to medications (Rumi *et al.* 2005) and possibly with psychotherapy.

Unconventional treatment alternatives

Deep brain stimulation and vagus nerve stimulation could be alternatives to patients who have failed medications, TMS, and ECT.

Clinical pearls of therapeutic wisdom

The Food and Drug Administration (FDA) letter to Neuronetics (October 7, 2008) stated, "FDA concludes that this device (NeuroStar), and substantially equivalent devices of this generic type, should be classified into class II…under the generic name, Transcranial magnetic stimulation system." FDA identifies this generic type of device as: 21 CFR 882.5805. "A transcranial magnetic stimulation system is a device intended for the treatment of major depressive disorder (MDD) that non-invasively delivers repetitive pulsed magnetic fields of sufficient magnitude to induce neural action potentials in the patient's cerebral cortex to treat the symptoms of MDD without inducing seizure."

It is important to emphasize that the FDA has determined that the NeuroStar TMS system is indicated for the treatment of major depressive disorder in adult patients who have failed to achieve satisfactory improvement from one prior antidepressant medication at or above the minimal effective dose and duration in the current episode. In other words, on-label treatment is for unipolar nonpsychotic patients who have failed one prior trial of antidepressant medication in the current episode. The use of the NeuroStar device in all other patients is at present considered "off label."

Also, FDA regulations require the use of TMS by prescription only. This means that it must be prescribed by a licensed MD or another professional with prescriptive authority (e.g., NP with advanced training in TMS and a written collaborative agreement with an MD experienced in TMS). Its use must be supervised by a licensed physician. The person who operates the TMS device directly must have the training, medical education, and experience to do so safely and effectively. BCLS training and management of an accidental seizure are basic requirements recommended for this person.

The FDA does not regulate the medical practice and physicians make clinical decisions regarding patient care, chosen according to their training and experience, consistent with the current medical practice and standards of care, and evidence-based medical literature and expert consensus.

Future directions

TMS is a technique that has already proven to be useful as a diagnostic and neurophysiological tool, as well as a therapeutic alternative for some patients.

There are several attempts to maximize its therapeutic efficacy profile. One approach is to use bilateral stimulation (with rapid frequency to the left DLPFC and low frequency to the right DLPFC). Sequential stimulation has already been tried with promising results (Fitzgerald *et al.* 2006).

Different coil shapes and sizes are also being tried to target deeper brain regions and await controlled trials to test their usefulness (Levkovitz *et al.* 2007).

The use of TMS as a means of inducing therapeutic seizures similar to those induced by ECT (Lisanby *et al.* 2001, Hoy and Fitzgerald 2010, Kayser *et al.* 2011), albeit with a much cleaner cognitive side-effects profile (McClintock *et al.* 2011), is another broad road that is under intense investigation.

Finally, new TMS devices are being developed which offer the possibility of changing and testing other parameters, such as pulse shape and width (Peterchev *et al.* 2011), offering newer opportunities for brain modulation and treatment.

References

Avery, D.H., Isenberg, K.E., Sampson, S.M. *et al.* (2008). Transcranial magnetic stimulation in the acute treatment of major depressive disorder: Clinical response in an open-label extension trial. *Journal of Clinical Psychiatry*, 69, 441–451.

Belmaker, B., Fitzgerald, P., George, M.S. *et al.* (2003). Managing the risks of repetitive transcranial stimulation. *CNS Spectrums*, 8, 489.

Burt, T., Lisanby, S.H., and Sackeim, H.A. (2002). Neuropsychiatric applications of transcranial magnetic stimulation: A meta-analysis. *International Journal of Neuropsychopharmacology*, 5, 73–103.

Couturier, J.L. (2005). Efficacy of rapid-rate repetitive transcranial magnetic stimulation in the treatment of depression: A systematic review and meta-analysis. *Journal of Psychiatry and Neuroscience*, 30, 83–90.

Fitzgerald, P.B., Benitez, J., De Castella, A. *et al.* (2006). A randomized, controlled trial of sequential bilateral repetitive transcranial magnetic stimulation for treatment-resistant depression. *American Journal of Psychiatry*, 163, 88–94.

Holtzheimer, P.E., III, Russo, J., and Avery, D.H. (2001). A meta-analysis of repetitive transcranial magnetic stimulation in the treatment of depression. *Psychopharmacological Bulletin*, 35, 149–169.

Hoy, K.E. and Fitzgerald, P.B. (2010). Introducing magnetic seizure therapy: A novel therapy for treatment resistant depression. *Australian and New Zealand Journal of Psychiatry*, 44, 591–598.

Janicak, P.G., O'Reardon, J.P., Sampson, S.M. *et al.* (2008). Transcranial magnetic stimulation in the treatment of major depressive disorder: A comprehensive summary of safety experience from acute exposure, extended exposure, and during reintroduction treatment. *Journal of Clinical Psychiatry*, 69, 222–232.

Joffe, R., Sokolov, S., and Streiner, D. (1996). Antidepressant treatment of depression: A metaanalysis. *Canadian Journal of Psychiatry*, 41, 613–616.

Kayser, S., Bewernick, B.H., Grubert, C. *et al.* (2011). Antidepressant effects, of magnetic seizure therapy and electroconvulsive therapy, in treatment-resistant depression. *Journal of Psychiatric Research*, 45, 569–576.

Levkovitz, Y., Roth, Y., Harel, E.V., Braw, Y., Sheer, A., and Zangen, A. (2007). A randomized controlled feasibility and safety study of deep transcranial magnetic stimulation. *Clinical Neurophysiology*, 118, 2730–2744.

Lisanby, S.H., Schlaepfer, T.E., Fisch, H.U., and Sackeim, H.A. (2001). Magnetic seizure therapy of major depression. *Archives of General Psychiatry*, 58, 303–305.

Lisanby, S.H., Husain, M.M., Rosenquist, P.B. *et al.* (2009). Daily left prefrontal repetitive transcranial magnetic stimulation in the acute treatment of major depression: Clinical predictors of outcome in a multisite, randomized controlled clinical trial. *Neuropsychopharmacology*, 34, 522–534.

Martin, J.L., Barbanoj, M.J., Schlaepfer, T.E., Thompson, E., Perez, V., and Kulisevsky, J. (2003). Repetitive transcranial magnetic stimulation for the treatment of depression: Systematic review and meta-analysis. *British Journal of Psychiatry*, 182, 480–491.

Martin, J.L., Barbanoj, M.J., Schlaepfer, T.E. *et al.* (2002). Transcranial magnetic stimulation for treating depression. *Cochrane Database of Systematic Reviews*, 2, CD003493.

McClintock, S.M., Tirmizi, O., Chansard, M., and Husain, M.M. (2011). A systematic review of the neurocognitive effects of magnetic seizure therapy. *International Review of Psychiatry*, 23, 413–423.

McNamara, B., Ray, J.L., Arthurs, O.J., and Boniface, S. (2001). Transcranial magnetic stimulation for depression and other psychiatric disorders. *Psychological Medicine*, 31, 1141–1146.

Moncrieff, J., Wessely, S., and Hardy, R. (1998). Meta-analysis of trials comparing antidepressants with active placebos. *British Journal of Psychiatry*, 172, 227–231; discussion 232–234.

Moncrieff, J., Wessely, S., and Hardy, R. (2004). Active placebos versus antidepressants for depression. *Cochrane Database of Systematic Reviews*, 1, CD003012.

O'Reardon, J.P., Solvason, H.B., Janicak, P.G. *et al.* (2007). Efficacy and safety of transcranial magnetic stimulation in the acute treatment of major depression: A multisite randomized controlled trial. *Biological Psychiatry*, 62, 1208–1216.

Peterchev, A.V., Murphy, D.L., and Lisanby, S.H. (2011). Repetitive transcranial magnetic stimulator with controllable pulse parameters. *Journal of Neural Engineering*, 8, 036016.

Rosa, M.A. and Lisanby, S.H. (2012). Somatic treatments for mood disorders. *Neuropsychopharmacology*, 37, 102–116.

Rossi, S., Hallett, M., Rossini, P.M., and Pascual-Leone, A. (2009). Safety, ethical considerations, and application guidelines for the use of transcranial magnetic stimulation in clinical practice and research. *Clinical Neurophysiology*, 120, 2008–2039.

Rumi, D.O., Gattaz, W.F., Rigonatti, S.P. *et al.* (2005). Transcranial magnetic stimulation accelerates the antidepressant effect of amitriptyline in severe depression: A double-blind placebo-controlled study. *Biological Psychiatry*, 57, 162–166.

Schlaepfer, T.E., George, M.S., and Mayberg, H. (2010). WFSBP guidelines on brain stimulation treatments in psychiatry. *World Journal of Biological Psychiatry*, 11, 2–18.

Wassermann, E.M. (1998). Risk and safety of repetitive transcranial magnetic stimulation: report and suggested guidelines from the International Workshop on the Safety of Repetitive Transcranial Magnetic Stimulation, June 5–7, 1996. *Electroencephalography and Clinical Neurophysiology*, 108, 1–16.

Chapter

26

Chronotherapeutics
Light therapy, wake therapy, and melatonin

Michael Terman and Jiuan Su Terman

Introduction

Antidepressant chronotherapy uses light, dark, and sleep interventions that impact the circadian timing system. The human hypothalamic inner clock is genetically programmed to time a cycle that deviates from 24 hours, with outputs to a host of physiological endpoints. Primary examples are body temperature, sleep and wakefulness, and cortisol and melatonin hormone production. The clock conforms to the solar day by sensing the pattern of light and darkness, creating cohesive temporal organization of physiological function. Multiple factors can disturb this harmony, however, among them sleep disturbance, work schedules, seasonal changes in day length, and artificial lighting. Sleeping out of synchrony with the circadian clock is closely tied to mood disorders (Wirz-Justice et al. 2009a). The goal of chronotherapy is to bring the ensemble of external and internal cycles into alignment.

Light therapy

Light therapy, first explored in the late 1970s (Kripke et al. 1983, Rosenthal et al. 1984) is the first somatic antidepressant treatment to have been born of a biological hypothesis rather than discovered by serendipity in the course of drug testing or brain stimulation (Wirz-Justice et al. 2004). The hypothesis arose from the observation of photoperiodism in animals – for example, seasonal variation in reproductive behavior tied to the length of the night and the duration of pineal melatonin production. There seemed to be a parallel in unipolar and bipolar patients who show more depression in winter than summer. It was plausible to hypothesize that daylight manipulations would affect mood state. By lengthening the day (shortening the night) with artificial light exposure, there were rapid remissions from winter depression (Rosenthal et al. 1984, Terman et al. 1989b).

Hotly debated for several years, a placebo explanation was hard to rule out, since, by definition, the active treatment is visible. Four kinds of controls provided supporting evidence, equating for subjects' expectations: dim or colored light vs. bright white light; brief vs. longer sessions; evening vs. morning light exposure; and a nonphotic, inert comparator treatment using deactivated or low-density negative air ionizers (Wirz-Justice, 1998).

Light therapy has seen increasing use in clinical practice, often in conjunction with antidepressant medication, but also as monotherapy. At the start of citalopram treatment, for example, augmentation with light therapy can expedite improvement (Benedetti et al. 2003) and prevent relapse under drug maintenance (Martiny et al. 2004). Light therapy is useful not only for seasonal affective disorder, but also for nonseasonal chronic, recurrent, bipolar, premenstrual, and gestational depression (Terman, 2007). The treatment protocol is similar in all cases.

Light therapy devices and the mode of administration are unregulated, however. This has made it popular for unsupervised self-treatment, with the attendant liabilities of unskilled, arbitrary dosing, unsupervised combination with drug treatment, absence of monitoring, and risky outcome. Inappropriate administration can exacerbate depression and sleep disturbance, and trigger adverse events such as headache, nausea, and agitation. Clinical guidance is important. Although the protocol is not complicated, it requires that clinicians learn the principles of circadian timing in order to supervise effectively.

Clinical Handbook for the Management of Mood Disorders, ed. J. John Mann, Patrick J. McGrath, and Steven P. Roose.
Published by Cambridge University Press. © Cambridge University Press 2013.

Wake therapy

That a night of sleep deprivation resulted in immediately improved mood state was first reported by a patient in the 1960s who would ride her bicycle all night to lift her depression (Schulte, 1966). Hundreds of cases have since been studied, with a majority showing improvement after a single night awake – *the fastest turnaround known to psychiatry* (Wirz-Justice *et al.* 1999). Rapid relapse upon recovery sleep, however, made the protocol useless in clinical practice.

The key, discovered 30 years later, was the application of two new chronotherapeutic methods immediately following nights of sleep deprivation (now rechristened *wake therapy*): *morning light therapy* coupled with *earlier recovery sleep* (also called sleep phase advance) (Wirz-Justice *et al.* 2009b). The combined protocol is termed *triple chronotherapy*. The overnight remission was sustained, and the course of inpatient treatment completed in a week or less, with durable maintained response.

Benedetti (2007) provides a comprehensive review of the components of triple chronotherapy, their efficacy in various patient populations, and their neurochemical, anatomical, and genetic mechanisms of action, which parallel the action of antidepressant drugs, but on an accelerated time course. For example, Wu *et al.* (2009) found that depression in bipolar patients was significantly improved relative to a medication control group after a single night awake followed by 3 days of phase-advanced recovery sleep and morning light therapy. At the 7-week endpoint, 63% of patients maintained remission. Similar results were obtained for patients with unipolar depression who began duloxetine treatment with a course of three wake therapy nights interspersed with earlier recovery sleep and initiation of daily morning light therapy, compared with a medicated control group that engaged in daily exercise (Martiny *et al.* 2012).

An earlier study of bipolar depression that combined wake and light therapy without sleep phase advance found 57% maintained remission after 9 months in patients without a history of drug resistance, but a far lower success rate of 17% in drug-resistant cases (Benedetti *et al.* 2005). Two studies of bipolar (Benedetti *et al.* 2001) and unipolar (Voderholzer *et al.* 2003) patients without light therapy demonstrated the benefit of the sleep phase advances across 3 nights following a single night of wake therapy, with remission sustained at the end of the 7-day hospital stay.

Melatonin

Above and beyond its role in photoperiodism, this hormone – a nocturnal product of the pineal gland – is temporally associated with sleep, although it does not trigger sleep in the same sense as pharmaceutical hypnotics (Wirz-Justice and Armstrong, 1996). Use of melatonin as a hypnotic shortly before bedtime is generally ineffective because it overlaps pineal melatonin production.

Recent research on melatonin administered before pineal production begins has revealed its potent function as a *chronobiotic* that acts directly on the circadian timing system to shift the internal clock earlier when taken in the afternoon or evening. When administered early in the morning, it shifts the clock later in a symmetrical fashion (Lewy *et al.* 1998, Burgess *et al.* 2008). Exogenous melatonin serves essentially as a complement to timed light administration, but without direct antidepressant effect. For patients with major sleep phase delays, the combination of low-dose melatonin in the evening with light therapy in the morning can expedite the course of treatment (Terman and Terman, 2010a, Figure 149–4).

Light therapy

Figure 26.1 outlines diagnostic steps, dosing strategy, and treatment management.

Preparatory diagnostics

Before beginning light therapy, triple chronotherapy, or melatonin administration, the clinician needs to estimate circadian rhythm status and its relation to the current sleep pattern – information key to all the procedures.

Circadian phase assessment

Although impractical for clinical use, the laboratory standard for circadian phase determination is *pineal melatonin onset*, obtained by saliva sampling over several hours before habitual sleep onset, and analyzed by radioimmunoassay. As an expedient, a 19-item chronotype questionnaire (Terman *et al.* 2001) is used to assess the daily pattern of behavior changes that reflect the underlying circadian rhythm. The chronotype score provides an estimate of melatonin onset, with a large effect size of about $r = 0.75$ (Terman and Terman, 2010a). The chronotype score range of

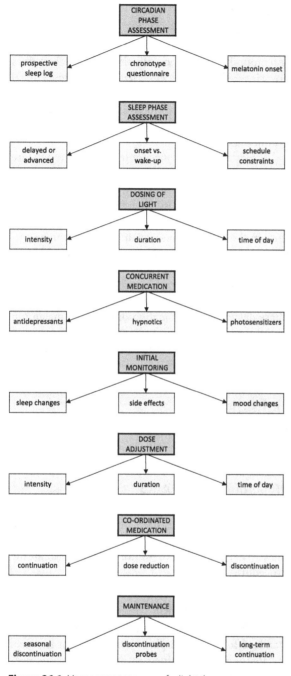

Figure 26.1 Management sequence for light therapy administration

advances – about 8.5 hours after melatonin onset. The questionnaire is most easily completed on the Web (Terman and White, 2003), which provides instant scoring and interpretation, and a printout summary for the patient to bring to the appointment. A patient's score may fall at any point along the spectrum of early to late chronotype – it need not be at the late end to use morning light therapy. (An exception is for unusual patients with advanced sleep phase disorder who fall asleep in the evening with final awakening in the middle of the night.)

Sleep phase assessment

Mere description of the generalized sleep pattern is often uninformative, with distorted retrospective generalizations (even for the past week) that are not useful for setting the schedule of light therapy. For 7 to 10 days before the appointment, the patient prepares a daily sleep log in graphic format (Wirz-Justice *et al.* 2009b, Appendix 5) that can be quickly reviewed in the office. The clinician notes and discusses the reasons for variability in sleep onset, night-time interruptions, duration, wake-up time, and napping. For example, extended weekend sleep may result from forced early awakening on workdays. Late bedtime may be the consequence of evening activities, meals, and light exposure, with sleep debt that accumulates toward the weekend.

Sleep timing in depressed patients may be advanced or delayed relative to the 11 PM to 7 AM norm. The delay tendency is seen most frequently in seasonal, atypical, and bipolar depression. The determination of sleep phase is easily confounded by depressive hypersomnia, when the patient goes to sleep far earlier than when in remission, awakens far later, or both. Late wake-up requires caution: light therapy should not begin more than 1 hour before current wake-up time, or it may exacerbate the delayed sleep pattern.

Although the circadian clock heavily influences sleep timing, actual bedtime is complicated by social pressures, work schedules, medications, … and depression itself. Since the efficacy of light therapy is anchored to circadian timing, chronotype is key to establishing the treatment schedule. But the clinician needs to reconcile mismatches of the sleep pattern with the patient's chronotype, and sometimes coach sleep hygiene in preparation for light therapy.

16 to 84 corresponds to a melatonin onset range of 6 PM to 12 AM (higher score, earlier onset). The score is used to specify the optimum time to begin morning light therapy and promote circadian rhythm phase

Table 26.1 A patient's response to variations in intensity, duration, and timing of light therapy

Light intensity/Condition	Session duration	Session time of day	Depression severity score[a]
Baseline	–	–	41
2500 lux	2 hours	Evening	43
2500 lux	2 hours	Morning	8[b]
2500 lux	1 hour	Morning	15
2500 lux	30 minutes	Morning	33
10 000 lux	30 minutes	Evening	33
10 000 lux	30 minutes	Morning	2[b]
Final withdrawal	–	–	37

[a] *Structured Interview for the Hamilton Depression Rating Scale – Seasonal Affective Disorder Version* (SIGH-SAD) (Williams *et al.* 2002). This instrument has been updated as the *Structured Interview for the Hamilton Depression Rating Scale with Atypical Depression Supplement* (SIGH-ADS) (Williams and Terman, 2003).
[b] Meets remission criteria (at least 50% improvement to a SIGH-SAD score of 8 or less).

Dosing and timing strategy

Light

The three major dosing parameters that comprise the treatment regimen – which are mutually interactive – are light intensity, exposure duration, and the circadian time of the daily session. Circadian time is specified as the interval between evening melatonin onset and the start time of the morning light therapy session. As a generalization, higher light intensity – measured as illuminance in lux – requires shorter exposure duration. The circadian rhythm and antidepressant effects of these lighting parameters are strongly modulated by the time of day of treatment, with the impact waning after the early morning hours.

In contrast to common drug-dosing strategy, light therapy does not require increments from the low end of dosing range to find the optimum level for individual patients. Because of the favorable side-effect profile, quicker progress is made by starting in the middle range and working in either direction, as the case dictates. A common starting point is 10 000 lux white light, the highest level that has been verified for safety and efficacy, in 30-minute sessions. Duration is then adjusted downward (as far as 10 minutes) if there are side effects, or upward (as far as 60 minutes) if progress is slow. If the patient experiences glare sensations or other visual discomfort at 10 000 lux, the level can be reduced as low as 2500 lux by varying the distance of the light box from the eyes, but this will require compensatory lengthening of session duration.

A single-case research example demonstrates the effect of dosing manipulations, which have been verified in group studies (Terman *et al.* 1989b, Terman *et al.* 1990). The 28-year-old patient had experienced a multi-year, unmedicated history of fall–winter depression, which remitted with euthymia in spring and summer. She underwent a series of 10-day light therapy and withdrawal phases throughout the winter, in which the intensity, duration, and time of treatment were varied in a randomized sequence. Light intensity was 2500 or 10 000 lux; session duration, 30 minutes to 2 hours; with morning sessions upon habitual awakening or evening timing 2 hours before bedtime. When she showed a positive response in any condition, she discontinued treatment and the next condition was delayed until relapse occurred. Table 26.1 summarizes the results.

As morning session duration decreased from 2 hours to 30 minutes at 2500 lux – the intensity used in the earliest clinical trials (Terman *et al.* 1989b) – the antidepressant effect waned. And regardless of intensity, evening light was not beneficial.

The dosing strategy for light is more cautious for bipolar I than for bipolar II and unipolar disorders, given the risk of switching. Switches to mania are exceedingly rare for patients using lithium or other stabilizing medication – although one study has noted mixed states that resolved with reductions in light dose (Sit *et al.* 2007). A bipolar I patient may begin at 7000 lux for 10 minutes at midday. If tolerated, the session can be moved earlier, the duration lengthened, and the light intensity increased to 10 000 lux.

Light therapy in seasonal, nonseasonal, and bipolar depression appears most effective when administered about 8.5 hours after evening melatonin onset, shortly after awakening (Terman *et al.* 2001). The chronotype questionnaire estimates melatonin onset and specifies the time of the morning light therapy session (as specified in the printout summary). For example, session time for a low chronotype score of 35 would be 7:30 AM, while a score of 55 would shift the session earlier to 6:15 AM (Terman and White, 2003). For patients who sleep longer than 7 hours, the treatment schedule requires earlier wake-up; in some cases, the need for sleep is reduced as the antidepressant response emerges, while in others the patient compensates with earlier bedtime. The treatment time may seem too early to manage for some patients, in which case it can be delayed for up to an hour. However, treatment should never be started *earlier* than the time specified by the questionnaire result, because – falling into the circadian night period – it risks a countertherapeutic *delay* in circadian rhythms, similar to what occurs with evening light exposure. Patients with irresistible late awakening can gradually shift the morning light session earlier as the circadian phase advances take hold.

For patients with late insomnia – waking far too early, as in the classic melancholic pattern – the priority after wake-up is to *restrict* light stimulation, with light therapy delayed to later in the morning. The same is true for patients with enforced early awakening due to their work schedule. In both cases, it is useful to wear blue-blocking glasses (see the section on Resources) to reduce the countertherapeutic effect of prematurely early light exposure, and not to remove the glasses until light therapy would have been scheduled. (Unlike sunglasses, the blue-blockers maintain clear visibility.)

If the patient is already at work when light therapy is scheduled, treatment may need to be postponed. It can begin on weekends or days off as a boost toward phase-advancing the circadian rhythm. Adjustment can be expedited with microdose, controlled-release melatonin, and blue-blockers in the evening hours before bedtime (see section on Melatonin as a chronobiotic, below). Daily light therapy can then begin when wake-up adjusts to the targeted circadian time.

Medication

There are few contraindications to the use of light therapy, which is compatible with most psychiatric medications. As a rule, we do not alter the drug regimen when starting light therapy, but rather wait to see if there is distinct improvement after introducing the treatment. If a patient is on an established medication regimen, it should not be tapered or discontinued in preparation for light therapy. (Note, however, that hypnotic or sedating psychotropic drugs can impose a sleep pattern that presents a problem for scheduling light therapy according to the circadian clock (see below).) If improvement under light therapy is dramatic, it is reasonable to consider drug tapering. Sometimes discontinuation is possible, while other times the dose can be reduced. Frequently, in cases of polypharmacy, drugs suspected of inaction can be dropped with others maintained.

Antidepressants

Case evidence demonstrates that patients who have discontinued antidepressant medication because of nonresponse can then respond to light therapy, while partially responsive or drug-resistant patients can respond in full with adjunctive light therapy (Papatheodorou and Kutcher, 1995, Beauchemin *et al.* 1997, Terman, 2007). Patients often seek to reduce their medication burden if light therapy works, but lacking clinical trials, clinicians often prefer to maintain combination treatment.

Frequently, patients seek light therapy, or the clinician may suggest it, because ongoing medications have been inadequate, the sleep pattern is obviously delayed, or there is extreme difficulty awakening, suggestive of a circadian rhythm disturbance. On the other side of the coin, if light therapy shows only partial benefit – especially after attempts at increased session duration and timing – medication can be added, with the caution that it may interact with light therapy and require lower dosing than otherwise.

When medication is indicated, light therapy can serve as a booster at drug start-up, accelerating improvement until the delayed drug effect sets in. At that point, light therapy might be discontinued (Martiny *et al.* 2012). While some patients perceive the morning light session as a schedule burden (and would prefer medication if effective), others enjoy the routine (quiet time, e-mail time, newspaper time, breakfast time), and are relieved to be free of medication.

Drug-naïve patients who show rapid, lasting remission with light therapy demonstrate that monotherapy can succeed, as exemplified by numerous studies of winter depression that excluded the use of antidepressant drugs (Terman *et al.* 1989, Wirz-Justice, 1998). In our experience, about 30% of patients seeking chronotherapy at our clinic have never used antidepressants, and we withhold that option until light therapy has been tested.

Hypnotics

Hypnotic medication complicates the dosing strategy for light therapy because it forces sleep out of synchrony with the circadian activity/rest rhythm. While early insomnia can have multiple causes including anxiety and depression, it often arises from delayed circadian rhythms. The patient might fall asleep easily at 2 AM, for example, but is pressured to sleep earlier because of the workday schedule. Chronotype estimates and sleep log data are distorted by the masking effect of hypnotics, which interferes with optimum scheduling of light therapy.

Patients want to be freed of hypnotics, but tapering usually is infeasible as preparation for morning light therapy. If, under hypnotic medication, the patient sleeps from 11 PM to 7 AM, pineal melatonin onset at the start of the circadian night might occur well after sleep onset, and the circadian signal for awakening might occur well after 7 AM. Light therapy upon awakening – in the middle of the circadian night – would further delay the rhythm, magnifying the problem. Short of abandoning light therapy, it can be scheduled later in the morning and gradually moved earlier until the sensation of sleepiness precedes taking the sleeping pill. At that point, the medication taper can begin with lower risk of insomnia relapse.

Photosensitizers

Several medications – psychiatric and nonpsychiatric – are known to induce damaging photosensitization of the skin, retina, or lens at the short-wavelength, violet-blue end of the visible spectrum – a major component of white light. This effect differs from ultraviolet photosensitization, which is controlled by the diffusion filter on the light box. Blue photosensitizers include the following drug groups: neuroleptic, porphyrin, psoralen, antiarrhythmic, antimalarial, and antirheumatic. In addition, St. John's Wort (*Hypericum*) photosensitizes in the longer-wavelength, green spectral range. When such photosensitizing drugs cannot be replaced with a benign alternative, light therapy should be avoided.

Treatment management

Initial monitoring

Light therapy often has accelerated action compared with the rate of response to antidepressant drugs. This creates a need for frequent clinical monitoring in the week or two after start-up. Apart from side effects seen in about 5% of cases (mainly mild nausea, headache, and agitation; Terman and Terman, 1999), the clinician needs to look for the emergence of awakening more than 30 minutes before the scheduled light therapy session. Such early awakening indicates too large of a circadian rhythm phase advance, and can lead to increased sleep debt, or a bipolar switch, and greatly concern the patient even if mood is improving.

Changes in mood state and sleep can occur within a day, so the standard schedule of office visits will not serve. To ensure vigilance, the patient continues the daily sleep log prepared for the initial evaluation, noting the light therapy session times, medications, and mood and energy ratings. The form is e-mailed or faxed to the doctor's office as frequently as twice a week to detect major sleep disruption, resumption of sleep after the light therapy session, or labile mood. The patient also submits log updates immediately if there is any sudden change. This initial feedback is critical for making rapid adjustments of the three dosing variables – intensity, duration, and time of day. The patient is instructed not to change these conditions without consulting, and to avoid inadvertent overdose. For example, unless instructed otherwise, patients with initial positive response may start extending session duration and become overexcited.

Dosing and timing adjustment

If the depression does not improve, session duration can be increased from 30 to 45 minutes, and then to 60 minutes, but not faster than every 4 days. If there are adverse effects, the first move is a reduction in session duration, a switch to lower light intensity, or both. Intensity level may be switchable on the device, or the screen can be moved farther from the eyes. The distance factor is sensitive, since lux falls off rapidly – not linearly – with distance from the light source.

Adjusting the time of day of the light therapy session is more of a challenge than adjusting intensity or duration, because there is no direct information about changes in circadian rhythm phase once treatment has begun. We aim for solid sleep until 15 minutes or less before the scheduled session. If the patient starts waking far earlier, the session should be delayed about an hour. This may be difficult if the patient needs to leave hours beforehand, in which case reducing session duration (e.g., from 30 to 20 minutes) or light intensity (e.g., from 10 000 to 2500 lux) may suffice.

When dealing with a very late sleep pattern, the aim to is move wake-up and the light therapy session toward a normal sleep/wake pattern. Often this can be achieved with 30-minute steps earlier, every 3 to 5 days, with complete adjustment in 2 weeks or less. If the progression earlier is too fast, it may trigger a relapse into the delayed state. In such cases, the process needs to start again with a slower progression.

Clearly, management of time of day of treatment requires that the patient comply with the schedule, noting "real" (rather than ideal) times of treatment on the log, and avoiding day-to-day variations as much as possible. In the absence of self-control it is difficult for the clinician to guide timing adjustments. The first few days of light therapy are often the hardest, especially when the patient finds earlier waking not the priority of moment. Encourage the patient that this challenge will pass as the treatment effect sets in. When convenient – and especially when oversleeping seems uncontrollable – it helps to have a family member monitor waking for the light therapy session for the first week.

Maintenance

Every patient asks how long it will be necessary to continue treatment once there is a positive response. For winter depression, the answer – from experienced patients who have continued with self-treatment – is fairly clear: the end of April at northerly US latitudes, by which time most people are waking up to daylight (Terman *et al.* 1994). The exception is for patients who historically show unusually early spontaneous remission (for example, in February, as the solstice period ends), or those who break the cycle with a vacation south in March.

There is little downside to attempting discontinuation of light therapy, since resuming the treatment rapidly recaptures the effect. Tapering is unnecessary, and does not improve outcome. Within the winter depression season, if a patient achieves complete remission, it becomes important to know whether a weekend or a week away from light therapy is possible without slumping or relapse. This has been tested early in the season following initial response in a 1-week trial (Terman *et al.* 1994). Some patients slumped noticeably within a day, most showed a relapse into a major depressive episode within a week, and a small number coasted as long as 3 weeks before relapse, but not longer. Ultimately, a maintenance schedule is needed.

The required dose of light can vary within an episode, and patients learn to sense changing needs

without guidance. January and February are usually the most difficult months, even when the seasonal relapse occurred earlier in the fall. Long after the supervised start-up period, patients may sense, for example, that 30 minutes at 10 000 lux at 6:30 AM is losing effectiveness, with noticeable fatigue and malaise short of relapse. By switching to 45-minute sessions, the slump immediately resolves. By mid-March, 45 minutes may feel "too much," with onset of sleep interruptions and morning irritability. Switching back to 30 minutes can fix the problem in a few days.

The ultimate goal of light therapy is intelligent self-treatment. The clinician cannot be there to micromanage.

Patients with nonseasonal depression who have responded to light therapy should maintain treatment for at least 2 months before attempting discontinuation. Again, resumption is simple, and it should not wait for a relapse, but rather an anticipatory slump. Patients sometimes "forget" their light therapy and fall back into depression within 3 days, to the point that they do not "remember" to resume treatment. Family members should watch out for such lapses and take initiative – the patient may no longer be in active contact with the clinician.

Of course, the clinician may have to be contacted when such relapses occur. It is very difficult to make specific recommendations without a current assessment of the sleep/wake pattern. The best one can advise is resuming the same schedule as before the treatment lapse. This may not be optimal, because sleep, circadian rhythm phase, or both may have drifted into a new pattern – with respect to time of day as well as to each other. Thus, patients should maintain their logs for at least half a year. Some have logged for years; they find it fascinating and instructive. To quote one, "When things fall apart and I'm in a state of confusion, I look back into my logs to see how we handled this in the past, and that works."

Triple chronotherapy

Light therapy has been used successfully with hospitalized patients in conjunction with standard medications and electroconvulsive therapy when the latter have produced insufficient improvement (Terman, 2007). On admission, prospective sleep logs will be unavailable, so decisions for timing must be made from the interview evaluation of the sleep pattern and

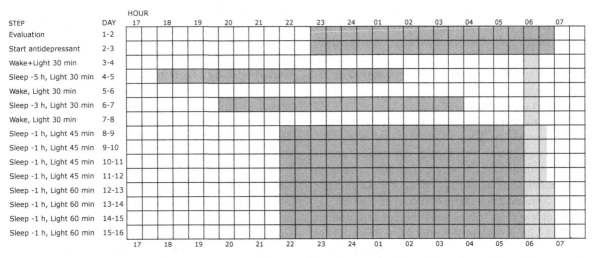

Figure 26.2 Inpatient protocol for a three-cycle sequence of wake therapy, light therapy, and sleep phase advance. The need for repeated wake therapy depends on the speed of improvement, and can be limited to one or two cycles if there is rapid remission. Dark gray spaces, sleep; light gray spaces, light therapy

the chronotype score. Importantly, the staff need to allow the patient to maintain the habitual sleep pattern regardless of the unit's standard lights-out and lights-on schedule, withhold early-morning vital signs when the patient is still asleep, and allow flexible mealtimes. The staff also need to begin an observational sleep log to guide dosing adjustments of light therapy. Alert patients can begin a self-report log.

Light therapy on the hospital unit is just one of a set of chronotherapeutic techniques that together can form the primary intervention. The elaborated protocol is termed *triple chronotherapy*, and includes:

- *Wake therapy*. Patients stay awake through the night, which can present a challenge. (See Wirz-Justice *et al.* 2009b for tips on avoiding sleep.) When the morning arrives, it becomes easier to remain awake because the circadian clock has signaled daytime wakefulness. The objective is for patients to remain awake up to 34 hours or longer despite accumulating sleep deprivation.
- *Recovery sleep with phase advance*. Toward the end of the day, but several hours *before* their usual bedtime, they go to sleep, compensating for their sleep loss the night before. Then, after sleeping about 8 hours, they wake up earlier, in the second half of the night
- *Light therapy*. Starting on the morning after the first wake therapy night, they do 30 minutes of light therapy, scheduled 60 minutes earlier than their baseline wake-up time.

The primary manipulation is *wake therapy* (less enthusiastically termed sleep deprivation), which has long been known to produce overnight remission of depression in a majority of hospitalized patients with bipolar or unipolar depression (Wirz-Justice and van den Hoofdakker, 1999). Although this is the fastest known therapeutic reversal of clinical state known to psychiatry, it comes with a liability: the next night's recovery sleep is likely to produce a relapse. By itself, then, wake therapy is not clinically useful.

Triple chronotherapy was developed to forestall the next day relapse and facilitate an enduring remission within a week. The initial response is maintained with daily light therapy starting at the end of the first wake therapy night, and a progression of earlier recovery sleep periods that converge on a normal sleep pattern over the week. Figure 26.2 outlines the protocol.

At entry, the patient is allowed to sleep habitual hours. Timing of the chronotherapies is anchored to habitual sleep time and the chronotype score. Treatment begins with a night of wake therapy followed by the first light therapy session, and light therapy continues each morning. Bedtime the next day is 5 hours earlier than normally (a sleep phase advance), with wake-up during the second half of the night, and light therapy in the morning. The remaining protocol varies individually, based on remission, partial improvement, nonresponse, worsening, or relapse following transient remission. With partial or no improvement, the patient receives a second night of wake therapy followed by sleep 3 hours before habitual bedtime. If necessary, the patient receives a third night of wake therapy followed by sleep starting 1 hour before habitual bedtime. Light exposure duration is increased in 15-minute steps, up to 60 minutes if response continues to fall short of remission.

Concurrent medication during triple chronotherapy is discretionary, though lithium magnifies the success rate in patients with bipolar depression, and is highly recommended (Benedetti *et al.* 2001). Antipsychotic medication blocks the effect of wake therapy, and is contraindicated (Wirz-Justice *et al.* 2009b).

A single cycle of triple chronotherapy can produce such rapid improvement that after a few more days of observation the patient can be discharged. Others may need a second or third cycle of wake therapy – but the expected course of acute treatment can be completed within a week. The risk of bipolar switching, about 5%, is no higher than for serotonergic antidepressants (Wirz-Justice *et al.* 2009b). Duration of remission – up to 9 months or longer – compares favorably with standard treatment (Benedetti *et al.* 2005). Maintained light therapy has yet to be tested in controlled studies, but in principle it should reinforce the remission.

Case vignette: triple chronotherapy at an accelerated pace

Mr. B, aged 21, a patient of John F. Gottlieb, MD (Northwestern University), was a college student who experienced his first manic episode as a freshman after flying across time zones on winter vacation. He recovered in hospital. Later that year, he fell into depression, and was drinking, keeping irregular sleep hours, and ultimately not getting out of bed.

He began a course of triple chronotherapy – not in hospital, but supervised by clinic staff in a Chicago hotel suite. At entry, he scored 29 points on the SIGH-ADS scale (Williams and Terman, 2003). A rotation of nurses and graduate assistants stayed with him throughout the wake therapy phases, beginning with admission at 11 PM. Later, he recollected the experience (Terman and McMahan, 2012), "It was rough. It was really hard to do. I drank coffee, and I had cigarette breaks, and I was splashing water on my face." Starting the next morning, he used a 10 000-lux light box for 30 minutes at 7:30 AM, the time specified by his chronotype score (Terman and White, 2003). Recovery sleep began the next evening at 6 PM. He was awakened at 1 AM, with next sleep at 8 PM to 3 AM, and bedtime the following day at 10 PM (the target bedtime for maintenance).

"It was cool, the way it shocked my system. It started working a lot faster than I thought it would. I realized that I was feeling better in 24 hours. I was surprised I would be going home (so soon)." (His wake therapy monitors noted improvement in 18 hours.) He left in complete remission, with a SIGH-ADS score of 2.

Mr. B continued light therapy after discharge. "I know it's a big deal about wake-up time, and I always wake up at the same time and I try to be very good about that. I do the lights every morning (except sometimes). Sometimes I don't. If I've not done it for a few days, I'm a little more sluggish. But if I'm late for work in the morning, I only do 10 minutes instead of half an hour – but 10 minutes helps."

Melatonin as a chronobiotic

Hormone production and circadian timing

Pineal melatonin is produced on a nocturnal cycle triggered by the internal circadian clock, which in turn is synchronized to the day/night cycle by appropriately timed light exposure. The hypothalamic suprachiasmatic nuclei (SCN), home to the circadian pacemaker, are rich with melatonin receptors, creating a negative feedback loop (SCN/pineal/SCN) that stabilizes the body's rhythms. For late chronotypes – as we often see in depressive illness with early insomnia and difficulty awakening – the SCN-onset signal to the pineal gland occurs hours later than the norm, with sleep delayed another 2 hours. While the average onset of melatonin production is about 9:30 PM, patients can show onsets well past midnight – indeed, as late as early morning.

Considering the close association of melatonin production and sleep, it is not surprising that synthetic tablet melatonin (and recently developed pharmacologic agonists) have been used as sleep promoters, although not very effectively. The major reason for this failure is timing shortly before bedtime (as when using hypnotics). With endogenous pineal production having started far earlier than tablet ingestion, the hormone is already in circulation, and the exogenous dose has limited additional effect.

The circadian feedback loop holds the key to the solution. For tablet supplementation to expedite sleep onset, it must be taken hours before spontaneous pineal production, when the daytime hormone level is at or near zero. The SCN responds by shifting its cycle toward the time of tablet ingestion. Optimum timing to achieve this effect is about 6 hours before current sleep onset (Lewy *et al.* 1998). Typical over-the-counter doses (0.5 to 5 mg), however, place far more hormone into the bloodstream than the pineal itself produces, and if taken 6 hours before bedtime can have a rapid hypnotic effect. Furthermore, controlled-release formulations at such high dose bleed over into the next day with a risk of hangover.

The therapeutic "microdose" regimen

The solution is to use a controlled-release microdose of melatonin 6 hours before bedtime. It binds to SCN receptors without producing sleepiness. As the circadian cycle shifts earlier, sleep onset also shifts, relieving the insomnia. The action is *chronobiotic* rather than hypnotic or soporific. The optimum physiologic dose is about 0.2 mg (see section on Resources). There is no perceptible sensation after taking the tablet, and the formulation ensures early-morning washout.

The endogenous melatonin cycle is intimately connected to the day/night pattern of light exposure, and thus to light therapy. Light therapy at the end of the circadian night serves to shift the internal clock earlier. Microdose melatonin acts the same way, but in *antiphase* with light – displaced by about 12 hours. It shifts the clock earlier when taken in the *evening*. In cases of extreme delayed chronotype – for example, with sleep onset at 3 AM – the combination of evening melatonin and morning light therapy can expedite response. The interval between presleep melatonin and morning light should not be shorter than 11 hours. As sleep moves earlier, melatonin and light administration can be moved earlier as an ensemble. After achieving a normalized sleep pattern, melatonin usually can be discontinued and the positive effect maintained with light therapy alone.

As a night-time hormone and physiological signal of darkness, melatonin circulates in the retina to support scotopic vision in dim light; exposure to bright light after taking the tablet can cause retinal photosensitization, while also working against the therapeutic circadian phase-advancing effect. Therefore, several additional measures are important after taking the melatonin tablet in the evening:

- Bright evening room and screen light (computer, screen reader, television) is contraindicated because it acts on the circadian cycle to delay rather than advance the sleep cycle. Room light fixtures should be placed on dimmers to allow visual comfort without excess illumination. Without dimming, low-color-temperature, soft-white bulbs rated at 2700 or 3000 K should be used. Computer displays should be controlled by a software program that reduces short-wavelength exposure while maintaining sharp visibility (see section on Resources). Screen-reader and television screen brightness should be reduced to the lowest comfort level.
- If going into bright artificial light, the action of melatonin can be protected by wearing blue-blocking glasses, whether singly or as fitovers on prescription glasses (see section on Resources).
- Caffeine should be avoided.
- Strenuous physical activity (for example, gym workouts) should be avoided.
- Dinner should be completed at least 3 hours before bedtime.

Future directions

Dawn simulation

Morning light therapy, with its antidepressant and circadian phase-shifting effects, is like walking outside into the sun after waking up. In fact, however, the action of morning light begins even earlier, during the twilight period preceding sunrise, when we are usually still asleep. Brought into the bedroom by lighting technology, the simulation of dawn triggers the same responses as post-awakening light therapy.

As we have seen, light exposure during the evening and morning has opposite effects on the circadian rhythm. Evening light leads to a delay, and morning light to an advance. Importantly, these effects are magnified when light is presented at different points during the night. (By "night," we mean the interval between sunset and sunrise, including the twilights.) As night-time progresses, phase delays to light exposure increase. Then at a certain point toward the end of the night, the process reverses, and light exposure leads to the largest *advance* shifts in the circadian cycle. This ability to phase advance then gradually tapers off as the morning hours proceed. Therefore, to achieve equivalent phase advances, less light is needed before we wake up than later in the morning.

The graded circadian response to light at different times of day suggested to us that a mimic of dawn illumination in the bedroom, while the patient still sleeps, could produce an antidepressant response similar to post-awakening bright light therapy (Terman *et al.* 1989a). Our translucent, closed eyelids still transmit light to the retina.

We devised a bedroom apparatus to simulate a gradual springtime dawn with sunrise around 6 AM, while it remained dark outside in midwinter. Depressed mood improved within 1 to 2 weeks, even when patients slept through until the artificial sunrise. In parallel, their melatonin cycle shifted earlier. We replicated these effects in controlled trials, with no significant difference from post-awakening bright light therapy in an independent group (Terman and Terman, 2006, 2010b).

These findings led to a spate of untested commercial "dawn alarm clocks" that differ, however, from the clinical trial device by presenting a narrow field illumination at the side of the bed, which is easily missed by turning away on the pillow. Such alarm clocks have no demonstrated efficacy. A key to successful dawn simulation is broad-field diffuse illumination from *above* the bed. Such a system can be configured from current commercial components – a programmable controller coupled with an overhanging incandescent fixture that projects diffuse light toward the pillow (see section on Resources). Development of an integrated unit is underway. Initial installations will be installed in a group of residential facilities for the elderly, in Switzerland (Terman and McMahan, 2012).

Optimum dosing parameters have yet to be established for the rate of increase of the dawn signal from darkness and the overall level of the dawn signal compared to outdoor levels. The data show that an attenuated dawn signal is sufficient, rising at sunrise to standard room light level of about 300 lux.

Potential advantages of dawn simulation are its automated presentation during sleep, which eliminates the need to reserve a morning period for light therapy. It is useful also for patients vulnerable to drug photosensitization and those suffering retinal degenerative diseases for which bright light exposure is contraindicated. A disadvantage is for bed partners who want or need to sleep later than the simulated dawn.

Antimanic light protection

Switching to hypomania or mania is a common springtime event even in patients without seasonal affective disorder. This implicates the seasonal increase of early morning light exposure. A study of patients who had undergone long-term lithium therapy found reduced retinal sensitivity to light (reversible, not pathologic) – as if they were wearing "pharmacologic sunglasses" (Wirz-Justice *et al.* 1997). In an exploratory antimanic intervention, patients were restricted to a dark bedroom for 14 hours, and symptoms abated within the session – a time course similar to that when using antipsychotic medication (Barbini *et al.* 2005).

Exposure to short-wavelength light in the violet to blue-green range may contribute to manic switching. This is the same spectral range that has maximal effect on the circadian-timing system. Phase advances – accompanied by early awakening – have long been associated with mania. In an exploratory test, we have had patients in both euphoric and agitated manic states wear blue-blocking glasses (see section on Resources) throughout their waking hours, while maintaining standard sleep hours in a dark bedroom. They were calmed within one day. Controlled trials are still pending, but there is little downside to wearing blue-blockers as an adjunct to standard care.

Clinical pearls

- Bright light therapy acts in three inter-related ways: as an acute energizer, as a circadian rhythm phase-shifter, and as an antidepressant.
- Light exposure upon awakening acts to reduce early insomnia, stabilize irregular sleep patterns, and discourage oversleeping. Excessive light exposure in the evening, and light in the bedroom at night, has the opposite effect.
- The circadian timing system responds as if it were night to filtered light that eliminates the short-wavelength, blue range of the visible spectrum.
- A night awake can immediately terminate a depressive episode. Starting the next day, morning light therapy and earlier bedtime protect against relapse.
- For patients with a delayed sleep pattern, low-dose melatonin taken hours before sleep can act synergistically with morning light therapy

to reset circadian rhythms and expedite the antidepressant response.

Resources

The professional organization for clinicians using and learning chronotherapy is the Society for Light Treatment and Biological Rhythms (http://www.sltbr.org), which offers a CME course at its annual meeting. The nonprofit Center for Environmental Therapeutics (http://www.cet.org) offers the following resources:

- Recommended chronotherapy products (light box, dawn simulation system, blue-blocker glasses, blue-blocking computer screen software, and microdose melatonin).
- Guides to ocular safety and light box design standards.
- Online questionnaires for seasonality, chronotype, and depression severity, with personalized feedback.
- Clinical assessment instruments from the Columbia group (including structured interviews for depression and hypomania; diagnosis of chronotype, seasonality, and atypical depression; treatment-emergent effects; a sleep log; and a structured eye exam).
- A privacy-protected discussion forum for clinicians, at http://www.chronotherapeutics.org.

Patients value background understanding when entering chronotherapy, because of its novelty. For a layperson's overview of the literature and procedures, with interview-based case reports, see Terman and McMahan (2012).

Acknowledgment and disclosure

The authors' research was supported by grants from the National Institute of Mental Health and the New York State Science and Technology Foundation. They have no personal financial interest in any of the commercial products described herein. Michael Terman is president of the Center for Environmental Therapeutics.

References

Barbini, B., Benedetti, F., Colombo, C. et al. (2005). Dark therapy for mania: A pilot study. Bipolar Disorders, 7, 98–101.

Beauchemin, K.M. and Hays, P. (1997). Phototherapy is a useful adjunct in the treatment of depressed patients. Acta Psychiatrica Scandinavica, 95, 424–427.

Benedetti, F., Barbini, B., Campori, E. et al. (2001). Sleep phase advance and lithium to sustain the antidepressant effect of total sleep deprivation in bipolar depression: New findings supporting the internal coincidence model? Journal of Psychiatric Research, 35, 323–329.

Benedetti, F., Colombo C., Pontiggia, A. et al. (2003). Morning light treatment hastens the antidepressant effect of citalopram: A placebo-controlled trial. Journal of Clinical Psychiatry, 64, 648–653.

Benedetti, F., Barbini, B., Fulgosi, M.C. et al. (2005). Combined total sleep deprivation and light therapy in the treatment of drug-resistant bipolar depression: Acute response and long-term remission rates. Journal of Clinical Psychiatry, 66, 1535–1540.

Benedetti, F., Barbini, B., Colombo, C. et al. (2007). Chronotherapeutics in a psychiatric ward. Sleep Medicine Reviews, 11, 509–522.

Burgess, H.J., Revell, V.L., and Eastman, C.I. (2008). A three pulse phase response curve to three milligrams of melatonin in humans. Journal of Physiology, 586, 639–647.

Kripke, D.F., Risch, S.C., and Janowsky, D. (1983). Bright white light alleviates depression. Psychiatry Research, 10, 105–112.

Lewy, A.J., Bauer, V.K., Ahmed, S. et al. (1998). The human phase response curve (PRC) to melatonin is about 12 hours out of phase with the PRC to light. Chronobiology International, 15, 71–83.

Martiny K., Lunde M., Simonsen, C, et al. (2004). Relapse prevention by citalopram in SAD patients responding to 1 week of light therapy: A placebo-controlled study. Acta Psychiatrica Scandinavica, 109, 230–234.

Martiny, K., Refsgaard, E., Lund, V. et al. (2012). Nine-week randomized trial comparing a chronotherapeutic intervention (wake and light therapy) to exercise in major depression. Journal of Clinical Psychiatry, 73, 1234–1242.

Papatheodorou, G. and Kutcher S. (1995). The effect of adjunctive light therapy on ameliorating breakthrough depressive symptoms in adolescent-onset bipolar disorder. Journal of Psychiatry and Neuroscience, 20, 226–232.

Rosenthal, N.E., Sack, D.A., Gillin, J.C. et al. (1984). Seasonal affective disorder: A description of the syndrome and preliminary findings with light therapy. Archives of General Psychiatry, 41, 72–80.

Schulte, W. (1966). Kombinierte psycho- und pharmakotherapie bei melancholikern. In Kranz, H. and Petrilowitsch, N., eds., Probleme der Pharmakopsychiatrischen Kombinations und

Langzeitbehandlung. Basel: Rothenberger Gespräch, Karger, 160–169.

Sit, D., Wisner, K.L., Hanusa, B.H. *et al.* (2007). Light therapy for bipolar disorder: A case series in women. *Bipolar Disorders*, 9, 918–927.

Terman, J.S., Terman, M., and Amira, L. (1994). One-week light treatment of winter depression at its onset: The time course of relapse. *Depression*, 2, 20–31.

Terman, J.S., Terman, M., Schlager, D. *et al.* (1990). Efficacy of brief, intense light exposure for treatment of winter depression. *Psychopharmacology Bulletin*, 26, 3–11.

Terman, J.S., Terman, M., Lo, E.S. *et al.* (2001). Circadian time of morning light administration and therapeutic response in winter depression. *Archives of General Psychiatry*, 58, 69–75.

Terman, M. (2007). Evolving applications of light therapy. *Sleep Medicine Reviews*, 11, 497–507.

Terman, M. and White, T. (2003). *Automated Morningness-Eveningness Questionnaire* (AutoMEQ) [online]. New York: New York State Psychiatric Institute. Available: http://www.cet.org (accessed April 15, 2012).

Terman, M. and Terman, J.S. (1999). Bright light therapy: side effects and benefits across the symptom spectrum. *Journal of Clinical Psychiatry*, 60, 799–808.

Terman, M. and Terman, J.S. (2006). Controlled trial of naturalistic dawn simulation and negative air ionization for seasonal affective disorder. *American Journal of Psychiatry*, 163, 2126–2133.

Terman, M. and Terman, J.S. (2010a). Light therapy. In Krieger, M.H., Roth, T., and Dement, W.C., eds., *Principles and Practice of Sleep Medicine, Fifth Edition*, St. Louis: Elsevier/Saunders, 1682–1695.

Terman, M. and Terman, J.S. (2010b). Circadian rhythm phase advance with dawn simulation treatment for winter depression. *Journal of Biological Rhythms*, 25, 297–301.

Terman, M. and McMahan, I. (2012). *Chronotherapy: Resetting Your Inner Clock to Boost Mood, Alertness, and Quality Sleep*. New York: Avery/Penguin.

Terman, M., Terman, J.S., and Ross, D.C. (1998). A controlled trial of timed bright light and negative air ionization for treatment of winter depression. *Archives of General Psychiatry*, 55, 875–882.

Terman, M., Schlager, D., Fairhurst, S. *et al.* (1989a). Dawn and dusk simulation as a therapeutic intervention. *Biological Psychiatry*, 25, 966–970.

Terman, M., Terman, J.S., Quitkin, F.M. *et al.* (1989b). Dosing dimensions of light therapy: Duration and time of day. In Silverstone, T. and Thompson, C., eds., *Seasonal Affective Disorder*. London: Clinical Neuroscience Publishers, 187–204.

Terman, M., Terman, J.S., Quitkin, F.M. *et al.* (1989c). Light therapy for seasonal affective disorder: A review of efficacy. *Neuropsychopharmacology*, 2, 1–22.

Terman, M., Rifkin, J.B., Jacobs, J. *et al.* (2001). *Morningness-Eveningness Questionnaire (revised)* [online]. New York: New York State Psychiatric Institute. Available: http://www.cet.org (accessed April 15, 2012).

Voderholzer, U., Valerius, G., Schaerer, L. *et al.* (2003). Is the antidepressive effect of sleep deprivation stabilized by a three day phase advance of the sleep period? A pilot study. *European Archives of Psychiatry and Clinical Neuroscience*, 253, 68–72.

Williams, J.B.W. and Terman, M. (2003). *Structured Interview Guide for the Hamilton Depression Rating Scale with Atypical Depression Supplement (SIGH-ADS)* [online]. New York: New York State Psychiatric Institute. Available: http://www.cet.org (accessed April 15, 2012).

Williams, J.B.W., Link, M.J., Rosenthal, N.E. *et al.* (2002). *Structured Interview Guide for the Hamilton Depression Rating Scale – Seasonal Affective Disorder Version (SIGH-SAD)*. Also, SIGH-SAD-SR (self-rating version) [online]. New York: New York State Psychiatric Institute. Available: http://www.cet.org (accessed April 15, 2012).

Wirz-Justice, A. (1998). Beginning to see the light. *Archives of General Psychiatry*, 55, 861–862.

Wirz-Justice, A. and Armstrong, S.M. (1996). Melatonin: Nature's soporific? *Journal of Sleep Research*, 5, 137–141.

Wirz-Justice, A. and van den Hoofdakker, R.H. (1999). Sleep deprivation in depression: What do we know, where do we go? *Biological Psychiatry*, 46, 445–453.

Wirz-Justice, A., Bromundt, V., and Cajochen, C. (2009a). Circadian disruption and psychiatric disorders: The importance of entrainment. *Sleep Med Clinics*, 4, 273–284.

Wirz-Justice, A., Benedetti, F., and Terman, M. (2009b). *Chronotherapeutics for Affective Disorders: A Clinician's Manual for Light and Wake Therapy*. Basel: Karger.

Wirz-Justice, A., Remé, C., Prune, A. *et al.* (1997). Lithium decreases retinal sensitivity, but this is not cumulative with years of treatment. *Biological Psychiatry*, 41, 743–746.

Wirz-Justice, A., Terman, M., Oren, D.A. *et al.* (2004). Brightening depression. *Science*, 303, 467–469.

Wu, J.C., Kelsoe, J.R., Schachat, C. *et al.* (2009). Rapid and sustained antidepressant response with sleep deprivation and chronotherapy in bipolar disorder. *Biological Psychiatry*, 66, 298–301.

Chapter 27

Ketamine in treatment-resistant depression

Kyle A.B. Lapidus and Sanjay J. Mathew

Introduction

Major depressive disorder (MDD) is a common, debilitating illness, and often responds incompletely to standard treatments. Despite advances in medication development, treatment-resistant depression (TRD) remains a major clinical problem. Although many patients with MDD achieve clinical response (defined as 50% improvement in core depressive symptoms) with initial antidepressant treatment, one-third to one-half of patients fail to respond despite adherence to treatments of adequate dose and duration (Fava and Davidson, 1996). Patients who have failed to respond to two successive treatments experience very low (10–20%) remission rates with subsequent treatment and high relapse rates if they do remit, while no single pharmacotherapy has shown significantly superior efficacy in this group (Rush *et al.* 2006, 2009). Clearly, there is a significant public health need for development of new therapies for TRD that address persistent mood symptoms, promote sustained remission, and improve quality of life. A second limitation of existing marketed antidepressants is the delay of weeks in attaining maximal antidepressant response. Ketamine, an anesthetic agent used for more than 40 years, is showing promise in the effort to identify rapidly acting therapies for patients with TRD (Covvey *et al.* 2011).

This chapter begins with an overview of the scientific rationale for the development of new therapeutic approaches. The next section reviews ketamine's history, basic and clinical pharmacology, and administration methods. We then review the scientific evidence to date for ketamine efficacy in patients with TRD. Finally, side effects of ketamine, including impact on hemodynamics and neurocognition are discussed.

Limitations of drug therapies and rationale for glutamate modulation in TRD

Although ongoing neuroscience research continues to create models that often elucidate novel antidepressant mechanisms and therapeutic targets, there have been few significant innovations and no paradigm-shifting "breakthrough" antidepressant drugs in several decades (Mathew, 2008, Mathew *et al.* 2008, Koo *et al.* 2010, Vialou *et al.* 2010). All currently approved antidepressant drugs (with the exception of the melatonergic agent agomelatine, approved in Europe) target monoaminergic neurotransmission, focusing on mechanisms identified decades ago. Unfortunately, research into new molecular targets (e.g., corticotropin-releasing factor (CRF) antagonists, neurokinin (NK) antagonists, signal transduction regulators such as phosphodiesterase inhibitors, etc.) has not yet produced effective new antidepressant treatments (Mathew *et al.* 2008). Somewhat surprisingly, as of early 2012, the olanzapine–fluoxetine combination (OFC) remains the only pharmacotherapy with US FDA approval for the specific indication of "treatment-resistant depression," defined by inadequate response to two different antidepressants in the current episode (Trivedi *et al.* 2009). Electroconvulsive therapy (ECT) has been widely used for decades as a highly effective acute antidepressant treatment in patients with severe depression who have failed to respond to antidepressant medications. However, its use is limited by the requirement for general anesthesia and cognitive side effects.

Glutamate is an amino acid critical for cellular metabolism, is the most abundant excitatory neurotransmitter, and is found throughout the brain; glutamate has been shown to play critical roles in synaptic plasticity, learning, and memory. Additionally, glutamate has neurotrophic effects and has been implicated in neurodevelopment and degeneration. *In vivo* brain-imaging data, post-mortem investigations, and gene expression studies all suggest that glutamatergic dysfunction plays a potentially important role in the pathophysiology of major depression (Sanacora *et al.* 2008). Imaging studies using magnetic resonance spectroscopy (MRS) have demonstrated abnormalities in regional concentrations of the amino acid neurotransmitters glutamate, glutamine, and GABA in patients with MDD (Auer *et al.* 2000, Rosenberg *et al.* 2005). Additional MRS data suggest that TRD is associated with more severe amino acid neurotransmitter abnormalities than more nontreatment-resistant MDD (Price *et al.* 2009b). *In vivo* brain glutamate abnormalities are consistent with alterations in peripheral blood and CSF glutamate levels, as well as post-mortem studies of NMDA receptors (Hashimoto, 2009).

Glutamatergic transmission is tightly regulated by a system that includes synthesis and packaging into vesicles, release, binding to a variety of receptors, scaffolding and signaling proteins, and excitatory amino acid transporters (Sanacora *et al.* 2008). Glutamate receptors can be broadly divided into ionotropic (directly passing ions) and metabotropic (exerting effects through signal transduction) types. In humans, ionotropic glutamate receptors nonselectively channel cations when activated; the major ionotropic glutamate receptor types include α-amino-3-hydroxy-5-methyl-4-isoxazole propionic acid receptors (AMPAR), kainate receptors (KAR), and *N*-methyl-D-aspartate receptors (NMDAR) (Machado-Vieira *et al.* 2009). Metabotropic glutamate receptors act through G-proteins and are also divided into three major groups with multiple sub-types. Despite glutamate's ubiquity, the variety of glutamate receptor sub-types and sub-units provide an opportunity for specific modulation. In addition to drugs used for other disorders, several glutamatergic agents are approved for neuropsychiatric disorders (for example, memantine, riluzole, and lamotrigine), though none is specifically indicated for depression. However, these glutamatergic drugs have demonstrated efficacy in modulating mood, and lamotrigine carries an indication for bipolar maintenance treatment, where it prevents both manic and depressive episodes.

Moreover, the glutamate-release inhibitor, riluzole, has also shown promise for treating depression. This FDA-approved medication for amyotrophic lateral sclerosis (ALS) demonstrated antidepressant properties in clinical studies of patients with major depression and particularly TRD (Zarate *et al.* 2004, Sanacora *et al.* 2007). Studies targeting AMPAR and metabotropic glutamate receptors are ongoing.

To date, most reported glutamatergic clinical trials in depression have focused on NMDAR modulators. Substantial preclinical evidence suggests that NMDAR antagonists have antidepressant properties, and that chronic administration of traditional monoamine-based antidepressants regulates NMDAR expression and function (Paul *et al.* 1994, Pittaluga *et al.* 2007). In addition to ketamine, several sub-type-selective NMDAR antagonists (e.g., NR2A, NR2B) are in the early stages of investigation for TRD. The first report of a randomized, placebo-controlled trial adjunctive administration of the NR2B antagonist CP-101,606, demonstrated rapid and sustained antidepressant efficacy (Preskorn *et al.* 2008).

Overview of ketamine

History and indications

Ketamine, the chiral arylcyclohexamine (RS)-2-(*O*-chlorophenyl)-2-methylamino cyclohexanone, is a noncompetitive NMDA antagonist (Reich and Silvay, 1989). First synthesized by Parke-Davis in the early 1960s, the dissociative anesthetic, ketamine, was developed to provide surgical anesthesia with more rapid recovery and less severe psychotomimetic effects than phencyclidine (PCP) (White *et al.* 1982). Ketamine is approved by the FDA for three indications: (1) as the sole anesthetic agent for surgical procedures that do not require skeletal muscle relaxation, (2) for induction of anesthesia prior to administration of other general anesthetic agents, and (3) to supplement low-potency agents, such as nitrous oxide. Anesthesia induction is often performed using IV doses in the range of 1–4.5 mg/kg. Ketamine is also used off-label for other applications in sedation and analgesia. Ketamine consistently affects EEG activity, including reduction of alpha and increase of beta, delta, and theta activity. Mild hypertonicity, mild respiratory suppression, and bronchodilation, with generally preserved airway patency but with increased salivary and broncheo-tracheal secretions are also observed (Reich and Silvay, 1989).

Pharmacology

Although ketamine is considered primarily to act at the NMDAR–PCP binding site as an antagonist, its pharmacological profile is complex, and affinity for other receptors has been demonstrated. Beyond direct antagonism of NMDAR, modulation of alternate receptors may contribute to ketamine's effect on mood and cognition. Ketamine's metabolism produces two major products, norketamine (NK), the initial, predominant metabolite, and dehydronorketamine (DHNK), a minor, inactive metabolite. NK is a noncompetitive NMDAR antagonist and contributes to ketamine analgesia.

Ketamine, like the NMDA antagonists 2-amino-5-phosphonovalerate (APV) and 2-amino-7-phosphonoheptanoate (APH), incompletely reduced glutamate- and aspartate-induced depolarizing responses in slices of rat cortex (Harrison and Simmonds, 1985). Each of these antagonists reduced responses to NMDA selectively, without impacting the action of quisqualate or kainate.

Ketamine has also been reported to exert cholinergic effects, inhibiting nicotinic ACh receptor activation, while also raising ACh levels by inhibiting acetylcholinesterase (Cohen et al. 1974, Lodge et al. 1982, Weber et al. 2005). The affinity for M1 muscarinic receptors is certain; though ketamine was not shown to affect stimulation-induced calcium changes, ketamine's pK_i of 45μM is in a clinically relevant range (Hirota et al. 2002). Ketamine's interactions with adrenergic receptors has also been demonstrated with K_d 3.4 mM at α_1 and K_d 0.35 mM at β_2 receptors; though less pronounced than other interactions, these may contribute to ketamine's hemodynamic effects (Bevan et al. 1997).

Of opioid receptor sub-types, ketamine has highest affinity for μ (K_i 26.8 μM) with lower affinity for σ and κ (K_i 66.0 and 85.2 μM, respectively) and lowest affinity for δ receptors (K_i 101 μM)(Smith et al. 1987). In vitro studies of ketamine's analgesic effects suggest that ketamine may act in a clinically relevant range as a low affinity μ opioid agonist (IC_{50} 14.8 μM without sodium) (Smith et al. 1980). However, the affinity was reduced only approximately sixfold with the addition of sodium, suggesting that ketamine may also have some opiate antagonist properties. Although

ketamine's affinity for the NMDA receptor is higher (IC_{50} 0.4–7 μM), these data suggest that effects on opioid receptors are likely relevant at anesthetic concentrations.

Ketamine and its metabolites can affect monoaminergic transmission by inhibiting transport of serotonin, norepinephrine, and dopamine (Smith et al. 1981). In addition, ketamine and its metabolites were found to inhibit monoamine deamination. Ketamine's potency at D_2 receptors (K_i 55 nM) was reported to be higher than for NMDA receptors (K_i 3100 nM) when human receptors are expressed in cultured hamster cells, though human PET studies have shown variable impact on D2 receptor availability or dopamine release (Seeman et al. 2005).

Although ketamine has not been reported to selectively affect GABA-B receptors, some preclinical data and a human single photon emission computed tomography (SPECT) study suggest that ketamine modulates GABA-A activity (Lin et al. 1992, Salmi et al. 2005, Heinzel et al. 2008). In addition, ketamine acts at a variety of ion channels, inhibiting veratridine-stimulation-induced Na^+ uptake with an IC_{50} >200 μM, while interacting with the Ca^{2+} ATPase to block Ca^{2+} influx and stimulate efflux (Allaoua and Chicheportiche, 1989). Importantly, ketamine inhibits HCN1 at clinically relevant concentrations with an EC_{50} of approximately 10 μM (Chen et al. 2009).

Enantiomers

Ketamine has a chiral center at the C-2 carbon of the cyclohexanone ring, resulting in two enantiomers (Reich and Silvay, 1989). In the USA, ketamine is only approved and is administered as a 1:1 racemic mixture of S(+) and R(-) configurations. However, S-ketamine was approved in Europe in 1998 and is available for medical use in Finland, Germany, Denmark, Iceland, and the Netherlands, with indications for induction and maintenance of general anesthesia, supplementation of regional anesthesia, and analgesia in emergency medicine.

S-ketamine binds with 3–4 times higher affinity for the NMDAR–PCP binding site than R-ketamine (Vollenweider et al. 1997a). S-ketamine's superior potency at the intended site of action offers the possibility that use of this agent may provide comparable clinical benefits with fewer adverse effects (Paul et al. 2009). However, S-ketamine also demonstrates higher potency for other receptors: 1–2 times more potent at ACh receptors and 2–3 times more potent at opioid receptors than R-ketamine (Finck and Ngai, 1982, Lodge *et al.* 1982). These affinity differences may underlie reported tolerability differences between the racemate and S-ketamine, although more comparative research is needed.

Routes of administration

Ketamine administration may include intravenous (IV), intramuscular (IM), intranasal (IN), intrarectal, epidural, subcutaneous, transdermal, intra-articular, sub-lingual, and oral routes. Bioavailability differs greatly between routes because ketamine undergoes extensive first-pass metabolism (Clements *et al.* 1982, Malinovsky *et al.* 1996, Yanagihara *et al.* 2003). After IV administration, the highest ketamine bioavailability, following IM administration, has been reported at 93%. A preliminary study of IM ketamine in depression has been reported, along with a suggestion that this method results in a higher and more rapid peak ketamine level (Glue *et al.* 2011). Because of low oral bioavailability (approximately 15–20%), this method of administration has not been widely used. However, oral administration has also been associated with higher levels, relative to other methods, of the active metabolite, norketamine. Although this metabolite has analgesic properties, interindividual metabolic differences, bitter taste, lack of indication, and no commercially available preparation for this route have led to recommendations for avoiding this method (Blonk *et al.* 2010). Sub-lingual and intrarectal bioavailability estimates are in the range of 30%. However, rectal administration has shown promise in children, and has been used as premedication in this context.

Intranasal or IN ketamine bioavailability has been reported at approximately 25–50%. This variability depends in part on the amount of administered dose that is swallowed by the patient. Because ketamine is indicated for anesthesia, IN ketamine has been most widely used for this purpose, particularly in children. IN ketamine administration was first reported in a randomized controlled trial, that demonstrated efficacy in children undergoing dental procedures (Abrams *et al.* 1993). Case studies and several randomized controlled trials have since demonstrated IN ketamine's safety and efficacy as anesthetic or premedication in pediatric populations for surgical, dental, and imaging procedures (Weksler *et al.* 1993, Louon and Reddy, 1994, Diaz, 1997, Weber *et al.* 2003, Roelofse *et al.* 2004).

In adults, an open-label trial of IN ketamine also suggested efficacy for aura in individuals with familial hemiplegic migraine (Kaube *et al.* 2000). Safety and efficacy of IN ketamine were also demonstrated in 20 adults with chronic pain in a randomized, double-blind, placebo-controlled study (Carr *et al.* 2004). A study of S-ketamine in 16 adults with neuropathic pain provides further evidence for efficacy of IN administration (Huge *et al.* 2010).

Ketamine in TRD
Single dose

The efficacy of ketamine in depression was first reported in 2000. This study included nine patients, eight with unipolar depression and one bipolar, at Yale University School of Medicine, and found rapid antidepressant effects following a single IV ketamine dose (Berman *et al.* 2000). In this randomized, double-blind, crossover study, subjects received a 40-minute infusion of ketamine (0.5 mg/kg) or saline, separated by at least 1 week. Ketamine treatment improved depressive symptoms relative to saline, indicated by significant decreases in Hamilton Rating Scale for Depression-25 item (HRSD-25) scores within 4 hours. Progressive reductions in HRSD-25 scores were seen 24, 48, and 72 hours after infusion and one subject's symptoms did not return to baseline for 2 weeks until additional antidepressant treatment was reinitiated. Four of the eight subjects who received ketamine responded (50% decrease in HRSD-25) within 72 hours, while only one of eight experienced a similar decrease after receiving saline. However, ketamine infusion also led to psychotomimetic effects, significantly increasing Brief Psychiatric Rating Scale (BPRS) scores, particularly the positive symptoms sub-scale. Additionally, subjects reported elevations in feelings of "high" on a Visual Analog Scale (VAS-High). These symptoms resolved within 2 hours and were not correlated with changes in depression ratings, which continued to decrease for several days after the psychotomimetic symptoms resolved.

In addition to the magnitude of improvement and durability of benefit, the time course of response in this study was impressive. While the beneficial effects of ketamine did not appear to be related to induction of euphoria, psychotomimetic side effects may have compromised the blind. However, analysis of individual HRSD-25 items suggested that ketamine specifically reduced depressed mood, suicidal ideation, helplessness, and worthlessness.

These findings were replicated in a larger study of 18 patients at the Mood Disorders Unit of the National Institute of Mental Health (NIMH) in 2004–2005 (Zarate *et al.* 2006). Though all patients in this replication study had TRD (with ≥2 treatment failures), this study's design otherwise was essentially identical to the first study: randomized, saline placebo-controlled, double-blind, crossover with subjects receiving IV ketamine (0.5 mg/kg) or saline infusion over 40 minutes. The results of the two studies were similar. Depressive symptoms, assessed with HRSD-21, were significantly reduced within 2 hours. Ketamine's effect size was very large after 1 day ($d = 1.46$; 95% confidence interval, 0.91–2.01) and moderate to large at 1 week ($d = 0.68$; 95% confidence interval, 0.13–1.23). One day after infusion, 12 (71%) of the 17 patients who received ketamine met response criteria (≥50% reduction in HRSD-21), while five (29%) met remission criteria (HRSD-21 ≤ 7). None of the patients met response or remission criteria at this time-point after receiving placebo. Benefits were well maintained for many patients; six subjects met response criteria 1 week after infusion, while benefits were maintained for at least 2 weeks in two patients. No serious adverse events were identified and psychotomimetic effects resolved within 2 hours of ketamine treatment.

These two studies indicated that a single subanesthetic dose of IV ketamine could elicit a rapid and sustained antidepressant response in patients with MDD or even TRD. However, addressing concerns about psychotomimetic side effects and longer-term durability of response remained important goals. Lamotrigine reduces the presynaptic glutamate release proposed to underlie ketamine's psychotomimetic effects. In healthy volunteers, lamotrigine had previously been reported to decrease ketamine-induced perceptual abnormalities and to limit BPRS increases (Anand *et al.* 2000). Lamotrigine also reduced dissociative symptoms and cognitive impairment without significantly altering ketamine-induced mood effects. Also, several pilot studies indicated that riluzole could provide antidepressant efficacy (Zarate *et al.* 2004, 2005, Sanacora *et al.* 2007). Therefore, investigators at Mount Sinai Medical Center designed a trial to optimize safety and extend time to relapse (Mathew *et al.* 2010). This study included other glutamatergic agents with potentially synergistic mechanisms, lamotrigine and riluzole, in addition to ketamine.

In this randomized controlled trial, a single dose of lamotrigine (300 mg) or placebo was administered 2 hours prior to open-label IV ketamine (0.5 mg/kg over 40 minutes). Twenty-six medically healthy subjects with TRD participated and 17 (65%) met response criteria (≥50% reduction in Montgomery–Asberg Depression Rating Scale [MADRS]) 24 hours post-ketamine, and 13 (50%) met remission criteria (MADRS ≤ 9). Fourteen patients (54%) met response criteria at 72 hours and were then entered into the continuation phase. This consisted of a 4-week randomized, placebo-controlled, double-blind, flexible-dose trial of riluzole (100–200 mg/d). Time to relapse and MADRS scores at completion did not differ significantly between patients treated with riluzole or placebo. On day 32, 1/6 (17%) subjects treated with riluzole met response criteria, compared with 4/8 (50%) treated with placebo meeting response criteria. Though the additional glutamatergic treatments did not provide additional benefit, the response rate to ketamine confirmed the previous findings. The negative findings for lamotrigine may be partly explained by the low rate of adverse psychotomimetic effects including no positive symptoms, only 3/26 subjects experiencing small increases in BPRS, and few experiencing high or very high CADSS scores (4/13 (31%) treated with placebo vs. 3/13 (23%) for lamotrigine). Similarly, small sample size may explain the failure of riluzole to separate from placebo for relapse prevention. Larger placebo-controlled studies testing riluzole and other relapse-prevention strategies are in progress (NCT00088699 and NCT01441505).

Another trial of riluzole continuation following single dose, open-label, IV ketamine (0.5 mg/kg over 40 minutes) was recently performed at the NIMH (Ibrahim *et al.* 2011). The initial response to ketamine was reported, and suggested that ketamine may provide benefit even in patients who had previously failed to respond to ECT. This study enrolled 42 patients, including 23 with TRD, but no prior ECT exposure, and 17 who failed an adequate trial of ECT. Both groups demonstrated significant improvement in depressive symptoms at 230 minutes and the proportion of patients meeting response criteria (50% reduction in MADRS scores) did not differ significantly between groups. Group differences noted included higher baseline scores in the ECT-resistant group and a larger effect size in the non-ECT-resistant group. Dissociative symptoms did not differ significantly between the two groups and resolved within 2 hours.

Repeated dose

One potential method for extending the antidepressant efficacy of ketamine includes repeated dosing after initial response. Repeated-dose protocols are commonly used for ECT in TRD, and ketamine has been repeatedly dosed in chronic pain conditions. The first trial of repeated ketamine dosing in TRD was an open-label administration of six infusions over 12 days and included 10 participants with a lifetime mean of eight antidepressant failures and response (≥50% reduction in MADRS, n = 9) 1 day following the initial dose of ketamine (aan het Rot *et al.* 2010). Each administration included 0.5 mg/kg given over 40 minutes with continuous monitoring in an inpatient setting. The schedule was designed to resemble the beginning of an acute course of ECT (Monday–Wednesday–Friday for 2 weeks). Following the sixth infusion, mood symptoms were assessed at follow-up visits, scheduled twice weekly for 4 weeks or until relapse. Relapse was defined as MADRS >50% of the preketamine baseline and >20 for two consecutive visits or a Clinical Global Impression-Improvement scale (CGI-I) score of 6 ("much worse") at any visit. Minimal psychotic symptoms (assessed by BPRS) and transient dissociative symptoms in only three patients were detected. All nine patients who responded to the initial dose maintained response throughout the 2-week course. The mean MADRS decrease from baseline following the sixth infusion was 85%. Despite the absence of other antidepressant medications, response was maintained in all nine patients throughout the 12 days of ketamine infusions. Mean time to relapse after completion of infusions was 19 days, but varied considerably from 6 days to >3 months, despite no use of other antidepressant medication (Murrough *et al.* 2011). Beyond reported efficacy, this study demonstrated the safety of repeated-dose IV ketamine for TRD. Drug-seeking behavior was not seen during the trial or follow-up period. In addition, cognitive deficits exceeding those at baseline were not reported. Because of small sample size and lack of control group, these safety and efficacy data require confirmation.

Repeated-dose, open-label IM ketamine administration has also been performed in a small group of patients with bipolar depression (Glue *et al.* 2011). This study included ascending doses, initially 0.5 mg/kg, followed by 0.7 and 1.0 mg/kg. The initial treatment at the lowest dose had only minimal effect on mood symptoms, while the higher doses resulted in greater improvements. In one of the two reported cases, remission was reported, though complete time course of response and time to remission were not reported. However, this study gave preliminary evidence for safety as all doses were tolerated and side effects, including light-headedness, and dissociative symptoms were similar to those reported for IV ketamine.

In addition to piloting multiple-dose IM ketamine for depression, these authors suggest that the pharmacokinetics of IM administration may be superior to other delivery methods because of higher peak ketamine levels. While this model and the data presented from a small case series are preliminary, this study motivates additional studies using alternative routes of administration and multiple ketamine doses.

In summary, ketamine administration has been associated with response rates of ≥50% in multiple studies with a total of approximately 100 patients with major depression and TRD. Beyond its efficacy in a difficult-to-treat group, the rapidity of onset of ketamine's antidepressant effects with mood improvement occurring within several hours distinguishes ketamine from conventional antidepressant drugs, though rapid response has also been reported with other somatic treatments. Moreover, the mood benefit of ketamine may persist for days to weeks, and repeated dosing, in some cases, has been shown to extend this benefit to several months.

Impact on suicidal ideation and related cognition

Investigation of which depressive symptoms respond to single- or multiple-dose ketamine treatment suggested that ketamine may target suicidal cognition. Analysis of TRD patients' response to IV ketamine (0.5 mg/kg over 40 minutes) in either single- or multiple-dose trials performed at Mount Sinai demonstrated that both explicit and implicit measures of suicidal cognition were decreased within 24 hours of infusion, and that this benefit persisted throughout the treatment course for patients who received multiple dose (Price *et al.* 2009a). Implicit suicidality was assessed and followed using a computer-based instrument, the Implicit Association Test (IAT). This test measures how tightly an individual associates words based on response latency, and another IAT had previously shown promise for self-harm assessment (Nock and Banaji, 2007). The MADRS suicide item (MADRS-SI) and Beck Scale for Suicidal Ideation (SSI) were used to assess explicit suicidal ideation. Although this group was not highly suicidal, each of these measures responded to ketamine. However, they were significantly correlated with each other, and the MADRS-SI change did not survive correcting for co-variance of the nonsuicide-related MADRS items, suggesting that the reduction in suicidal ideation was mediated by overall reduction in depression. Rapid reduction in suicidal ideation was also reported in a trial of open-label infusion of ketamine (0.5 mg/kg over 40 minutes) in TRD performed at the NIMH (DiazGranados et al. 2010). This patient population had a higher level of suicidal ideation at baseline including 10 of 33 total with SSI $\geq$ 4. All patients in this group had SSI $<$ 4 within 80 minutes of infusion. In the larger group, significant decreases in suicidal ideation, assessed by SSI and suicide items from depression scales, were found within 40 minutes of infusion and persisted for 4 hours after ketamine administration. Open-label administration of a bolus of ketamine (0.2 mg/kg over 1–2 minutes), given in an emergency department at Yale, was found to rapidly reduce suicidal ideation and depressive symptoms (Larkin and Beautrais, 2011). Mean MADRS in this group of 14 patients was reduced from 40.8 at baseline to 11.5 at 4 hours after the bolus and response persisted for 7 days in all patients and for 10 days in all but one patient who was lost to follow-up on day 8. Decreases in mean MADRS-SI were also found, from 3.9 at baseline to below 1 at 40 minutes and all subsequent time-points assessed to day 10. The open-label use of ketamine to reduce suicidal ideation has also been discussed in a palliative care setting (Thangathurai and Mogos, 2011). The Yale study also raises the question as to the optimal ketamine dose required for antidepressant action, and suggests that it may be lower than the commonly used 0.5 mg/kg given IV over 40 minutes.

Neural mechanisms of antidepressant efficacy

Current understanding of MDD includes changes in a network of prefrontal, sub-cortical, and limbic brain regions. Depressive symptom severity has been associated with impaired frontal cortical regulation/activity and increased sub-cortical and limbic activity (Erk et al. 2010). Monoamine, amino acid, neuropeptide, and neuroendocrine-related neurotransmitters are thought to regulate emotion through effects on these circuits (Krishnan and Nestler, 2010). Ketamine is hypothesized to exert antidepressant effects by altering the function of these mood-regulating circuits by directly affecting glutamate activity and indirectly, through other neurochemical systems. Specifically, ketamine is hypothesized to shift the balance of neural activity from sub-cortical and limbic structures that process emotion toward cortical regulatory structures, including medial and dorsal regions of the prefrontal cortex (PFC).

Animal studies have demonstrated that ketamine increases excitatory glutamatergic transmission in cortical regions (Vollenweider and Kometer, 2010). In healthy human subjects, ketamine-induced increases in brain metabolic activity with marked increases in frontal cortical regions (i.e., PFC, anterior cingulate cortex [ACC]) have been identified through use of PET and [18F]fluorodeoxyglucose (FDG) (Brier et al. 1997, Vollenweider et al. 1997b). In 13 MDD patients, antidepressant treatment was found to increase and normalize PFC metabolism, suggesting that these metabolic changes may be central to relief of depression (Kennedy et al. 2001). However, studies using functional magnetic resonance imaging (fMRI) data failed to demonstrate these metabolic increases, instead finding ketamine prevented fear-imagery-induced metabolic decreases in limbic and sub-cortical regions, including the amygdala (Abel et al. 2003). This provides evidence that ketamine may exert antidepressant effects via reducing the activation of limbic regions in addition to frontal effects.

Investigation of how ketamine affects neurocircuitry in MDD is in the early stages, with few published studies. However, two magnetoencephalography (MEG) studies have demonstrated correlations between ACC activity and ketamine antidepressant response (Salvadore et al. 2009, 2010). One study found abnormal increases in ACC activity for MDD subjects who were exposed to fearful stimuli; these increases correlated with antidepressant response to IV ketamine and were proposed as a biomarker for treatment response (Salvadore et al. 2009). The second reported an inverse correlation between ACC activation in a working memory task and response, and also found that connectivity between ACC and amygdala inversely correlated with response (Salvadore et al. 2010).

Proton MRS was used to investigate how ketamine affects amino acid transmitter (e.g., glutamine, glutamate, GABA) levels in the occipital cortex of MDD patients, though no differences from placebo were found (Valentine *et al.* 2011). This study replicated previous findings of ketamine efficacy in a group of 10 MDD subjects, but failed to detect differences between ketamine and placebo from baseline to 3 and 48 hours after administration.

Signaling pathways beyond the NMDA receptor have recently gained attention for understanding the mechanism of ketamine's rapid antidepressant action. The mammalian target of rapamycin (mTOR) pathway is rapidly activated by ketamine and leads to increased synaptic signaling proteins and increased density and maturation of spine synapses in rodent PFC (Li *et al.* 2010). AMPA and mTOR activity were necessary for ketamine's effects on synapses and behavior. This study further extends prior research indicating that ketamine efficacy involves AMPA signaling, along with neurotrophic factors and neuroplasticity (Duman and Monteggia, 2006, Maeng *et al.* 2008, Murrough and Charney, 2010). Taken together, these results increase understanding of ketamine's mechanism beyond simply affecting NMDA receptors, and provide additional targets for research and therapeutics development.

Side effects

Hemodynamic changes

Since the early use of ketamine in anesthesia, blood pressure changes have been documented with IV or IM administration (Bovill *et al.* 1971). Although increases on the order of 30 mmHg have been reported, in the dose range used for depression most blood pressure changes are absent or of smaller magnitude. These changes are generally manageable with adequate monitoring and medication treatment is rarely indicated. Although ketamine is negatively inotropic when acting directly on myocardium, this does not explain the hemodynamic effects usually seen in clinical practice (Gelissen *et al.* 1996). Additional hemodynamic effects include increased heart rate, intraventricular pressure, and cardiac output, which are likely mediated through central autonomic effects (Tweed *et al.* 1972). However, these are less frequently of clinical concern and in fact ketamine is considered favorably in hemodynamically compromised patients (Morris *et al.* 2009). At doses used in MDD, hypertension as well as tachycardia and bradycardia have been reported. However, these side effects have resolved within hours after infusion and have not resulted in serious adverse events in single- or repeated-dose trials.

Cognitive function

Acute effects

Beyond acute dissociative and psychotomimetic symptoms, cognitive effects of ketamine have been investigated. These investigations were partly motivated by animal studies demonstrating the importance of NMDAR function in long-term potentiation and memory acquisition, concerns regarding potential for NMDA antagonist-mediated neurotoxicity, and use of ketamine to model symptoms of schizophrenia (Olney *et al.* 1991, Jeutovic-Todorovic *et al.* 2001). Ketamine administration in healthy volunteers was shown to acutely impair spatial and verbal learning, while retrieval remained intact (Rowland *et al.* 2005). Other studies found sub-anesthetic doses of ketamine to impair attention, recognition, and recall in healthy volunteers, and confirmed that deficits were related to encoding rather than retrieval (Malhotra *et al.* 1996, Hetem *et al.* 2000). Similar acute impairments have been reported in recreational users of ketamine and other illicit drugs (Curran and Morgan, 2001). However, in healthy volunteers, cognitive impairments following an acute dose of ketamine resolved within 3 days of drug administration, with no residual deficits (Morgan *et al.* 2004a).

Chronic effects

Although preclinical data suggest chronic effects of ketamine, in humans there is little data regarding cognitive effects of chronic ketamine administration. Much of the available information on chronic ketamine use involves small groups of poly-drug-abusing subjects (Curran and Morgan, 2000). The largest study performed to date investigated neurocognitive effects of chronic ketamine use in 150 participants in a 1-year longitudinal study (Morgan *et al.* 2010). This population included five groups: healthy and poly-drug-using controls, along with frequent, infrequent, and currently abstinent ketamine users. Cognitive impairments were found in frequent ketamine users, who self-administered ketamine more than four times weekly. Although frequent users exhibited impaired recognition and working memory, these effects were not seen in infrequent or remitted users, suggesting that recovery may occur rapidly upon discontinuation of abuse. In contrast, a longer-term follow-up study of illicit ketamine users found recovery of semantic memory, but ongoing impairment of episodic memory 3 years after reduction or cessation of ketamine use (Morgan *et al.* 2004b). Conflicting results and other limitations of the available data (e.g., few studies with small sample sizes, heterogenous designs, and inconsistent administration routes and protocols) indicate a pressing need for further studies to clarify the impact of ketamine on cognition in longer-term prospective, controlled trials (Morgan and Curran, 2006).

Summary and future directions

Although ketamine's pharmacology and safety has long been explored in the context of its utility in anesthesia and analgesia, understanding ketamine's antidepressant effect requires further investigation. Ketamine is known to antagonize NMDAR function, but probing downstream mechanisms (e.g., effects on glutamate, signal transduction, dendritic spines, and neuroprotection) remains an area of active focus. At present it is unclear which of these effects are critical for the rapid and sustained improvements in depression of some patients in clinical trials. Additionally, understanding of the benefits obtained remains challenging in light of concerns about study design (i.e., many saline-controlled crossover studies), small sample sizes, and broader safety and efficacy concerns. The data for repeated-dose ketamine is even more limited, with no adequately controlled randomized trials published to date. Although ketamine therapy remains largely experimental, the significant efficacy, particularly in severely treatment-resistant patients, coupled with the rapidity of response suggest that ketamine may offer new promise for depression treatment.

Currently, research is underway to optimize dosing, explore alternate delivery routes, prevent relapse, and understand mechanisms of ketamine's antidepressant action. In addition to efficacy, safety concerns such as hemodynamic and cognitive impact, along with psychotomimetic effects, will need to be addressed or accounted for in risk–benefit assessments for ketamine therapy of MDD.

References

aan het Rot, M., Collin, K.A., Murrough, J.W. *et al.* (2010). Safety and efficacy of repeated-dose intravenous ketamine for treatment-resistant depression. *Biological Psychiatry*, 67, 139–145.

Abel, K.M., Allin, M.P.G., Kuchrska-Pietura K. *et al.* (2003). Ketamine alters neural processing of facial emotion recognition in healthy men: An fMRI study. *NeuroReport*, 14, 387–391.

Abrams, R., Morrison, J.E., Villasenor, A. *et al.* (1993). Safety and effectiveness of intranasal administration of sedative medications (ketamine, midazolam, or sufentanil) for urgent brief pediatric dental procedures. *Anesthesia Progress*, 40, 63–66.

Allaoua, H. and Chicheportiche, R. (1989). Anaesthetic properties of phencyclidine (PCP) and analogues may be related to their interaction with Na+ channels. *European Journal of Pharmacology*, 163, 327–335.

Anand, A., Charney, D.S., Oren, D.A. *et al.* (2000). Attenuation of the neuropsychiatric effects of ketamine with lamotrigine: support for hyperglutamatergic effects of N-methyl-D-aspartate receptor antagonists. *Archives of General Psychiatry*, 57, 270–276.

Auer, D.P., Putz, B., Kraft, E. *et al.* (2000). Reduced glutamate in the anterior cingulate cortex in depression: An in vivo proton magnetic resonance spectroscopy study. *Biological Psychiatry*, 47, 305–313.

Berman, R.M., Cappiello, A., Anand, A. *et al.* (2000). Antidepressant effects of ketamine in depressed patients. *Biological Psychiatry*, 47, 351–354.

Bevan, R.K., Rose, M.A., and Duggan, K.A. (1997). Evidence for direct interaction of ketamine with alpha 1- and beta 2-adrenoceptors. *Clinical and Experimental Pharmacology and Physiology*, 24, 923–926.

Blonk, M.I., Koder., B.G., van den Bemt, P.M.L.A. *et al.* (2010). Use of oral ketamine in chronic pain management: A review. *European Journal of Pain*, 14, 466–472.

Bovill, J.G., Clarke, R.S., Davis, E.A., and Dundee, J.W. (1971). Some cardiovascular effects of ketamine in man. *British Journal of Pharmacology*, 41, 411P–412P.

Breier, A., Malhotra, A.K., Pinals, D.A. *et al.* (1997). Association of ketamine-induced psychosis with focal activation of the prefrontal cortex in healthy volunteers. *American Journal of Psychiatry*, 154, 805–811.

Carr, D.B., Goudas, L.C., Denman, W.T. *et al.* (2004). Safety and efficacy of intranasal ketamine for the treatment of breakthrough pain in patients with chronic pain: A randomized, double-blind, placebo-controlled, crossover study. *Pain*, 108, 17–27.

Chen, X., Shu, S., and Bayliss, D.A. (2009). HCN1 channel subunits are a molecular substrate for hypnotic actions of ketamine. *Journal of Neuroscience*, 29, 600–609.

Clements, J.A., Nimmo, W.S., and Grant, I.S. (1982). Bioavailability, pharmacokinetics, and analgesic activity of ketamine in humans. *Journal of Pharmaceutical Science*, 71, 539–542.

Cohen, M.G., Chan, S.L., Bhargava, H.N. *et al.* (1974). Inhibition of mammalian brain acetylcholinesterase by ketamine. *Biochemical Pharmacology*, 23, 1647–1652.

Covvey, J.R., Crawford, A.N., and Lowe, D.K. (2011). Intravenous ketamine for treatment-resistant major depressive disorder. *Annals of Pharmacotherapy*, 46, 117–123.

Curran, H.V. and Morgan, C. (2000). Cognitive, dissociative and psychotogenic effects of ketamine in recreational users on the night of drug use and 3 days later. *Addiction*, 95, 575–590.

Curran, H.V. and Monaghan, L. (2001). In and out of the K-hole: a comparison of the acute and residual effects of ketamine in frequent and infrequent ketamine users. *Addiction*, 96, 749–760.

Diaz, J.H. (1997). Intranasal ketamine preinduction of paediatric outpatients. *Paediatric Anaesthesia*, 7, 273–278.

DiazGranados, N., Ibrahim, L.A., Brutsche, N.E. *et al.* (2010). Rapid resolution of suicidal ideation after a single infusion of an N-methyl-D-aspartate antagonist in patients with treatment-resistant major depressive disorder. *Journal of Clinical Psychiatry*, 71, 1605–1611.

Duman, R.S. and Monteggia, L.M. (2006). A neurotrophic model for stress-related mood disorders. *Biological Psychiatry*, 59, 1116–1127.

Erk, S., Mikschl, A., Stier, S. *et al.* (2010). Acute and sustained effects of cognitive emotion regulation in major depression. *Journal of Neuroscience*, 30, 15726–15734.

Fava, M. and Davidson, K.G. (1996). Definition and epidemiology of treatment-resistant depression. *Psychiatric Clinics of North America*, 19, 179–200.

Finck, A.D. and Ngai, S.H. (1982). Opiate receptor mediation of ketamine analgesia. *Anesthesiology*, 56, 291–297.

Gelissen, H.P., Epema, A.H., Henning, R.H. *et al.* (1996). Inotropic effects of propofol, thiopental, midazolam, etomidate, and ketamine on isolated human atrial muscle. *Anesthesiology*, 84, 397–403.

Glue, P., Gulati, A., Le Nedelec, M. *et al.* (2011). Dose- and exposure-response to ketamine in depression. *Biological Psychiatry*, 70, e9–10; author reply e11–12.

Harrison, N.L. and Simmonds, M.A. (1985). Quantitative studies on some antagonists of *N*-methyl D-aspartate in slices of rat cerebral cortex. *British Journal of Pharmacology*, 84, 381–391.

Hashimoto, K. (2009). Emerging role of glutamate in the pathophysiology of major depressive disorder. *Brain Research Reviews*, 61, 105–123.

Heinzel, A., Steinke, R., Poeppel, T.D. *et al.* (2008). S-ketamine and GABA-A-receptor interaction in humans: An exploratory study with I-123-iomazenil SPECT. *Human Psychopharmacology*, 23, 549–554.

Hetem, L.A., Danion, J.M., Diemunsch, P. *et al.* (2000). Effect of a subanesthetic dose of ketamine on memory and conscious awareness in healthy volunteers. *Psychopharmacology (Berlin)*, 152, 283–288.

Hirota, K., Hashimoto, Y., and Lambert, D.G. (2002). Interaction of intravenous anesthetics with recombinant human M1-M3 muscarinic receptors expressed in chinese hamster ovary cells. *Anesthesia and Analgesia*, 95, 1607–1610, table of contents.

Huge, V., Lauchart, M., Magerl, W. *et al.* (2010). Effects of low-dose intranasal (S)-ketamine in patients with neuropathic pain. *European Journal of Pain*, 14, 387–394.

Ibrahim, L., DiazGranados, N., Luckenbaugh, D.A. *et al.* (2011). Rapid decrease in depressive symptoms with an N-methyl-d-aspartate antagonist in ECT-resistant major depression. *Progress in Neuropsychopharmacology and Biological Psychiatry*, 35, 1155–1159.

Jevtovic-Todorovic, V., Wozniak, D.F., Benshoff, N.D. *et al.* (2001). A comparative evaluation of the neurotoxic properties of ketamine and nitrous oxide. *Brain Research*, 895, 264–267.

Kaube, H., Herzon, J., Kaufer, T. *et al.* (2000). Aura in some patients with familial hemiplegic migraine can be stopped by intranasal ketamine. *Neurology*, 55, 139–141.

Kennedy, S.H., Evans, K.R., Kruger, S. *et al.* (2001). Changes in regional brain glucose metabolism measured with positron emission tomography after paroxetine treatment of major depression. *American Journal of Psychiatry*, 158, 899–905.

Ketamine Hydrochloride Injection, USP. *Package Insert.*

Koo, J.W., Russo, S.J., Ferguson, D. *et al.* (2010). Nuclear factor-kappaB is a critical mediator of stress-impaired neurogenesis and depressive behavior. *Proceedings of the National Academy of Sciences USA*, 107, 2669–2674.

Krishnan, V. and Nestler, E.J. (2010). Linking molecules to mood: new insight into the biology of depression. *American Journal of Psychiatry*, 167, 1305–1320.

Li, N., Lee, B., Liu, R. *et al.* (2010). mTOR-dependent synapse formation underlies the rapid antidepressant effects of NMDA antagonists. *Science*, 329, 959–964.

Lin, L.H., Chen, L.L., Zirrolli, J.A. *et al.* (1992). General anesthetics potentiate gamma-aminobutyric acid actions on gamma-aminobutyric acid A receptors expressed by Xenopus oocytes: Lack of involvement of intracellular calcium. *Journal of Pharmacology and Experimental Therapeutics*, 263, 569–578.

Larkin, G.L. and Beautrais, A.L. (2011). A preliminary naturalistic study of low-dose ketamine for depression and suicide ideation in the emergency department. *International Journal of Neuropsychopharmacology*, 14, 1127–1131.

Lodge, D., Anis, N.A., and Burton, N.R. (1982). Effects of optical isomers of ketamine on excitation of cat and rat spinal neurones by amino acids and acetylcholine. *Neuroscience Letters*, 29, 281–286.

Louon, A. and Reddy, V.G. (1994). Nasal midazolam and ketamine for paediatric sedation during computerised tomography. *Acta Anaesthesiologica Scandinavica*, 38, 259–261.

Machado-Vieira, R., Manji, H.K., and Zarate, C.A. (2009). The role of the tripartite glutamatergic synapse in the pathophysiology and therapeutics of mood disorders. *Neuroscientist*, 15, 525–539.

Maeng, S., Zarate, C.A. Jr., Du J. *et al.* (2008). Cellular mechanisms underlying the antidepressant effects of ketamine: Role of alpha-amino-3-hydroxy-5-methylisoxazole-4-propionic acid receptors. *Biological Psychiatry*, 63, 349–352.

Malhotra, A.K., Pinals, D.A., Weingartner, H. *et al.* (1996). NMDA receptor function and human cognition: the effects of ketamine in healthy volunteers. *Neuropsychopharmacology*, 14, 301–307.

Malinovsky, J.M., Servin, F., Cozian, A. *et al.* (1996). Ketamine and norketamine plasma concentrations after i.v., nasal and rectal administration in children. *British Journal of Anaesthesia*, 77, 203–207.

Mathew, S.J. (2008). Treatment-resistant depression: recent developments and future directions. *Depression and Anxiety*, 25, 989–992.

Mathew, S.J., Manji, H.K., and Charney, D.S. (2008). Novel drugs and therapeutic targets for severe mood disorders. *Neuropsychopharmacology*, 33, 2080–2092.

Mathew, S.J., Murrough, J.W., aan het Rot, M. *et al.* (2010). Riluzole for relapse prevention following intravenous ketamine in treatment-resistant depression: A pilot randomized, placebo-controlled continuation trial. *International Journal of Neuropsychopharmacology*, 13, 71–82.

Morgan, C.J. and Curran, H.V. (2006). Acute and chronic effects of ketamine upon human memory: A review. *Psychopharmacology*, 188, 408–424.

Morgan, C.J., Muetzelfeldt, L., and Curran, H.V. (2010). Consequences of chronic ketamine self-administration upon neurocognitive function and psychological wellbeing: a 1-year longitudinal study. *Addiction*, 105, 121–133.

Morgan, C.J., Mofeez, A., Brander, B. *et al.* (2004a). Ketamine impairs response inhibition and is positively reinforcing in healthy volunteers: A dose-response study. *Psychopharmacology*, 172, 298–308.

Morgan, C.J., Monaghan, L., and Curran, H.V. (2004b). Beyond the K-hole: A 3-year longitudinal investigation of the cognitive and subjective effects of ketamine in recreational users who have substantially reduced their use of the drug. *Addiction*, 99, 1450–1461.

Morris, C., Perris, A., Klein, J. *et al.* (2009). Anaesthesia in haemodynamically compromised emergency patients: Does ketamine represent the best choice of induction agent? *Anaesthesia*, 64, 532–539.

Murrough, J.W. and Charney, D.S. (2010). Cracking the moody brain: Lifting the mood with ketamine. *Nature Medicine*, 16, 1384–1385.

Murrough, J.W., Perez, A.M., Mathew, S.J. *et al.* (2011). A case of sustained remission following an acute course of ketamine in treatment-resistant depression. *Journal of Clinical Psychiatry*, 72, 414–415.

Nock, M.K. and Banaji, M.R. (2007). Assessment of self-injurious thoughts using a behavioral test. *American Journal of Psychiatry*, 164, 820–823.

Olney, J.W., Labruyere, J., Wang., G. *et al.* (1991). NMDA antagonist neurotoxicity: Mechanism and prevention. *Science*, 254, 1515–1518.

Paul, I.A., Nowak, G., Layer, R.T. *et al.* (1994). Adaptation of the *N*-methyl-D-aspartate receptor complex following chronic antidepressant treatments. *Journal of Pharmacology and Experimental Therapeutics*, 269, 95–102.

Paul, R., Schaaff, N., Padberg, F. *et al.* (2009). Comparison of racemic ketamine and S-ketamine in treatment-resistant major depression: Report of two cases. *World Journal of Biological Psychiatry*, 10, 241–244.

Pittaluga, A., Raiteri, L., Longordo, F. *et al.* (2007). Antidepressant treatments and function of glutamate ionotropic receptors mediating amine release in hippocampus. *Neuropharmacology*, 53, 27–36.

Preskorn, S.H., Baker, B., Kolluri, S. *et al.* (2008). An innovative design to establish proof of concept of the antidepressant effects of the NR2B subunit selective *N*-methyl-D-aspartate antagonist, CP-101,606, in patients with treatment-refractory major depressive disorder. *Journal of Clinical Psychopharmacology*, 28, 631–637.

Price, R.B., Nock., M.K., Charney, D.S. *et al.* (2009a). Effects of intravenous ketamine on explicit and implicit measures of suicidality in treatment-resistant depression. *Biological Psychiatry*, 66, 522–526.

Price, R.B., Shungu, D.C., Mao, X. *et al.* (2009b). Amino acid neurotransmitters assessed by proton magnetic resonance spectroscopy: Relationship to treatment resistance in major depressive disorder. *Biological Psychiatry*, 65, 792–800.

Reich, D.L. and Silvay, G. (1989). Ketamine: An update on the first twenty-five years of clinical experience. *Candian Journal of Anaesthiology*, 36, 186–197.

Roelofse, J.A., Shipton, E.A., De La Harpe, C.J. *et al.* (2004). Intranasal sufentanil/midazolam versus ketamine/midazolam for analgesia/sedation in the pediatric population prior to undergoing multiple dental extractions under general anesthesia: A prospective, double-blind, randomized comparison. *Anesthesia Progress*, 51, 114–121.

Rosenberg, D.R., Macmaster, F.P., Mirza, Y. *et al.* (2005). Reduced anterior cingulate glutamate in pediatric major depression: A magnetic resonance spectroscopy study. *Biological Psychiatry*, 58, 700–704.

Rowland, L.M., Astur, R.S., Jung, R.E. *et al.* (2005). Selective cognitive impairments associated with NMDA receptor blockade in humans. *Neuropsychopharmacology*, 30, 633–639.

Rush, A.J., Trivedi, M.H., Wisniewski, S.R. *et al.* (2006). Acute and longer-term outcomes in depressed outpatients requiring one or several treatment steps: A STAR*D report. *American Journal of Psychiatry*, 163, 1905–1917.

Rush, A.J., Warden, D., Wisniewski, S.R. *et al.* (2009). STAR*D: Revising conventional wisdom. *CNS Drugs*, 23, 627–647.

Salmi, E., Langsjo, J.W., Aalto, S. *et al.* (2005). Subanesthetic ketamine does not affect 11C-flumazenil binding in humans. *Anesthesia and Analgesia*, 101, 722–725, table of contents.

Salvadore, G., Corwell, B.R., Colon-Rosario, V. *et al.* (2009). Increased anterior cingulate cortical activity in response to fearful faces: A neurophysiological biomarker that predicts rapid antidepressant response to ketamine. *Biological Psychiatry*, 65, 289–295.

Salvadore, G., Cornwell, B.R., Sambataro, F. *et al.* (2010). Anterior cingulate desynchronization and functional connectivity with the amygdala during a working memory task predict rapid antidepressant response to ketamine. *Neuropsychopharmacology*, 35, 1415–1422.

Sanacora, G., Kendell, S.F., Levin, Y. *et al.* (2007). Preliminary evidence of riluzole efficacy in antidepressant-treated patients with residual depressive symptoms. *Biological Psychiatry*, 61, 822–825.

Sanacora, G., Zarate, C.A., Krystal, J.H. *et al.* (2008). Targeting the glutamatergic system to develop novel, improved therapeutics for mood disorders. *Nature Reviews Drug Discovery*, 7, 426–437.

Seeman, P., Ko, F., and Tallerico, T. (2005). Dopamine receptor contribution to the action of PCP, LSD and ketamine psychotomimetics. *Molecuar Psychiatry*, 10, 877–883.

Seeman, P., Guan, F.C., and Hirbec, H. (2009). Dopamine D2High receptors stimulated by phencyclidines, lysergic acid diethylamide, salvinorin A, and modafinil. *Synapse*, 63, 698–704.

Smith, D.J., Pekoe, G.M., Martin, L.L. *et al.* (1980). The interaction of ketamine with the opiate receptor. *Life Sciences*, 26, 789–795.

Smith, D.J., Azzaro, A.J., Zaldivar, S.B. *et al.* (1981). Properties of the optical isomers and metabolites of ketamine on the high affinity transport and catabolism of monoamines. *Neuropharmacology*, 20, 391–396.

Smith, D.J., Bouchal, R.L., deSanctis, C.A. *et al.* (1987). Properties of the interaction between ketamine and opiate binding sites in vivo and in vitro. *Neuropharmacology*, 26, 1253–1260.

Thangathurai, D. and Mogos, M. (2011). Ketamine alleviates fear, depression, and suicidal ideation in terminally ill patients. *Journal of Palliative Medicine*, 14, 389.

Trivedi, M.H., Thase, M.E., Osuntokun, O. *et al.* (2009). An integrated analysis of olanzapine/fluoxetine combination in clinical trials of treatment-resistant depression. *Journal of Clinical Psychiatry*, 70, 387–396.

Tweed, W.A., Minuck, M., and Mymin, D. (1972). Circulatory responses to ketamine anesthesia. *Anesthesiology*, 37, 613–619.

Valentine, G.W., Mason, G.F., Gomez, R. *et al.* (2011). The antidepressant effect of ketamine is not associated with changes in occipital amino acid neurotransmitter content as measured by [(1)H]-MRS. *Psychiatry Research*, 191, 122–127.

Vialou, V., Robison, A.J., Laplant, Q.C. *et al.* (2010). DeltaFosB in brain reward circuits mediates resilience to stress and antidepressant responses. *Nature Neuroscience*, 13, 745–752.

Vollenweider, F.X. and Kometer, M. (2010). The neurobiology of psychedelic drugs: Implications for the treatment of mood disorders. *Nature Reviews Neuroscience*, 11, 642–651.

Vollenweider, F.X., Leenders, K.L., Oye, I. *et al.* (1997a). Differential psychopathology and patterns of cerebral glucose utilisation produced by (S)- and (R)-ketamine in healthy volunteers using positron emission tomography (PET). *European Neuropsychopharmacology*, 7, 25–38.

Vollenweider, F.X., Leenders, K.L., Scharfetter, C. *et al.* (1997b). Metabolic hyperfrontality and psychopathology in the ketamine model of psychosis using positron emission tomography (PET) and [18F]fluorodeoxyglucose (FDG). *European Neuropsychopharmacology*, 7, 9–24.

Weber, F., Wulf, H., and El Saeidi, G. (2003). Premedication with nasal s-ketamine and midazolam provides good conditions for induction of anesthesia in preschool children. *Canadian Journal of Anaesthesia*, 50, 470–5.

Weber, M., Motin, L., Gaul, S. *et al.* (2005). Intravenous anaesthetics inhibit nicotinic acetylcholine receptor-mediated currents and Ca^{2+} transients in rat intracardiac ganglion neurons. *British Journal of Pharmacology*, 144, 98–107.

Weksler, N., Ovadia, L., Muati, G. *et al.* (1993). Nasal ketamine for paediatric premedication. *Canadian Journal of Anaesthesia*, 40, 119–121.

White, P.F., Way, W.L., and Trevor, A.J. (1982). Ketamine – its pharmacology and therapeutic uses. *Anesthesiology*, 56, 119–136.

Yanagihara, Y., Ohtani, M., Kariya, S. *et al.* (2003). Plasma concentration profiles of ketamine and norketamine after administration of various ketamine preparations to healthy Japanese volunteers. *Biopharmaceutics and Drug Disposition*, 24, 37–43.

Zarate, C.A., Jr., Payne, J.L., Quiroz, J. *et al.* (2004). An open-label trial of riluzole in patients with treatment-resistant major depression. *American Journal of Psychiatry*, 161, 171–174.

Zarate, C.A., Jr., Quiroz, J., Singh, J.B. *et al.* (2005). An open-label trial of the glutamate-modulating agent riluzole in combination with lithium for the treatment of bipolar depression. *Biological Psychiatry*, 57, 430–432.

Zarate, C.A., Jr., Singh, J.B., Carlson, P.J. *et al.* (2006). A randomized trial of an N-methyl-D-aspartate antagonist in treatment-resistant major depression. *Archives of General Psychiatry*, 63, 856–864.

Chapter 28

Brain imaging

Martin J. Lan and Ramin V. Parsey

Introduction

Neuroimaging allows for *in vivo* measurements of biological differences in the brain tissue of patients with mood disorders. As such, it offers unique tools to investigate the pathophysiology of the disorders. A large number of neuroimaging studies have been performed to date that investigate mood disorders, and this chapter will summarize the most promising and reproduced findings. Neuroimaging research may one day lead to a sensitive and specific test to diagnose the different mood disorders. Better detection of these disorders may allow for earlier and more accurate clinical interventions for patients. Such a test may also help predict whether or not a patient will respond to a particular medication or type of psychotherapy before patients undergo treatment trials. Imaging may also be used to track the biological effect of an antidepressant or to evaluate the effects of new drugs in development; for example, to determine their optimal dose range.

In the current clinical care of mood disorders, neuroimaging is used only to rule out any neurological causes of mood symptoms. Head computer tomography (CT) scans are routinely ordered for this purpose when patients have their first severe depressive or manic episode. Structural brain magnetic resonance imaging (MRI) can also be ordered if there are clinical reasons to suspect a neurological etiology that can only be detected by MRI. Using these tools, cerebrovascular accidents, CNS malignancy, demyelinating disease, or CNS infections may be ruled out as alternative causes of a mood disorder. Otherwise, no neuroimaging tests are currently used in the diagnosis or treatment of mood disorders.

Overview of imaging modalities

MRI has been used extensively to study mood disorders. Structural MRI assesses the molecular property of water molecules in order to delineate the morphology of different brain regions that have different tissue compositions. White matter, gray matter, and cerebrospinal fluid all have different water composition, and they are therefore distinct on MRI images. In functional MRI, the proton signal from hemoglobin is used to measure blood oxygen level dependence (BOLD) signal, an indirect measure of neural activity. Brain activity stimulates more local blood flow and a higher average level of deoxygenated hemoglobin, which is detected by the MRI. Differences in BOLD signal are relatively subtle. Although the changes may be statistically different, the fold differences are often less than 1% between groups. With another MRI technique, magnetic resonance spectroscopy (MRS), levels of other molecules in the brain, such as *N*-acetyl aspartate, can be measured. Like BOLD, these molecules have a low signal relative to water. Another MRI technique, diffusion weighted or diffusion tensor MRI, measures the diffusivity of water in the brain. This signal reflects both the organization of cells within the brain tissue and the microstructure of the cells in that brain region. White matter tracts, for example, can be delineated with the technique.

In positron emission tomography (PET) and single photon emission computer tomography (SPECT), radiolabeled molecules are injected that bind to targets such as receptors, enzymes, or transporters. The extent of radiotracer binding to proteins in the brain allows for quantitation of those molecules. The two techniques differ in the type of radiotracers they

Clinical Handbook for the Management of Mood Disorders, ed. J. John Mann, Patrick J. McGrath, and Steven P. Roose.
Published by Cambridge University Press. © Cambridge University Press 2013.

use. PET is more expensive, but offers greater spatial resolution.

Structural neuroimaging studies of bipolar disorder

There have been close to 100 studies published that have reported structural changes in the brain tissue of patients with bipolar disorder when compared to healthy control subjects. These have employed both head CT and brain MRI scans. The most robust and reproducible findings include larger lateral ventricles when compared to control subjects and increased rates of white matter hyperintensities on MRI than control subjects. These findings are neither sensitive nor specific for the disorder. Many bipolar patients do not have either of these effects and both of these effects are seen in a number of other conditions.

Based on two recent meta-analyses, the average lateral ventricles of a patient with bipolar disorder are between 17 and 27% larger than that of the average healthy control subject (Kempton *et al.* 2008, Arnone *et al.* 2009). The difference in volume has been found not to be dependent on age of the patient, age of onset of their disorder, gender of the patient, or duration of disorder. The cause of the increase in volume is unknown but likely reflects a change in the brain tissue surrounding the ventricles. Whether it is due to a decrease in glial cells, neuronal density, cell volume, or all three is unknown. A similar scale increase in volume of the lateral ventricles is seen with major depressive disorder when compared to control subjects. Schizophrenia patients have 26–35% larger lateral ventricle volume levels compared with bipolar disorder (Kempton *et al.* 2008, Arnone *et al.* 2009).

The rate of white matter hyperintensities has been found to be approximately 2.5 times that of healthy control subjects. White matter hyperintensities are lesions that are detected on a particular type of MRI scan, T_2 weighted and fluid attenuated inversion recovery (FLAIR) scans of the brain. A number of pathophysiological processes can cause this finding, including ischemia, gliosis, edema, or demyelination. It is unknown what causes this increased rate in bipolar disorder. The hyperintensities are found most frequently in the deep white matter tissue. Hyperintensities have also been found with increased frequency with advancing age in the general population and in subjects with cardiovascular risk factors. The increased rate in bipolar patients, however, has been shown to

be independent of age and cardiovascular risk factors. These lesions may be indicative of a pathophysiological process occurring in the white matter as part of bipolar disorder. They are also found with higher rates in major depressive disorder and neurodegenerative disorders such as Huntington's disease (Beyer *et al.* 2009).

Other structural changes have been reported in the literature but have not been as reliably reproduced. Decreased global brain volume, decreased volume of the prefrontal cortex, increased volume of the globus pallidus, and decreased corpus callosum volume have all been reported in bipolar patients. These volumetric studies may have been affected by the finding that lithium treatment increases the gray matter volume of the brain (Emsell and McDonald, 2009).

Diffusion tensor imaging has also shown differences in organization of the white matter when compared to control subjects. Decreased fractional anisotropy in white matter located between the prefrontal cortex and sub-cortical areas have been reproducibly reported. Decreased anisotropy has also reproducibly been reported in the corpus callosum of adult bipolar patients. Two tract-based spatial statistics (TBSS) analyses have shown increased fractional anisotropy, however, in the frontal cortex. Although more work is needed to evaluate the reproducibility of these results, the data may indicate white matter abnormalities in bipolar disorder. For example, decreased fractional anisotropy could be caused by a number of pathologic processes, including abnormal connections of neurons or increased inflammation (Heng *et al.* 2010, Mahon *et al.* 2010).

Functional neuroimaging studies of bipolar disorder

The functional activation pattern of the brain during the different mood states of bipolar disorder has been studied using fMRI and PET. A variety of cognitive tests have been employed to evaluate how the brain functions in these mood states when compared to control subjects. Even when patients show no differences in performance outcomes on these tasks, differences in neural activation patterns have been found using neuroimaging. The two main areas of functioning that the tasks have investigated include executive functioning and emotional reactivity. Abnormalities of these functions characterize much of the psychopathology in bipolar disorder. Broadly, these data show alterations in functioning of the prefrontal cortex, the anterior limbic areas (particularly the anterior cingulate and the amygdala), the thalamus, and the striatum of bipolar patients (Strakowski *et al.* 2005a, Pan *et al.* 2009). Unlike structural MRI studies, combining the data from these studies is problematic because they generally use different tasks that the subjects perform.

The continuous performance task, the nonemotionally laden Stroop interference task and the n-back working memory task, all challenges of executive function, have provoked differences in bipolar patients. Most studies have reported changes in activation within the prefrontal cortex, some increased (Adler *et al.* 2004) and some decreased by tasks (Gruber *et al.* 2004, Kronhaus *et al.* 2006), even in euthymic bipolar patients when compared to healthy control subjects. A number of other regions have been reported to be altered in euthymic patients, including sub-regions of the cingulate and the basal ganglia (Strakowski *et al.* 2005b). These data may suggest that bipolar patients experience unemotional stimuli with more emotional valence than healthy control subjects. Manic patients, when compared to healthy control subjects have been shown to have decreased neural activation within the prefrontal cortex during executive tasks (Blumberg *et al.* 1999, Sax *et al.* 1999).

The neural response to emotionally laden stimuli has also been studied in patients with bipolar disorder. Reading words or seeing faces with emotional expressions are the most common stimuli. Differences in subcortical limbic activity have been reported in patients when compared to healthy control subjects. The effect has been demonstrated in euthymic patients (Malhi *et al.* 2005, Wessa *et al.* 2007, depressed subjects (Sheline *et al.* 2001), and manic patients (Chen *et al.* 2006). These data suggest that the subcortical limbic system may be more sensitive to emotional stimuli that are in contrast to the patient's current mood state, but that the sensitivity also remains in the euthymic state. Changes in the prefrontal cortex activation have also been reported as altered during tasks where patients are exposed to emotionally laden stimuli in the euthymic (Gruber *et al.* 2004), manic (Altshuler *et al.* 2005), and depressed state (Malhi *et al.* 2004). Together, these studies indicate an alteration in the limbic–cortical–striatal–pallidal–thalamic circuitry in bipolar disorder (Sheline, 2003).

PET studies have reported changes in metabolic rates in brain tissue when the subjects are at a resting mental state. When bipolar patients representing all three mood states were investigated together,

decreased activity in a number of prefrontal subregions was found when compared to healthy control subjects (al-Mousawi *et al.* 1996). Depressed patients have been reported to have decreased subgenual prefrontal cortex activity when compared to controls and manic patients have shown increased activity in the same region (Blumberg *et al.* 2000, Drevets *et al.* 2008). Depressed bipolar patients have also shown increased sub-cortical activity in the striatum, thalamus, and amygdale when compared to control subjects. Euthymic bipolar patients have been shown to have increased anterior cingulate activity and decreased prefrontal cortex activity when compared to control subjects at rest. These studies have been performed on small groups of patients and require further repetition (Gonul *et al.* 2009).

Molecular neuroimaging studies of Bipolar disorder

To date, fewer than a dozen molecular neurotransmitter PET studies have been published on patients with bipolar disorder. The data show significant changes in targets involved with monoamine neurotransmission in bipolar patients. The serotonin 1A receptor was reported to be increased in the forebrain of depressed bipolar patients but unchanged in medicated euthymic patients (Sullivan *et al.* 2009, Sargent *et al.* 2010). Serotonin 2A receptors were reported to be lower in frontal, temporal, parietal, and occipital lobes in manic bipolar patients when compared with healthy controls. Changes in serotonin transporter levels have been reported, but the results contradict each other (Ichimiya *et al.* 2002, Cannon *et al.* 2006, Oquendo *et al.* 2007). Dopamine D1 receptors are decreased in the frontal cortex but not in the striatum of bipolar patients. Dopamine D2 receptors are not changed in bipolar disorder except when psychotic features are present. With psychotic features, they are increased to a similar degree as in schizophrenia (Gonul *et al.* 2009). These studies add to pharmacologic data to suggest that monoamine neurotransmitter systems are likely involved in the pathophysiology of bipolar disorder.

Magnetic resonance spectroscopy has also been used to study molecular differences in the brain of bipolar patients. n-acetyl aspartate (NAA), has been found to be lower in the hippocampus, orbital, and prefrontal cortex of patients with bipolar disorder when compared to healthy control subjects (Yildiz-Yesiloglu and Ankerst, 2006). A greater Glx signal has also been reported in bipolar disorder, consistent with an alteration in glutamine and glutamate signaling (Yuksel and Ongur, 2010). Although the significance of this change is unknown, it is consistent with a neuronal pathology in the disorder involving fewer GABA neurons post-mortem. Several studies using ^{31}P magnetic resonance imaging have shown alterations in the frontal lobe of bipolar patients in all three mood states. Changes in sugar metabolism or phospholipids content shifts could account for the differences in ^{31}P signal (Yildiz et al. 2001).

Structural neuroimaging studies of major depressive disorder

MRI and CT scans have been used to identify changes in brain morphology in major depressive disorder. Several meta-analyses have been performed to identify the most robust and reproducible structural changes across the different studies. The most recent meta-analysis assessed 255 published studies (Kempton et al. 2011). The most robust findings included larger lateral ventricle volumes (about 22% larger than healthy control patients), greater cerebrospinal fluid volume, and smaller volume of hippocampus and gyrus rectus. An increased rate of MRI hyperintensities was also found, primarily in the sub-cortical gray matter. None of these changes are specific to major depression and studies showing no changes in each of these regions have been published. A number of other brain regions have been reported to be smaller in major depressive disorder, but these differences are less robust or reproducible. These include smaller frontal lobe, the basal ganglia (caudate, putamen, and globus pallidus), and thalamus (Soares and Mann, 1997, Hamilton et al. 2008, Koolschijn et al. 2009).

The significance of the smaller hippocampal volume in major depressive disorder remains unclear. The volume has been shown to be somewhere between 4% and 10% smaller than that of healthy control subjects and is bilateral (Videbech and Ravnkilde, 2004, Cole et al. 2011). It has been reported in first-onset cases of major depression. It may prove to be a potentially neurotoxic effect of chronic stress that many depressed patients experience. Consistent with this theory, when rodents are exposed to repeated electrical shocks or confinement, a model of human chronic stress, a decrease in hippocampal volume

has been found (Warner-Schmidt and Duman, 2006). Increases in lateral ventricle size and CSF volume indicate more widespread decreases in brain volume than just hippocampal changes. Bipolar disorder, in contrast to major depression, has not shown reproducible decreases in hippocampal volumes.

The rate of MRI white matter hyperintensities has been found to be less when compared to patients with bipolar disorder. They have been found more commonly in the periventricular region in major depressive disorder as opposed to the deep white matter as in bipolar disorder. The smaller volume and increased rates of white matter hyperintensities may be evidence for a pathologic process in the brain tissue of older patients with major depressive disorder (Kempton et al. 2011).

Functional neuroimaging studies of major depressive disorder

Functional MRI, PET, and SPECT have all been utilized to identify regions of the brain that are differentially activated in major depressive disorder when compared to healthy control subjects. Most studies find differences between the two groups. A consistent, localized region that can account for the pathology has not been determined, but data point to several circuits that are likely altered in the disorder.

A number of studies have evaluated the resting state of the brain, a state that is elicited by having subjects not think about anything in particular while in the scanner. These studies have primarily used PET and SPECT imaging. A recent meta-analysis of these studies (Fitzgerald et al. 2008) reported lower activity in depressed patients in the pregenual anterior and posterior cingulate, the bilateral middle frontal gyri, the insula, and the left superior temporal gyrus. The areas that showed higher resting activity included thalamus, caudate, the left superior frontal, and the right middle frontal gyri. Another meta-analysis found higher resting state activation in the ventromedial prefrontal cortex, the left ventral striatum, and the left thalamus and decreases in the left postcentral gyrus, the left fusiform gyrus, and the left insula, relative to control subjects (Kuhn and Gallinat, 2011). If regions do have altered activity at rest during major depression, therefore, the regions of differential activity are broad and subtle. The relatively consistent reports of alterations in metabolism in the prefrontal cortex provided the theoretical basis for targeting this area with transmagnetic stimulation (TMS), a treatment recently approved by the Food and Drug Administration for major depressive disorder.

Differences relative to control subjects have also been identified when patients perform different cognitive tasks within the scanner. The activation of the amygdale has been consistently reported as greater during major depression, both in activity and duration. Studies of amygdale function have primarily used functional MRI where subjects and control subjects are exposed to stimuli with negative valence. This increase in activity is generally mood congruent, limited primarily to when patients are in depressive episodes (Savitz and Drevets, 2009).

A recent meta-analysis reported consistent changes in activity within the dorsolateral prefrontal cortex while patients performed a number of different tasks (Fitzgerald et al. 2006). The direction of change was not found to be consistent, however, with some reports of increased activation and some reports with decreased activation. Some also reported changes just on the right side and others just on the left. There were a variety of tasks used, including cognitive tasks such as verbal fluency and arithmetic, and emotional activation tasks. Direct comparisons were therefore difficult to make. These data added to the resting state reports to point to the dorsolateral prefrontal cortex as a target of TMS to treat major depressive disorder.

Altered correlation of activity between the frontal lobe and the amygdale has been reported during functional MRI studies of patients with major depressive disorder. This decoupling of activity has been reported during exposure to stimuli with both negative and positive valences and during a working memory task. This disco-ordination may underlie the mood dysregulation that occurs as part of major depressive disorder (Savitz and Drevets, 2009).

Several studies have also reported decreased activation patterns of the subgenual prefrontal cortex with major depression at rest. This area is thought to co-ordinate executive function with emotional states. Not all studies have verified this finding, however (Drevets et al. 2008).

Molecular neuroimaging studies of major depressive disorder

Most molecular studies using PET neuroimaging have investigated changes in proteins related to the monoamine neurotransmitter systems. Serotonin 1A receptors are of clinical interest because they function as autoreceptors that regulate serotonin release and postsynaptic signaling in the brain. The receptors are also affected by treatment with selective serotonin reuptake inhibitors, the primary treatment of depression. A number of PET studies have shown differences in 5-HT_{1A} binding levels in brain with major depressive disorder. When the arterial input function is used to normalize the data, 5-HT_{1A} binding is higher in patients with major depressive disorder. Studies reported lower binding but only when the cerebellum has been used as a reference region, a less reliable approach (Parsey, 2010). Antidepressant treatment may also affect findings (Parsey et al. 2006a). 5-HT_{2A} receptor binding is reported to be higher, lower or unchanged in major depressive disorder when compared to control subjects (Meyer et al. 1999). We found lower transporter binding in MDD (Parsey et al. 2006b), although this has not been consistently reported (Meyer et al. 2004, Cannon et al. 2006).

Dopamine D1 receptor binding is lower in major depressive disorder using different PET radiotracers for the receptors in two studies (D'Haenen and Bossuyt, 1994, Cannon et al. 2009). Most studies have reported no differences in dopamine D2 receptors in the brain using either PET or SPECT (Parsey et al. 2001, Montgomery et al. 2007, Hirvonen et al. 2008) and have not reported consistent alterations of dopamine transporter binding (Meyer et al. 2001, Brunswick et al. 2003). Monoamine oxidase A has also been found to be higher in level in patients with major depressive disorder than healthy control subjects (Meyer et al. 2006). This increase was found to correlate with outcomes after 6 months of treatment but not short-term treatment with SSRIs (Meyer et al. 2009).

The most robust findings using MRS in major depressive disorder include lower GABA levels within the occipital cortex and several subsections of the prefrontal cortex. Lower Glx signal, which reflects quantities of both glutamate and glutamine, have also been consistently reported in multiple regions of the brain. When glutamine and glutamate are distinguished using MRS, glutamine is the metabolite most consistently reduced. These data represent further evidence that metabolic rate in the brain is altered in depression and may signal a shift in excitatory and inhibitory neurotransmission (Yuksel and Ongur, 2010, Hasler and Northoff, 2011).

Prediction of treatment response in major depressive disorder

A number of neuroimaging studies have attempted to identify a signal that would predict whether patients with major depression would respond to either a particular medication or psychotherapy treatment. These data may prove to be the first steps towards using neuroimaging to limit trial and error during the treatment of patients with mood disorders.

A number of studies have investigated whether smaller hippocampal volume in depressed patients predicts whether patients are less responsive to treatment. In general, smaller hippocampal volume predicts worse clinical outcome. Hsieh et al., for example, studied 60 elderly patients at baseline and after 12 weeks of treatment for depression (Hsieh et al. 2002). The patients with the lowest 25% of hippocampal volumes were less likely to respond to treatment than those with the largest 25% of hippocampal volume. Similarly, one study found an association with smaller hippocampal volumes and recurrence of major depressive episodes over a year period (Kronmuller et al. 2008), and another showed the lower volume to be associated with lower rate of remission over a 1 year period (Frodl et al. 2004). When patients were studied for 8 weeks of treatment prospectively, remitted patients had larger hippocampi than nonremitters in one study (MacQueen et al. 2008), although this result was limited to female patients in another study (Vakili et al. 2000). If smaller hippocampal volume proves to be a signal that predicts more treatment resistance, more robust treatments such as antidepressant combination or even ECT may be warranted earlier in these patients' treatment.

Brain metabolic rates have been evaluated using ^{18}F fluorodeoxyglucose PET imaging to identify metabolic patterns that are predictive of treatment response. Mayberg et al. reported decreases in metabolic activity in limbic and striatal areas and increases in metabolic activity in brainstem and dorsal cortical areas in patients who responded to medication response (Mayberg et al. 2000). This study was limited by modest subject numbers. Similarly, Milak et al. identified a cluster of activity in the globus maxima of the midbrain whose decrease in metabolic activity corresponded to remission from depressive symptoms after 3 months (Milak et al. 2009). Brockmann et al. used SPECT to identify a large region of the brain that included the prefrontal, subgenual anterior cingulate

and temporal cortices that had increased activity in patients who responded to antidepressant treatment after 4 weeks (Brockmann et al. 2009). These results require replication.

Changes in levels of proteins related to the serotonin signaling system have also been reported to be correlated to response to antidepressant treatment. Parsey et al. reported that MDD patients who did not remit after year of antidepressant treatment had higher pretreatment brain 5-HT$_{1A}$ autoreceptor binding compared with those who did remit (Parsey et al. 2006a). Miller et al. from the same group reported that lower pretreatment serotonin transporter (5-HTT) binding in the midbrain, amygdale, and anterior cingulate cortex predicted patients who did not remit from depression after treatment with antidepressants when compared to patients who did remit (Miller et al. 2008).

Limitations of neuroimaging in mood disorders

Both bipolar disorder and major depressive disorder are likely heterogeneous conditions with different molecular, cellular, genetic, or environmental causes that produce the same clinical phenotype of the disorder. If etiological heterogeneity exists, any imaging signatures that correspond to each of these etiologies would be lost in the studies to date, as the patients are classified by the DSM-IV symptom criteria only. As we learn more about the etiology of each disorder, imaging studies may be tailored to study the potential sub-types.

Clinical variability also exists within each disorder. Based on the current diagnostic criteria for major depression, for example, two patients can both have depression but share just one symptom of the disorder. Some patients may have had one mood episode only whereas others have recurring episodes. Some patients may also have had significant past psychological trauma. Most imaging studies to date do not account for these clinical differences. Although most studies account for variation in demographic variables such as age and sex, other demographic factors, such as patients' past exposure to psychiatric medications, are often not accounted for. Genetic differences are also rarely considered.

Heterogeneity in techniques among different imaging studies provides another limitation. Tasks that are performed by subjects in functional MRI studies vary from study to study. Similarly, PET studies utilize a range of molecular probes that may not be directly comparable. Differences in processing of the neuroimaging signals also contribute to variability. Both MR and PET images need to be normalized in order to compare images, accounting for natural variability in the morphology of brains. The method that is used in this process can have an impact on the final comparisons. Similarly, some studies normalize PET data to arterial input function of the radiotracer injected where others normalize the data to reference region of the brain, a difference that can affect the final result which assumes the reference region is not altered in MDD or affected by the treatment. Some imaging studies use a "region of interest" approach, focusing on only regions of the brain of biological interest; other studies use a more exploratory approach, considering all areas of the brain based solely on clusters of activity. Combining and repetition of analyses is important in order to assess the robustness of the results, but variability of techniques limits this process.

Future directions

Technical advances in neuroimaging techniques may allow for new questions to be asked into the biological underpinnings of mood disorders and may be used to predict responses to treatments. New radiotracers for PET neuroimaging and new tasks for functional neuroimaging are two advances that are within our current technological capabilities. Novel imaging analysis methods may allow MRI, PET, or SPECT to delineate imaging signatures that have not yet been observed. Because PET is used in multiple fields of clinical practice and because its data yield absolute values, we believe it holds the most promise for future clinical use. Whole new brain imaging modalities may be invented which will allow new questions to be asked into the etiology of the disorders. Data from other fields may also allow new questions to be asked using existing imaging techniques. Hopefully there will soon be a clinically useful imaging signature that will help diagnose and treat patients with mood disorders more accurately.

References

Adler, C.M., Holland, S.K. *et al.* (2004). Changes in neuronal activation in patients with bipolar disorder during performance of a working memory task. *Bipolar Disorders*, 6, 540–549.

al-Mousawi, A.H., Evans, N. *et al.* (1996). Limbic dysfunction in schizophrenia and mania: A study using 18F-labelled fluorodeoxyglucose and positron emission tomography. *British Journal of Psychiatry*, 169, 509–516.

Altshuler, L., Bookheimer, S. *et al.* (2005). Increased amygdala activation during mania: a functional magnetic resonance imaging study. *American Journal of Psychiatry*, 162, 1211–1213.

Arnone, D., Cavanagh, J. *et al.* (2009). Magnetic resonance imaging studies in bipolar disorder and schizophrenia: Meta-analysis. *British Journal of Psychiatry*, 195, 194–201.

Beyer, J.L., Young, R. *et al.* (2009). Hyperintense MRI lesions in bipolar disorder: a meta-analysis and review. *Int Rev Psychiatry*, 21, 394–409.

Blumberg, H.P., Stern, E. *et al.* (1999). Rostral and orbital prefrontal cortex dysfunction in the manic state of bipolar disorder. *American Journal of Psychiatry*, 156, 1986–1988.

Blumberg, H.P., Stern, E. *et al.* (2000). Increased anterior cingulate and caudate activity in bipolar mania. *Biological Psychiatry*, 48, 1045–1052.

Brockmann, H., Zobel, A. *et al.* (2009). The value of HMPAO SPECT in predicting treatment response to citalopram in patients with major depression. *Psychiatry Research*, 173, 107–112.

Brunswick, D.J., Amsterdam, J.D. *et al.* (2003). Greater availability of brain dopamine transporters in major depression shown by [99m Tc]TRODAT-1 SPECT imaging. *American Journal of Psychiatry*, 160, 1836–1841.

Cannon, D.M., Ichise, M. *et al.* (2006). Serotonin transporter binding in bipolar disorder assessed using [11C]DASB and positron emission tomography. *Biological Psychiatry*, 60, 207–217.

Cannon, D.M., Klaver, J.M. *et al.* (2009). Dopamine type-1 receptor binding in major depressive disorder assessed using positron emission tomography and [11C]NNC-112. *Neuropsychopharmacology*, 34, 1277–1287.

Chen, C.H., Lennox, B. *et al.* (2006). Explicit and implicit facial affect recognition in manic and depressed states of bipolar disorder: a functional magnetic resonance imaging study. *Biological Psychiatry*, 59, 31–39.

Cole, J., Costafreda, S.G. *et al.* (2011). Hippocampal atrophy in first episode depression: A meta-analysis of magnetic resonance imaging studies. *Journal of Affective Disorders*, 134, 483–487.

D'Haenen, H.A. and Bossuyt, A. (1994). Dopamine D2 receptors in depression measured with single photon emission computed tomography. *Biological Psychiatry*, 35, 128–132.

Drevets, W.C., Savitz, J. *et al.* (2008). The subgenual anterior cingulate cortex in mood disorders. *CNS Spectrums*, 13, 663–681.

Emsell, L. and McDonald, C. (2009). The structural neuroimaging of bipolar disorder. *International Review of Psychiatry*, 21, 297–313.

Fitzgerald, P.B., Oxley, T.J. *et al.* (2006). An analysis of functional neuroimaging studies of dorsolateral prefrontal cortical activity in depression. *Psychiatry Research*, 148, 33–45.

Fitzgerald, P.B., Laird, A.R. *et al.* (2008). A meta-analytic study of changes in brain activation in depression. *Human Brain Mapping*, 29, 683–695.

Frodl, T., Meisenzahl, E.M. *et al.* (2004). Hippocampal and amygdala changes in patients with major depressive disorder and healthy controls during a 1-year follow-up. *Journal of Clinical Psychiatry*, 65, 492–499.

Gonul, A.S., Coburn, K. *et al.* (2009). Cerebral blood flow, metabolic, receptor, and transporter changes in bipolar disorder: The role of PET and SPECT studies. *International Review of Psychiatry*, 21, 323–335.

Gruber, S.A., Rogowska, J. *et al.* (2004). Decreased activation of the anterior cingulate in bipolar patients: An fMRI study. *Journal of Affective Disorders*, 82, 191–201.

Hamilton, J.P., Siemer, M. *et al.* (2008). Amygdala volume in major depressive disorder: A meta-analysis of magnetic resonance imaging studies. *Molecular Psychiatry*, 13, 993–1000.

Hasler, G. and Northoff, G. (2011). Discovering imaging endophenotypes for major depression. *Molecular Psychiatry*, 16, 604–619.

Heng, S., Song, A.W. *et al.* (2010). White matter abnormalities in bipolar disorder: Insights from diffusion tensor imaging studies. *Journal of Neural Transmission*, 117, 639–654.

Hirvonen, J., Karlsson, H. *et al.* (2008). Striatal dopamine D2 receptors in medication-naive patients with major depressive disorder as assessed with [11C]raclopride PET. *Psychopharmacology (Berl)*, 197, 581–590.

Hsieh, M.H., McQuoid, D.R. *et al.* (2002). Hippocampal volume and antidepressant response in geriatric depression. *International Journal of Geriatric Psychiatry*, 17, 519–525.

Ichimiya, T., Suhara, T. *et al.* (2002). Serotonin transporter binding in patients with mood disorders: A PET study with [11C](+)McN5652. *Biological Psychiatry*, 51, 715–722.

Kempton, M.J., Geddes, J.R. *et al.* (2008). Meta-analysis, database, and meta-regression of 98 structural imaging studies in bipolar disorder. *Archives of General Psychiatry*, 65, 1017–1032.

Kempton, M.J., Salvador, Z. *et al.* (2011). Structural neuroimaging studies in major depressive disorder: Meta-analysis and comparison with bipolar disorder. *Archives of General Psychiatry*, 68, 675–690.

Koolschijn, P.C., van Haren, N.E. *et al.* (2009). Brain volume abnormalities in major depressive disorder: A meta-analysis of magnetic resonance imaging studies. *Human Brain Mapping*, 30, 3719–3735.

Kronhaus, D.M., Lawrence, N.S. *et al.* (2006). Stroop performance in bipolar disorder: Further evidence for abnormalities in the ventral prefrontal cortex. *Bipolar Disorders*, 8, 28–39.

Kronmuller, K.T., Pantel, J. *et al.* (2008). Hippocampal volume and 2-year outcome in depression. *British Journal of Psychiatry*, 192, 472–473.

Kuhn, S. and Gallinat, J. (2011). Resting-state brain activity in schizophrenia and major depression: a quantitative meta-analysis. *Schizophrenia Bulletin*.

MacQueen, G.M., Yucel, K. *et al.* (2008). Posterior hippocampal volumes are associated with remission rates in patients with major depressive disorder. *Biological Psychiatry*, 64, 880–883.

Mahon, K., Burdick, K.E. *et al.* (2010). A role for white matter abnormalities in the pathophysiology of bipolar disorder. *Neuroscience Biobehavioral Reviews*, 34, 533–554.

Malhi, G.S., Lagopoulos, J. *et al.* (2005). An emotional Stroop functional MRI study of euthymic bipolar disorder. *Bipolar Disorders*, 7, 58–69.

Malhi, G.S., Lagopoulos, J. *et al.* (2004). Cognitive generation of affect in bipolar depression: An fMRI study. *Europen Journal of Neuroscience*, 19, 741–754.

Mayberg, H.S., Brannan, S.K. *et al.* (2000). Regional metabolic effects of fluoxetine in major depression: Serial changes and relationship to clinical response. *Biological Psychiatry*, 48, 830–843.

Meyer, J.H., Kapur, S. *et al.* (1999). Prefrontal cortex 5-HT2 receptors in depression: An [18F]setoperone PET imaging study. *American Journal of Psychiatry*, 156, 1029–1034.

Meyer, J.H., Kruger, S. *et al.* (2001). Lower dopamine transporter binding potential in striatum during depression. *NeuroReport*, 12, 4121–4125.

Meyer, J.H., Houle, S. *et al.* (2004). Brain serotonin transporter binding potential measured with carbon

11-labeled DASB positron emission tomography: effects of major depressive episodes and severity of dysfunctional attitudes. *Archives of General Psychiatry*, 61, 1271–1279.

Meyer, J.H., Ginovart, N. *et al.* (2006). Elevated monoamine oxidase a levels in the brain: An explanation for the monoamine imbalance of major depression. *Archives of General Psychiatry*, 63, 1209–1216.

Meyer, J.H., Wilson, A.A. *et al.* (2009). Brain monoamine oxidase A binding in major depressive disorder: Relationship to selective serotonin reuptake inhibitor treatment, recovery, and recurrence. *Archives of General Psychiatry*, 66, 1304–1312.

Milak, M.S., Parsey, R.V. *et al.* (2009). Pretreatment regional brain glucose uptake in the midbrain on PET may predict remission from a major depressive episode after three months of treatment. *Psychiatry Research*, 173, 63–70.

Miller, J.M., Oquendo, M.A. *et al.* (2008). Serotonin transporter binding as a possible predictor of one-year remission in major depressive disorder. *Journal Psychiatric Research*, 42, 1137–1144.

Montgomery, A.J., Stokes, P. *et al.* (2007). Extrastriatal D2 and striatal D2 receptors in depressive illness: Pilot PET studies using [11C]FLB 457 and [11C]raclopride. *Journal of Affective Disorders*, 101, 113–122.

Oquendo, M.A., Hastings, R.S. *et al.* (2007). Brain serotonin transporter binding in depressed patients with bipolar disorder using positron emission tomography. *Archives of General Psychiatry*, 64, 201–208.

Pan, L., Keener, M.T. *et al.* (2009). Functional neuroimaging studies of bipolar disorder: Examining the wide clinical spectrum in the search for disease endophenotypes. *International Review of Psychiatry*, 21, 368–379.

Parsey, R.V. (2010). Serotonin receptor imaging: clinically useful? *Journal of Nuclear Medicine*, 51, 1495–1498.

Parsey, R.V., Oquendo, M.A. *et al.* (2001). Dopamine D(2) receptor availability and amphetamine-induced dopamine release in unipolar depression. *Biological Psychiatry*, 50, 313–322.

Parsey, R.V., Oquendo, M.A. *et al.* (2006a). Altered serotonin 1A binding in major depression: A [carbonyl-C-11]WAY100635 positron emission tomography study. *Biological Psychiatry*, 59, 106–113.

Parsey, R.V., Hastings, R.S. *et al.* (2006a). Lower serotonin transporter binding potential in the human brain during major depressive episodes. *American Journal of Psychiatry*, 163, 52–58.

Sargent, P.A., Rabiner, E.A. *et al.* (2010). 5-HT(1A) receptor binding in euthymic bipolar patients using positron emission tomography with [carbonyl-

(11)C]WAY-100635. *Journal of Affective Disorders*, 123, 77–80.

Savitz, J.B. and Drevets, W.C. (2009). Imaging phenotypes of major depressive disorder: Genetic correlates. *Neuroscience*, 164, 300–330.

Sax, K.W., Strakowski, S.M. *et al.* (1999). Frontosubcortical neuroanatomy and the continuous performance test in mania. *American Journal of Psychiatry*, 156, 139–141.

Sheline, Y.I. (2003). Neuroimaging studies of mood disorder effects on the brain. *Biological Psychiatry*, 54, 338–352.

Sheline, Y.I., Barch, D.M. *et al.* (2001). Increased amygdala response to masked emotional faces in depressed subjects resolves with antidepressant treatment: an fMRI study. *Biological Psychiatry*, 50 651–658.

Soares, J.C. and Mann, J.J. (1997). The anatomy of mood disorders–review of structural neuroimaging studies. *Biological Psychiatry*, 41, 86–106.

Strakowski, S.M., Adler, C.M. *et al.* (2005a). Abnormal FMRI brain activation in euthymic bipolar disorder patients during a counting Stroop interference task. *American Journal of Psychiatry*, 162, 1697–1705.

Strakowski, S.M., DelBello, M.P. *et al.* (2005b). The functional neuroanatomy of bipolar disorder: A review of neuroimaging findings. *Molecular Psychiatry*, 10, 105–116.

Sullivan, G.M., Ogden, R.T. *et al.* (2009). Positron emission tomography quantification of serotonin-1A receptor binding in medication-free bipolar depression. *Biological Psychiatry*, 66, 223–230.

Vakili, K., Pillay, S.S. *et al.* (2000). Hippocampal volume in primary unipolar major depression: A magnetic resonance imaging study. *Biological Psychiatry*, 47, 1087–1090.

Videbech, P. and Ravnkilde, B. (2004). Hippocampal volume and depression: A meta-analysis of MRI studies. *American Journal of Psychiatry*, 161, 1957–1966.

Warner-Schmidt, J.L. and Duman, R.S. (2006). Hippocampal neurogenesis: Opposing effects of stress and antidepressant treatment. *Hippocampus*, 16, 239–249.

Wessa, M., Houenou, J. *et al.* (2007). Fronto-striatal overactivation in euthymic bipolar patients during an emotional go/nogo task. *American Journal of Psychiatry*, 164, 638–646.

Yildiz, A., Sachs, G.S. *et al.* (2001). 31P Nuclear magnetic resonance spectroscopy findings in bipolar illness: A meta-analysis. *Psychiatry Research*, 106, 181–191.

Yildiz-Yesiloglu, A. and Ankerst, D.P. (2006). Neurochemical alterations of the brain in bipolar disorder and their implications for pathophysiology: a systematic review of the in vivo proton magnetic resonance spectroscopy findings. *Progress in Neuropsychopharmacology and Biological Psychiatry*, 30, 969–995.

Yuksel, C. and Ongur, D. (2010). Magnetic resonance spectroscopy studies of glutamate-related abnormalities in mood disorders. *Biological Psychiatry*, 68, 785–794.

Chapter

29

Pharmacogenetics and mood disorders

Gonzalo Laje and Francis J. McMahon

Introduction

Pharmacogenetics is concerned with the impact of individual genetic variation on the outcome of treatment. Treatment outcomes can be defined in many ways, including symptom reduction, remission, and adverse events. One major goal of pharmacogenetics is to better match medications with patients to maximize efficacy while minimizing or eliminating adverse events. This goal is particularly relevant in the treatment of mood disorders, where there is great variability in individual treatment outcomes. In psychiatry – as in much of medicine – the choice of treatment is still largely a question of clinical judgment. Solid pharmacogenetic information could substantially improve this process and may lead to better outcomes.

The term "pharmacogenetics" is often used interchangeably with "pharmacogenomics," which emphasizes the application of genetic technologies to new and existing drugs. Genetic markers that can help predict treatment outcomes have long been sought, but so far only a few tests have come into clinical use. The anticoagulant drug, warfarin, is one example: since about 40% of the difference in individual dosing is attributable to variation in a few genes (Wadelius *et al.* 2005), the FDA now provides dosing guidelines based on genetic test results. As genomic technologies have advanced rapidly over the past decade, the number of FDA-recognized pharmacogenetic tests has grown. As of 2012, the FDA mentions pharmacogenetic markers in the official label of 32 drugs used commonly for mental illness (Table 29.1). One of these, a genetic marker for serious adverse events that can occur during treatment with carbamezepine, is highly clinically relevant for psychiatry and is discussed in detail below.

Traditionally, pharmacogenetic variation has been separated into two main classes: (1) drug absorption, distribution, metabolism, and excretion (ADME or pharmacokinetic effects) and (2) drug action (pharmacodynamic effects). This remains a useful heuristic, but oversimplifies the picture for many drugs. Pharmacokinetic and -dynamic effects are often closely intertwined, and some of the major sources of individual variation in psychiatric treatment outcomes, such as drug tolerability and treatment adherence, do not fit neatly into these traditional classes.

In this chapter, we will review some of the key pharmacogenetic considerations in the treatment of mood disorders. We will cover antidepressants and mood stabilizers. We will not discuss antipsychotic medications, even though they do play an important role in mood disorder treatment. So far, there are few pharmacogenetic markers of clinical significance for antipsychotics, but ongoing research is making some progress.

Methodological issues

Pharmacogenetic studies in psychiatry are still in a relatively early stage of development. The strategies employed have evolved from candidate gene studies, where one or more genes are studied due to their hypothesized role in a trait of interest, to genome-wide association studies (GWAS). GWAS take advantage of genetic markers strategically distributed in the genome to reflect common genetic variation in almost all known genes – and even the large stretches of DNA between genes that presumably serve a regulatory function (Figure 29.1). Both approaches have strengths and weaknesses. While candidate gene studies benefit from focus on one or a few genes, our limited understanding of the pathophysiology of neuropsychiatric disorders and of gene function in the brain make the selection of candidate genes very challenging. The GWAS covers a large proportion of

Clinical Handbook for the Management of Mood Disorders, ed. J. John Mann, Patrick J. McGrath, and Steven P. Roose.
Published by Cambridge University Press. © Cambridge University Press 2013.

Table 29.1 FDA pharmacogenomics labeling for drugs with psychiatric indications

Drug	Label sections
	HLA-B*1502
Carbamazepine	Boxed warning, warnings and precautions
Phenytoin	warnings
	UCD
Valproic Acid	Contraindications, precautions, adverse reactions
	CYP2C19
Citalopram	Drug interactions, warnings
Diazepam	Drug interactions, clinical pharmacology
Fluvoxamine	Drug interactions
Modafinil	Drug interactions
	CYP2C9
Fluvoxamine	Drug interactions
Aripiprazole	Clinical pharmacology, dosage and administration
Atomoxetine	Dosage and administration, warnings and precautions, drug interactions
Citalopram	Drug interactions
Clomipramine	Drug interactions
Clozapine	Drug interactions, clinical pharmacology
Desipramine	Drug interactions
Doxepin	Precautions
Fluoxetine	Warnings, precautions, clinical pharmacology
Fluvoxamine	Drug interactions
Iloperidone	Clinical pharmacology, dosage and administration, drug interactions, specific populations, warnings, precautions
Imipramine	Drug interactions
Modafinil	Drug interactions
Nefazodone	Drug interactions
Nortriptyline	Drug interactions
Paroxetine	Clinical pharmacology, drug interactions
Perphenazine	Clinical pharmacology, drug interactions
Pimozide	Warnings, precautions, contraindications, dosage and administration
Protriptyline	Precautions
Risperidone	Drug interactions, clinical pharmacology
Thioridazine	Precautions, warnings, contraindications
Trimipramine	Drug interactions
Venlafaxine	Drug interactions

Adapted from: Table of pharmacogenomic biomarkers in drug labels (http://www.fda.gov/drugs/scienceresearch/researchareas/pharmacogenetics/ucm083378.htm, US Food and Drug Administration, accessed March 2012).

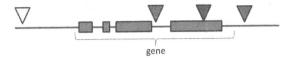

Exons, which encode amino acids in the gene product

SNPs reflecting nearby functional genetic variants

Other common SNPs that may or may not regulate nearby gene(s)

Figure 29.1 Some common forms of genetic variation. Genes typically comprise exons, which encode amino acids, introns, which lie between exons, and regulatory regions at each end. Single nucleotide polymorphisms (SNPs) used in genetic association studies are rarely functional themselves, but may reflect nearby functional variants. SNPs in regions flanking genes may or may not play a regulatory role, e.g., in gene expression

discriminate changes that result from the illness or its treatment from those that are truly etiologic.

Each individual's genome varies considerably. The variants themselves are referred to as *alleles*; there are several common and many less common alleles present in the population at each gene (Figure 29.1). Single nucleotide polymorphisms (SNPs) are common (>1%) single base-pair changes that occur throughout the genome. There appears to be one SNP for every 2–3 thousand base-pairs of DNA. SNPs are convenient to study, but usually impact gene function only indirectly. Single base-pair changes that are less common are usually referred to as single nucleotide variants (SNVs). SNVs sometimes occur in and near genes, where they can have a large impact on function.

Variations that affect more than one base-pair include repeat polymorphisms, insertion/deletion polymorphisms (indels), and copy number variants (CNVs). Repeat polymorphisms typically consist of two to many base-pair units of DNA that are repeated, often imperfectly, several times at the same position on a chromosome. Well-known repeat polymorphisms include the triplet (3-bp) repeats that, when expanded, cause Huntington's disease and fragile X syndrome. The best-known indel is the 44-bp polymorphism that affects expression of the serotonin transporter gene and has been associated with a large range of neuropsychiatric traits. CNVs are a more recently discovered form of genetic variation, involving large segments of chromosomes that are deleted or duplicated. CNVs are quite common and do not always cause disease, but certain CNVs have been associated with schizophrenia, autism, or other developmental

known genes, but at the cost of a larger burden of multiple comparisons. Thus GWAS usually require samples of at least 1000 to detect modest effects (OR < 2). Large samples are a key element of robust findings in these studies (Ioannidis *et al.* 2003). Gene expression studies are another approach, but may be limited by access to relevant tissue (e.g., particular groups of neurons) and can suffer from a confusion of cause with consequence: unlike studies of inherited genetic variation, most gene expression studies cannot confidently brain disorders, suggesting that CNVs may have important functional impacts. All of these forms of genetic variation are typically passed from parents to offspring, but can also arise spontaneously – so-called *de novo* events. CNVs are particularly subject to *de novo* variation and can even vary from cell to cell within the same individual, a phenomenon known as somatic mosaicism.

The course of illness and severity may also impact pharmacogenetic studies in important ways. Spontaneous remission, placebo effects, and acquired treatment resistance are all major concerns. Pharmacogenetic studies may also need to consider elements that are unique to the drug(s) used, such as time to effect, tolerability, and drug adherence. For example, several studies have shown that variation in the gene encoding the serotonin transporter (SLC6A4) may be more important in antidepressant tolerability than in response per se (Hu *et al.* 2007, Murphy *et al.* 2004). In this context, the field of psychiatric pharmacogenetics is still developing consensus definitions, particularly of treatment outcome and adverse effects. Without such definitions, replication studies and meta-analyses are difficult to interpret.

Another aspect of human variation important for pharmacogenetic studies is ethnic diversity. Genetic ancestry is often reflected in recognized racial or ethnic differences in response to a variety of medications. Some of these differences reflect differences in the frequencies of particular alleles in genes encoding enzymes involved in drug metabolism or immune proteins. For example, an allele of the major histocompatibility locus HLA that is common in individuals of Southeast Asian ancestry confers a five- to tenfold increased risk of Stevens–Johnson syndrome after exposure to carbamazepine (see below).

Work over the past several years has focused on the role of common genetic variation, where differences in large groups of individuals can be discerned. The advent of ultra-high throughput sequencing technology is now moving the focus toward rarer forms of genetic variation. We are beginning to recognize that each individual carries about 10 000 functionally relevant genetic variants, many of which are unique to that person or their close relatives (Lupski *et al.* 2011). This fact will add an important new dimension to pharmacogenetic studies in the near future, potentially allowing a truly personalized approach to treatment. The rapidly falling cost of large-scale sequencing will soon make it practical to generate a complete genomic sequence as a standard part of each patient's medical record. When we learn how to interpret all this information – what genetic variation affects what medication in what way – then pharmacogenetic findings will for the first time be directly translatable to the clinic. This milestone will also pose an enormous challenge to clinicians, who will need to interpret this large quantity of data to determine the best path for each individual patient toward optimal treatment outcomes (Winner *et al.* 2010).

Antidepressants

There have been a number of small studies aimed at finding genetic markers of antidepressant treatment outcome. However, most of the findings have not been replicated in larger cohorts. Several such cohorts have been developed over the past decade. The Sequenced Treatment Alternatives to Relieve Depression sample (STAR*D) remains the largest pharmacogenetic study of major depression carried out to date, with close to 2000 outpatients with major depression who provided DNA samples. The Genome-based Therapeutic Drugs for Depression (GENDEP) study has assembled a sample of over 700 outpatients with major depression in Europe and the United Kingdom. The Munich Antidepressant Response Signature (MARS) study has generated DNA and outcome data on over 300 inpatients and outpatients with major depression or a depressive episode of bipolar disorder.

Patients with major depression are often ill in many ways. Studies such as STAR*D have identified clinical variables associated with poorer outcome, such as frequency and severity of concomitant medical illness, and anxious depression (Trivedi *et al.* 2006). Other variables such as personality disorders, and alcohol and drug use, among others, have relevance for antidepressant treatment outcome (reviewed in Serretti *et al.* 2008). To the extent that these factors vary across samples, different findings may emerge. The samples included in the large pharmacogenetic study cohorts were meant to represent "typical" patients, rather than major depression in its purest form.

Symptomatic improvement

Antidepressant treatment response does not have a universally agreed definition. Many studies use different assessment methods and different criteria for good outcomes. Furthermore, remission in MDD can occur spontaneously and the placebo response rate can be as high as 40% in controlled trials (Khan *et al.* 2003). It can thus be difficult to demonstrate that antidepressants are effective – except in relatively severe depression (Fournier *et al.* 2010). Variablility in treatment adherence, medication tolerability, and many typically unmeasured variables – such as adverse life events – pose further complications. While we would ideally have quantitative, biological measures of response, the field has instead needed to work with relatively arbitrary, clinical measures.

Four groups across the US have tested outcomes in the STAR*D sample. All have focused on Level 1, where all study participants received citalopram as their sole antidepressant treatment for up to 12 weeks. Although the main outcomes were treatment response and remission, each study was different, defining these outcomes somewhat differently. Major differences across studies can be seen for minimum required treatment duration, whether and how drug tolerability was considered, primary outcome measure (self- or clinician-rated Quick Inventory of Depression Symptoms, the QIDS16), and duration of any improvement.

The GENDEP study (Uher *et al.* 2010), the only one of these studies expressly designed for pharmacogenetics, recruited patients from multiple sites across Europe. Patients were treated with escitalopram or nortriptyline. Outcome was based on change in the Montgomery–Asberg Depression Rating Scale (MADRS) score from baseline to week 12.

MARS (Ising *et al.* 2009) defined three outcome phenotypes: early partial response after up to 3 weeks of treatment, along with response and remission after 5 weeks of treatment. All MARS participants were enrolled as inpatients, in contrast to STAR*D and GENDEP, which enrolled only outpatients.

Candidate genes

The serotonin transporter (SLC6A4)

If the serotonin transporter (SLC6A4) is the most studied gene in psychiatry, a functional polymorphism in its promoter region (known as the linked polymorphic region or LPR), is the most studied genetic marker. As the proximal target for SSRIs, the most widely prescribed class of antidepressants, this gene is an obvious pharmacodynamic candidate for association studies. Variation in the LPR seems to affect gene expression in important ways (Rasmussen and Werge, 2007), and additional alleles have also

been characterized functionally. Multiple small studies and a subsequent meta-analysis by Serretti *et al.* (2007) suggested an association with antidepressant outcome – but with some inconsistencies.

Three different publications tested genetic variation in SLC6A4 for association with treatment outcome in STAR*D (Hu *et al.* 2007, Kraft *et al.* 2007, Mrazek *et al.* 2008), with somewhat divergent results. Kraft *et al.* reported no association between citalopram treatment response or remission and any of 10 genetic markers they studied (Kraft *et al.* 2007). Hu *et al.* also found no association with symptomatic improvement, but did detect an association with drug tolerability: carriers of the S or L_G alleles reported more side effects (Hu *et al.* 2007), consistent with some previous studies (Murphy *et al.* 2004). Mrazek *et al.* (2008) did not consider tolerability, but divided the STAR*D sample into four self-described ethnic groups, and sequenced the entire SLC6A4 gene in 60 individuals from each group. This study concluded that there was an association between SLC6A4 and remission during citalopram treatment, but only in "white nonHispanic" participants. The most recent meta-analysis, which included all previous studies, STAR*D, and a number of unpublished studies, found no association between SLC6A4 and antidepressant treatment outcome (Taylor *et al.* 2010).

How does this all make sense? Overall, it seems likely that genetic variation in SLC6A4 does play some role in antidepressant treatment outcome, but the effect is modest and variable – and drug tolerability seems to be a major factor. Although several SLC6A4 genetic assays are commercially available, current evidence does not support their use in clinical decision-making.

The cytochrome p450 system

Genes that regulate the metabolism of antidepressant drugs could also have a significant impact on response and tolerability. Many drugs, including the majority of antidepressants, are metabolized by the liver through the cytochrome P450 pathway and its enzymatic sub-groups (reviewed in Black, 2007). Genes such as CYP2D6, CYP1A2, CYP3A4, and CYP2C19 have been well studied and characterized, but their clinical utility in the management of mood disorders has so far been limited (Berg *et al.* 2007).

Peters *et al.* (2008) studied common genetic variation in CYP2D6, CYP2C19, CYP3A4, and CYP3A5, among others. They found no association with citalopram treatment outcomes in the STAR*D sample. Some other studies have found statistically significant effects of certain alleles in certain groups (Huezo-Diaz *et al.* 2011, Mrazek *et al.* 2011), but the effect sizes have been small, suggesting that most patients would not benefit clinically from genetic testing.

Serotonin 2A receptor (HTR2A)

Two large candidate gene studies performed in the STAR*D sample implicated markers near the genes encoding the serotonin 2A receptor (HTR2A) and the glutamate receptor sub-unit KA1 in citalopram treatment outcome (McMahon *et al.* 2006, Paddock *et al.* 2007). The association was detected for treatment response, remission, and change in QIDS-C16, although the effect sizes were small. Some subsequent studies have also found evidence of association between HTR2A markers and antidepressant outcome in major depression and generalized anxiety disorder, but the implicated markers and alleles have not been consistent (Uher *et al.* 2009, Kishi *et al.* 2010, Lucae *et al.* 2010, Lohoff *et al.* 2011), although Smith *et al.* (2012) found the HTR2A C1354T poly-morphism was associated with remission on paroxetine in MDD. More studies of HTR2A in large samples are needed to clarify its potential role in antidepressant outcome.

GRIK4

The STAR*D sample also showed evidence of association between citalopram treatment outcome and the gene encoding the glutamate receptor KA1 sub-unit, GRIK4. (McMahon *et al.* 2006, Paddock *et al.* 2007). The homozygous carriers of both the HTR2A and GRIK4 response-associated alleles were 23% less likely to be citalopram nonresponders than participants with neither of these alleles, but the area under the curve (AUC) expressing the probability of correctly identifying a responder from a random pair of participants was only 0.58, suggesting these two markers have very small predictive value. Replication studies have yielded mixed results (Horstmann *et al.* 2010, Perlis *et al.* 2010). Further study of GRIK4 may be warranted, even though its pharmacogenetic significance is unclear.

FKBP5

The FKBP5 gene encodes a chaperone protein important for fine-tuning of the HPA axis. An association between genetic variants in this gene and antidepressant treatment and recurrence of MDD was first described by Binder *et al.* (2004). This gene is a good candidate based on its relevance to pathways in the hypothalamic pituitary adrenal axis (HPA axis). Leckman *et al.* (2008) replicated these findings in the STAR*D sample, with a modest effect size. Further support was seen in a small cohort of German patients (Kirchheiner *et al.* 2008), but not in a Han Chinese sample. The signal in FKBP5 can now be considered to be replicated. Additional studies of large samples with prospective follow-up are needed to establish clinical significance.

Brain-derived neurotrophic factor (BDNF)

BDNF is a member of the neurotrophin family and is involved in neuronal growth and plasticity. Variation in BDNF has been thought to play a role in the etiology of affective disorders and the mediation of antidepressant treatment response. Expression of BDNF may also be modified by antidepressant treatment (Saarelainen *et al.* 2003). A functional nonsynonymous single nucleotide polymorphism (SNP) causing an amino acid substitution of valine to methionine has been identified in codon 66 (val66met; rs6265) (Ventriglia *et al.* 2002, Egan *et al.* 2003).

The BDNF val66met polymorphism has been at the center of antidepressant treatment outcome studies, with some positive (Choi *et al.* 2006) and some negative (Anttila *et al.* 2007) results. The largest study found no evidence of association in STAR*D or in a smaller German sample (Domschke *et al.* 2009). More comprehensive studies in larger samples are needed to clarify whether BDNF plays an important role in antidepressant treatment outcome.

The phosphodiesterase (PDE) family

PDE1A and PDE11A are two genes from the large phosphodiesterase family. These genes are reasonable candidates because they metabolize cyclic adenosine monophosphate (cAMP), which indirectly regulates expression of BDNF (Nair and Vaidya, 2006). In 2006 Wong *et al.* published a report linking variation in PDE1A and PDE11A to antidepressant treatment outcome in a Mexican American population (n = 284) (Wong *et al.* 2006).

Two replication attempts were conducted in STAR*D, the first one by Teranishi *et al.* (2007) and the second by Cabanero *et al.* (2009). Neither report found evidence of association with markers in PDE11A, PDE9A, or PDE1A, either in the whole sample or in the Hispanic sub-set, but larger studies of Hispanic patients are needed.

ABCB1

Another pharmacokinetic gene, ABCB1, also known as MDR1 (multi-drug resistance 1) encodes a glyco-protein expressed in the gut, liver, kidney, and at the blood–brain barrier, where it affects brain concentrations of some antidepressants.

One study found that several polymorphisms in ABCB1 were associated with outcome of antidepressant treatment in patients given drugs shown to be substrates of ABCB1 in knockout mice (Uhr et al. 2008). So far, two studies have supported these findings (Sarginson et al. 2010, Lin et al. 2011), and two have not (Peters et al. 2008, Perlis et al. 2010). Further studies are needed to clarify how important ABCB1 may be in antidepressant treatment.

The rapid advance of genotyping technology has now rendered candidate gene studies largely obsolete, but the candidate gene studies that have already been done have been valuable. These studies have shown that common genetic variation in several genes may be related to treatment outcomes, but no finding can yet be considered to be widely replicated and clinically significant. We probably have not yet studied all of the relevant candidates, but genome-wide studies, reviewed below, are beginning to move toward this goal with increasing speed and efficiency.

Genome-wide association studies (GWAS)

GWAS are a relatively new kind of genetic study that take advantage of large numbers of highly informative genetic markers (usually SNPs), spread across each chromosome. GWAS compare genetic marker frequencies in two groups (cases vs. controls, responders vs. nonresponders, etc.), under the assumption that differences reflect important variation in nearby genes. A typical GWAS tests between 500 000 and 2 million SNPs. With so many tests, thresholds for statistical significance have to be set high: a p-value $< 5 \times 10^{-8}$ is the generally accepted threshold for genome-wide significance.

Three antidepressant outcome studies have implemented genome-wide approaches to detect common variation associated with antidepressant response: STAR*D (n = 1953) (Garriock et al. 2010), MARS (n = 339) (Ising et al. 2009), and GENDEP (n = 706) (Uher et al. 2010). These studies are all very different in design, genotyping platform used, sample size, and outcome measures. None of the reported findings were genome-wide significant.

The results reported from STAR*D were based on Level 1, where all participants were treated with citalopram. Two main phenotypes were derived: response and remission. No genome-wide significant results were found, but Garriock et al. (2010) highlighted SNPs near the genes encoding ubiquitin protein ligase E3C (UBE3C), bone morphogenic protein 7 (BMP7), and RAR-related orphan receptor alpha (RORA).

The MARS study (Ising et al. 2009) used the three outcome phenotypes described above. No genome-wide significant signals were detected. Top hits included markers near the gene encoding cadherin-17 (CDH17), that were associated with early partial response, and two markers near the ephrin type-B receptor 1 gene (EPHB1), associated with early partial response, response, and remission.

The GENDEP study (Uher et al. 2010) also found no genome-wide significant results, but highlighted two markers near the gene encoding interleukin-11 (IL11), associated with nortriptyline response, and one marker near the uronyl 2-sulphotransferase gene (UST), associated with citalopram response.

The lack of overlap in findings between these studies is obvious. It probably reflects the differences in samples, treatments, and outcome measures. Limited statistical power is another major issue, since few of the samples studied so far have been large enough to ensure that small effects would be found. Larger, more uniform samples are needed.

Adverse events

Adverse events occur with all pharmacological treatments. Severe adverse events must be avoided if possible, but even mild adverse events can reduce treatment adherence and lead to discontinuation. Most modern antidepressants are quite safe, but early identification of the minority of patients who might suffer an adverse event during treatment could have a big impact on treatment choice and monitoring. Two groups of antidepressant-associated adverse events have been studied in large samples: treatment-emergent suicidal ideation (TESI) and sexual dysfunction.

Treatment-emergent suicidal ideation (TESI)

Suicidal ideation is an uncommon symptom that can emerge during antidepressant treatment, and is highlighted by a "Black Box Warning" on the labeling of all antidepressants sold in the USA, describing the risk of treatment-emergent suicidality in younger patients (FDA, 2005). Importantly, the word "suicidality" here refers to thoughts of death or suicide, not actual suicidal behavior. TESI phenotypes have been studied in the STAR*D, MARS, and GENDEP cohorts. While the phenotype definitions vary somewhat, all are based on the emergence or worsening of suicidal thoughts or behavior during antidepressant treatment.

TESI is a good example of the problem known as "confounding by indication:" the recognition during treatment of a symptom already known to be characteristic of the condition being treated. Suicidal thoughts and behavior are common in depression, and suicidal behavior is actually substantially decreased in patients receiving antidepressants, compared to depressed patients taking a placebo. The concern about TESI rests on a small, but statistically significant excess of suicidal ideation in depressed patients assigned to active drug in randomized trials.

Three studies of TESI in the STAR*D sample have been published. In a candidate gene study of the cyclic adenosine monophosphate response element binding protein (CREB1), Perlis et al. (2008) reported two SNPs and two 5-SNP haplotypes associated with clinician-rated TESI in STAR*D, but only in men (Perlis et al. 2007). Subsequently, Laje et al. (2007) screened SNPs in 68 candidate genes. They found that markers near genes encoding two different glutamate receptors, GRIA3 and GRIK2, were associated with self-rated TESI. Later, GRIA3 and GRIK2 were also found to be associated with clinician-rated TESI in the MARS sample, but the markers and alleles were different (Menke et al. 2008). A small GWAS was also performed in a sub-set of the STAR*D cohort, implicating the genes PAPLN and IL28RA (Laje et al. 2009). Although these findings are of scientific interest, they appear to have low sensitivity for identifying patients at risk for TESI in a clinical setting.

The MARS group also conducted a genome-wide TESI study in their inpatient cohort (Menke et al. 2012). Using a phenotype definition similar to that employed in the STAR*D sample, the MARS investigators found a comparable rate of TESI in their sample (8.1%, compared to 6.3% in STAR*D). No markers achieved genome-wide significance in this small sample, but there was some support for the previous findings implicating GRIA3 and GRIK2, as noted above. The top hit was an intergenic marker ~300 kb from the 3' end of the RORA gene. Markers near this same

gene were previously reported to be associated with symptomatic improvement in the STAR*D sample (see above).

Genetic predictors of TESI were also studied by the GENDEP group using both a candidate gene and a genome-wide approach (Perroud et al. 2009, 2012). Their phenotype definition, however, departed from previous definitions of TESI in that it also included participants who experienced an "increase" in suicidal ideation from baseline. The candidate gene study found some support for a role of BDNF and its receptor, NTRK2 (Perroud et al. 2009). The GWAS reported no genome-wide significant findings, highlighting a marker located ~30 kb downstream of the gene encoding guanine deaminase, GDA (Perroud et al. 2012).

TESI remains an important issue in antidepressant treatment, but the genetic studies so far have failed to find consistent evidence of predictive markers. Larger sample sizes and meta-analytic approaches may clarify the picture in the future. TESI may not be under substantial genetic control, but if it is, clinically meaningful genetic markers should exist, and could play an important role in management of depressed patients.

Sexual dysfunction

Sexual dysfunction (SD) is major contributor to treatment nonadherence among patients treated with SSRIs. So far there has been one pharmacogenetic study of SD, based on self-reports of erectile dysfunction, decreased libido, or anorgasmia during citalopram treatment in Level 1 of the STAR*D trial. The results highlighted several genes encoding glutamate receptors (GRIA3, GRIK2, GRIA1, and GRIN3A) (Perlis et al. 2009b). There have been no attempts to replicate these results in an independent sample.

Mood stabilizers

Lithium

Lithium remains a mainstay in the treatment of bipolar disorder, and may also have a role in the treatment of recurrent major depression. Lithium response can be measured over time, and reliable instruments have been developed (Grof et al. 2002). The heritability of lithium response has not yet been determined – and would be very difficult to demonstrate with the twin study design typically used to establish heritability. However, some studies have indicated that responsiveness to lithium is a strongly familial trait (Grof *et al.* 2002).

In view of these facts, lithium response should be a promising target for pharmacogenetic studies. Lithium response can mean different things. One could consider the relatively acute antimanic effects of lithium, the antidepressant effects of lithium when given adjunctively, or the longer-term effects of chronic lithium treatment. For the latter, distinctions can be drawn between relapse, reduction in the number of episodes over time, and reduction in the duration or severity of episodes, when they occur. For each of these, further distinctions can be made between manic and major depressive episodes. Most published studies have focused on prevention of relapse.

Several candidate gene studies have been published. Most highlight well-studied genes such as the serotonin transporter (SLC6A4), but some focus on other genes (for review see McCarthy *et al.* 2010). Like many candidate gene findings, few have been replicated in independent samples (Smith *et al.* 2010).

Another way to understand how lithium may interact with genetic variation is to study genes whose expression is altered by lithium treatment. Several such studies have been published (Brandish *et al.* 2005, Popkie *et al.* 2010, Yu *et al.* 2011), but there is little agreement across studies at the gene level, perhaps owing to substantial methodological differences. One analysis suggests that many studies are consistent at the level of a biological pathway, where several or many genes interact to affect a physiologic process (Gupta *et al.* 2011). A major limitation of gene expression studies is the difficulty of studying lithium effects in brain cells *in vitro*. This limitation may be surmountable in the near future by use of induced pluripotent stem cell technology, which allows neurons and glia to be derived from nonneural cells (e.g., skin cells) obtained from living volunteers (Brennand *et al.* 2011).

To date, two genome-wide association studies of lithium response have been published. The first and largest study, known as the Systematic Treatment Enhancement Program for Bipolar Disorder (STEP-BD), followed over 1000 patients with bipolar disorder over a period of about 2 years each (Perlis *et al.* 2009a). STEP-BD was not designed as a pharmacogenetic study, but close to 500 patients were treated with lithium. When "time to recurrence" was taken

as the outcome, no significant genetic associations were detected, although suggestive signals in a region spanning the gene encoding the AMPA glutamate receptor, GRIA2, were found, and markers in the same region were also associated with positive lithium response in a second sample.

The second study was carried out in Sardinia, where long-term follow-up of a genetically homogeneous population is possible (Squassina *et al.* 2010). No significant genetic associations were detected in a sample of over 200 patients. The strongest association signal was near the gene encoding the amiloride-sensitive cation channel 1, ACCN1, but the clinical or biological importance of this gene is unclear.

That the two GWAS of lithium response published so far did not yield convergent findings is not surprising, given the relatively small sample sizes and methodological differences between the two studies. Larger samples are needed, along with a uniform and reliable method of scoring lithium response. The Consortium on Lithium Genetics (ConLiGen), a multi-site study that aims to assemble a large, uniformly phenotyped sample for GWAS analysis, is currently underway (Schulze *et al.* 2010).

Adverse events limit the use of lithium in many patients. These include thyroid disease and renal disease (typically reduced creatinine clearance, which can be serious in some patients). Yet many patients take lithium for years without experiencing these problems. This observation suggests that individuals vary in their risk for lithium-related adverse events. If genetic variation contributes to this variation in risk, and genetic markers can be found, then these might yield important clues to the underlying pathophysiology and form the basis of genetic tests with clinical predictive value for these severe adverse effects. To our knowledge, no human genetic studies of lithium-related adverse events have been published to date. Such studies would be challenging, given the relative rarity of these events in the population, but could be accomplished, for example, with a registry-based retrospective case-control design.

Carbamazepine

Anticonvulsant medications play an important adjunctive role in the treatment of bipolar disorder and related conditions. It has long been recognized that a small minority of patients treated with anti-convulsant medications develop a localized rash or a more severe, generalized cutaneous reaction, known as Stevens–Johnson syndrome (SJS), or toxic epidermal necrolysis. SJS is a serious condition, with substantial mortality (5%).

In 2004, Chung et al. (2004) reported that patients of Han Chinese ancestry who developed SJS after exposure to carbamazepine were more likely to carry the human leukocyte antigen (HLA) marker known as HLA-B*1502 (Chung et al. 2004). This marker, which is common in persons of Asian ancestry, conferred a substantially increased risk of SJS (odds ratios around 5) in people exposed to carbamazepine. This finding was quickly confirmed in other Asian populations. Soon thereafter, the US Food and Drug Administration changed the carbamazepine labeling to recommend HLA testing in patients of Asian ancestry (Ferrell and McLeod, 2008). Subsequent studies in other nonAsian populations also reported similar findings, although the HLA-B*1502 is uncommon outside Asia (McCormack et al. 2011).

It is recommended that all patients of Asian ancestry who are under consideration for carbamazepine therapy be screened for HLA-B*1502 before commencing treatment. It is not clear that such screening is indicated in people of nonAsian ancestry, but a prior or family history of hypersensitivity or other skin reactions after exposure to anticonvulsants may indicate patients at higher risk who could benefit from screening.

Conclusions

The next decade will likely bring significant progress for pharmacogenetics in psychiatry. Although clinically useful pharmacogenetic tests derived from common variants are so far very limited, pharmacogenetics can contribute to improving our understanding of the underlying mechanisms of mood disorders and their treatment. New genome sequencing methods are beginning to offer a view not only of common variation but also of rare variants with a much larger impact on gene function. Studies based on these approaches are expected to give a new dimension to pharmacogenetics in the near future, potentially moving toward a truly personalized form of treatment, which considers both rare and common genetic differences among individuals, along with other person-specific factors, in planning treatment. This is the next step toward more effective medications, fewer adverse events, and a reduction in the burden of mood disorders for patients and society.

References

Anttila, S., Huuhka, K., Huuhka, M. et al. (2007). Interaction between 5-HT1A and BDNF genotypes increases the risk of treatment-resistant depression. *Journal of Neural Transmission*, 114, 1065–1068.

Berg, A.O., Piper, M., Armstrong, K. et al. (2007). Recommendations from the EGAPP Working Group: testing for cytochrome P450 polymorphisms in adults with nonpsychotic depression treated with selective serotonin reuptake inhibitors. *Genetics in Medicine*, 9, 819–825.

Binder, E.B., Salyakina, D., Lichtner, P. et al. (2004). Polymorphisms in FKBP5 are associated with increased recurrence of depressive episodes and rapid response to antidepressant treatment. *Nature Genetics*, 36, 1319–1325.

Black, J.L., III, O'Kane, D.J., and Mrazek, D.A. (2007). The impact of CYP allelic variation on antidepressant metabolism: A review. *Expert Opinion on Drug Metabolism and Toxicology*, 3, 21–31.

Brandish, P.E., Su, M., Holder, D.J. et al. (2005). Regulation of gene expression by lithium and depletion of inositol in slices of adult rat cortex. *Neuron*, 45, 861–872.

Brennand, K.J., Simone, A., Jou, J. et al. (2011). Modelling schizophrenia using human induced pluripotent stem cells. *Nature*, 473, 221–225.

Cabanero, M., Laje, G., Tera-Wadleigh, S., and McMahon, F.J. (2009). Association study of phosphodiesterase genes in the Sequenced Treatment Alternatives to Relieve Depression sample. *Pharmacogenetics and Genomics*, 19, 235–238.

Choi, M.J., Kang, R.H., Lim, S.W., Oh, K.S., and Lee, M.S. (2006). Brain-derived neurotrophic factor gene polymorphism (Val66Met) and citalopram response in major depressive disorder. *Brain Research*, 1118, 176–182.

Chung, W.H., Hung, S.I., Hong, H.S. et al. (2004). Medical genetics: A marker for Stevens–Johnson syndrome. *Nature*, 428, 486.

Domschke, K., Lawford, B., Laje, G. et al. (2009). Brain-derived neurotrophic factor (BDNF) gene: No major impact on antidepressant treatment response. *International Journal of Neuropsychopharmacology*, 13, 93–101.

Egan, M.F., Kojima, M., Callicott, J.H. et al. (2003). The BDNF val66met polymorphism affects activity-dependent secretion of BDNF and human memory and hippocampal function. *Cell*, 112, 257–269.

FDA (2005). *Antidepressant Use in Children, Adolescents and Adults* [online] Avalabel. http://www.fda.gov/cder/drug/antidepressants/default.htm (accessed March 2012).

Ferrell, P.B., Jr. and McLeod, H.L. (2008). Carbamazepine, HLA-B*1502 and risk of Stevens–Johnson syndrome and toxic epidermal necrolysis: US FDA recommendations. *Pharmacogenomics*, 9, 1543–1546.

Fournier, J.C., DeRubeis, R.J., Hollon, S.D. *et al.* (2010). Antidepressant drug effects and depression severity: A patient-level meta-analysis. *Journal of the American Medical Association*, 303, 47–53.

Garriock, H.A., Kraft, J.B., Shyn, S.I. *et al.* (2010). A genomewide association study of citalopram response in major depressive disorder. *Biological Psychiatry*, 67, 133–138.

Grof, P., Duffy, A., Cavazzoni, P. *et al.* (2002). Is response to prophylactic lithium a familial trait? *The Journal of Clinical Psychiatry*, 63, 942–947.

Gupta, A., Schulze, T.G., Nagarajan, V. *et al.* (2011). Interaction networks of lithium and valproate molecular targets reveal a striking enrichment of apoptosis functional clusters and neurotrophin signaling. *Pharmacogenomics Journal*, 12, 328–341.

Horstmann, S., Lucae, S., Menke, A. *et al.* (2010). Polymorphisms in GRIK4, HTR2A, and FKBP5 show interactive effects in predicting remission to antidepressant treatment. *Neuropsychopharmacology*, 35, 727–740.

Hu, X.Z., Rush, A.J., Charney, D. *et al.* (2007). Association between a functional serotonin transporter promoter polymorphism and citalopram treatment in adult outpatients with major depression. *Archives of General Psychiatry*, 64, 783–792.

Huezo-Diaz, P., Perroud, N., Spencer, E. *et al.* (2011). CYP2C19 genotype predicts steady state escitalopram concentration in GENDEP. *Journal of Psychopharmacology*, 26, 398–407.

Ioannidis, J.P., Trikalinos, T.A., Ntzani, E.E., and Contopoulos-Ioannidis, D.G. (2003). Genetic associations in large versus small studies: An empirical assessment. *Lancet*, 361, 567–571.

Ising, M., Lucae, S., Binder, E.B. *et al.* (2009). A genomewide association study points to multiple loci that predict antidepressant drug treatment outcome in depression. *Archives of General Psychiatry*, 66, 966–975.

Khan, A., Detke, M., Khan, S.R., and Mallinckrodt, C. (2003). Placebo response and antidepressant clinical trial outcome. *Journal of Nervous and Mental Disease*, 191, 211–218.

Kirchheiner, J., Lorch, R., Lebedeva, E. *et al.* (2008). Genetic variants in FKBP5 affecting response to antidepressant drug treatment. *Pharmacogenomics*, 9, 841–846.

Kishi, T., Fukuo, Y., Yoshimura, R. *et al.* (2010). Pharmacogenetic study of serotonin 6 receptor gene with antidepressant response in major depressive disorder in the Japanese population. *Human Psychopharmacology*, 25, 481–486.

Kraft, J.B., Peters, E.J., Slager, S.L. *et al.* (2007). Analysis of association between the serotonin transporter and antidepressant response in a large clinical sample. *Biological Psychiatry*, 61, 734–742.

Laje, G., Paddock, S., Manji, H. *et al.* (2007). Genetic markers of suicidal ideation emerging during citalopram treatment of major depression. *American Journal of Psychiatry*, 164, 1530–1538.

Laje, G., Allen, A.S., Akula, N. *et al.* (2009). Genome-wide association study of suicidal ideation emerging during citalopram treatment of depressed outpatients. *Pharmacogenetics and Genomics*, 19, 666–674.

Lekman, M., Laje, G., Charney, D. *et al.* (2008). The FKBP5-gene in depression and treatment response: An association study in the Sequenced Treatment Alternatives to Relieve Depression (STAR*D) cohort. *Biological Psychiatry*, 63, 1103–1110.

Lin, K.M., Chiu, Y.F., Tsai, I.J. *et al.* (2011). ABCB1 gene polymorphisms are associated with the severity of major depressive disorder and its response to escitalopram treatment. *Pharmacogenetics and Genomics*, 21, 163–170.

Lohoff, F.W., Aquino, T.D., Narasimhan, S. *et al.* (2011). Serotonin receptor 2A (HTR2A) gene polymorphism predicts treatment response to venlafaxine XR in generalized anxiety disorder. *Pharmacogenomics Journal*, e-pub ahead of print, doi: 10.1038/tpj.2011.47.

Lucae, S., Ising, M., Horstmann, S. *et al.* (2010). HTR2A gene variation is involved in antidepressant treatment response. *European Neuropsychopharmacology*, 20, 65–68.

Lupski, J.R., Belmont, J.W., Boerwinkle, E., and Gibbs, R.A. (2011). Clan genomics and the complex architecture of human disease. *Cell*, 147, 32–43.

McCarthy, M.J., Leckband, S.G., and Kelsoe, J.R. (2010). Pharmacogenetics of lithium response in bipolar disorder. *Pharmacogenomics*, 11, 1439–1465.

McCormack, M., Alfirevic, A., Bourgeois, S. *et al.* (2011). HLA-A*3101 and carbamazepine-induced hypersensitivity reactions in Europeans. *New England Journal of Medicine*, 364, 1134–1143.

McMahon, F.J., Buervenich, S., Charney, D. *et al.* (2006). Variation in the gene encoding the serotonin 2A receptor is associated with outcome of antidepressant treatment. *American Journal of Human Genetics*, 78, 804–814.

Menke, A., Lucae, S., Kloiber, S. *et al.* (2008). Genetic markers within glutamate receptors associated with antidepressant treatment-emergent suicidal ideation. *American Journal of Psychiatry*, 165, 917–918.

Menke, A., Domschke, K., Czamara, D. *et al.* (2012). Genome-wide association study of antidepressant treatment-emergent suicidal ideation. *Neuropsychopharmacology*, 37, 797–807.

Mrazek, D.A., Rush, A.J., Biernacka, J.M. *et al.* (2008). SLC6A4 variation and citalopram response. *American Journal of Medical Genetics, B*: 150B, 341–351.

Mrazek, D.A., Biernacka, J.M., O'Kane, D.J. *et al.* (2011). CYP2C19 variation and citalopram response. *Pharmacogenetics and Genomics*, 21, 1–9.

Murphy, G.M., Jr., Hollander, S.B., Rodrigues, H.E., Kremer, C., and Schatzberg, A.F. (2004). Effects of the serotonin transporter gene promoter polymorphism on mirtazapine and paroxetine efficacy and adverse events in geriatric major depression. *Archives of General Psychiatry*, 61, 1163–1169.

Nair, A. and Vaidya, V.A. (2006). Cyclic AMP response element binding protein and brain-derived neurotrophic factor: Molecules that modulate our mood? *Journal of Bioscience*, 31, 423–434.

Paddock, S., Laje, G., Charney, D. *et al.* (2007). Association of GRIK4 with outcome of antidepressant treatment in the STAR*D cohort. *American Journal of Psychiatry*, 164, 1181–1188.

Perlis, R.H., Fijal, B., Dharia, S., Heinloth, A.N., and Houston, J.P. (2010). Failure to replicate genetic associations with antidepressant treatment response in duloxetine-treated patients. *Biological Psychiatry*, 67, 1110–1113.

Perlis, R. H., Purcell, S., Fava, M. *et al.* (2007). Association between treatment-emergent suicidal ideation with citalopram and polymorphisms near cyclic adenosine monophosphate response element binding protein in the STAR*D study. *Archives of General Psychiatry*, 64, 689–697.

Perlis, R.H., Dennehy, E.B., Miklowitz, D.J. *et al.* (2009a). Retrospective age at onset of bipolar disorder and outcome during two-year follow-up: Results from the STEP-BD study. *Bipolar Disorders*, 11, 391–400.

Perlis, R.H., Laje, G., Smoller, J.W. *et al.* (2009b). Genetic and clinical predictors of sexual dysfunction in citalopram-treated depressed patients. *Neuropsychopharmacology*, 34, 1819–1828.

Perroud, N., Aitchison, K.J., Uher, R. *et al.* (2009). Genetic predictors of increase in suicidal ideation during antidepressant treatment in the GENDEP project. *Neuropsychopharmacology*, 34, 2517–2528.

Perroud, N., Uher, R., Ng, M.Y. *et al.* (2012). Genome-wide association study of increasing suicidal ideation during antidepressant treatment in the GENDEP project. *Pharmacogenomics Journal*, 12, 68–77.

Peters, E.J., Slager, S.L., Kraft, J.B. *et al.* (2008). Pharmacokinetic genes do not influence response or

tolerance to citalopram in the STAR*D sample. *PLoS One*, 3, e1872.

Popkie, A.P., Zeidner, L.C., Albrecht, A.M. *et al.* (2010). Phosphatidylinositol 3-kinase (PI3K) signaling via glycogen synthase kinase-3 (Gsk-3) regulates DNA methylation of imprinted loci. *Journal of Biological Chemistry*, 285, 41337–41347.

Rasmussen, H.B. and Werge, T.M. (2007). Novel procedure for genotyping of the human serotonin transporter gene-linked polymorphic region (5-HTTLPR) – a region with a high level of allele diversity. *Psychiatric Genetics*, 17, 287–291.

Saarelainen, T., Hendolin, P., Lucas, G. *et al.* (2003). Activation of the TrkB neurotrophin receptor is induced by antidepressant drugs and is required for antidepressant-induced behavioral effects. *Journal of Neuroscience*, 23, 349–357.

Sarginson, J.E., Lazzeroni, L.C., Ryan, H.S. *et al.* (2010). ABCB1 (MDR1) polymorphisms and antidepressant response in geriatric depression. *Pharmacogenetics and Genomics*, 20, 467–475.

Schulze, T.G., Alda, M., Adli, M. *et al.* (2010). The International Consortium on Lithium Genetics (ConLiGen): An initiative by the NIMH and IGSLI to study the genetic basis of response to lithium treatment. *Neuropsychobiology*, 62, 72–78.

Serretti, A., Kato, M., and Kennedy, J.L. (2008). Pharmacogenetic studies in depression: A proposal for methodologic guidelines. *Pharmacogenomics Journal*, 8, 90–100.

Serretti, A., Kato, M., De, R.D., and Kinoshita, T. (2007). Meta-analysis of serotonin transporter gene promoter polymorphism (5-HTTLPR) association with selective serotonin reuptake inhibitor efficacy in depressed patients. *Molecular Psychiatry*, 12, 247–257.

Smith, D.J., Evans, R., and Craddock, N. (2010). Predicting response to lithium in bipolar disorder: A critical review of pharmacogenetic studies. *Journal of Mental Health*, 19, 142–156. Original Article: Willeie, M.J.V., Smith, G., Day, R.K. *et al.* (2009). Polymorphisms in the SLC6A4 and HTRZA genes influence treatment outcome following antidepresssant therapy. *The Pharmacogenetics Journal*, 9, 61–70.

Squassina, A., Piccardi, P., Del Zompo, M. *et al.* (2010). NRG1 and BDNF genes in schizophrenia: An association study in an Italian case-control sample. *Psychiatry Research*, 176, 82–84.

Taylor, M.J., Sen, S., and Bhagwagar, Z. (2010). Antidepressant response and the serotonin transporter gene-linked polymorphic region. *Biological Psychiatry*, 68, 536–543.

Teranishi, K.S., Slager, S.L., Garriock, H. *et al.* (2007). Variants in PDE11A and PDE1A are not associated with citalopram response. *Molecular Psychiatry*, 12, 1061–1063.

Trivedi, M.H., Rush, A.J., Wisniewski, S.R. *et al.* (2006). Evaluation of outcomes with citalopram for depression using measurement-based care in STAR*D: Implications for clinical practice. *American Journal of Psychiatry*, 163, 28–40.

Uhr, M., Tontsch, A., Namendorf, C. *et al.* (2008). Polymorphisms in the drug transporter gene ABCB1 predict antidepressant treatment response in depression. *Neuron*, 57, 203–209.

Uher, R., Huezo-Diaz, P., Perroud, N. *et al.* (2009). Genetic predictors of response to antidepressants in the GENDEP project. *Pharmacogenomics Journal*, 9, 225–233.

Uher, R., Perroud, N., Ng, M.Y. *et al.* (2010). Genome-wide pharmacogenetics of antidepressant response in the GENDEP project. *American Journal of Psychiatry*, 167, 555–564.

Ventriglia, M., Bocchio Chiavetto, L., Benussi, L. *et al.* (2002). Association between the BDNF 196 A/G

polymorphism and sporadic Alzheimer's disease. *Molecular Psychiatry*, 7, 136–137.

Wadelius, M., Chen, L.Y., Downes, K. *et al.* (2005). Common VKORC1 and GGCX polymorphisms associated with warfarin dose. *Pharmacogenomics Journal*, 5, 262–270.

Winner, J.G., Goebert, D., Matsu, C., and Mrazek, D.A. (2010). Training in psychiatric genomics during residency: A new challenge. *Academic Psychiatry*, 34, 115–118.

Wong, M.L., Whelan, F., Deloukas, P. *et al.* (2006). Phosphodiesterase genes are associated with susceptibility to major depression and antidepressant treatment response. *Proceedings of the National Academy of Sciences USA*, 103, 15124–15129.

Yu, Z., Ono, C., Sora, I., and Tomita, H. (2011). Effect of chronic lithium treatment on gene expression profile in mouse microglia and brain dendritic cells. *Japanese Journal of Psychopharmacology*, 31, 101–102.

Chapter

30

Electrophysiological predictors of clinical response to antidepressants

Gerard E. Bruder, Craig E. Tenke, and Jürgen Kayser

Introduction

Electrophysiological measures are important tools for assessing brain function, which have found their main clinical use in neurology for assessment of epilepsy, coma, and integrity of neural circuits. They include the electroencephalogram (EEG) and evoked or event-related potentials (ERPs). Electrophysiological measures have the advantage of being noninvasive (i.e., no radioactive or magnetic field exposure), economical, and provide continuous millisecond by millisecond recordings of brain electrical activity. Although their temporal resolution far exceeds that of fMRI and PET, electrophysiological measures have more limited spatial resolution. The use of electrophysiological measures in psychiatry has largely been in the research domain or to measure and document seizure activity during electroconvulsive therapy (ECT). Promising findings reviewed in this chapter point to a potential wider clinical role in mood disorders and their treatment.

The EEG is typically measured using electrodes placed on the scalp (e.g., using an elastic electrode cap). Clinical EEG recordings have traditionally been used in psychiatry to screen for brain disorders or to monitor cortical activity during ECT or sleep. A description of the neural basis of the EEG and applications of clinical EEG is available in the textbook by Niedermeyer and Lopes Da Silva (2004). Digital recording and analysis of EEG has made possible quantitative measures, which usually involves doing a Fast Fourier Transform (FFT) to measure the amplitude (power) of the EEG spectrum within frequency ranges in the classical delta (1–4 Hz), theta (4–8 Hz), alpha (8–13 Hz), and beta (13–30 Hz) bands. Although quantitative EEG measures may have some value for the differential diagnosis of dementia and depression (Hughes and John,

1999), their clinical utility as an adjunct for psychiatric diagnosis has not been demonstrated. There is, however, a growing literature suggesting that quantitative EEG measures in the theta and alpha bands, obtained prior to treatment of mood disorders or soon after it begins, predict subsequent clinical response to antidepressants.

Evoked potentials or ERPs, which are averaged EEG epochs time-locked to the onset of stimuli or other discrete events, have been widely used in clinical and research settings. For instance, evoked potentials that occur in the first 12 ms after onset of clicks are used clinically to assess hearing in infants and for assessment of brainstem lesions and multiple sclerosis. ERPs occurring about 100–200 ms after the onset of tones (N1 and P2 potentials) are indicative of early sensory or attentional processing, and later ERPs (most notably the P3 potential) provide neurophysiologic correlates of cognitive processing. Numerous studies have found a reduction of the P3 potential in depressed patients, which is consistent with evidence of cognitive deficits in depression (see Bruder et al. 2012b for a review of ERP studies in depression). This reduction is greatest in patients having a melancholic or psychotic depression, and clinical improvement is accompanied by an increase in P3 amplitude. P3 reduction is not, however, specific to depression, but occurs in other neuropsychiatric disorders, and is therefore not of value for diagnostic purposes. A more promising finding from a clinical perspective has been evidence of a relationship between early auditory ERPs (N1, P2) and response to SSRI antidepressants.

This chapter focuses selectively on EEG and ERP findings that have raised hopes for the application of electrophysiological measures as clinical aids for selecting the most appropriate course of treatment for depressed patients.

Clinical Handbook for the Management of Mood Disorders, ed. J. John Mann, Patrick J. McGrath, and Steven P. Roose. Published by Cambridge University Press. © Cambridge University Press 2013.

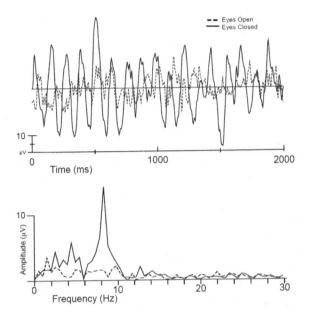

Figure 30.1 Top portion shows alpha oscillations during 2 s sample of eyes-closed EEG (solid lines) and alpha blocking with eyes open (dashed lines). Bottom portion gives the corresponding frequency spectra with peak amplitude in alpha band in the eyes-closed condition, but not in the eyes-open condition

EEG alpha power and asymmetry in depression

The alpha rhythm (8–13 Hz) is an oscillatory EEG pattern that is maximal when an individual is in a relaxed, wakeful state with eyes closed, but is reduced (blocked) when the individual becomes alert or when visual processes are engaged by opening the eyes (see Figure 30.1). Alpha is thought of as an idling rhythm and is inversely related to cortical activity as indexed by PET measures of cerebral blood flow (Cook *et al.* 1998) or fMRI measures of blood oxygen level dependent (BOLD) signal in posterior regions where alpha is greatest (Feige *et al.* 2005). EEG alpha has been used as an index of relative cortical deactivation, with greater alpha (less activation) being found in depressed patients than healthy controls (Polack and Schneider 1990, Debener *et al.* 2000, Grin-Yatsenko *et al.* 2010, Kemp *et al.* 2010). Studies have also reported abnormal, regional hemispheric asymmetry of alpha, with depressed patients showing relatively less activity over left frontal (Gotlib *et al.* 1998, Henriques and Davidson, 1991, Kemp *et al.* 2010, Stewart *et al.* 2010) or right parietal regions (Bruder *et al.* 1997, Reid *et al.* 1998, Kentgen *et al.* 2000, Kemp *et al.* 2010, Stewart *et al.* 2011).

There have, however, been conflicting alpha asymmetry findings for depressed patients. Thibodeau *et al.* (2006) reviewed findings of frontal alpha asymmetry in depression and examined a number of possible moderator variables that could help account for inconsistent findings. The moderate effect size for frontal alpha asymmetry differences between depressed patients and controls (Cohen's $d = 0.54$) and low test–retest reliability of frontal alpha asymmetry in depressed patients (Debener *et al.* 2000) might also contribute to inconsistencies. While Debener *et al.* found higher test–retest reliability of parietal asymmetry in depressed patients, their study and others (e.g., Schaffer *et al.* 1983, Henriques and Davidson, 1991) did not find reduced right parietal activity in depression. Heller *et al.* (1995) suggested that this may be due to the opposing effects of anxiety or anxious arousal on parietal alpha asymmetry. They hypothesized that anxious arousal, such as seen in panic disorders, is associated with right parietotemporal hyperactivation, whereas depression is associated with right parietotemporal hypoactivation. Evidence supporting this hypothesis was found in a study examining the effect of co-morbidity of depressive and anxiety disorders on regional alpha asymmetry (Bruder *et al.* 1997). Patients having a major depressive disorder (MDD) and co-morbid anxiety disorders, primarily panic disorder or social phobia, showed an alpha asymmetry indicative of relatively greater activity over right frontal and parietal sites, whereas patients having "pure" major depression showed less activity over right than left parietal sites, but no frontal asymmetry. Thus, co-morbidity of depressive and anxiety disorders may heighten abnormal frontal alpha asymmetry favoring right over left hemisphere activity, but counteract the tendency for depressed patients to show reduced right posterior activity.

As part of a multi-generational study (Weissman *et al.* 2005), offspring of depressed probands who are at risk for depressive disorders also showed an EEG alpha asymmetry indicative of relatively less right posterior activity (Bruder *et al.* 2005). Moreover, anatomical MRI findings in this high-risk study revealed an association between risk for depression and cortical thinning across lateral parietal, posterior temporal, and frontal cortices of the right hemisphere (Peterson *et al.* 2009). Alpha power was found to correlate inversely with cortical thickness among individuals in this study, particularly over the right posterior region, suggesting that EEG evidence of reduced cortical activity was associated with increased cortical thinning (Bruder *et al.* 2012a). Self-ratings of depression severity in adults having MDD also correlated inversely with PET measures of glucose metabolism in dorsal areas of prefrontal, occipital, temporal, and parietal cortex, predominantly in the right hemisphere (Milak *et al.* 2010).

In summary, abnormalities of EEG alpha power and asymmetry have been found in depressed patients. Although there have been conflicting findings, alpha asymmetry abnormalities may represent biological traits associated with risk for developing a depressive disorder.

Alpha power and asymmetry in antidepressant responders and nonresponders

A likely contributor to inconsistent alpha asymmetry findings is the clinical and biological heterogeneity of depression. One approach for reducing this heterogeneity is to divide a sample of unmedicated depressed patients into those who subsequently respond favorably to a specific antidepressant and those who do not respond. Patients who respond to an antidepressant with a specific mode of action, e.g., an SSRI, may share a common biological substrate not present in nonresponders. Findings of pretreatment EEG differences between responders and nonresponders also have potential clinical utility for identifying predictors of clinical response, and personalizing treatment for individual patients.

There is good agreement that pretreatment EEG alpha may differentiate patients who respond to antidepressants from those who do not. Ulrich *et al.* (1986) found increased alpha over occipital sites in depressed patients who eventually responded to amitriptyline and they suggested that there are two sub-types of depression having different pathophysiology and response to antidepressants. Prichep *et al.* (1993), using cluster analysis of neurometric EEG features to identify clusters of patients having distinctive EEG profiles, similarly found evidence for two sub-groups among 27 patients having an obsessive compulsive disorder. About 82% of members of a sub-group with increased relative alpha power in frontal and temporal regions responded well to an SSRI antidepressant, while only 20% of members

of a second cluster with increased relative theta power were treatment responders. This neurometric technique was also used by Suffin and Emory (1995) in a study of 54 depressed patients treated with an SSRI or tricyclic antidepressant and they found 86% of treatment responders to have increased relative alpha power in frontal and occipital regions. In a study of 29 patients having a unipolar depressive disorder who were treated with a tricyclic antidepressant, Knott *et al.* (1996) found that greater pretreatment relative alpha in responders than nonresponders did not reach a conventional level of statistical significance. In summary, these early studies suggest that increased alpha power, which was originally identified in depressed patients by Polack and Schneider (1990), is particularly likely to be found among depressed patients who respond to an SSRI or tricyclic antidepressant, although the predictive value of this measure needs further study to make it clinically useful.

We confirmed the value of alpha power in predicting clinical response to an SSRI and also found a difference in posterior alpha asymmetry between responders and nonresponders (Bruder *et al.* 2008). Resting EEG scalp potentials were measured from 28 electrodes (nose reference) in 18 depressed patients before and after about 12 weeks of treatment with fluoxetine, and 18 matched healthy controls were also tested. Treatment responders (n = 11) showed significantly greater alpha power when compared to nonresponders (n = 7) and controls, with the largest difference at occipital sites where alpha was greatest. As shown in Figure 30.2, greater alpha power in responders than nonresponders was present across the pretreatment and post-treatment sessions and there was no change in alpha following SSRI treatment. Test–retest reliability of alpha power was high at both frontal and posterior sites ($r \geq 0.92$), and is comparable to that found for healthy adults for retest periods over 1 year (Smit *et al.* 2005). Elevated alpha has also been found in depressed patients in a euthymic state (Pollock and Schneider, 1989), which suggests that it reflects a stable biological trait in patients who respond favorably to antidepressants. Responders in our study also differed from nonresponders in alpha asymmetry at occipital sites, with responders having greater alpha (less activation) over right than left occipital cortex and nonresponders showing the opposite asymmetry. The difference in alpha asymmetry between SSRI responders and nonresponders is consistent with our prior findings (Bruder *et al.* 2001),

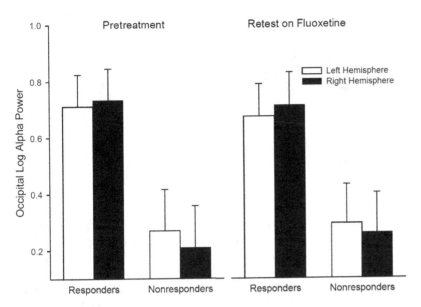

Figure 30.2 Mean log alpha power (± SEM) over right and left posterior sites for responders and nonresponders before treatment and after 12 weeks of treatment on fluoxetine (nose-referenced EEG)

and did not change following treatment (Figure 30.2). Test–retest correlations were, however, lower for alpha asymmetry ($r \geq 0.63$ at frontal and posterior sites), which agrees with the lower test–retest correlations of alpha asymmetry for healthy adults (Hagemann *et al.* 2005). To examine the value of alpha power and asymmetry at occipital sites for predicting clinical response to an SSRI, the average scores for healthy adults were used as a cutoff for dividing patients into those who were greater or less than normal. Both alpha power and asymmetry showed reasonable positive predictive value (i.e., response rate $\geq 72\%$ for patients predicted to be responders), but lower negative predictive value (i.e., nonresponse rate $\geq 56\%$ for those predicted to be nonresponders).

A recent study (Tenke *et al.* 2011) was designed to confirm the predictive value of EEG alpha amplitude and asymmetry in an independent sample of patients. Resting EEG was recorded with eyes open and eyes closed prior to treatment in a larger sample of depressed patients ($n = 41$) and in healthy controls ($n = 41$). This study extended our prior study in several respects. First, the predictive value of alpha was examined, not only for patients receiving an SSRI, but also those receiving dual treatment with an SSRI plus a noradrenaline/dopamine reuptake inhibitor (NDRI; bupropion) or a serotonin/noradrenaline reuptake inhibitor (SNRI; duloxetine or venlafaxine). Second, to improve the spatial resolution of spectral topographies, EEG was recorded from a dense array of

recording electrodes (67 channels) and current source density (CSD) measures were used to reduce volume conduction from distal sites, and avoid problems associated with selection of a reference electrode. CSD measures are reference-free and indicate the strength of underlying radial current generators (Tenke and Kayser, 2005, Kayser and Tenke, 2006, Nunez and Srinivasan, 2006). Third, CSD measures were quantified using frequency principal components analysis (fPCA) to derive empirically based frequency bands. Two factors corresponding to alpha sub-bands were examined: a high-alpha factor (10.5 Hz peak) and a low alpha/theta (9.0 Hz peak), which included activity usually classified as theta (4–8 Hz).

Significant differences in alpha were found between treatment responders ($n = 28$) and nonresponders ($n = 13$), which were particularly evident for the eyes-closed condition and were seen broadly across the low and high alpha bands. Figure 30.3a shows the condition-dependent topographies, averaged across the low and high alpha bands, for patients who responded to treatment (Clinical Global Improvement rating of "much or very much improved"), nonresponders, and healthy controls. Nonresponders had significantly less alpha than responders and controls over posterior regions where alpha was maximal for each group. The marked difference in alpha between responders and nonresponders was present for patients who received monotherapy with an SSRI or dual therapy (Figure 30.3b). It was seen at

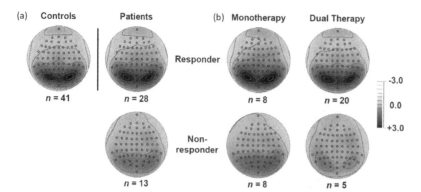

Figure 30.3 (a) Condition-dependent (eyes closed minus eyes open) topographies of alpha (average across high and low alpha factors using CSD-transformed EEG) for controls, responders, and nonresponders. Alpha reduction in nonresponders is most marked over posterior sites (bottom of maps). (b) Corresponding condition-dependent alpha topographies for patients treated with a monotherapy or dual therapy. Both nonresponder groups showed marked alpha reduction compared to responders

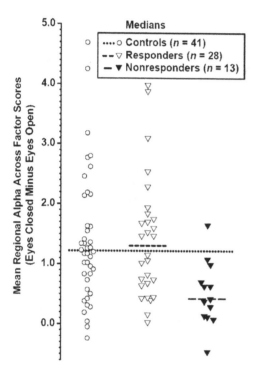

Figure 30.4 Scatterplot of mean condition-dependent (eyes closed minus eyes open) posterior alpha for controls, responders, and nonresponders. The median for healthy controls (dotted line) was used as the cutoff for predicting treatment response

posterior sites over each hemisphere and there was no significant difference in alpha asymmetry among groups.

The value of alpha for predicting treatment response was examined by classifying patients as to whether they had alpha above the median for healthy controls (predicted to be responders) or less than the median for controls (predicted to be nonresponders). As shown in Figure 30.4, alpha had high positive predictive value of 93.3, with 14 of 15 patients with alpha above median for controls responding to

treatment, and high specificity of 92.3 (percentage of nonresponders predicted to be nonresponders), but lower sensitivity of 50.0 (percentage of responders who were predicted to be responders) and negative predictive value of 46.1. Thus, depressed patients who have prominent condition-dependent posterior alpha are predicted to respond to serotonergic antidepressants with a high degree of confidence. However, half of responders had alpha below the median for controls and were not predicted to be responders. It is possible that a sizable portion of these responders may be placebo responders or not true drug responders. There was also no evidence for differential prediction of clinical response to an SSRI as opposed to dual therapy targeting both serotonergic and nonserotonergic neurotransmitters. Moreover, the early studies reviewed above suggest that alpha is not specific for predicting response to an SSRI but also predicts response to a tricyclic antidepressant. In contrast to our prior study (Bruder *et al.* 2008), treatment response was not related to hemispheric asymmetry of alpha. Although the reason for this lack of replication is unknown, alpha asymmetry is less reliable than alpha power and may be more influenced by a number of moderator variables.

In summary, EEG alpha power may be useful when it predicts good response because about 90% of those cases with prominent alpha will indeed be medication responders, but about half of cases where poor response is predicted will actually turn out to be medication responders.

Theta power in responders and nonresponders

Several studies have reported EEG differences between antidepressant responders and nonresponders in the lower frequency theta band (4–8 Hz). Knott *et al.* (1996) examined the value of both pretreatment EEG and changes during acute treatment for predicting response to imipramine. EEG from 16 electrodes was recorded in 29 depressed patients with eyes closed while they pressed a hand-held button. Response to 4 weeks of treatment with imipramine was defined as greater than 50% reduction in HAM-D ratings. Relative theta power, i.e., the percentage of theta relative to total absolute power across the delta, theta, alpha, and beta bands, was less in responders than nonresponders prior to treatment, and responders exhibited greater increase in theta 3 hours after the first dose and after 2 weeks. Thus, both baseline theta and changes during acute treatment may predict subsequent clinical response. In studies using the neurometric EEG approach (Prichep *et al.* 1993, Suffin and Emory, 1995), patients having either a depressive disorder or OCD with increased relative theta power were nonresponders to antidepressants. More recently, Iosifescu *et al.* (2009) measured EEG from frontotemporal electrodes (F7, F8, A1, A2 referenced to Fpz) in depressed patients before and 1 week after starting 8 weeks of open treatment with an SSRI or venlafaxine. EEG was recorded while patients counted backwards from 1000 to keep them alert. Relative theta power was lower in treatment responders (HAM-D reduction ≥ 50%) than in nonresponders and predicted response with an accuracy of 63% (64% sensitivity and 62% specificity). Relative theta after 1 week of treatment showed comparable differences between responders and nonresponders. The unusual electrode montage used by Iosifescu *et al.* (2009), however, makes their findings difficult to interpret and compare with conventional EEG studies. In contrast to the above studies, Spronk *et al.* (2011) reported that *higher* absolute theta power at a midline frontal site (Fz; linked-mastoids reference) predicted improvement of depression after 8 weeks of open-label treatment with predominantly SSRI or SNRI antidepressants. Among 25 patients having a MDD, higher theta power was associated with greater decrease in HAM-D ratings.

In summary, there is conflicting evidence as to whether lower or higher theta power predicts favorable response to an SSRI or other antidepressants. Differences in study procedures (e.g., EEG recording site or reference electrode), medication, or EEG analyses (e.g., use of relative as opposed to absolute theta measures) might account for the difference in theta findings. The use of low resolution electromagnetic tomography analysis (LORETA; Pascual-Marqui *et al.* 1994) to measure theta activity localized to the region of the anterior cingulate cortex (ACC) has yielded more consistent predictions of treatment response.

LORETA measures of theta and treatment response

Mayberg *et al.* (1997) were first to report that PET measures of glucose metabolism in the rostral ACC predicted response to antidepressants. Pizzagalli (2011) recently reviewed studies using neuroimaging (PET, fMRI, SPECT) or EEG measures supporting the hypothesis that increased activity or metabolism in rostral ACC predicts response to a wide range of treatments for depression (including various antidepressants, sleep deprivation, and rTMS). EEG evidence comes from three studies using the LORETA source localization technique to infer the distributed current density attributable by this model to the region of the rACC. Pizzagalli *et al.* (2001) recorded resting EEG from 28 electrodes in 18 patients having MDD and 18 healthy controls. Clinical response to 4–6 months of treatment with nortriptyline was assessed using the Beck Depression Inventory (BDI). Although most patients (n = 16) were responders, they used a median split of BDI ratings to compare patients having better or worse responses to treatment. Patients having a better response showed greater theta (6.5–8.0 Hz; eyes closed), localized by LORETA to the region of the rACC. There was a significant correlation between pretreatment theta activity and BDI scores, consistent with the hypothesis that higher rACC activity is associated with greater improvement in depression. A subsequent study by Mulert *et al.* (2007) compared resting EEG (eyes closed) of responders (≥50% reduction in HAM-D) and nonresponders to 4 weeks of treatment with either citalopram (seven responders, four nonresponders) or reboxetine (three responders, six nonresponders). Responders had greater pretreatment theta activity (6.5–8 Hz), again localized by LORETA to the rACC when compared to nonresponders, and there was a significant correlation of pretreatment theta and improvement in depression after treatment, which replicates the findings of Pizzagalli *et al.* (2001). In the first double-blind, placebo-controlled study to examine the relationship of pretreatment EEG and antidepressant response, Korb *et al.* (2009) used LORETA to localize theta activity (4–7 Hz) to the same rACC region as specified by Pizzagalli *et al.* (2001).

Patients who responded to either fluoxetine or venlafaxine (n = 22) had greater theta than nonresponders (n = 15), whereas there was no difference between placebo responders (n = 15) and nonresponders. They report that rACC activity had a sensitivity of 64% and a specificity of 67% for predicting treatment response. Results for midline frontal theta using conventional EEG measures were consistent with the above findings, but did not attain statistical significance.

In summary, EEG measures of resting midline frontal theta, as quantified by LORETA, predict clinical response to a variety of antidepressants, but the sensitivity and specificity may be too modest at this stage to be of use to the clinician. Also, the LORETA technique involves a number of assumptions, and localizing generators underlying surface potentials is difficult and subject to problems because an infinite number of theoretical generators in the brain can yield the same scalp potentials.

Cordance and antidepressant response index

Cook *et al.* (1999) did not find pretreatment differences in relative theta power between responders and nonresponders to 8 weeks of treatment with fluoxetine, but did find differences in "cordance," a measure that integrates relative and absolute theta power. Although the biophysical basis of cordance is not clear (Tenke and Kayser, 2005), it has been reported to be positively correlated with PET scan measures of cortical perfusion (Leuchter *et al.* 1999). Based on pretreatment measures of EEG cordance, 24 patients were retrospectively divided into concordant or discordant groups depending on the type of association of absolute and relative power in theta band. Patients in the concordant group had a robust response to fluoxetine, while the discordant group did not. In a subsequent study (Cook *et al.* 2002), they did not, however, find a significant difference in the numeral value of cordance at baseline between responders (HAM-D ≤ 10 after 8 weeks of treatment) and nonresponders to fluoxetine or venlafaxine. They did find a difference in the change of prefrontal cordance after 1 week of treatment, with responders showing a decrease in cordance not seen in nonresponders or placebo responders. The decreased cordance predicted treatment response with a sensitivity of 69% and a specificity of 75%. Independent studies (Bares *et al.* 2007, 2008) replicated

this relationship between early change in prefrontal cordance and clinical response in patients treated with a variety of antidepressants. Also, among 18 treatment-resistant depressed patients who received 4 weeks of treatment with bupropion, responders (≥50% reduction of MADRS) differed from nonresponders in showing higher baseline prefrontal cordance and a decrease after 1 week of treatment (Bares *et al.* 2010). In summary, studies indicate that a reduction of cordance after 1 week of treatment is predictive of clinical response to SSRI, SNRI, or NDRI antidepressants. However, there is less agreement as to the value of pretreatment cordance for predicting treatment response, and the biophysical basis of cordance remains unknown.

Iosifescu *et al.* (2009) developed an Antidepressant Treatment Response (ATR) index, which is derived from a weighted combination of theta and alpha power at baseline and after 1 week of treatment, and is recorded from frontotemporal sites (Fpz, FT7, FT8, A1, A2). Initial studies showed promise of the ATR index for predicting response to an SSRI or venlafaxine, but not placebo (Iosifescu *et al.* 2009, Hunter *et al.* 2011). In a multi-site BRITE-MD study (Leuchter *et al.* 2009a, b), resting EEG of patients having a MDD was recorded at baseline and after 1 week of treatment with escitalopram. Patients were then randomly assigned to continue on escitalopram, switch to bupropion, or a combination of both antidepressants. Responders to escitalopram had significantly higher ATR index than nonresponders. A threshold value selected to maximize classification of responders and nonresponders predicted response with 58% sensitivity and 91% specificity. These values are comparable to those reported by Tenke *et al.* (2011) for alpha power, and indicate that about half of escitalopram responders would not be predicted to be responders. Escitalopram responders differed from bupropion responders in ATR index. Patients with high ATR values were more likely to respond to escitalopram than those with low ATR values, whereas patients with low ATR values who were switched to bupropion were more likely to respond to bupropion alone than those who remained on escitalopram. While the ATR index may be of value in differential prediction of response to antidepressants, a replication using the same ATR algorithm and threshold cutoff is needed to independently confirm these findings. Also, since the ATR index is based on an atypical electrode montage and a complex proprietary algorithm, it is not clear what high or low ATR scores mean or what their relation is to standard EEG measures of theta or alpha. While the limited electrode montage may be an advantage for clinical applications, the frontal sites (Fpz, FT7, FT8) could be problematic because they are near known sources of artifact from the eyes and facial musculature.

In summary, both cordance and ATR measures, based on baseline EEG and changes after 1 week of treatment, show promise as predictors of clinical response to SSRI, SNRI, or NDRI antidepressants. These are, however, complex proprietary measures, which makes it difficult to independently replicate findings and limits their value as biomarkers of treatment response.

Clinical and theoretical implications of EEG findings in depression

Resting EEG measures of alpha and theta have potential for clinical application because they are relatively easy to measure and have high reliability. Two measures obtained *before* treatment appear to have particular potential for predicting response to antidepressants. Alpha over posterior brain regions and midline frontal theta, localized using LORETA inverse model to rACC, were found to be greater in antidepressant responders than nonresponders. Pizzagalli (2011) suggested that the default mode network may explain the relation between resting rACC activity and treatment response. Activity in the default network, including rACC, posterior cingulate, lateral parietal and temporal cortex, and other structures, is greatest during resting states and decreases during processing of external stimuli. Pizzagalli postulated that increased resting rACC activity in treatment responders may be linked to introspective or adaptive self-referential processing, which is thought to involve the default network. This hypothesis also suggests a possible interpretation of increased resting alpha in responders. Greater alpha in responders is more evident with eyes closed than open and is maximal over the lateral parietal cortex (Tenke *et al.* 2011), which is a region in the default mode network. Moreover, Tenke *et al.* found a trend for the difference between responders and nonresponders to be greatest for a "low alpha factor" having a bandwidth that overlaps the theta band typically used in LORETA measures of rACC activity (6.5–8 Hz). Increased resting alpha and rACC theta activity in treatment responders could

therefore both be related to default network activity. A study is now underway to test this hypothesis.

A reduction of frontal cordance in theta band after 1 week of antidepressant treatment also appears to be predictive of antidepressant response. Most recently, an ATR index, which uses theta and alpha measures at baseline and after 1 week of antidepressant, was developed to maximize predictions. The ATR index shows promise not only for predicting response to an SSRI or SNRI, but also differential response to an SSRI vs. an NDRI antidepressant. A critical problem with the ATR index is that its algorithm and cutoffs were derived in studies to maximize predictions and it is therefore in need of independent replications. Further research using multiple EEG measures, i.e., resting alpha, theta, LORETA rACC, cordance, ATR index, is needed to evaluate their relative merits as predictors of treatment response, and to determine how these measures relate to each other. Of greatest clinical value would be measures that can make differential prediction of response to antidepressants with different mechanisms of action or to nonpharmacological treatments, e.g., cognitive behavior therapy.

Auditory-evoked potentials and treatment response

Although there are reports relating amplitude of auditory ERPs (e.g., N1, P2) and antidepressant response (Vandoolaeghe *et al.* 1998, Spronk *et al.* 2011, Bruder *et al.* 2012b), the most replicated finding has come for loudness dependency of auditory-evoked potentials (LDAEPs). Increases in tone intensity from 60 to 100 dB are known to result in a monotonic increase in N1 and P2 amplitude. In an ongoing study, we measured ERPs of 64 healthy adults to 1000 Hz tones (40 ms duration; 1600–2000 ms ISI) while they sat quietly with eyes fixed on a cross. Figure 30.5 shows CSD waveforms with peaks corresponding to N1 and P2 potentials. N1, which was maximal at central electrode sites (C3/C4), showed the expected monotonic increase in amplitude with increasing tone intensity from 60 to 100 dB.

Hegerl and Juckel (1993) reviewed evidence suggesting that the slope of the function relating tone loudness and N1–P2 amplitude provides a noninvasive indicator of serotonergic activity. They suggest that serotonergic neurons originating in the dorsal raphé modulate activity in auditory cortex by providing a stable, tonic-firing rate. Low-firing rate of serotonergic

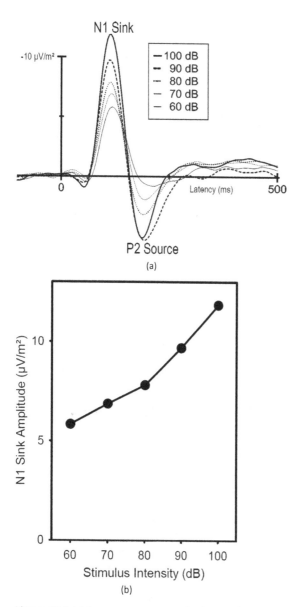

Figure 30.5 (a) Average current source density waveforms at C3/C4 sites for 64 healthy adults showing peaks corresponding to N1 and P2. (b) LDAEP function showing increase in tangential N1 with increasing intensity of tones

neurons is related to strong loudness dependency, i.e., a steep increase in N1–P1 amplitude with increasing tone loudness, whereas high-firing rate is related to weak loudness dependency, i.e., only a small increase in N1–P2 with increasing loudness (Hegerl *et al.* 2001). Direct evidence of an inverse relationship between serotonergic activity in dorsal raphé and LDAEP was found in recordings from primary auditory cortex of cats (Juckel *et al.* 1999). A recent review did not find

strong support for the utility of LDAEP as a marker of central serotonin function, but did conclude that LDAEP shows promise as a predictor of response to antidepressants (O'Neill *et al.* 2008a).

Depressed patients with low serotonergic activity, as evidenced by pronounced LDAEP prior to treatment, respond better to SSRI antidepressants compared to patients with high serotonergic activity, as evidenced by weak LDAEP (Paige *et al.* 1994, Gallinat *et al.* 2000, Hegerl *et al.* 2001, Lee *et al.* 2005). Although Paige *et al.* (1995) found a similar difference in LDAEP between a small sample of responders (n = 4) vs. nonresponders (n = 4) to an NDRI antidepressant (bupropion), more recent studies suggest that LDAEP may differentially predict clinical response to serotonergic and noradrenergic antidepressants. Among 16 patients having MDD, stronger pretreatment loudness dependency of N1 was associated with greater reduction in depression following 3–4 weeks of treatment with the SSRI citalopram (Linka *et al.* 2004). In contrast, in 14 patients tested before treatment with a noradrenaline reuptake inhibitor (NRI), reboxetine, *smaller* loudness dependency of N1 was associated with greater improvement in depression (Linka *et al.* 2005). In the first study in which depressed patients were randomly assigned to treatment with either the citalopram or reboxetine, Mulert *et al.* (2007) measured LDAEP for current source distribution (latency window of 60–240 ms) localized using LORETA to the primary auditory cortex. SSRI responders (n = 7) showed significantly stronger LDAEP when compared to SSRI nonresponders (n = 4), whereas NRI responders (n = 3) did not differ significantly from NRI nonresponders (n = 6). Stronger LDAEP was associated with greater improvement in depression following citalopram treatment ($r = 0.71$), whereas weaker LDAEP tended to be associated with greater improvement in depression following reboxetine treatment ($r = -0.54$).

LDAEP has not, however, been associated with the clinical state of depressed patients or levels of central serotonergic neurotransmission. Thus, studies have *not* found a change in LDAEP following treatment with SSRI or other antidepressants (Paige *et al.* 1994, 1995, Gallinat *et al.* 2000, Linka *et al.* 2009). Also, acute enhancement of serotonin levels by administrating an SSRI to healthy adults has not yielded consistent findings. A double-blind, placebo-controlled study in healthy adults found a decrease in LDAEP during acute administration of a single dose of the SSRI citalopram, which would be expected given an increase in central serotonin (Nathan *et al.* 2006). This change in LDAEP was not replicated in a study in which healthy females received an intravenous infusion of citalopram or placebo (Uhl *et al.* 2006) or in a study measuring LDAEP during administration of sertraline or escitalopram (Guille *et al.* 2008). Moreover, acute depletion of serotonin in healthy adults during administration of tryptophan did not alter LDAEP (O'Neill *et al.* 2008b, Dierks *et al.* 1999, Debener *et al.* 2002).

In summary, studies have found that LDAEP predicts clinical response to an SSRI and may be of value for differential prediction of response to an NRI antidepressant. LDAEP may represent a stable trait that is not readily altered by changes in clinical state or serotonin levels.

Conclusions

The findings reviewed in this chapter indicate that certain electrophysiologic measures of brain activity are predictive of clinical response to antidepressants. The most promising EEG predictors are resting alpha and theta with eyes closed. Specific measures derived from the EEG, e.g., current source density, cordance, LORETA, ATR index, have all shown value as predictors, but further research is needed to compare their physiological interpretability and relative merits. Auditory-evoked potential measures of loudness dependency (LDAEP) also predict response to antidepressants. A variety of different measures have been used to assess LDAEP, including scalp potentials, LORETA, and dipole source analyses of N1, P2, or N1–P2 differences. To the extent that EEG and LDAEP measures are uncorrelated and separately predictive, their combined use could lead to models with clinically relevant predictive power.

Several points are important for developing and evaluating electrophysiological predictors of treatment response. First, measures that are stable indicators with good test–retest reliability are likely to be of most value for predicting clinical response in individual patients. Resting EEG alpha and theta potentials have demonstrated high test–retest reliability (generally ≥0.90) in both healthy adults (Smit *et al.* 2005) and depressed patients (Allen *et al.* 2004, Bruder *et al.* 2008). Auditory-evoked potentials likewise have high reliability in healthy adults and depressed patients. Hensch *et al.* (2008), in reviewing prior studies and their study of 166

healthy adults, reported reliability of the LDAEP function to generally be in the region of 0.70 to 0.80. Comparable LDAEP reliabilities have been found for depressed patients retested after antidepressant treatment (Gallinat *et al.* 2000, Linka *et al.* 2009). Less is known, however, about the test–retest reliability of EEG cordance, LORETA rACC, or ATR measures, which are derived from alpha and theta scalp potentials. Assessment of reliability is particularly important for measures, such as the ATR index, that depend on assessing changes in EEG between baseline and 1 week of treatment. Second, to be of clinical value, measures should have high sensitivity and specificity for predicting treatment response. The EEG measures reviewed in this chapter generally had only moderate sensitivity (50 to 70% of responders correctly predicted to be responders) and somewhat higher specificity (60 to 90% of nonresponders correctly predicted to be nonresponders). Studies of LDAEP have generally reported average data for small samples with no indication of sensitivity or specificity. Third, the typical procedure for determining the predictive value of a measure is to choose a cutoff or threshold value above which patients are predicted to be responders. There are quantitative procedures available to aid in choosing a cutoff, e.g., receiver operating characteristic (ROC) curve, but there is no guarantee that a cutoff established in a given study will work for a new sample of patients. Another approach is to use the median value for healthy adults as the cutoff, for example, with the rationale being that responders have higher than normal values and nonresponders lower values (e.g., Tenke *et al.* 2011). Normative data for a large sample of healthy adults could then be developed for a given population. Fourth, electrophysiologic measures would ideally be predictive of treatment response to a specific class of antidepressants with known pharmacologic profile, e.g., SSRI, and be of value for differential prediction of treatment response. Some EEG measures, e.g., LORETA measures of rACC activity, are clearly not specific, but predict response to a wide range of treatments. There are, however, preliminary indications that the ATR index and LDAEP may differentially predict response to SSRI and NDRI or NRI antidepressants. Fifth, ease of application of predictors in clinical settings is a critical issue. For instance, it would not be efficient to use a large array of electrodes in the clinic. It should, however, be possible to record resting EEG or LDAEP with a small number of well-targeted electrodes and use computer algorithms to predict response for individual patients. A multi-site BRITE-MD study (Leuchter *et al.* 2009b) using the ATR index was conducted with this in mind, but further studies to replicate their findings are needed before it could be recommended for clinical use.

Lastly, it may be too optimistic to expect any one electrophysiologic measure to provide sufficiently accurate predictions of clinical response. A recent review by Alhaj *et al.* (2011) referred to evidence that combining various EEG or ERP measures may improve prediction. For instance, Mulert *et al.* (2007) suggested that a resting EEG measure, using LORETA to infer rACC activity, might be useful as a first step to identify a sub-group of depressed patients who are *not* likely to respond to standard antidepressants and, if response is likely, LDAEP could be used for differential prediction of response to a SSRI or NRI antidepressant. Moreover, neuropsychological tests and neuroimaging measures (PET or MRI scans) may also contribute to prediction of treatment response. An ongoing NIMH initiative "Establishing Moderators and Biosignatures of Antidepressant Response in Clinical Care" (EMBARC; M. Trivedi and P. McGrath, Principal Investigators) is a multi-site, double-blind study examining the value of resting EEG, LDAEP, MRI (structural and functional), and neurocognitive tests for differential prediction of clinical response to an SSRI vs. placebo. The aim is to begin to evaluate whether combined use of the best predictors in these domains could ultimately serve as biosignatures for personalizing antidepressant treatment.

References

Alhaj, H., Wisniewski, G., McAllister-Williams, R.H. *et al.* (2011). The use of the EEG in measuring therapeutic drug action: Focus on depression and antidepressants. *Journal of Psychopharmacology*, 25, 1175–1191.

Allen, J.J., Urry, H.L., Hitt, S.K. *et al.* (2004). The stability of resting frontal electroencephalographic asymmetry in depression. *Psychophysiology*, 41, 269–280.

Bares, M., Brunosvsky, M., Kopecek, M. *et al.* (2007). Changes in QEEG prefrontal cordance as a predictor of response to antidepressants in patients with treatment resistant depressive disorder: A pilot study. *Journal of Psychiatric Research*, 41, 319–325.

Bares, M., Brunovsky, M., Kopecek, M. *et al.* (2008). Early reduction in prefrontal theta QEEG cordance value predicts response to venlafaxine treatment in patients with resistant depressive disorder. *European Psychiatry*, 23, 350–355.

Bares, M., Brunovsky, M. Novak, T. *et al.* (2010). The change of prefrontal QEEG theta cordance as a predictor of response to bupropion treatment in patients who had failed to respond to previous antidepressant treatments. *European Neuropsychopharmacology*, 20, 459–466.

Bruder, G.E., Stewart, J.W., Tenke, C.E. *et al.* (2001). Electroencephalographic and perceptual asymmetry differences between responders and nonresponders to an SSRI antidepressant. *Biological Psychiatry*, 48, 416–425.

Bruder, G.E., Tenke, C.E., Warner, V. *et al.* (2005). Electroencephalographic measures of regional hemispheric activity in offspring at risk for depressive disorders. *Biological Psychiatry*, 57, 328–335.

Bruder, G.E., Sedoruk, J.P., Stewart, J.W. *et al.* (2008). Electroencephalographic alpha measures predict therapeutic response to a selective serotonin reuptake inhibitor antidepressant: Pre- and post-treatment findings. *Biological Psychiatry*, 63, 1171–1177.

Bruder, G.E., Bansal, R., Tenke, C.E. *et al.* (2012a). Relationship of resting EEG with anatomical MRI measures in individuals at high and low risk for depression. *Human Brain Mapping*, 33, 1325–1333.

Bruder, G.E., Kayser, J., and Tenke, C.E. (2012b). Event-related brain potentials in depression: Clinical, cognitive and neurophysiologic implications. In Luck, S.J. and Kappenman, E.S., eds., *The Oxford Handbook of Event-Related Potential Components*. New York: Oxford University Press, 563–592.

Cook, I.A., O'Hara, R., Uijtdehaage, S.H. *et al.* (1998). Assessing the accuracy of topographic EEG mapping for determining local brain function. *Electroencephalography and Clinical Neurophysiology*, 107, 408–414.

Cook, I.A., Leuchter, A.F., Witte, E. *et al.* (1999). Neurophysiologic predictors of treatment response to fluoxetine in major depression. *Psychiatry Research*, 85, 263–273.

Cook, I.A., Leuchter, A.F., Morgan, M. *et al.* (2002). Early changes in prefrontal activity characterize clinical responders to antidepressants. *Neuropsychopharmacology*, 27, 120–131.

Debener, S., Beauducel, A., Nessler, D. *et al.* (2000). Is resting anterior EEG alpha asymmetry a trait marker for depression? Findings for healthy adults and clinically depressed patients. *Neuropsychobiology*, 41, 31–37.

Debener, S., Strobel, A., Kurschner, K. *et al.* (2002). Is auditory evoked potential augmenting/reducing affected by acute tryptophan depletion? *Biological Psychology*, 59, 121–133.

Dierks, T., Barta, S., Demisch, L. *et al.* (1999). Intensity dependence of auditory evoked potentials (AEPs) as biological marker for cerebral serotonin levels: Effects of tryptophan depletion in healthy subjects. *Psychopharmacology*, 146, 101–107.

Feige, B., Scheffler, K., Esposito, F. *et al.* (2005). Cortical and subcortical correlates of electroencephalographic alpha rhythm modulation. *Journal of Neurophysiology*, 93, 2864–2872.

Gallinat, J., Bottlender, R., Juckel, G. *et al.* (2000). The loudness dependency of the auditory evoked N1/P2-component as a predictor of the acute SSRI response in depression. *Psychopharmacology*, 148, 404–411.

Gotlib, I.H., Ranganath, C., and Rosenfeld, P. (1998). Frontal EEG alpha asymmetry, depression, and cognitive functioning. *Cognition and Emotion*, 12, 449–478.

Grin-Yatsenko, V.A., Baas, I., Ponomarev, V.A. *et al.* (2010). Independent component approach to the analysis of EEG recordings at early stages of depressive disorders. *Clinical Neurophysiology*, 121, 281–289.

Guille, V., Croft, R.J., O'Neill, B.V. *et al.* (2008). An examination of acute changes in serotonergic neurotransmission using the loudness dependence measure of auditory cortex evoked activity: Effects of citalopram, escitalopram and sertraline. *Human Psychopharmacology*, 23, 231–241.

Hagemann, D., Hewig, J., Seifert, J. *et al.* (2005). The latent state-trait structure of resting EEG asymmetry: Replication and extension. *Psychophysiology*, 42, 740–752.

Heller, W., Etienne, M.A., and Miller, G.A. (1995). Patterns of perceptual asymmetry in depression and anxiety: Implications for neuropsychological models of emotion and psychopathology. *Journal of Abnormal Psychology*, 104, 327–333.

Henriques, J.B. and Davidson, R.J. (1991). Left frontal hypoactivation in depression. *Journal of Abnormal Psychology*, 100, 535–545.

Hensch, T., Herold, U., Diers, K. *et al.* (2008). Reliability of intensity dependence of auditory-evoked potentials. *Clinical Neurophysiology*, 119, 224–236.

Hergerl, U. and Juckel, G. (1993). Intensity dependence of auditory evoked potentials as an indicator of central serotonergic neurotransmission: A new hypothesis. *Biological Psychiatry*, 33, 173–187.

Hergerl, U., Gallinat, J., and Juckel, G. (2001). Event-related potentials: do they reflect central serotonergic neurotransmission and do they predict clinical response to serotonin agonists? *Journal of Affective Disorders*, 62, 93–100.

Hughes, J.R. and John, E.R. (1999). Conventional and quantitative electroencephalography in psychiatry. *Journal of Neuropsychiatry and Clinical Neurosciences*, 11, 190–207.

Hunter, A.M., Cook, I.A., Greenwald, S.D. *et al.* (2011). The antidepressant treatment response index and treatment outcomes in a placebo-controlled trial of fluoxetine. *Journal of Clinical Neurophysiology*, 28, 478–482.

Iosifescu, D.V., Greenwald, S., Devlin, P. *et al.* (2009). Frontal EEG predictors of treatment outcome in major depressive disorder. *European Neuropsychopharmacology*, 19, 772–777.

Juckel, G., Hegerl, U., Molnar, M. *et al.* (1999). Auditory evoked potentials reflect serotonergic neuronal activity: a study in behaving cats administered drugs acting on 5-HT1A autoreceptors in the dorsal raphe nucleus. *Neuropsychopharmacology*, 21, 710–716.

Kayser, J. and Tenke, C.E. (2006). Principal components analysis of Laplacian waveforms as a generic method for identifying ERP generator patterns: I. Evaluation with auditory oddball tasks. *Clinical Neurophysiology*, 117, 348–368.

Kayser, J. and Tenke, C.E. (2010). In search of the Rosetta Stone for scalp EEG: Converging on reference-free techniques. *Clinical Neurophysiology*, 121, 1973–1975.

Kemp, A.H., Griffiths, K., and Felmingham, K.L. (2010). Disorder specificity despite comorbidity: Resting EEG alpha asymmetry in major depressive disorder and post-traumatic stress disorder. *Biological Psychology*, 85, 350–354.

Kentgen, L.M., Tenke, C.E., Pine, D.S. *et al.* (2000). Electroencephalographic asymmetries in adolescents with major depression: Influence of comorbidity with anxiety disorders. *Journal of Abnormal Psychology*, 109, 797–802.

Knott, V.J., Telner, J.I., Lapierre, Y.D. *et al.* (1996). Quantitative EEG in the prediction of antidepressant response to imipramine. *Journal of Affective Disorders*, 39, 175–184.

Korb, A.S., Hunter, A.M., Cook, I.A. *et al.* (2009). Rostral anterior cingulate cortex theta current density and response to antidepressants and placebo in major depression. *Clinical Neurophysiology*, 120, 1313–1319.

Lee, T.W., Yu, Y.W., and Chen, T.J. (2005). Loudness dependence of the auditory evoked potential and response to antidepressants in Chinese patients with major depression. *Journal of Psychiatry and Neuroscience*, 30, 202–205.

Leuchter, A.F., Uitjdehaage, S.H., Cook, I.A. *et al.* (1999). Relationship between brain electrical activity and cortical perfusion in normal subjects. *Psychiatry Research*, 90, 125–140.

Leuchter, A.F., Cook, I.A., Gilmer, W.S. *et al.* (2009a). Effectiveness of a quantitative electroencephalographic biomarker for predicting differential response or remission with escitalopram and bupropion in major depressive disorder. *Psychiatry Research*, 169, 132–138.

Leuchter, A.F., Cook, I.A., Marangell, L.B. *et al.* (2009b). Comparative effectiveness of biomarkers and clinical indicators for predicting outcomes of SSRI treatment in Major Depressive Disorder: Results of the BRITE-MD study. *Psychiatry Research*, 169, 124–131.

Linka, T., Müller, B.W., Bender, S. *et al.* (2004). The intensity dependence of the auditory evoked N1 component as a predictor of response to citalopram treatment in patients with major depression. *Neuroscience Letters*, 367, 375–378.

Linka, T., Müller, B.W., Bender, S. *et al.* (2005). The intensity dependence of auditory evoked ERP components predicts responsiveness to reboxetine treatment in major depression. *Pharmacopsychiatry*, 38, 139–143.

Linka, T., Sartory, G., Wiltfang, J. *et al.* (2009). Treatment effects of serotonergic and noradrenergic antidepressants on the intensity dependence of auditory ERP components in major depression. *Neuroscience Letters*, 463, 26–30.

Mayberg, H.S., Brannan, S.K., Mahurin, R.K. *et al.* (1997). Cingulate function in depression: A potential predictor of treatment response. *NeuroReport*, 8, 1057–1061.

Milak, M.S., Keilp, J., Parsey, R.V. *et al.* (2010). Regional brain metabolic correlates of self-reported depression severity contrasted with clinical ratings. *Journal of Affective Disorders*, 126, 113–124.

Mulert, C., Juckel, G., Brunnmeier, M. *et al.* (2007). Prediction of treatment response in major depression: Integration of concepts. *Journal of Affective Disorders*, 98, 215–225.

Nathan, P.J., Segrave, R., Phan, K.L. *et al.* (2006). Direct evidence that acutely enhancing serotonin with the selective serotonin reuptake inhibitor citalopram modulates the loudness dependence of the auditory evoked potential (LDAEP) marker of central serotonin function. *Human Psychopharmacology*, 21, 47–52.

Niedermeyer, E. and Lopes Da Silva, F.H. (2004). *Electroencephalography: Basic Principles, Clinical Applications and Related Fields, Fifth Edition.* Philadelphia: Lippincott, Williams and Wilkins.

Nunez, P.L. and Srinivasan, R. (2006). *Electric Fields of the Brain: The Neurophysics of EEG.* New York: Oxford University Press.

O'Neill, B.V., Croft, R.J., and Nathan, P.J. (2008a). The loudness dependence of the auditory evoked potential (LDAEP) as an in vivo biomarker of central serotonergic function in humans: Rationale, evaluation and review of findings. *Human Psychopharmacology*, 23, 355–370.

O'Neill, B.V., Guille, V., Croft, R.J. *et al.* (2008b). Effects of selective and combined serotonin and dopamine depletion on the loudness dependence of the auditory evoked potential (LDAEP) in humans. *Human Psychopharmacology*, 23, 301–312.

Paige, S.R., Fitzpatrick, D.F., Kline, J.P. *et al.* (1994). Event-related potential amplitude/intensity slopes predict response to antidepressants. *Neuropsychobiology*, 30, 197–201.

Paige, S.R., Hendricks, S.E., Fitzpatrick, D.F. *et al.* (1995). Amplitude/intensity functions of auditory event-related potentials predict responsiveness to bupropion in major depressive disorder. *Psychopharmacology Bulletin*, 31, 243–248.

Pascual-Marqui, R.D., Michel, C.M., and Lehmann, D. (1994). Low resolution electromagnetic tomography: A new method for localizing electrical activity in the brain. *International Journal of Psychophysiololgy*, 18, 49–65.

Peterson, B.S., Warner, V., Bansal, R. *et al.* (2009). Cortical thinning in persons at increased familial risk for major depression. *Proceedings of the National Academy of Science USA*, 106, 6273–6278.

Pizzagalli, D.A. (2011). Frontocingulate dysfunction in depression: toward biomarkers of treatment response. *Neuropsychopharmacology*, 36, 183–206.

Pizzagalli, D., Pascual-Marqui, R.D., Nitschke, J.B. *et al.* (2001). Anterior cingulate activity as a predictor of degree of treatment response in major depression: Evidence from brain electrical tomography analysis. *American Journal of Psychiatry*, 158, 405–415.

Pollock, V.E. and Schneider, L.S. (1989). Topographic electroencephalographic alpha in recovered depressed elderly. *Journal of Abnormal Psychology*, 98, 268–273.

Pollock, V.E. and Schneider, L.S. (1990). Topographic quantitative EEG in elderly subjects with major depression. *Psychophysiology*, 27, 438–444.

Prichep, L.S., Mas, F., Hollander, E. *et al.* (1993). Quantitative electroencephalographic subtyping of obsessive-compulsive disorder. *Psychiatry Research*, 50, 25–32.

Reid, S.A., Duke, L.M., and Allen, J.J.B. (1998). Resting frontal electroencephalographic asymmetry in depression: Inconsistencies suggest the need to identify mediating factors. *Psychophysiology*, 35, 389–404.

Schaffer, C.E., Davidson, R.J., and Saron, C. (1983). Frontal and parietal electroencephalogram asymmetry in depressed and nondepressed subjects. *Biological Psychiatry*, 18, 753–762.

Smit, D.J., Posthuma, D., Boomsma, D.I. *et al.* (2005). Heritability of background EEG across the power spectrum. *Psychophysiology*, 42, 691–697.

Spronk, D., Arns, M., Barnett, K.J. *et al.* (2011). An investigation of EEG, genetic and cognitive markers of treatment response to antidepressant medication in patients with major depressive disorder: A pilot study. *Journal of Affective Disorders*, 128, 41–48.

Stewart, J.L., Bismark, A.W., Towers, D.N. *et al.* (2010). Resting frontal EEG asymmetry as an endophenotype for depression risk: Sex-specific patterns of frontal brain asymmetry. *Journal of Abnormal Psychology*, 119, 502–512.

Stewart, J.L., Towers, D.N., Coan, J.A. *et al.* (2011). The oft-neglected role of parietal EEG asymmetry and risk for major depressive disorder. *Psychophysiology*, 48, 82–95.

Suffin, S.C. and Emory, W.H. (1995). Neurometric subgroups in attentional and affective disorders and their association with pharmacotherapeutic outcome. *Clinical Electroencephalography*, 26, 76–83.

Tenke, C.E. and Kayser, J. (2005). Reference-free quantification of EEG spectra: combining current source density (CSD) and frequency principal components analysis (fPCA). *Clinical Neurophysiology*, 116, 2826–2846.

Tenke, C.E., Kayser, J., Manna, C.G. *et al.* (2011). Current source density measures of electroencephalographic alpha predict antidepressant treatment response. *Biological Psychiatry*, 70, 388–394.

Thibodeau, R., Jorgensen, R.S., and Kim, S. (2006). Depression, anxiety, and resting frontal EEG asymmetry: A meta-analytic review. *Journal of Abnormal Psychology*, 115, 715–729.

Uhl, I., Gorynia, I., Gallinat, J. *et al.* (2006). Is the loudness dependence of auditory evoked potentials modulated by the selective serotonin reuptake inhibitor citalopram in healthy subjects? *Human Psychopharmacology*, 21, 463–471.

Ulrich, G., Renfordt, E., and Frick, K. (1986). The topographical distribution of alpha-activity in the resting EEG of endogenous-depressive inpatients with and without clinical-response to pharmacotherapy. *Pharmacopsychiatry*, 19, 272–273.

Vandoolaeghe, E., van Hunsel, F., Nuyten, D. *et al.* (1998). Auditory event related potentials in major depression: Prolonged P300 latency and increased P200 amplitude. *Journal of Affective Disorders*, 48, 105–113.

Weissman, M.M., Wickramaratne, P., Nomura, Y. *et al.* (2005). Families at high and low risk for depression: A 3-generation study. *Archives of General Psychiatry*, 62, 29–36.

Chapter

31

Prospects for the future of mood disorder therapeutics

Patrick J. McGrath, Steven P. Roose, and J. John Mann

Overview

In the foreseeable future, mood disorders will assume increasing importance in the future of medicine. Because of their high prevalence, early onset, and frequently chronic courses, unipolar mood disorders have been shown to be associated with functional impairment comparable to chronic medical disorders like diabetes and coronary artery disease (Wells *et al.* 1989). Further, the co-morbidity of depression with chronic diseases causes more ill health compared to depression alone, a chronic disease alone, or even the combination of other chronic diseases. (Moussavi *et al.* 2007). For example, a major determinant of outcome post-myocardial infarction, post-stroke, and in epilepsy is the presence of untreated major depression. These characteristics make mood disorders one of the most disabling illnesses worldwide, in both developed and underdeveloped nations. According to the World Health Organization, unipolar depression will become the second ranked condition in terms of impairment in quality of life and ability to function productively in society in the year 2020 (Murray and Lopez, 1996). The high level of impairment and consequent societal burden appear likely to trigger increasing attention to enhancement of therapeutics to mitigate this illness burden at a personal level and as a societal burden. That effort will influence health care policy and strategies as governments in all developed nations seek to rationalize their health care expenditures. Clearly, concentrating research resources on highly disabling disorders is an important strategy, as they in turn, in addition to benefiting patients, will have the largest effect on the secondary costs of impaired social and vocational functioning. The realization of the amount of economic and societal burden caused by psychiatric disorders in general, and mood disorders

in particular, is likely to have an impact on the organization and funding of health care in all societies. Just as econometric analyses have shown that health care systems actually save money by offering treatment for attention deficit hyperactivity disorder (ADHD) (Matza *et al.* 2005), so may similar analyses point to a cost advantage to providing excellent treatment for mood disorder (Von Korff *et al.* 1998), which is not what is typically provided today, even in the most comprehensive health care systems.

Clinical

DSM-5

Publication of the fifth edition of the *Diagnostic and Statistical Manual of Mental Disorders* (DSM-5) in May 2013 will undoubtedly change, and hopefully improve, the diagnostic framework for mood disorders in incremental, but meaningful ways, as summarized in Chapter 2. The DSM is already seeking to replace conventional descriptive syndromal diagnoses with diagnoses based on a more fundamental understanding of pathogenesis and pathobiology, and this trend seems likely to continue and accelerate with deepening neuroscience research.

Encouraging progress has been made in utilizing our current nosology, which might be expected to continue. Evidence has been presented showing that the correct diagnosis of bipolar disorder is now being made considerably earlier in the course of illness, potentially leading to earlier intervention with appropriate treatments rather than no treatment or the prescription of antidepressants without mood stabilizers, which has too often been the norm heretofore (Post *et al.*).

A bold and different approach to nosology is contained in the National Institute of Mental Health (NIMH) Strategic Plan, which calls for the development of new ways of classifying psychopathology based on dimensions of observable behavior and neurobiological measures. As promulgated by the NIMH, The Research Domain Criteria project (RDoC) has been launched by NIMH to implement this strategy (Insel *et al.* 2010), "In brief, the effort is to define basic dimensions of functioning (such as fear circuitry or working memory) to be studied across multiple units of analysis, from genes to neural circuits to behaviors, cutting across disorders as traditionally defined. The intent is to translate rapid progress in basic neurobiological and behavioral research to an improved integrative understanding of psychopathology and the development of new and/or optimally matched treatments for mental disorders." The large overlap of the population with unipolar mood disorders with those of anxiety, somatoform, and eating disorders, provides a perfect example of how it appears that there may be neurobiologic mechanisms shared to some degree by all of these disorders. Moreover, understanding of the pathophysiology of one set of disorders may shed light on all of the disorders. NIMH established an internal working group in the Spring of 2009 to put in place both a structure and a process toward this end. The various domains of functioning are being defined by an ongoing series of consensus workshops with input from the research community. NIMH has stated that it anticipates that "research grants employing this new experimental classification will represent an increasingly large share of its funding portfolio in coming years."

Controversial extent of bipolar spectrum disorders

There has been considerable controversy over the correct diagnosis for patients with mood disorder associated with the lifetime occurrence of hypomanic symptoms which are sub-threshold for the diagnosis of bipolar disorder. Epidemiologic studies by Angst and others (Angst *et al.* 2002, 2003) have shown that the occurrence of hypomanic symptoms is much more common than has been recognized previously. There has been considerable attention paid to this, arguing that such patients actually have a form of bipolar disorder and are inappropriately treated with antidepressant medication, which is thought to exacerbate mood cycling (Akiskal and Mallya, 1987, Akiskal, 2002, 2007) Further, it is argued that since bipolar depression has been shown in placebo-controlled studies to be unresponsive to some antidepressant medications, antidepressants may prove to be helpful in this population. Some others have gone further, declaring that a "bipolar spectrum" exists which includes depressed patients who might never have had hypomanic symptoms, but share some of the features of bipolar depression such as early onset, chronic illness, bipolar family history, and reversed vegetative symptoms such as overeating and oversleeping. That position may be too extreme, but certainly further research on how to classify those with sub-clinical manic symptoms might yield both a clearer nosologic categorization for these patients, and also a more evidence-based therapeutic algorithm.

Biologic

Genetic

Extrapolating from the accelerating accumulation of knowledge of the biology of psychiatric disorders over the last several decades, it is easy to anticipate that this trend will continue and that such knowledge will define the molecular pathways whereby genes and environment affect the risk for mood disorders. While twin and adoption studies have incontrovertibly shown that a genetic diathesis is a major risk factor for the development of mood disorders, currently there are no genes that have been validated at the genome-wide level and shown to be etiologic in depression. From studies of the genetics of other complex disorders, that is disorders which do not show simple Mendelian inheritance patterns, it has become clear that such disorders are generally not associated with a few genes of large effect, but rather caused by many alleles of small to moderate effect, or by many rare variants of large effect. This means that the discovery of such genes by genome-wide association studies requires sample sizes in the multiple tens of thousands, far beyond what has been collected so far for psychiatric disorder. Such large studies are better able to both detect rare genes of large effect, and gene–gene or gene–environment interactions, which smaller sample studies conducted to date have not been able to, that survive the threshold for the false discovery rate. Finally, epigenetic studies of factors affecting the expression of candidate genes, that may mediate environmental effects, and can sometimes be transmissible across generations, are needed to complement genotyping in order to more fully explain the basis for the genetic predisposition to mood disorder and environmental influences which interact with the genome.

Progress in understanding the genetics of depression will have enormous consequences for the diagnosis, classification, and treatment of these disorders. Identification of the relevant genetic alleles will ultimately allow testing of those apparently at risk for mood disorder to identify those with an actual risk increase. This will potentially allow screening for risk and the development of either early intervention strategies, or better, of preventative treatment strategies. If there are multiple, possible genetic, signatures of predisposition, as seems likely, this would have the consequence of there being multiple pathophysiologic pathways to the final common syndrome. This would imply that individual pathways might be associated with differing responses to treatment and that treatment for the individual could be prescribed using this knowledge, a paradigm called "personalized medicine."

Proteomics

Proteomics is the study of proteins as they are expressed in tissues, in terms of identity, heterogeneity, and amounts. For example, there are hundreds of proteins in the human plasma that have known roles in intercellular signaling and in the regulation of tissue and organ function. While it is in its infancy, such studies have already characterized a protein expression signature of central nervous system disorders like Alzheimer's disease (Ray *et al.* 2007), and there are early efforts to apply such strategies to mood disorders. Modern proteomic methods, allowing the simultaneous quantification of many hundreds of circulating proteins in a small sample of human blood, clearly will be an attractive area for research in the quest to be able to distinguish individual disease sub-groups, select specific treatments, and monitor treatment response.

Imaging

As summarized by Lan and Parsey in Chapter 28 on imaging, it is clear that technical advances in neuroimaging techniques are to be expected and may provide data to allow the prediction of response to

treatment. In addition to new radiotracers for PET neuroimaging, new tasks are being devised for functional neuroimaging to capture information clinically relevant to the selection and prescription of treatment. While PET imaging has been hampered by the need for specific radiotracers for targets of interest, the fact that it provides absolute values of brain activity and more importantly, data on levels of key proteins such as neurotransmitter receptors, transporters, enzymes, and even signal transduction components, means it can characterize neurotransmitter systems. PET can also assist drug development by measuring occupancy by new candidate drugs of their target site to allow estimation of the optimal dose range.

The discovery that high risk of major depression is associated with areas of cortical thinning demonstrable on simple structural MRI imaging across multiple generations has been a landmark discovery (Peterson *et al.* 2009). This means that in the future, individuals at high risk can potentially be identified early in life, the factors provoking the emergence of syndromal depression identified, and for the first time, strategies developed to prevent the emergence of syndromal mood disorder. Such early intervention could lead to mitigation of the enormous societal burden of mood disorders and the associated morbidity and mortality they cause.

Electrophysiology

Electrophysiology, primarily in the form of electroencephalographic recording, has shown significant promise in application to mood disorder therapeutics (see Chapter 30). Traditional EEG recording, quantitated with modern techniques like evoked-potential and low-resolution EEG tomographic analysis (Pizzagalli *et al.* 2006), holds the promise in the near future of conveniently and noninvasively estimating activation in both cortical and sub-cortical neural circuits. This may allow the development of a biosignature of response to antidepressant therapy, perhaps allowing differentiation of patients likely to respond to specific pharmacotherapies or to specific psychotherapeutic treatment.

Multi-dimensional clinical neuroscience

An important intellectual trend is that the rapidly advancing technologies of quantitative neuroscience and molecular genetics appear to be making enormous progress toward demonstrating a neurobiological substrate of mood disorder. One example of this trend is the recent awarding of a collaborative NIMH grant entitled "Establishing Moderators/Mediators for a Biosignature of Antidepressant Response in Clinical Care" – EMBARC (http://embarc.utsouthwestern.edu). This project is a pioneering study to use the most sophisticated techniques of MRI imaging, quantitative electrophysiology, together with behavioral testing and clinical phenotyping to begin to develop a biological signature to enable antidepressant medication treatment to be prescribed based on biological testing prior to treatment. The hope is that this will be a first step toward biologically based mood disorder therapeutics, personalized to the individual patient.

Glutamatergic medications

The past five decades have brought multiple classes of antidepressant medications of differing pharmacologic profile, but all having in common their potential to alter neurotransmission by monoamines and/or indolamines. The two most recent such classes introduced have been the selective serotonin reuptake inhibitors (SSRI) and the selective serotonin-norepinephrine reuptake inhibitors (SNRI). The best available research suggests that while these medications are clearly effective, they have a large overlap in spectrum of efficacy with previous classes of antidepressants. Further, despite vigorous treatment with these and other available antidepressants, only barely more than half of patients beginning treatment for major depressive disorder achieve remission, despite lengthy treatment and multiple medication trials.

The serendipitous observation that ketamine, a glutamatergic medication that is an NMDA receptor antagonist and long used in higher dosage as an anesthetic, is rapidly effective even in erstwhile treatment-resistant depression, creates the possibility of more effective and fast-acting pharmacotherapy targeting the glutamatergic system (Zarate et al. 2006; see Chapter 27). Currently research is underway to explore the mechanism of ketamine antidepressant action in depression, and pharmaceutical companies have developed a series of compounds that are designed to have effects similar to ketamine, that is, antagonism of the NMDA receptor, without the potentially toxic psychotomimetic effects of ketamine and

without the necessity to administer the medication parenterally. Should these efforts be successful, they might result in antidepressant medications which are effective for patients unresponsive to typical uptake inhibitor antidepressant medication and which have a rapid onset of action like ketamine (Mathew et al. 2005).

Deep brain stimulation

Pioneering work by Dr. Helen Mayberg's group and others has shown that deep brain stimulation has the potential to alleviate severe depression which has been resistant to treatment with all other available modalities (Mayberg et al. 2005, Mayberg 2009). While this work is in its infancy, it has clearly demonstrated a proof of principal that regional sub-cortical brain stimulation, already well established in the treatment of epilepsy and Parkinson's disease, has evidence of efficacy for depression. Refining the optimal location for electrode placement and stimulus parameters is an area of active investigation and promises to produce treatments for the substantial sub-group of patients for whom conventional therapeutics are ineffective. Further, the enhanced knowledge of brain circuit activation relevant to depression illness will further advance the basic understanding of the pathophysiology of these disorders.

Chronobiology

Promising interventions, including methods for stabilizing the benefits of sleep deprivation or partial sleep deprivation, by the use of phototherapy, are being investigated as novel therapeutic agents. As discussed in Chapter 26 by Terman, innovative use of chronotherapy has been reported to be effective in otherwise treatment-resistant mood disorders. The field of chronobiology of mood disorders is quite new and is clearly promising for the future. Being able to mitigate mood disorders by the manipulation of the circadian rhythm with light exposure or with low-toxicity pharmacologic interventions like melatonin, if effective, might be expected to have broad acceptance by patients and be free of many of the adverse effects associated with current pharmacotherapy.

Complementary and alternative medicine

Complementary and alternative medicine (CAM) therapeutics for mood disorders has generated considerable interest, mainly because consumers voice a preference for such methods. This preference appears based on the perception that such methods are more "natural" and likely to cause fewer side effects than are conventional pharmaceuticals. The research establishment has followed this consumer preference with an increasing number of studies exploring these methods. Unfortunately, as summarized in Chapter 18 by Ramsey, Sublette, and Muskin, much of the evidence for the efficacy of these methods comes from uncontrolled clinical trials. While some of these studies are suggestive, there is little definitive evidence from controlled studies to support the efficacy of most treatments, with the exception of omega-3 fatty acid supplementation and St. John's wort. As of this time, research in CAM is in its infancy, but seems likely to develop further support from the NIMH and other funding agencies, ultimately progressing to including some demonstrably effective interventions in the conventional therapeutic portfolio and delineating their appropriate place in an evidence-based treatment algorithm. Ideally, this would also include reliable information concerning moderators of treatment outcome with any effective treatment strategy, that is, clinically determinable predictors of specific treatment outcome to enable clinicians to tailor treatment specific for an individual.

Augmentations

The clearly demonstrated benefit of second-generation antipsychotic medications (SGAs) supported the approval in the United States of several SGAs. The future is likely to include more work in this area, both in finding other effective SGAs and in development of medications or other strategies to counteract the detrimental metabolic effect of these medications (Papakostas and Shelton, 2008).

Psychotherapy

Previous research in the psychotherapy of mood disorders has mainly compared medication treatment and manualized psychotherapies such as cognitive behavior therapy and interpersonal psychotherapy head-to-head to test their relative overall efficacy (see Chapter 23). Newer work is likely to focus on ways to combine medication and psychotherapy practically to achieve the best possible outcome, but also theoretically, to better understand the domains of psychopathology most amenable to treatment

with each modality, and tailoring the modalities to augment one another's action. Like pharmacotherapy, psychotherapies in the future may be tailored to both the neurobiologic substrate in an individual case and to the experiential history of the individual. The pioneering observation that depression in patients with a history of childhood trauma responded better to the combination of pharmacotherapy and a specific structured psychotherapy (the cognitive behavioral analysis system of psychotherapy) than to pharmacotherapy alone is an example of the potential for individualizing treatment for specific groups of patients (Nemeroff et al. 2003) (never replicated and based on a questionable sub-set of patients). Examples of this include newer approaches utilizing behavioral activation psychotherapy for depression which may be more effective than the standardly used CBT approaches (Dimidjian et al. 2006). Current neurobiologic studies using fMRI to measure activation of the ventral striatum during reward and punishment tasks have suggested that depression is associated with impaired reward response, but not with a heightened sensitivity to negative reinforcement (Robinson et al. 2012). This might suggest that psychotherapies aimed at mitigating this lack of activation might be more useful than those aimed at diminution of avoidance. Even more interesting is the possibility that novel treatments like attention bias modification, explored as a behavioral training task in the laboratory to diminish anxiety in children with anxiety disorders, might be developed to target specific cognitive and behavioral abnormalities in patients with mood disorders (Eldar et al. 2012). Approaches like these, utilizing rapidly advancing insights from cognitive neuroscience, may enhance the therapeutic specificity of psychotherapy for individuals with mood disorders.

Long term

The history of science in medicine has amply shown that the ability to predict relevant scientific discoveries in the long term is abysmal. All we can state with confidence is that new discoveries will certainly be made, the most transformative of which will likely be completely unanticipated. The increasing emphasis on basic neuroscience research can be expected to yield new insights and understanding, which in turn will facilitate the development of new and more effective treatment alternatives for these disabling disorders.

References

Akiskal, H.S. (2002). The bipolar spectrum–the shaping of a new paradigm in psychiatry. *Current Psychiatry Reports*, 4, 1–3.

Akiskal, H.S. (2007). The emergence of the bipolar spectrum: validation along clinical-epidemiologic and familial-genetic lines. *Psychopharmacological Bulletin*, 40, 99–115.

Akiskal, H.S. and Mallya, G. (1987). Criteria for the "soft" bipolar spectrum: Treatment implications. *Psychopharmacological Bulletin*, 23, 68–73.

Angst, J., Gamma, A., and Lewinsohn, P. (2002). The evolving epidemiology of bipolar disorder. *World Psychiatry*, 1, 146–148.

Angst, J., Gamma, A., Benazzi, F. *et al.* (2003). Toward a re-definition of subthreshold bipolarity: Epidemiology and proposed criteria for bipolar-II, minor bipolar disorders and hypomania. *Journal of Affective Disorders*, 73, 133–146.

Dimidjian, S., Hollon, S.D., Dobson, K.S. *et al.* (2006). Randomized trial of behavioral activation, cognitive therapy, and antidepressant medication in the acute treatment of adults with major depression. *Journal of Consulting and Clinical Psychology*, 74, 658–670.

Eldar, S., Apter, A., Lotan, D. *et al.* (2012). Attention bias modification treatment for pediatric anxiety disorders: A randomized controlled trial. *American Journal of Psychiatry*, 169, 213–220.

Insel, T., Cuthbert, B., Garvey, M. *et al.* (2010). Research domain criteria (RDoC): Toward a new classification framework for research on mental disorders. *American Journal of Psychiatry*, 167, 748–751.

Mathew, S.J., Keegan, K., and Smith, L. (2005). Glutamate modulators as novel interventions for mood disorders. *Revista Brasileira de Psiquiatria*, 27, 243–248.

Matza, L.S., Paramore, C., and Prasad, M. (2005). A review of the economic burden of ADHD. *Cost Effective Resource Allocation*, 3, 5.

Mayberg, H.S. (2009). Targeted electrode-based modulation of neural circuits for depression. *Journal of Clinical Investigation*, 119, 717–725.

Mayberg, H.S.,Lozano, A.M., Voon, V. *et al.* (2005). Deep brain stimulation for treatment-resistant depression. *Neuron*, 45, 651–660.

Moussavi, S., Chatterji, S., Verdes, E. *et al.* (2007). Depression, chronic diseases, and decrements in health: Results from the World Health Surveys. *Lancet*, 370, 851–858.

Murray, C.J. and Lopez, A.D. (1996). Evidence-based health policy: Lessons from the Global Burden of Disease Study. *Science*, 274, 740–743.

Nemeroff, C.B., Heim, C.M., Thase, M.E. *et al.* (2003). Differential responses to psychotherapy versus pharmacotherapy in patients with chronic forms of major depression and childhood trauma. *Proceedings of the National Academy of Sciences USA*, 100, 14293–14296.

Papakostas, G.I. and Shelton, R.C. (2008). Use of atypical antipsychotics for treatment-resistant major depressive disorder. *Current Psychiatry Reports*, 10, 481–486.

Peterson, B.S., Warner, V., Bansal, R. *et al.* (2009). Cortical thinning in persons at increased familial risk for major depression. *Proceedings of the National Academy of Sciences USA*, 106, 6273–6278.

Pizzagalli, D.A., Peccoralo, L.A., Davidson, R.J., and Cohen, J.D. (2006). Resting anterior cingulate activity and abnormal responses to errors in subjects with elevated depressive symptoms: A 128-channel EEG study. *Human Brain Mapping*, 27, 185–201.

Post, R.M., Leverich, G.S., Kupka, R.W. *et al.* (2010). Early-onset bipolar disorder and treatment delay are risk factors for poor outcome in adulthood. *Journal of Clinical Psychiatry*, 71, 864–872.

Ray, S., Britschgi, M., Herbert, C. *et al.* (2007). Classification and prediction of clinical Alzheimer's diagnosis based on plasma signaling proteins. *Nature Medicine*, 13, 1359–1362.

Robinson, O.J., Cools, R., Carlisi, C.O., Sahakian, B.J., and Drevets, W.C. (2012). Ventral striatum response during reward and punishment reversal learning in unmedicated major depressive disorder. *American Journal of Psychiatry*, 169, 152–159.

Von Korff, M., Katon, W., Bush, T. *et al.* (1998). Treatment costs, cost offset, and cost-effectiveness of collaborative management of depression. *Psychosomatic Medicine*, 60, 143–149.

Wells, K.B., Stewart, A., Hays, R.D. *et al.* (1989). The functioning and well-being of depressed patients. Results from the Medical Outcomes Study. *Journal of the American Medical Association*, 262, 914–919.

Zarate, C.A., Jr., Singh, J.B., Carlson, P.J. *et al.* (2006). A randomized trial of an N-methyl-D-aspartate antagonist in treatment-resistant major depression. *Archives of General Psychiatry*, 63, 856–864.

Index